Eighth Edition

SAUER'S
MANUAL OF SKIN DISEASES

Eighth Edition

SAUER'S
MANUAL OF SKIN DISEASES

John C. Hall, M.D.

Primary Staff
St. Luke's Hospital
Trinity Hospital

Lecturer of Medicine
University of Missouri-Kansas City School of Medicine

Teaching Staff
Department of Pediatric Dermatology
Children's Mercy Hospital

Clinician
Kansas City Free Health Clinic
Kansas City, Missouri

With 13 Contributing Authors

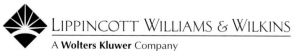

LIPPINCOTT WILLIAMS & WILKINS
A **Wolters Kluwer** Company
Philadelphia · Baltimore · New York · London
Buenos Aires · Hong Kong · Sydney · Tokyo

Acquisitions Editor: Richard Winters
Developmental Editor: Delois Patterson
Production Editor: Rosemary Palumbo
Manufacturing Manager: Tim Reynolds
Cover Designer: Karen Quigley
Compositor: Maryland Composition Company, Inc.

© 2000 by LIPPINCOTT WILLIAMS & WILKINS
227 East Washington Square
Philadelphia, PA 19106-3780 USA
LWW.com

Printed and bound in China

Library of Congress Cataloging-in-Publication Data

Hall, John C., 1947-
    Sauer's manual of skin diseases / John C. Hall ; with 13
contributing authors. — 8th ed.
        p.   cm.
    Rev. ed. of: Manual of skin diseases / Gordon C. Sauer, John C.
Hall. 7th ed. c1996.
    Includes bibliographical references and index.
    ISBN 0-7817-1629-2
    1. Skin—Diseases Handbooks, manuals, etc.   I. Sauer, Gordon C.
(Gordon Chenoweth), 1921-   Manual of skin diseases.   II. Title.
III. Title: Manual of skin diseases.
    [DNLM: 1. Skin Diseases.   WR   140   H177s   1999]
RL74.S25 1999
616.5—dc21
DNLM/DLC
for Library of Congress   99-26912
                                                                              CIP

Care has been taken to confirm the accuracy of the information presented and to describe generally accepted practices. However, the authors, editors, and publisher are not responsible for errors or omissions or for any consequences from application of the information in this book and make no warranty, expressed or implied, with respect to the currency, completeness, or accuracy of the contents of the publication. Application of this information in a particular situation remains the professional responsibility of the practitioner.

The authors, editors, and publisher have exerted every effort to ensure that drug selection and dosage set forth in this text are in accordance with current recommendations and practice at the time of publication. However, in view of ongoing research, changes in government regulations, and the constant flow of information relating to drug therapy and drug reactions, the reader is urged to check the package insert for each drug for any change in indications and dosage and for added warnings and precautions. This is particularly important when the recommended agent is a new or infrequently employed drug.

Some drugs and medical devices presented in this publication have Food and Drug Administration (FDA) clearance for limited use in restricted research settings. It is the responsibility of the health care provider to ascertain the FDA status of each drug or device planned for use in their clinical practice.

10 9 8 7 6 5 4 3 2 1

In memory of Clarence S. Livingood, M.D. *and William E. Hall,* Ph.D.,

to Susan R. Hall,

and to Gordon C. Sauer, M.D. *whose book this will always be.*

Contents

Contributing Authors

Francisco G. Bravo, M.D.
Assistant Professor
Department of Dermatology
Universidad Peruana Cayetano Heredia
Attending Physician
Dermatology Service
Instituto de Enfermedades Infecciosas y Tropicales
  Alexander Von Humboldt
Hospital Nacional Cayetano Heredia
Av. Honorio Delgado s/n, San Martin de Porres
Lima 31, Peru
Chapter 35, Tropical Diseases of the Skin

John C. Hall, M.D.
Primary Staff
St. Luke's Hospital
Trinity Hospital
Lecturer of Medicine
University of Missouri
Kansas City School of Medicine
Teaching Staff
Department of Pediatric Dermatology
Children's Mercy Hospital
Clinician
Kansas City Free Health Clinic
4400 Broadway, Suite 416
Kansas City, Missouri 64111

Warren R. Heymann, M.D.
Head
Division of Dermatology
Associate Professor
Department of Clinical Medicine
UMDNJ-Robert Wood Johnson Medical School at
  Camden
Cooper Hospital/University Medical Center
1 Cooper Plaza
Camden, New Jersey 08103
Chapter 26, The Skin and Internal Disease

Richard S. Kalish, M.D, Ph.D.
Associate Professor
Department of Dermatology
Health Sciences Center
State University of New York at Stony Brook
Stony Brook, New York 11794-8165
Chapter 10, Dermatologic Immunology

Thelda Kestenbaum, M.D.
Assistant Professor
Department of Medicine
Division of Dermatology
University of Kansas Medical Center
3901 Rainbow Boulevard
Kansas City, Kansas 66160
Chapters 27 and 28, Diseases Affecting the
  Hair and Diseases Affecting the Nails

Frank Custer Koranda, M.D.
Associate Clinical Professor
Department of Otolaryngology-Head and Neck
  Surgery
Division of Dermatology
University of Kansas Medical Center
Kansas City, Kansas
Staff Surgeon
Department of Otolaryngology-Head and Neck
  Surgery
St. Luke's Shawnee Mission
Georgetown Medical Building #148
8901 W. 74th Street
Shawnee Mission, Kansas 66204
Chapter 7, Fundamentals of Cutaneous
  Surgery

Robin M. Levin, M.D.
Chief Resident
Department of Dermatology
UMDNJ-Robert Wood Johnson Medical School at
  Camden
Cooper Hospital/University Medical Center
1 Cooper Plaza
Camden, New Jersey 08103
Chapter 26, The Skin and Internal Disease

Alejandro Morales, M.D.
Associate Professor
Department of Dermatology
Universidad Peruana Cayetano Heredia
Av. Honorio Delgado s/n
Chief
Instituto Dermatologica
El Bucare 551
La Molina
Lima 12, Peru
Chapter 35, Tropical Diseases of the Skin

Marianne N. O'Donoghue, M.D.
Associate Professor
Department of Dermatology
Rush Presbyterian–St. Luke's Medical Center
Chicago, Illinios
120 Oak Brook Center Mall
Oak Brook, Illinios 60523
Chapter 8, Cosmetics for the Physician

Neil S. Prose, M.D.
Associate Professor
Departments of Medicine (Dermatology) and
  Pediatrics
Duke University Medical Center
Durham, North Carolina 27710
Chapter 18, Cutaneous Diseases Associated
  with Human Immunodeficiency Virus

M. Joyce Rico, M.D.
Associate Professor
Department of Dermatology
New York University
550 First Avenue, H-100
Chief
Dermatology Service
New York VA Medical Center
423 East 23rd Street
New York, New York 10010
Chapter 18, Cutaneous Diseases Associated
  with Human Immunodeficiency Virus

Vidya Sharma, M.B.B.S., M.P.H., M.D.
Associate Professor
Department of Pediatrics
University of Missouri
Staff Physician
Department of Dermatology
Children's Mercy Hospital
Kansas City, Missouri 64108
Chapter 33, Pediatric Dermatology

Virginia P. Sybert, M.D.
Professor
Department of Medicine
University of Washington School of Medicine
Box 356524
Seattle, Washington 98195
Chapter 31, Genodermatoses

Kenneth R. Watson, D.O.
Department of Pathology
St. Luke's Hospital
4401 Wornall Road
Kansas City, Missouri 64111
Chapters 1 and 2, Structure of the Skin and
  Laboratory Procedures and Tests

Preface to the First Edition (abridged)

Approximately 15 percent of all patients who walk into the general practitioner's office do so for care of some skin disease or skin lesion. It may be for such a simple treatment as the removal of a wart, for the treatment of athlete's foot or for something as complicated as severe cystic acne. There have been so many recent advances in the various fields of medicine that the medical school instructor can expect his students to learn and retain only a small percentage of the material that is taught them. I believe that the courses in all phases of medicine, and particularly the courses of the various specialties, should be made as simple, basic and concise as possible. If the student retains only a small percentage of what is presented to him, he will be able to handle an amazing number of his walk-in patients. I am presenting in this book only the material that medical students and general practitioners must know for the diagnosis and the treatment of patients with common skin diseases. In condensing the material many generalities are stated, and the reader must remember that there are exceptions to every rule. The inclusion of these exceptions would defeat the intended purpose of this book. More complicated diagnostic procedures or treatments for interesting problem cases are merely frosting on the cake. This information can be obtained by the interested student from any of several more comprehensive dermatologic texts.

This book consists of two distinct but complementary parts: The first part contains the chapters devoted to the diagnosis and the management of the important common skin diseases. In discussing the common skin diseases, a short introductory sentence is followed by a listing of the salient points of each disease in outline form. All diseases of the skin have primary lesions, secondary lesions, a rather specific distribution, a general course which includes the prognosis and the recurrence rate of the diseases, varying subjective complaints, and a known or unknown cause. Where indicated, a statement follows concerning seasonal incidence, age groups affected, family and sex incidence, contagiousness or infectiousness, relationship to employment and laboratory findings. The discussion ends with a paragraph on differential diagnosis and treatment. Treatment, to be effective, has to be thought of as a chain of events. The therapy outlined on the first visit is usually different from the one given on subsequent visits or for cases that are very severe. The treatment is discussed with these variations in mind. The first part of the book concludes with a chapter on basic equipment necessary for managing dermatologic patients.

The second part consists of a very complete Dictionary–Index to the entire field of dermatology, defining the majority of rare diseases and the unusual dermatologic terms. The inclusion of this Dictionary–Index has a dual purpose. First, it enables me to present a concise first section on common skin diseases unencumbered by the inclusion of the rare diseases. Second, the Dictionary–Index provides rather complete coverage of all of dermatology for the more interested student. In reality, two books are contained in one.

Dermatologic nomenclature has always been a bugaboo for the new student. I heartily agree with many dermatologists that we should simplify the terminology, and that has been attempted in this text. Some of the changes are mine, but many have been suggested by others. However, after a diligent effort to simplify the names of skin diseases, one is left with the appalling fact that some of the complicated terms defy change. One of the main reasons for this is that all of our field, the skin, is visible to the naked eye. As a result, any minor alteration from normal has been scrutinized by countless physicians through the years and given countless names. The liver or heart counterpart of folliculitis ulerythematosa reticulata (ulerythema acneiform, atrophoderma reticulatum symmetricum faciei, atrophoderma vermiculatum) is yet to be discovered.

What I am presenting in this book is not specialty dermatology but general practice dermatology. Some of my medical educator friends say that only internal medicine, pediatrics, and obstetrics should be taught to medical students. They state that the specialized fields of medicine should be taught only at the internship, residency, or postgraduate level. That idea misses the very important fact that cases from all of the so-called specialty fields wander in to the general practitioner's office. The general practitioner must have some basic knowledge of the varied aspects of all of medicine so that he can properly take care of his general everyday practice. This basic knowledge must be taught in the undergraduate years. The purpose of this book is to complement such teaching.

Gordon C. Sauer, M.D.

Preface

Many new things have been added to the 8th edition of the *Manual of Skin Diseases*.

The Dictionary–Index has been completely revamped with many unnecessary items eliminated, and many new items added. For the first time in this book, or any American published dermatology textbook, a special section on Tropical Dermatology is included, which adds a great deal to the overall completeness of this text.

All chapters have been updated and new authors, who are experts in their field, have written the chapters on dermatopathology, immunodermatology, cutaneous manifestations of underlying diseases, the genetics of dermatology, and pediatric dermatology.

Updates of chapters from outstanding authors who have written previous chapters include: dermatology cosmetics, cutaneous diseases associated with immunodeficiency and fundamentals of cutaneous surgery and chapters on hair and nail disease.

Numerous new color photographs have been added to the text, which greatly enhance the dermatology diagnosis. It is often said that "a picture is worth a thousand words" and in no specialty is this more true than in dermatology.

I have kept most chapters in the basic proven structure that Dr. Sauer has been recognized for worldwide during his outstanding dermatology teaching career.

John C. Hall, M.D.

Acknowledgments

I have never enjoyed a task more than spending time with and learning from Dr. Sauer. From my earlier training days, I am forever indebted to Drs. Richard Q. Crotty and Clarence S. Livingood for the opportunity of a dermatology residency. I had the unique honor of having trained under Dr. Livingood and Edward A. Krull. Dr. Livingood taught me much about the science and the art of medicine. I feel that I have stood in the shadow of giants.

As brevity is the soul of wit, it is also the soul of the early understanding of a complex subject. An overview is more priceless at the onset of learning than a mountain of detail. To stir one's interest and curiosity about a field of scientific endeavor, one needs to see that field as a whole. Therein lies the true genius of Gordon Sauer.

Thanks to pathologist Ken Watson and to pharmacist Doug Albers, both whom have been of invaluable help both in producing this book and throughout my career. My family—Charlotte, Shelly, Kim, Brian, and Sam—and my office staff—Yolanda, Brandy, Christa, Pam, and Reta—have been unwavering in their support and patience. My parents, the late William E. Hall and Susan R. Hall, and my wife's parents, Arnold W. Peterson and the late Fern Marie Peterson, have given me endless encouragement.

I would like to acknowledge the diligent work of Yolanda Payton who was very instrumental in the revision and typing of the text. She was assisted by Brandy Del Debbio. My office manager, Christa Czysz, nurse, Pam Skripsky, and physician assistant, Reta Dodds, also made the publication a reality.

In the seven previous editions, further acknowledgements were made, but it would be redundant to repeat them here. Finally, a great deal of credit again goes to Lippincott Williams & Wilkins, especially to Richard Winters, Medical Editor. The book profited by my association with them.

For the most realistic presentation of skin diseases, color photography is essential. However, the cost of color reproduction is so great that it is almost impossible to enjoy the advantages of color figures and still keep the price of the book within the range where it will have the broadest appeal. This problem has been solved for the eighth edition of this book through the generosity of several pharmaceutical companies, which contributed the cost of the color figures credited to them. For this edition, the following drug companies contributed money for additional new color figures:

Dermik Laboratories
Galderma
Glaxo Wellcome, Inc.
Merck & Co., Inc.
Neutrogena Skin Care Institute
Norvartis Pharmaceutical
Ortho Pharmaceutical Corporation
Schering Corporation
Smith-Kline Beecham
Stiefel Laboratories

Chapters have been revised for this edition by Marianne O'Donoghue, M. Joyce Rico, Neil Prose, Frank C. Koranda, and Thelda Kestenbaum. All of these authors have contributed to other editions and I feel fortunate to have their expertise displayed again in this edition.

I also feel very fortunate to have added new chapter authors to this edition. They are Drs. Kenneth R. Watson, Richard S. Kalish, Virginia P. Sybert, Vidya Sharma, Francisco G. Bravo, and Alejandro Morales. Seldom has such an army of talented clinicians and authors been displayed in a text of this type and I am honored by their efforts. The labor and input of these knowledgeable contributors are greatly appreciated.

Dr. Sauer and I frequently hear from dermatologists and nondermatologists alike that this book is their first exposure to the study of skin diseases. The eighth edition and all preceding editions are a tribute to Dr. Sauer's ability to open up the specialty of dermatology to those who wish to use its magic to help in the care of their patients.

Eighth Edition

Sauer's
Manual of Skin Diseases

1

Structure of the Skin

Revised by Kenneth R. Watson, D.O.*

The skin is the largest organ of the human body. It is composed of tissue that grows, differentiates, and renews itself constantly. Because the skin is a barrier between the internal organs and the external environment, it is uniquely subjected to noxious external agents and is also a sensitive reflection of internal disease. An understanding of the cause and the effect of this complex interplay in the skin begins with a thorough understanding of the basic structure of this organ.

LAYERS OF THE SKIN

The skin is divided into three rather distinct layers. From the inside out, they are the subcutaneous tissue, the dermis, and the epidermis (Fig. 1-1).

Subcutaneous Tissue

The subcutaneous tissue serves as a receptacle for the formation and the storage of fat, is a locus of high dynamic lipid metabolism, and supports the blood vessels and the nerves that pass from the tissues beneath to the dermis above. The thickness of the subcutaneous fat varies from one area of the body to another. The subcutaneous

tissue constitutes the largest volume of adipose tissue in the body. Fat cells are derived from mesenchymal cells, as are fibroblasts. They are organized into lobules by fibrous septae, which contain most of the blood vessels, nerves, and lymphatics that nourish the skin.

Dermis

The dermis consists of connective tissue, cellular elements, and ground substance. It has a rich blood and nerve supply and contains pilosebaceous, apocrine, and eccrine structures. Anatomically, it is divided into two compartments. The first consists of thin collagen fibers, which are located beneath the epidermis (papillary dermis) and surrounding adnexal structures (periadnexal dermis). Together, the collagen fibers are regarded as a single unit called the adventitial dermis. This is an important unit because it is altered together with the adjacent epithelium in many inflammatory diseases. The second compartment, known as the reticular or deep dermis, is composed of thick collagen bundles and comprises the bulk of the dermis.

The *connective tissue* component of the dermis consists of collagen fibers, including reticulin fibers, and elastic fibers. These fibers contribute to the support and elasticity of the skin.

There are two different types of collagen that predominate in the dermis. Type I collagen forms

---

*Department of Pathology, St. Luke's Hospital, Kansas City, Missouri

1

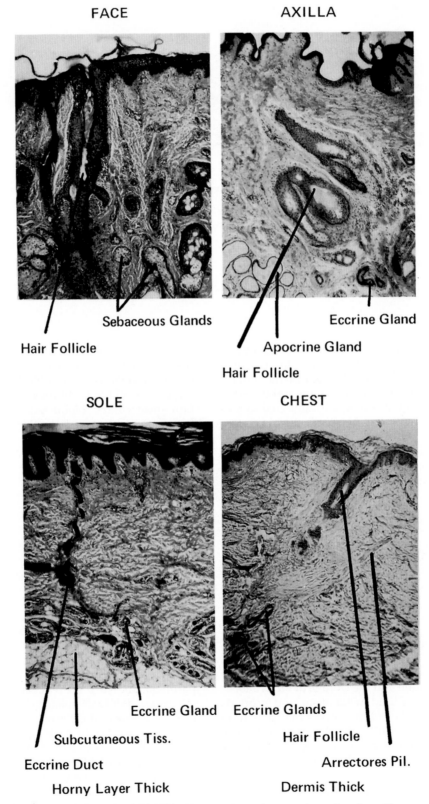

FACE

AXILLA

Sebaceous Glands

Hair Follicle

Eccrine Gland

Apocrine Gland

Hair Follicle

SOLE

CHEST

Eccrine Gland   Eccrine Glands

Subcutaneous Tiss.   Hair Follicle

Eccrine Duct   Arrectores Pil.

Horny Layer Thick   Dermis Thick

Figure 1-1.   Histology of the skin. Microscopic sections are shown from four different areas of the body. Note the variations in the histologic features, such as the thickness of the horny layer and the presence or absence of the three types of glands and the hair follicles. These photographs were taken at the same magnification. *(Dr. D. Gibson)*

the thick fibers in the reticular dermis. Type III collagen, also known as *reticulin*, forms the thin fibers within the papillary and periadnexal dermis. These reticulin fibers are not visible in hematoxylin and eosin-stained sections but can be identified with silver stains. They are abundant in certain pathologic conditions such as tuberculous granulomas, syphilis, sarcoidosis, and some mesodermal tumors. The proteins present in collagen fibers are responsible for nearly one fourth of a person's overall protein mass. If tannic acid or the salts of heavy metals, such as dichromates, are combined with collagen, the result is leather.

Elastic fibers are thinner than most collagen fibers and are entwined among them. They are composed of the protein elastin. Elastic fibers do not readily take up acidic or basic stains, such as hematoxylin and eosin, but they can be identified with Verhoeff–Van Gieson stain.

The *cellular elements* of the dermis include fibroblasts, endothelial cells, mast cells, and a variety of miscellaneous cells including muscle, nerve, and hematopoietic cells. The hematopoietic cells include histiocytes (macrophages), lymphocytes, and plasma cells that are present in the dermis under various pathologic conditions.

Fibroblasts form collagen and also produce ground substance. They are involved in immunologic and reparative processes and are increased in numerous skin disorders.

Mast cells arise from undifferentiated mesenchymal cells. They have intracytoplasmic basophilic metachromatic granules containing heparin and histamine. The normal skin contains relatively few mast cells, but their number is increased in many different skin conditions, particularly the itching dermatoses, such as *atopic eczema*, *contact dermatitis*, and *lichen planus*. In *urticaria pigmentosa* the mast cells may occur in tumor-like masses.

Histiocytes (macrophages) are present in only small numbers in the normal skin. However, in pathologic conditions they migrate to the dermis as tissue monocytes. They play a predominant role in the phagocytosis of the particulate matter and bacteria. Under special pathologic conditions they may form giant cells. They are also involved in the immune system by phagocytizing antigens.

Lymphocytes and plasma cells are found in only small numbers in normal skin but are significantly increased in pathologic conditions.

The *ground substance* of the dermis is a gel-like amorphous matrix not easily seen in routine sections, but it may be identified with colloidal iron and Alcian blue stains. It is of tremendous importance because it contains proteins, mucopolysaccharides, soluble collagens, enzymes, immune bodies, metabolites, and many other substances.

Epidermis

The epidermis is the most superficial of the three layers of the skin and averages in thickness about the width of the mark of a sharp pencil, or less than 1 mm. It contains several types of cells including keratinocytes, dendritic cells (melanocytes and Langerhans' cells), and Merkel cells.

The keratinocytes, or keratin-forming cells, are by far the most common and develop into four identifiable layers of the epidermis (Fig. 1-2). From inside out, they are as follows:

Basal layer
Spinous layer   } Living epidermis
Granular layer
Cornified layer   Dead end-product

The basal layer lies next to the dermis. The keratin-forming cells can be thought of as stem cells, which are capable of progressive maturation into cell forms higher in the epidermis. It normally requires 3 or 4 weeks for the epidermis to replicate itself by the process of division and differentiation. This cell turnover is greatly accelerated in such diseases as *psoriasis* and *ichthyosiform erythroderma*. In these diseases, the turnover rate may be as short as 2 to 3 days.

The spinous layer, or stratum malpighii, is made up of several layers of epidermal cells, chiefly of polyhedral shape. The cells of this layer are connected by intercellular bridges, which may be seen in routine sections.

The granular layer is composed of flatter cells containing protein granules called keratohyalin granules. In lichen planus, the granular cell layer is focally increased.

The outermost layer of the epidermis is the *cornified (horny) layer*. It is made up of stratified layers of dead keratinized cells that are constantly shedding (Fig. 1-3). The chemical protein in these cells is called keratin. It is capable of absorbing vast amounts of water. This is readily seen during bathing, when the skin of the palms and the soles becomes white, swollen, and wrinkled. The cornified layer provides a major barrier of protection for the body.

The normal oral mucous membrane does not have granular or cornified layers.

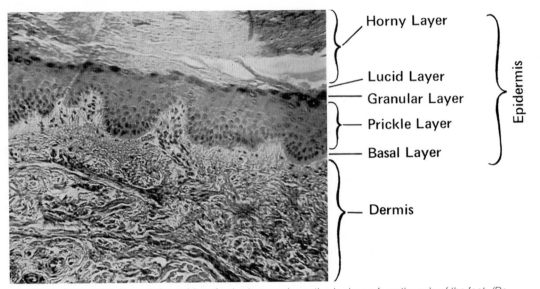

Figure 1-2. **Histology of the epidermis.** A microscopic section is shown from the sole of the foot. *(Dr. D. Gibson)*

The *melanin-forming cells*, or *melanocytes*, are sandwiched between the more numerous keratin-forming cells in the basal layer. These melanocytes are dopa-positive because they stain darkly after contact with a solution of levorotatory 3,4-dihydroxyphenylalanine, or *dopa*. This laboratory reaction closely simulates physiologic melanin formation in which the amino acid tyrosine is oxidized by the enzyme tyrosinase to form dopa. Dopa is then further changed, through a series of complex metabolic processes, to melanin.

Melanin pigmentation of the skin, whether increased or decreased, is influenced by many local

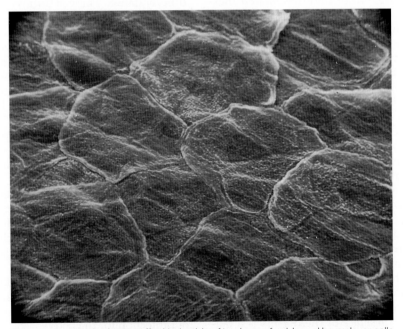

Figure 1-3. **Horny-layer cells.** Underside of top layer of epidermal horny layer cells on Scotch tape stripping is seen with Cambridge Mark II Stereoscan at 1000×. *(Drs. J. Arnold, W. Barnes, and G. Sauer)*

and systemic factors (see Chap. 24). Melanocyte-stimulating hormone from the pituitary is the most potent melanizing agent. Melanin is transferred from melanocytes to basal keratinocytes. Skin color is largely related to the amount of melanin present in basal cells.

Langerhans' cells are found scattered evenly throughout the epidermis. They are bone marrow-derived mononuclear cells. They are involved in cell-mediated hypersensitivity, antigen processing and recognition, stimulation of immune-competent cells, and graft rejection. Sunlight suppresses their immune functioning. Their number is decreased in certain skin diseases, such as psoriasis. Staining with membrane adenosine triphosphatase and monoclonal antibodies such as S-100 protein and CD-1 can be done for identification. By electron microscopy, they contain characteristic racket-shaped Birbeck granules.

Merkel's cells are normally located in the basal layer, although they are inconspicuous in routine sections. Ultrastructurally they contain dense core neurosecretory granules. They are assumed to function as a touch receptor. They give rise to primary neuroendocrine carcinoma of the skin (Merkel's-cell tumor).

VASCULATURE

A continuous arteriovenous meshwork perforates the subcutaneous tissues and extends into the dermis. Blood vessels of varying sizes are present in most levels and planes of the skin. In fact, the vascularization is so extensive that it has been postulated that its main function is to regulate heat and blood pressure of the body, with providing nutrition to the skin a secondary function. No blood vessels are present within the epidermis.

A special vascular body, the glomus, deserves mention. The glomus body is most commonly seen on the tips of the fingers and the toes, and under the nails. Each glomus body consists of a venous and arterial segment, called the *Sucquet-Hoyer canal*. This canal represents a short-circuit device that connects an arteriole with a venule directly, without intervening capillaries. The result is a marked increase in the blood flow through the skin. If this body grows abnormally, it forms an often painful, red, benign glomus tumor, commonly beneath the nail.

NERVE SUPPLY

The nerve supply of the skin consists of sensory nerves and motor nerves.

Sensory Nerves

The sensory nerves mediate the sensations of touch, temperature, and pain. The millions of terminal nerve endings, or Merkel's cell–neurite complexes, have more to do with the specificity of skin sensation than the better known, highly specialized nerve endings, such as the Vater-Pacini and Wagner-Meissner tactile corpuscles.

Itching is the most important presenting symptom of an unhappy patient. It may be defined simply as the desire to scratch. Itching apparently is a mild painful sensation that differs from pain in having a lower frequency of impulse stimuli. The release of proteinases (such as follows itch-powder application) may be responsible for the itch sensation. The pruritus may be of a pricking type or of a burning type and can vary greatly from one person to another. Sulzberger called those abnormally sensitive people "itchish," analogous to "ticklish." Itching can occur without any clinical signs of skin disease or from circulating allergens or local superficial contactants. The skin of atopic or eczema patients tends to be more itchy. Scratching makes the itching worse. This results in a perpetual itch-scratch cycle.

Motor Nerves

The involuntary sympathetic motor nerves control the sweat glands, arterioles, and smooth muscle of the skin. Adrenergic fibers carry impulses to the arrector pili muscles, which produce gooseflesh if they are stimulated. This is caused by traction of the muscle on the hair follicles to which it is attached. Cholinergic fibers if stimulated increase sweating and may cause a specific type of hives called *cholinergic urticaria* (see Chap. 12).

APPENDAGES

The appendages of the skin include both the cornified appendages (hairs and nails) and the glandular appendages.

Hairs

Hairs are produced by the hair follicles, which develop from germinative cells of the fetal epidermis. Because no new hair follicles are formed after birth, the different types of body hairs are manifestations of the effect of location, and of external and internal stimuli. Hormones are the most important internal stimuli influencing the various types of hair growth. This growth is cyclic, with a growing (anagen) phase and a resting (telogen) phase. The catagen cycle is the transition phase between the growing and resting stages and lasts only a few days. Ninety percent of the normal scalp hairs are in the growing (anagen) stage, and 10% are in the resting (falling out) stage, which lasts from 60 to 90 days. The average period of scalp hair growth ranges from 2 to 6 years. However, systemic stresses, such as childbirth, or systemic anesthesia may cause hairs to enter a resting stage prematurely. This *postpartum effect* or *postanesthetic effect* is noticed most commonly in the scalp when these resting hairs are depilated during combing or washing, and the thought of approaching baldness causes sudden alarm.

SAUER NOTES

1. Shaving of excess hair, as women do on their legs and thighs, does not promote more rapid growth of coarse hair. The shaved stubs appear more coarse, but if allowed to grow normally, the hairs appear and feel no different than before shaving.

2. The value of intermittent massage to stimulate scalp hair growth has not been proved.

3. Hair cannot turn gray overnight. The melanin pigmentation, which is distributed throughout the length of the nonvital hair shaft, takes weeks to be shed through the slow process of hair growth.

4. Heredity is the greatest factor predisposing to baldness, and an excess of male hormone may contribute to hair loss. Male castrates do not become bald.

5. The common male pattern baldness cannot be reversed by over-the-counter "hair restorers." Minoxidil solution (Rogaine), which is over-the-counter, is beneficial for a limited percentage of patients and finasteride (Propecia) pills are available by prescription.

TYPES

The adult has two main types of hairs: (1) the vellus hairs (lanugo hairs of the fetus) and (2) the terminal hairs. The vellus hairs ("peach fuzz") are the fine, short hairs of the body, whereas the terminal hairs are coarse, thick, and pigmented. The terminal hairs are developed most extensively on the scalp, brow, and extremities.

HAIR FOLLICLES

The hair follicle may be thought of as an invagination of the epidermis, with its different layers of cells. These cells make up the matrix of the hair follicle and produce the keratin of the mature hair. The protein synthesizing capacity of this tissue is enormous. At the rate of scalp hair growth of 0.35 mm per day, more than 100 linear feet of scalp hair is produced daily. The density of hairs in the scalp varies from 175 to 300 hairs per square centimeter. Up to 100 hairs may be normally lost daily.

Nails

The second cornified appendage, the nail, consists of a nail plate and the tissue that surrounds it. This plate lies in a nail groove, which like the hair follicle is an invagination of the epidermis. Unlike hair growth, which is periodic, nail growth is continuous. Nail growth proceeds at about one third of the rate of hair growth, or about 0.1 mm per day. It takes about 3 months to restore a removed fingernail and about three times that long for the regrowth of a new toenail. Nail growth can be inhibited during serious illnesses or in old age, increased through nail biting or occupational trauma, and altered because of hand dermatitis or systemic disease. Topical treatment of nail disturbances is very unsatisfactory, owing to the inaccessibility of the growth-producing areas.

Glandular Appendages

The three types of glandular appendages of the skin are the sebaceous glands, apocrine glands, and eccrine glands (Fig. 1-4).

The *sebaceous glands* are present everywhere on the skin, except the palms and the soles. In most areas they are associated with hair follicles. There are sebaceous glands that are not associated with hair follicles, such as the buccal mucosa

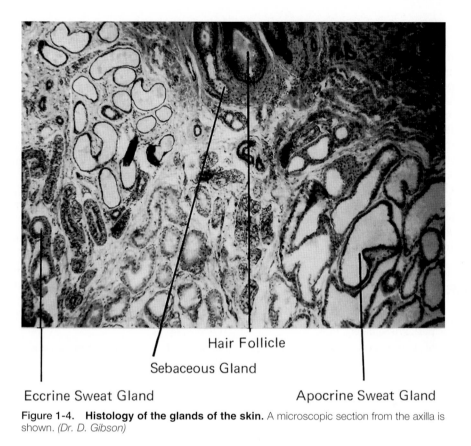

Hair Follicle

Sebaceous Gland

Eccrine Sweat Gland

Apocrine Sweat Gland

Figure 1-4. **Histology of the glands of the skin.** A microscopic section from the axilla is shown. *(Dr. D. Gibson)*

and vermillion border of the lip, nipple and areola of the breast, labia minora, and eyelids (Meibomian glands). They are holocrine glands, forming their secretions through the disintegration of the entire glandular cell. The secretion from these glands is evacuated through the sebaceous duct to a follicle that may contain either a large terminal hair or vellus hair. This secretion, known as sebum, is not under any neurologic control but is a continuous outflowing of the material of cell breakdown. The sebum covers the skin with a thin lipoidal film that is mildly bacteriostatic and fungistatic and retards water evaporation. The scalp and the face may contain as many as 1000 sebaceous glands per square centimeter. The activity of the gland increases markedly at the age of puberty, and, in certain people, it becomes plugged with sebum, debris, and bacteria to form the blackheads and the pimples of acne.

Apocrine glands are found in the axillae, genital region, breast, external ear canal (ceruminous glands), and eyelid (Moll's glands). They do not develop until the time of puberty. They consist of a coiled secretory gland located in the deep dermis or subcutaneous fat and a straight duct that usually empties into a hair follicle. The function of the secretions is unknown; however, they may act as pheromones. They are responsible for the production of body odor (the infamous "BO"). Any emotional stresses that cause adrenergic sympathetic discharge produce apocrine secretion. This secretion is sterile when excreted but undergoes decomposition when contaminated by bacteria from the skin surface, resulting in a strong and characteristic odor. The purpose of the many cosmetic underarm preparations is to remove these bacteria or block the gland excretion. The apocrine glands are involved in hidradenitis suppurativa. This inflammatory process results from follicular obstruction and retention of follicular products, which usually occur in patients with the acne–seborrhea complex.

Eccrine sweat glands are distributed everywhere on the skin surface, with the greatest concentration on the palms, soles, and forehead. They develop as a downgrowth from the primitive epidermis. They are composed of coiled secretory glands, a coiled duct, a straight duct, an intraepidermal coil, and an eccrine pore. The eccrine sweat glands and the vasculature of the skin serve in the maintenance of the stable internal body temperature, despite marked environmental temperature changes. They flood the skin surface with water for cooling, and the blood vessels dilate or constrict to dissipate or conserve body heat. Their prime stimulus is heat and their activity is under the control of the nervous system, usually through the hypothalamus. Both adrenergic and cholinergic fibers innervate the glands. Blockage of the eccrine ducts results in the disease known as *miliaria* (*prickly heat*). If eccrine glands are congenitally absent, as in *anhidrotic ectodermal dysplasia*, a life-threatening hyperpyrexia may develop.

BIBLIOGRAPHY

Ackerman BA. Histologic diagnosis of inflammatory skin diseases. Philadelphia, WB Saunders, 1978.

Barnhill RL. Textbook of dermatopathology. New York, McGraw-Hill, 1997.

Briggaman RA. Epidermal-dermal junction structure, composition, function and disease relationships. Prog Dermatol 1990;24(2):1.

Farmer RE, Hood AF. Pathology of the skin. Norwalk, CT, Appleton & Lange, 1990.

Fleischer AB. The clinical management of itching, therapeutic protocols for pruritis. Parthenon Publishing Group, 1998.

Goldsmith L. Physiology, biochemistry, and molecular biology of the skin. New York, Oxford University Press, 1991.

Hurwitz RM, Hood AF. Pathology of the skin, atlas of clinical-pathological correlation. Stamford, CT, Appleton & Lange, 1997.

Lever WE, Schaumburg-Lever G. Histopathology of the skin, ed 7. Philadelphia, JB Lippincott, 1990.

Murphy GF, Elder EE. Atlas of tumor pathology, non-melanocytic tumors of the skin. Washington, DC, Armed Forces Institute of Pathology, 1991.

Nickolof BJ. Dermal immune system. Boca Raton, FL, CRC Press, 1993.

Rosen T, Martin S. Atlas of black dermatology. Boston, Little, Brown and Company, 1981.

2

Laboratory Procedures and Tests

Revised by Kenneth R. Watson, D.O.*

In addition to the usual laboratory procedures used in the workup of medical patients, certain special tests are of importance in the field of dermatology. These include *skin tests*, *fungus examinations*, *biopsies*, and *immunologic diagnosis*. For special problems, additional testing methods are suggested in the sections on the various diseases.

SKIN TESTS

There are three types of skin tests:

- Intracutaneous
- Scratch
- Patch

The *intracutaneous tests* and the *scratch tests* can have two types of reactions: an *immediate wheal reaction* or a *delayed reaction*. The immediate wheal reaction develops to a maximum in 5 to 20 minutes. This type of reaction is elicited in testing for the cause of urticaria, atopic dermatitis, and inhalant allergies. This immediate wheal reaction test is seldom used for determining the cause of skin diseases.

The delayed reaction to intracutaneous skin testing is exemplified best by the tuberculin skin test. Tuberculin is available in two forms: as pu-

rified protein derivative and as a tuberculin tine test.

The purified protein derivative test is performed by using tablets that come in two strengths and by injecting a solution of either one intracutaneously. If there is no reaction after the test with the first strength, then the second strength may be employed.

The tuberculin tine test (Mantoux) is a simple and rapid procedure using OTK. Nine prongs, or tines, covered with OTK are pressed into the skin. If at the end of 48 or 72 hours there is more than 2 mm of induration at the site of any prong insertion, the test is positive.

Patch tests are used commonly in dermatology and offer a simple and accurate method of determining whether a patient is allergic to any of the testing agents. There are two different reactions to this type of test: a *primary irritant reaction* and an *allergic reaction*. The primary irritant reaction occurs in most of the population if they are exposed to agents (in appropriate concentrations) that have skin-destroying properties. Examples of these agents include soaps, cleaning fluids, bleaches, "corn" removers, and counterirritants. The allergic reaction indicates that the patient is more sensitive than normal to the agent being tested. This test reaction is idiosyncratic and not necessarily related to concentration or dose. It also shows that the patient has had a previous exposure to that agent or a cross-sensitizing agent.

*Department of Pathology, St. Luke's Hospital, Kansas City, Missouri

The technique of the patch test is simple, but the interpretation of the test is not. For example, consider a patient presenting with dermatitis on top of the feet. It is possible that shoe leather or some chemical used in the manufacture of the leather is causing the reaction. The procedure for a patch test is to cut out a 1/2-inch-square piece of the material from the inside of the shoe, moisten the material with distilled water, place it on the skin surface, and cover it with an adhesive band or some patch-test dressing. The patch test is left on for 48 hours. When the patch test is removed, the patient is considered to have a positive patch test if there is any redness, papules, or vesiculation under the site of the testing agent. Delayed reactions to allergens can occur, and, ideally, a final reading should be made after 96 hours (4 days), or, in other words, 2 days after the patch is removed.

The patch test can be used to make or confirm a diagnosis of poison ivy dermatitis, ragweed dermatitis, or contact dermatitis caused by medications, cosmetics, or industrial chemicals. Fisher (1995) and Adams (1990) compiled lists of chemicals, concentrations, and vehicles to be used for eliciting the allergic type of patch test reaction. Most tests can be performed very simply, however, as in the case of the shoe-leather dermatitis. One precaution is that the test must not be allowed to become wet in the 48-hour period.

A patch test kit, T.R.U.E. Test (Glaxo), includes ready-to-apply self-adhesive allergen tapes.

A method of testing for food allergy is to use the Rowe elimination diet. The procedure is to limit the diet to the following basic foods, which are known to be hypoallergenic: lamb, lemon, grapefruit, pears, lettuce, spinach, carrots, sweet potato, tapioca, rice and rice bread, corn sugar, maple syrup, sesame oil, gelatin, and salt. The patient is to remain on this basic diet for 5 to 7 days. At the end of that time, one new food can be added every 2 days. The following foods can be added early: beef, white potatoes, green beans, milk (along with butter and American cheese), and white bread with puffed wheat. If there is a flare-up of the dermatitis, which should occur

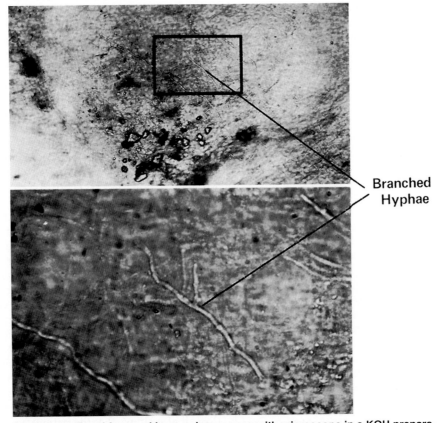

Branched Hyphae

Figure 2-1. Fungi from a skin scraping as seen with microscope in a KOH preparation. (*Top*) Low-power lens (100×) view. (*Bottom*) High-power lens (450×) view of area outlined above. (*Dr. D. Gibson*)

within 2 to 8 hours after ingestion of an offending food, the new food should be discontinued for the present. More new foods are added until the normal diet, minus the allergenic foods, is regained.

Keeping a "diet diary" of all foods, medicines, oral hygiene items, or anything injected or inhaled can sometimes be a retrospective way of identifying an allergen. The skin reaction usually occurs less than 8 hours after ingestion.

FUNGUS EXAMINATIONS

The KOH preparation is a simple office laboratory procedure for the detection of fungal organisms present in skin and nails. It is accomplished by scraping the diseased skin and examining the material with the microscope. The skin scrapings are obtained by abrading a scaly diseased area with a scalpel. If a blister is present, the underside of the blister is examined. The material is deposited on a glass slide and then covered with

20% aqueous potassium hydroxide solution and a coverslip. The preparation can be gently heated or allowed to stand at room temperature for 15 to 60 minutes. The addition of dimethyl sulfoxide to the KOH preparation eliminates the need to heat the specimen. A diagnostically helpful pale violet stain can be imparted to the fungi if the 20% KOH solution is mixed with an equal amount of Parker's Super Quink permanent blue-black ink. The slide is then examined microscopically for fungal organisms (Fig. 2-1).

For culture preparation, a portion of the material from the scraping can be implanted on several different types of agar including: mycobiotic agar, IMA inhibitory mold agar, BHI with blood, chloramphenicol, gentamicin agar, and Sabouraud's glucose agar. A white or variously colored growth is noted in approximately 1 to 3 weeks (Fig. 2-2). The species of fungus can be identified by morphology on the culture plate, biochemical characteristics, and microscopic morphology with a lacto-phenol cotton blue stain of a smear from the fungal colony.

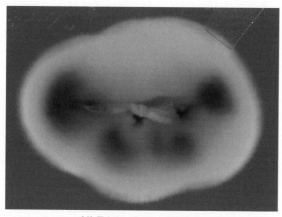

(A) Trichophyton rubrum

Figure 2-2. Fungus cultures: Subcultures grown on potato dextrose agar. *(St. Luke's Hospital)*

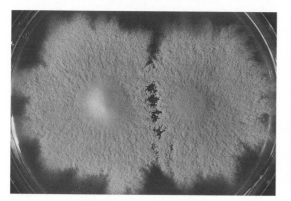

(B) Microsporum gypseum

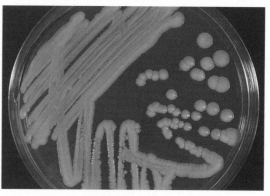

(C) Candida albicans

BIOPSIES

The biopsy and microscopic examination of a questionable skin lesion may be invaluable. The histologic appearance of many skin conditions may be diagnostic, particularly if correlated with the clinic findings. It is imperative that there be good communication between the physician performing the biopsy and the histopathologist. The instruments and materials needed to perform a skin biopsy are discussed in Chapter 7.

There are four principal techniques for performing skin biopsies: (a) surgical excision with suturing, (b) punch biopsy, (c) excision with scissors, and (d) shave biopsy. The decision in favor of one method depends on such factors as location of the biopsy, cosmetic result desired, depth of the disease being looked for, type of lesion to be removed (flat or elevated), and simplicity of technique. For example, vesicles should be completely excised in an attempt to keep the roof intact, and scalp biopsy specimens should extend into the subcutis to include the bulbs of terminal follicles.

SAUER NOTE

The skin biopsy specimen must include adequate tissue for proper interpretation by the pathologist.

Surgical Excision

The technique of performing surgical excision biopsies with suturing of the skin is well known. In general, this type of biopsy is performed if a good cosmetic result is desired and if the entire lesion is to be removed. The disadvantage is that this procedure is the most time-consuming of the three techniques, and it is necessary for the patient to return for removal of the sutures. It is important that a sharp scalpel be used to reduce compression artifact, and that care is taken not to crush the specimen with the forceps.

Punch Biopsy

Punch biopsies can be done rather rapidly, with or without suturing of the wound. A punch-biopsy instrument of appropriate size is needed. Disposable biopsy punches are available. A local anesthetic is usually injected at the site. The op-erator rotates the instrument until it penetrates to the subcutaneous level. The circle of tissue is then removed. Bleeding can be stopped with pressure or by the use of one or two sutures. An elliptical wound instead of a circular wound can be produced by stretching the skin perpendicular to the desired suture line before the punch is rotated. The resultant scar, after suturing, is neater. Punch biopsies may be inadequate for evaluation of vesiculobullous diseases and must be deep enough to include subcutaneous fat if used for diagnosis of panniculitis or tumors in a subcutaneous location. In most instances, pigmented lesions should not be punched unless they can be completely excised.

Scissors Biopsy

The third way to remove skin tissue for a biopsy specimen is to excise the piece with sharp pointed scissors and stop the bleeding with light electrosurgery, Monsel solution, or aluminum chloride solution. This latter procedure is useful for certain types of elevated lesions and in areas in which the cosmetic result is not too important. The greatest advantage of this procedure is the speed and the simplicity with which it can be done.

Shave Biopsy

A scalpel or razor blade can be used to slice off a lesion. This can be performed superficially or deeply. Hemostasis can be accomplished by pressure, light electrosurgery, Monsel solution, or aluminum chloride solution.

Biopsy Handling

The biopsy specimen must be placed in an appropriate fixture, usually 10% formalin. If the specimen tends to curl, it can be stretched out on a piece of paper or cardboard before fixing. Mailing specimens in formalin during winter may result in freezing artifact. This may be avoided by the addition of 95% ethyl alcohol, 10% by volume.

CYTODIAGNOSIS

The Tzanck test is useful in identifying bullous diseases such as pemphigus and vesicular virus eruptions (herpes simplex and herpes zoster). The technique and choice of lesions are important. For best results, select an early lesion. In the case of a blister, remove the top with a scalpel or sharp scissors. Blot the excess fluid with a gauze pad. Then gently scrape the floor of the blister with a scalpel blade. Try not to cause bleeding. Make a thin smear of the cells on a clean glass slide. If you are dealing with a solid lesion, squeeze the material between two slides. The slide may be air dried, but it can also be fixed by placing it in 95% ethanol for 15 seconds. Stain the slide with Wright-Giemsa stain, or hematoxylin and eosin.

In addition to skin testing, fungus examination, biopsies, and cytodiagnosis, there are certain tests for specific skin conditions that are discussed in connection with the respective diseases.

ADDITIONAL STUDIES

The deposition of immunoglobulin and complement may be detected by direct immunofluorescence. This is an extremely valuable technique for the diagnosis of lupus erythematosus and autoimmune bullous diseases. It is performed on a frozen section, and therefore the biopsy specimen must be received fresh or in Michel's solution.

Immunohistology is particularly helpful in the accurate diagnosis and classification of neoplasms. It is possible to identify specific antigens in a routinely processed tissue section by attaching a labeled antibody. For example, malignant melanoma may be identified using antibodies directed against S-100 protein and melanoma-specific antigen (HMB-45). Epithelial tumors are immunoreactive for cytokeratins, and malignant lymphoma for leukocyte common antigen.

DNA technology may be very useful. In situ hybridization allows recognition of specific DNA or RNA sequences using a gene probe in frozen or paraffin tissue sections. For example, a variety of different viruses, including herpes simplex, cytomegalovirus, and a human papillomavirus, can be identified using this technique.

The polymerase chain reaction is a technique that amplifies defined DNA sequences. It may be used to identify microorganisms and genetic diseases. It is so sensitive that false positive tests can occur from contamination.

ACKNOWLEDGMENT

I would like to acknowledge the assistance of Dr. Cindy Essmeyer and members of her staff, Marcella Godinez, M.T., Katrin Boese, M.T., and Tammy Thorne, M.T., in preparation of the section on fungus examination. I would also like to acknowledge Clint Gillespie, of Photographic Services, for the kodachromes.

BIBLIOGRAPHY

Skin Tests

Adams RM. Occupational skin disease. Orlando, FL, Grune & Stratton, 1990.

Fisher AA. Contact dermatitis, ed 4. Philadelphia, Lea & Febiger, 1995.

Fungus Examinations

Koneman EW, Roberts GD. Practical laboratory mycology, ed 3. Baltimore, Williams & Wilkins, 1985.

Isenberg HD, ed. Essential procedures for clinical microbiology. ASM Press, 1998.

(See Chap. 19 for additional references.)

Biopsies

Ackerman AB. Histopathologic diagnosis of inflammatory skin diseases. Philadelphia, Lea & Febiger, 1978:149.

Epstein E, Epstein E Jr. Skin surgery, ed 6. Philadelphia, WB Saunders, 1987.

Lever WF, Schaumburg-Lever G. Histopathology of the skin, ed 7. Philadelphia, JB Lippincott, 1990.

Immunodiagnosis

Vassileva S. Immunofluorescence in dermatology. Int J Dermatol 1990;332:153.

General References

Beare JM, Bingham EA. The influence of the results of laboratory and ancillary investigations in the management of skin disease. Int J Dermatol 1981;20:653. The authors conclude that the number of ancillary investigations required by an experienced clinician is quite extraordinarily small, including only biopsy, patch testing, sedimentation rate, and Wood's light.

Hurwitz RM, Hood AF. Pathology of the skin: Atlas of clinical–pathological correlation. Stamford, CT, Appleton & Lange, 1998.

3

Dermatologic Diagnosis

To aid in determining the diagnosis of a presenting skin problem, this chapter contains discussions of primary and secondary lesions and also of diagnosis by location. Included are lists of seasonal skin diseases, military dermatoses, and dermatoses of African-Americans.

PRIMARY AND SECONDARY LESIONS

No two skin diseases look alike, but most have some characteristic primary lesions, and it is important to examine the patient closely to find them. Commonly, however, the primary lesions have been obliterated by the secondary lesions of overtreatment, excessive scratching, or infection. Even in these cases, it is usually possible, by careful examination, to find some primary lesions at the edge of the eruption or on other, less irritated areas of the body (Figs. 3-1–3-3).

Combinations of primary and secondary lesions frequently occur as part of the clinical picture.

Primary Lesions

Descriptions of the basic primary lesions follow:

Macules are up to 1 cm and are circumscribed, flat discolorations of the skin. Examples: freckles, flat nevi.

Patches are larger than 1 cm and are circumscribed, flat discolorations of the skin. Examples: vitiligo, senile freckles, measles rash.

Papules are up to 1 cm and are circumscribed, elevated, superficial, solid lesions. Examples: elevated nevi, warts, lichen planus. A *wheal* is a type of papule that is edematous and transitory (present less than 24 hours). Examples: Hives, sometimes insect bites.

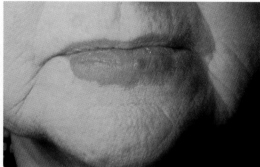

(*A*) Macule, on lip (port-wine hemangioma).

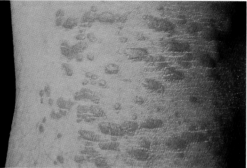

(*B*) Papules, on knee (lichen planus).

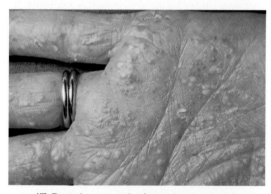

(*C*) Nodule, on lower eyelid (basal cell carcinoma).

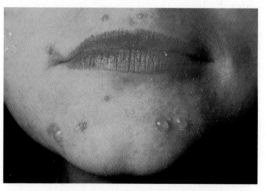

(*D*) Tumor, of abdomen (mixed hemangioma).

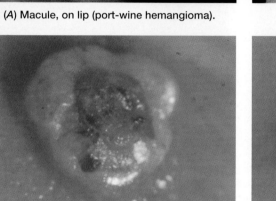

(*E*) Pustules, on palm (pustular psoriasis).

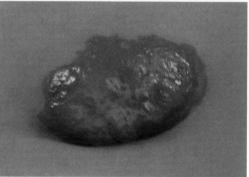

(*F*) Vesicles, on chin (pemphigus vulgaris).

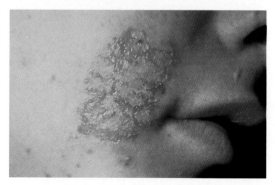

(*G*) Crust, on cheek (impetigo).

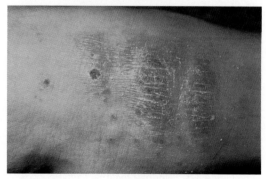

(*H*) Lichenification, on dorsum of ankle (localized neurodermatitis).

Figure 3-1. **Primary and secondary lesions.** *(Geigy Pharmaceuticals)*

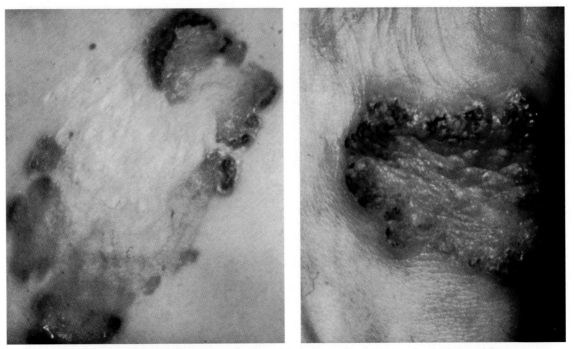

Figure 3-2. Nodular lesions. (*Left*) Grouped nodular lesions with central scarring (tertiary syphiloderm). (*Right*) Grouped warty, nodular lesions with central scarring (tuberculosis verrucosa cutis). (*Marion B. Sulzberger, Folia Dermatologica, No. 1, Geigy Pharmaceuticals*)

Plaques are larger than 1 cm and are circumscribed, elevated, superficial, solid lesions. Examples: mycosis fungoides, lichen simplex chronicus.

Nodules range to 1 cm and are solid lesions with depth; they may be above, level with, or beneath the skin surface. Examples:

nodular secondary or tertiary syphilis, basal cell cancers, xanthomas.

Tumors are larger than 1 cm and are solid lesions with depth; they may be above, level with, or beneath the skin surface. Examples: tumor stage of mycosis fungoides, larger basal cell cancers.

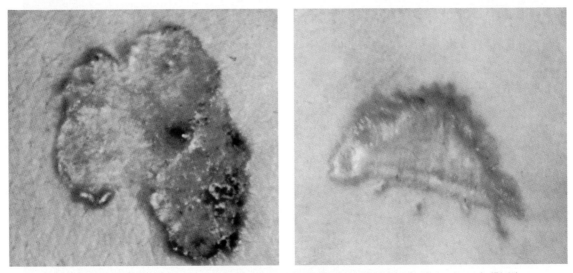

Figure 3-3. Nodular lesions. (*Left*) Polycyclic nodular lesion (superficial basal cell carcinoma). (*Right*) Keloid. (*Marion B. Sulzberger, Folia Dermatologica, No. 1, Geigy Pharmaceuticals*)

Vesicles range to 1 cm and are circumscribed elevations of the skin containing serous fluid. Examples: early chickenpox, zoster, contact dermatitis.

Bullae are larger than 1 cm and are circumscribed elevations containing serous fluid. Examples: pemphigus, second-degree burns.

Pustules vary in size and are circumscribed elevations of the skin containing purulent fluid. Examples: acne, impetigo.

Petechiae range to 1 cm and are circumscribed deposits of blood or blood pigments. Examples: thrombocytopenia and drug eruptions.

Purpura is a larger than 1 cm circumscribed deposit of blood or blood pigment in the skin. Examples: senile purpura and vasculitis.

Secondary Lesions

Secondary lesions include the following:

Scales are shedding, dead epidermal cells that may be dry or greasy. Examples: dandruff (greasy), psoriasis (dry).

Crusts are variously colored masses of skin exudates. Examples: impetigo, infected dermatitis.

Excoriations are abrasions of the skin, usually superficial and traumatic. Examples: scratched insect bites, scabies.

Fissures are linear breaks in the skin, sharply defined with abrupt walls. Examples: congenital syphilis, athlete's foot.

Ulcers are irregularly sized and shaped excavations in the skin extending into the dermis or deeper. Examples: stasis ulcers of legs, tertiary syphilis.

Scars are formations of connective tissue replacing tissue lost through injury or disease.

Keloids are hypertrophic scars beyond the borders of the original injury.

Lichenification is a diffuse area of thickening and scaling with resultant increase in the skin lines and markings.

Several combinations of primary and secondary lesions commonly exist on the same patient. Examples: *papulosquamous lesions* of psoriasis, *vesiculopustular lesions* in contact dermatitis, and *crusted excoriations* in scabies.

Special Lesions

Some primary lesions, limited to a few skin diseases, can be called *specialized lesions.*

Comedones or **blackheads** are plugs of whitish or blackish sebaceous and keratinous material lodged in the pilosebaceous follicle, usually seen on the face, the chest, or the back, rarely on the upper part of the arms. Example: acne.

Milia are whitish nodules, 1 to 2 mm in diameter, that have no visible opening onto the skin surface. Examples: in healed burn or superficial traumatic sites, healed bullous disease sites, or newborns.

Telangiectasias are dilated superficial blood vessels. Examples: spider hemangiomas, chronic radiodermatitis.

Burrows are very small and short (in scabies) or tortuous and long (in creeping eruption) tunnels in the epidermis.

In addition, distinct and often diagnostic changes in the nail plates and the hairs are discussed in the chapters relating to these appendages.

DIAGNOSIS BY LOCATION

A physician is often confronted with a patient with skin trouble localized to one part of the body (Figs. 3-4–3-7). The following list of diseases with special locations is meant to aid in the diagnosis of such conditions, but this list must not be considered all-inclusive. Generalizations are the rule, and many of the rare diseases are omitted. For further information concerning the particular diseases, consult the Dictionary–Index.

SAUER NOTES

In diagnosing a rather generalized skin eruption, the following three mimicking conditions must be considered first and ruled in or out by appropriate history or examination:

1. Drug eruption
2. Contact dermatitis
3. Infectious diseases, such as acquired immunodeficiency syndrome and secondary syphilis

Scalp: Seborrheic dermatitis, contact dermatitis, psoriasis, folliculitis, pediculosis, and hair loss due to the following: Male or female pattern, alopecia areata, tinea, chronic dis-

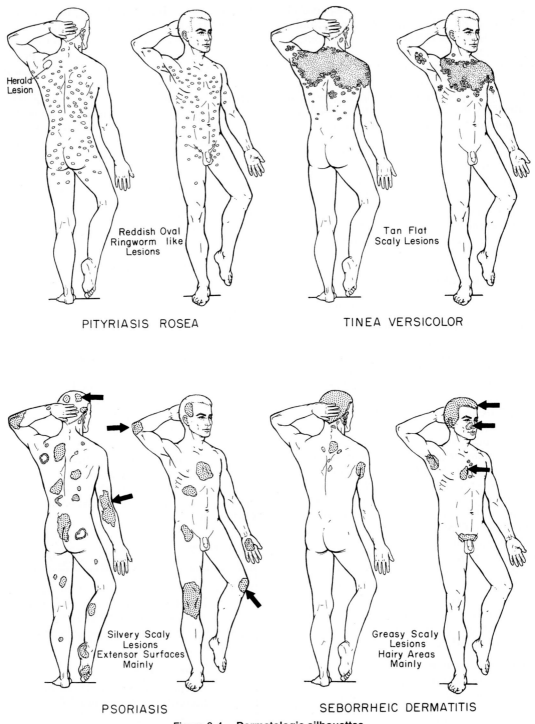

Herald
Lesion

Reddish Oval
Ringworm like
Lesions

Tan Flat
Scaly Lesions

PITYRIASIS ROSEA

TINEA VERSICOLOR

Silvery Scaly
Lesions
Extensor Surfaces
Mainly

Greasy Scaly
Lesions
Hairy Areas
Mainly

PSORIASIS

SEBORRHEIC DERMATITIS

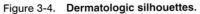

Figure 3-4. **Dermatologic silhouettes.**

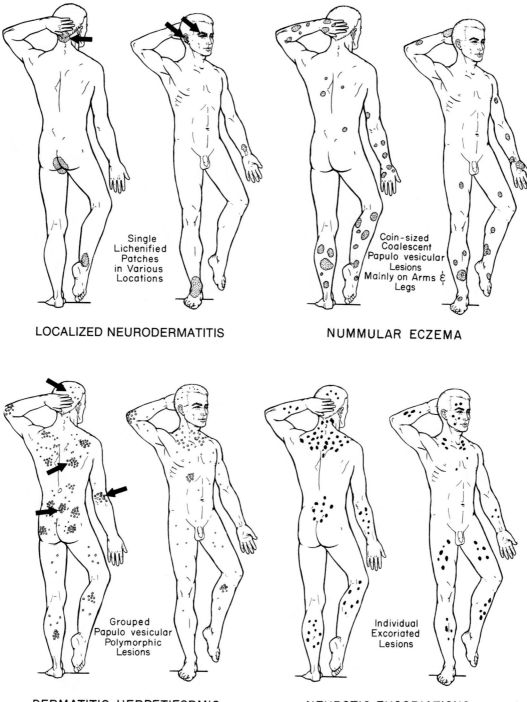

Single
Lichenified
Patches
in Various
Locations

LOCALIZED NEURODERMATITIS

Coin-sized
Coalescent
Papulo vesicular
Lesions
Mainly on Arms &
Legs

NUMMULAR ECZEMA

Grouped
Papulo vesicular
Polymorphic
Lesions

DERMATITIS HERPETIFORMIS

Individual
Excoriated
Lesions

NEUROTIC EXCORIATIONS

Figure 3-5. **Dermatologic silhouettes.**

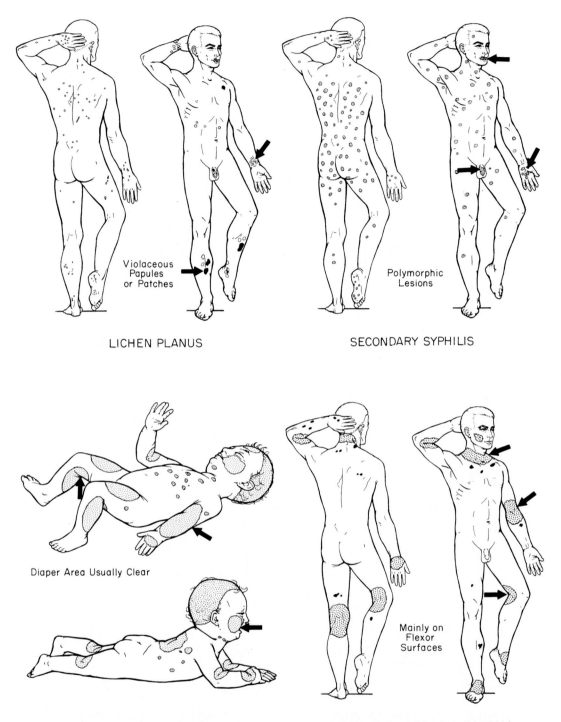

LICHEN PLANUS

Violaceous
Papules
or Patches

SECONDARY SYPHILIS

Polymorphic
Lesions

Diaper Area Usually Clear

INFANTILE FORM of ATOPIC ECZEMA

ADULT FORM of ATOPIC ECZEMA

Mainly on
Flexor
Surfaces

Figure 3-6. **Dermatologic silhouettes.**

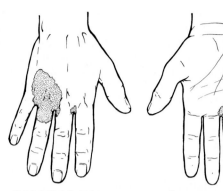

CONTACT DERMATITIS (Housewife)   DYSHIDROSIS or ID (Due to Tinea of Feet)

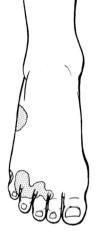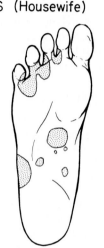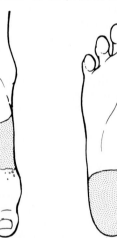

FUNGUS INFECTION   CONTACT DERMATITIS (Shoes)

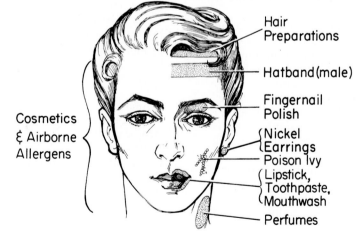

Hair
Preparations

Hatband (male)

Fingernail
Polish

Nickel
Earrings
Poison Ivy

Lipstick,
Toothpaste,
Mouthwash

Perfumes

Cosmetics
& Airborne
Allergens

CONTACT DERMATITIS

Figure 3-7. **Dermatologic silhouettes.**

coid lupus erythematosus, postpregnancy alopecia, alopecia areata, or trichotillomania.

Ears: Seborrheic dermatitis, psoriasis, atopic eczema, and actinic keratoses.

Face: Acne, rosacea, impetigo, contact dermatitis, seborrheic dermatitis, folliculitis, herpes simplex, lupus erythematosus, actinic keratoses, and dermatomyositis.

Eyelids: Contact dermatitis due to fingernail polish or hair sprays, seborrheic dermatitis, or atopic eczema.

Posterior neck: Neurodermatitis (lichen simplex chronicus), seborrheic dermatitis, psoriasis, or contact dermatitis, and acne keloidalis in African-Americans.

Mouth: Aphthae, herpes simplex, geographic tongue, syphilis, lichen planus, oral hairy leukoplakia, squamous cell cancer, and pemphigus.

Axillae: Contact dermatitis, seborrheic dermatitis, hidradenitis suppurativa, erythrasma, acanthosis nigricans, and Fox-Fordyce disease.

Chest and back: Tinea versicolor, pityriasis rosea, acne, seborrheic dermatitis, psoriasis, and secondary syphilis.

Groin and crural areas: Tinea infection, candidal infection, bacterial intertrigo, scabies, pediculosis, and granuloma inguinale.

Penis: Contact dermatitis, fixed drug eruption, condyloma acuminata, candidal balanitis, chancroid, herpes simplex, primary and secondary syphilis, scabies, and, balanitis xerotica obliterans.

Hands: Contact dermatitis, id reaction to fungal infection of the feet, atopic eczema, psoriasis, verrucae, pustular psoriasis, nummular eczema, erythema multiforme, secondary syphilis, and fungal infection.

Cubital fossae and popliteal fossae: Atopic eczema, contact dermatitis, and prickly heat.

Elbows and knees: Psoriasis, xanthomas, dermatomyositis, granuloma annulare, and, atopic eczema.

Feet: Fungal infection, primary or secondary bacterial infection, contact dermatitis from footwear or foot care, atopic eczema, verrucae, psoriasis, erythema multiforme, and secondary syphilis (soles of feet).

SEASONAL SKIN DISEASES

Certain dermatoses have an increased incidence in various seasons of the year. In a busy dermatologist's office, one sees "epidemics" of atopic eczema, pityriasis rosea, psoriasis, and winter itch, to mention only a few. Knowledge of this seasonal incidence is helpful from a diagnostic standpoint. It is sufficient simply to list these seasonal diseases here, because more specific information concerning them can be found elsewhere in this text. Remember that there are exceptions to every rule.

WINTER

Atopic eczema
Contact dermatitis of hands
Psoriasis
Seborrheic dermatitis
Nummular eczema
Winter itch and dry skin (xerosis)
Ichthyosis

SPRING

Pityriasis rosea
Erythema multiforme
Acne (flares)

SUMMER

Contact dermatitis due to poison ivy
Tinea of the feet and the groin
Candidal intertrigo
Miliaria or prickly heat
Impetigo and other pyodermas
Polymorphous light eruption
Insect bites
Tinea versicolor (noticed after suntan)
Darier's disease (uncommon)
Epidermolysis bullosa (uncommon)

FALL

Winter itch
Senile pruritus
Atopic eczema
Pityriasis rosea
Contact dermatitis due to ragweed
Tinea of the scalp (schoolchildren)
Acne (flares)

MILITARY DERMATOSES

Although the major part of the world is now at nominal peace, under the ravages of previous wars the lack of good personal hygiene, the lack of adequate food, and the presence of overcrowding, injuries, and pestilence resulted in the aggravation of any existing skin disease and an increased incidence of the following skin diseases:

Scabies
Pediculosis
Syphilis and other sexually transmitted diseases
Bacterial dermatoses
Tinea of the feet and the groin
Pyoderma
Miliaria

DERMATOSES OF AFRICAN-AMERICANS

The following skin diseases are seen with greater frequency in African-Americans than in Caucasians (Figs. 3-8 and 3-9):

Keloids
Dermatosis papulosa nigra (variant of seborrheic keratoses)

Pyodermas of legs in children
Pigmentary disturbances from many causes, both hypopigmented and hyperpigmented
Traumatic marginal alopecia (from braids and from heated irons used in hair straightening)
Seborrheic dermatitis of scalp, aggravated by grease on hair
Ingrown hairs of beard (pseudofolliculitis barbae)
Acne keloidalis nuchae
Annular form of secondary syphilis
Granuloma inguinale
Mongolian spots

On the other hand, certain skin conditions are rarely seen in African-Americans patients:

Squamous cell or basal cell carcinomas
Actinic keratoses
Psoriasis

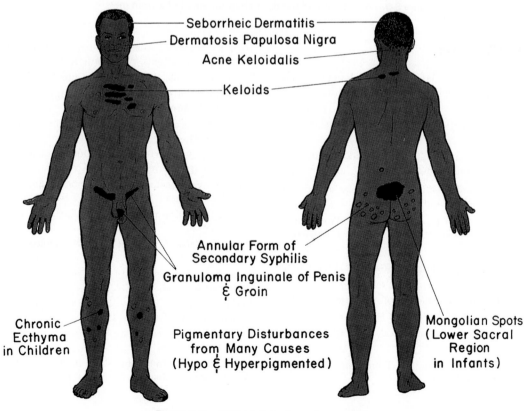

Figure 3-8.   **African-American dermogram.**

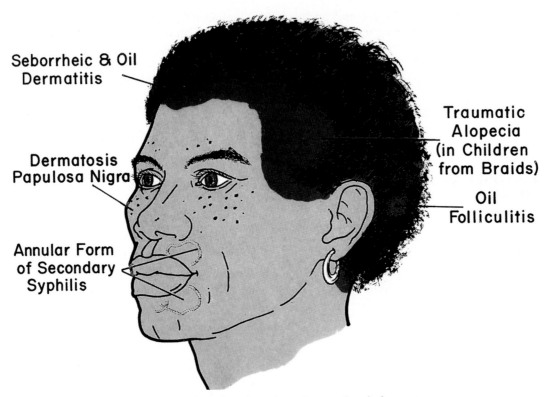

Seborrheic & Oil
Dermatitis

Traumatic
Alopecia
(in Children
from Braids)

Dermatosis
Papulosa Nigra

Oil
Folliculitis

Annular Form
of Secondary
Syphilis

Figure 3-9.   **African-American dermatogram, head of a woman.**

BIBLIOGRAPHY

Ackerman AB, Cockerell CJ. Cutaneous lesions: correlations from microscopic to gross morphologic features. Cutis 1986;37:137.

Ackerman AB, Cockerell CJ. Papules. Cutis 1986;37:242.

Archer CB. Black and white skin diseases: An atlas and text, ed 1. Blackwell Science, 1995.

Ashton R, Leppard B. Differential diagnosis in dermatology. Philadelphia, JB Lippincott, 1989.

Bouchier IAD, Ellis H, Fleming PR. New edition: French's index of differential diagnosis, ed 13. Butterworth-Heineman, 1996.

Callen, JP. Color atlas of dermatology, ed 1. Philadelphia, WB Saunders, 1993.

Callen, JP. Current practice of dermatology, ed 1. Stamford, CT, Appleton & Lange, 1995.

Eliot H, Ghatan Y. Dermatological differential diagnosis and pearls. Parthenon, 1998.

Johnson BL, Moy RL, White GM. Ethnic skin: Medical and surgical. St.Louis, Mosby, 1998.

Helm KF, Marks JG. Atlas of differential diagnosis in dermatology. Philadelphia, WB Saunders, 1998.

Kenney JA, ed. Black dermatology. Cutis 1983;32:334.

Lewis EJ, Dahl MV. On standard definitions 33 years hence. Arch Dermatol 1997;133.

Lynch PJ. Dermatology, ed 3. Baltimore, Williams & Wilkins, 1994.

McDonald CJ. Some thoughts on differences in black and white skin. Int J Dermatol 1976;15:427.

Murphy GF. Dermatopathology: A practical guide to common disorders, ed 1. Philadelphia, WB Saunders, 1995.

Reeves JRT. Clinical dermatology illustrated, ed 2. FA Davis, 1991.

Rosen T, Martin S. Atlas of black dermatology. Boston, Little, Brown, 1981.

Rotstein H. De Launey and Land: Principles and practice of dermatology, ed 3. 1993.

Shelley W, Shelley D. Advanced dermatologic diagnosis. Philadelphia, WB Saunders, 1992.

Steigleder, GK. Pocket atlas of dermatology, ed 2. New York, Theime, 1993.

Sybert VP. Skin manifestations in individuals of African or Asian descent. Pediatr Derm 1996;13:2.

4

Introduction to the Patient

After the usual conversation introducing yourself to the new patient, the following may transpire:

PHYSICIAN: What can I do for you, Mrs. Jones?

MRS. JONES: I have a bad breaking out on my hands.

PHYSICIAN: (*Writes on his chart under* Present Complaint, *"hand dermatitis"*) How long have you had this breaking out?

MRS. JONES: Well, I've had this before, but what I have now has been here for only 3 weeks.

PHYSICIAN: (*Writes, "duration, 3 weeks"*) When did you have this before, Mrs. Jones?

MRS. JONES: Let me see. I believe I had this twice before. The first time I had this breaking out was shortly after our marriage, and I thought that it had to do with the fact that I had my hands in soap and water more than before. It took about a month to heal up. I treated it with salves that I had at home. It certainly wasn't bad then. The next time I broke out it was a little bit worse. This was after my first

child was born. Johnny is 3 years old now. I suppose I should have expected my hands to break out again now because I just had my second baby 3 months ago.

PHYSICIAN: (*Finishes writing, "The patient states that she has had this eruption on two previous occasions. Home treatment only. Both eruptions lasted about 1 month. Present eruption attributed to care of baby born 3 months ago."*) Mrs. Jones, what have you been putting on your hands for this breaking out?

MRS. JONES: Let me take off my bandages, and I'll show you how my hands look.

PHYSICIAN: Let me help you with those bandages. However, I want to ask you a few more questions before I look at your hands.

MRS. JONES: Well, first I used a salve that I got over at the corner drugstore that said on the label it was good for athlete's foot. One of my neighbors told me that she used it for her hand trouble, and it had cured her hands. I don't think that her hands looked like mine, though, and I sort of feel that the salve made my hands worse. Then I decided I would burn out the infection, so I soaked my hands in some bleaching solution. This helped some with the itching, but it made the skin too dry. Then I remembered that you had given me some salve for Johnny's "infantigo," so I put some of that on. That softened up my hands but didn't seem to help with the itching. So here I am, Doctor.

PHYSICIAN: (*Writes, "Treated with athlete's foot Rx, bleach soaks, Johnny's impetigo Rx"*) How much itching are you having?

MRS. JONES: Well, my hands sting and burn when I get any soap and water on them, but I can sleep without them bothering me.

PHYSICIAN: (*Notes, "Mild itching"*) Are you taking any medicine by mouth now for anything? I even want to know about laxatives, vitamins, or aspirin. Have you had any shots recently?

MRS. JONES: No, I'm not taking any medicine.

PHYSICIAN: Now, are you sure?

MRS. JONES: Well I do take sleeping medicine at night occasionally, and, oh yes, I'm taking some reducing pills that Dr. Smith gave me about 2 months ago.

PHYSICIAN: (*Writes, "Drugs—takes sleeping medicine h.s. and reducing pills"*) Mrs. Jones, does anyone in your family have any allergies? Does anyone have any asthma, hay fever, or eczema? Your parents, brothers, sisters, children, other family members?

MRS. JONES: No, not that I can recall, Doctor.

PHYSICIAN: Have you ever had any of those conditions? Any asthma, hay fever, or eczema?

MRS. JONES: No, I haven't had any of those. Sometimes I have a little sinus trouble though.

PHYSICIAN: (*Writes, "No atopy in patient or family"*) Now, let me have a good look at those hands. I also want you to remove your shoes and hose so that I can get a good look at your feet. (*Examines the patient's hands and feet carefully*) Now, are you sure that you don't have this anywhere else, Mrs. Jones?

MRS. JONES: No, I am positive I don't, because I looked all over my skin this morning when I took a bath. However, I do have a mole on my back that I want you to look at, Doctor.

PHYSICIAN: Has it been bothering you recently?

MRS. JONES: Well, no, but my bra strap rubs it occasionally.

PHYSICIAN: (*Examines the mole on her back*) That certainly is a small mole, Mrs. Jones. It doesn't have any unusual color, and I see no reason for having it removed. It could be removed if you wish, but I don't think it is necessary.

MRS. JONES: Well, I don't want it removed if you don't think it is necessary. Now, what do you think about my hands?

PHYSICIAN: Let me make a few notes about what I saw and then I'll tell you about your hands and the treatment. (*Writes, "Physical exam: (1)*

A crusting, vesicular dermatitis is seen mainly in the webs of the fingers of both hands, worse on the right hand. There is no sharp border to the eruption. The nail of the right ring finger has several transverse furrows. The feet are clear. (2) In the midline of the upper back is a 3×3-mm flat, faintly brownish lesion. Diagnosis: (1) Contact dermatitis, probably due to excess soap and water. (2) Pigmented compound nevus.")

SAUER NOTES

As part of a good examination record, one should place in the patient's chart simple diagrams appropriately marked with the site, size, and configuration of growths, scars, rashes, and so on.

1. You need not be an artist to draw a face, a back, a chest, or a hand. You can also use a printed sticker or stamp of the site.

2. Mark in the lesions or configurations and note the size.

3. The value of these simple annotations is multiple. They benefit you, your patient, and, if necessary, your lawyer.

PHYSICIAN: Mrs. Jones, you have a very common skin condition, commonly called housewives' eczema or housewives' dermatitis. I feel sure that it is aggravated by having your hands in soap and water so many times a day. Most housewives don't even have enough time to dry their hands carefully every time they are wet. Some people appear to be more sensitive to soaps than others. It isn't a real allergy but just a sensitivity because the soap and the water have a tendency to remove the normal skin's protective oils and fats. Some of those blisters are infected, and we will have to take care of that infection along with the other irritation. Here is what we will do to treat your hands. (*Gives careful instructions to Mrs. Jones, particularly with regard to the hand soaks, the way the salve is to be applied, advice concerning avoidance of excess soap and water, the use of rubber and cotton gloves, and so on.*)

In this play-by-play description, a type of conversation that is repeated many times a month in any busy practitioner's office, I have attempted to show some of the basic points in history taking.

SAUER NOTES

A careful, thorough medical history from your patient is very important.

LOCAL TREATMENT HISTORY

Find out how much treatment and what kind of local treatment has been administered by the patient or by physicians. Many over-the-counter medications can aggravate a dermatosis.

SYSTEMIC DRUG HISTORY

Don't just ask, "Are you taking any medicines?" Ask, "Are you taking any medicine for *any* reason? Are you on birth control pills (if appropriate), are you on vitamins or sleeping pills, do you take aspirin or Tylenol, do you get any shots?" This history is important for two reasons. First, something about the patient can be learned from the drugs taken. For example, it is important to know if a person is taking insulin for diabetes or corticosteroids for arthritis. This information can well influence your treatment of the patient. Second, drugs can cause many skin eruptions, and your index of suspicion of a drug eruption will be higher if that information is consistently requested.

ALLERGY HISTORY

"Do you or did you ever have any asthma, hay fever, eczema, or migraine headaches?" A positive allergy history is important for two reasons. First, a family or a patient history of allergies can aid in making a diagnosis of atopic dermatitis. Second, if there is a positive allergy history, usually it can be predicted that the patient's skin disorder will respond more slowly to treatment than a similar dermatitis in a nonallergic patient. Patients with atopy are more "itchish."

A careful history is followed by a complete examination of the skin problem, and this, in turn, is followed by therapy, or what I prefer to call *management*. For good management of the patient, I have found it helpful to write out the diagnosis, other information, and instructions. Advantages to the patient and physician are multiple. The patient has an individualized short note about the diagnosis, cause (if known), what the physician can or cannot do (if there is no cure, as for atopic eczema or psoriasis, say so), and instructions about diet, bathing, therapy, and so on. For the physician, the advantage is that a copy can be kept in the patient's chart and used later to help refresh the patient's mind about instructions, or it could even be used advantageously in a medicolegal problem regarding information given to the patient.

Patient information pamphlets available from the American Academy of Dermatology, drug companies, and various disease-specific organizations are helpful especially when handed to the patient by the physician. Note in the chart that this was done.

A common way of arranging a medical record is called "SOAP." This stands for *subjective, objective, assessment, and plan*. Each chart should indicate a presenting complaint, a history of the present illness, a review of systems, past medical history, physical examination, a diagnosis with pertinent differential diagnoses, and a proposed plan of action. Regardless of what method of patient chart organization is used, a uniform complete medical record is mandatory in today's environment of managed care, medical legal hazards, insurance industry reimbursement issues, and Medicare and Medicaid mandates. Computer use can make some of these tasks faster, easier, and more accurate. Patient confidentiality is always to be kept in mind. Medical records need to be legible.

SAUER NOTES

When a patient is in the hospital, many people in white coats or with stethoscopes around their necks come and go. The visit of the dermatologic consultant (or others) may be forgotten in the confusion and misery of the hospital confinement.

There is a simple measure that should help the patient remember the dermatologist's visit: Leave your calling card or an instruction sheet where you write down your diagnosis and instructions. This card, or instruction sheet, has your name, address, and phone number. You can even write on the reverse some information you may wish to convey about the skin problem you were asked to see. And when your bill comes, the patient and family will have it as a reminder of your visit.

SAUER NOTES

The specialty of dermatology, like any medical field, needs good public relations efforts. Most important, we need to promote better public relations in our own sphere of influence.

1. We need to provide correct diagnoses, correct therapy, and proper management for the patient. This should be our most tangible public relations effort.

2. It is important to be a visible dermatologist. This can be accomplished by attending medical meetings and assuming offices in medical societies. There are also medical societies in surrounding communities that need speakers. When you begin practice, it helps to go from door to door, at least in your own office building, to meet the possible referring physicians face to face.

3. After you get a patient referred from another physician, do not fail to thank the physician. Write a note and include the diagnosis with a short description of your treatment.

4. A physician should provide services to the community. One can give medical talks to lay groups and can serve on civic committees.

5. Physicians should have courteous and competent personnel in the office. Pay attention to what goes on at your front desk.

5

Dermatologic Therapy

Many hundreds of medications are available for use in treating skin diseases. Most physicians, however, have only a few favorite prescriptions that are prescribed day in and day out. These few prescriptions may then be altered slightly to suit an individual patient or disease. For commonly used preparations, pretyped prescriptions save time and are legible.

Treatment of most of the common skin conditions is simpler to understand when the physician is aware of three basic principles:

1. The *type of skin lesion*, more than the cause, influences the kind of local medication used. The old adage, "If it's wet, use a wet dressing, and if it's dry, use an ointment," is true in most cases. For example, to treat a patient with an acute oozing, crusting dermatitis of the dorsum of the hand, whether due to poison ivy or soap, the physician should prescribe wet soaks. For a chronic-looking, dry, scaly patch of psoriasis on the elbow, an ointment is indicated because an aqueous lotion or a wet dressing would only be more drying. Bear in mind, however, that *the type of skin lesion can change rapidly under treatment*. The patient must be followed closely after beginning therapy. An acute oozing dermatitis treated with soaks can change, in 2 or 3 days, to a dry, scaly lesion that requires a cream or an ointment. Conversely, a chronic dry patch may become irritated with too strong therapy and begin to ooze.

2. The second basic principle in treatment is *never do any harm* and never overtreat. It is important for the physician to know which of the chemicals prescribed for local use on the skin are the greatest irritants and sensitizers. It is no exaggeration to say that the most commonly seen dermatitis is the *overtreatment contact dermatitis*. The overtreatment is often performed by the patient, who has gone to the neighborhood drugstore, or to a friend, and used any, and many, of the medications available for the treatment of skin diseases. It is certainly not unusual to hear the patient tell of using a strong athlete's foot salve for the treatment of the lesions of pityriasis rosea.

3. The third principle is to *instruct the patient adequately regarding the application of the medicine prescribed*. The patient does not have to be told how to swallow a pill but does have to be told how to put on a wet dressing. Most patients with skin disorders are ambulatory, so there is no nurse to help them. They are their own nurses. The success or the failure of therapy rests on adequate instruction of the patient or person responsible for the care. Even in hospitals, particularly when wet dressings or aqueous lotions are prescribed, it is wise for the physician to instruct the nurse regarding the procedure.

With these principles of management in mind, let us now turn to the medicine used. It is important to stress that we are endeavoring to present here only the most basic material necessary to treat most skin diseases. For instance, there are many solutions for wet dressings, but Burow's solution is our preference. Other physicians have preferences different from the drugs listed, and their choices are respected, but to list all of them will not serve the purpose of this book.

Two factors have guided us in the selection of medications presented in this formulary. First, the medication must be readily available in most drugstores; second, it must be a very effective medication for one or several skin conditions. The medications listed in this formulary also are listed in a complete way in the treatment section concerning the particular disease. Instructions for the use of the medications, however, are more nearly complete in this formulary.

FORMULARY

A particular topical medication is prescribed to produce a specific beneficial effect.

Effects of Locally Applied Drugs

Antipruritic agents relieve itching in various ways. Commonly used chemicals and strengths include menthol (0.25%), phenol (0.5%), camphor (2%), pramoxine hydrochloride 1%, and coal tar solution (liquor carbonis detergens [LCD]) (2% to 10%). These chemicals are added to various bases for the desired effect. Numerous safe and unsafe proprietary preparations for relief of itching are also available. The unsafe preparations are those that contain sensitizing antihistamines, benzocaine, and related "-caine" derivatives.

Keratoplastic agents tend to increase the thickness of the horny layer. Salicylic acid (1% to 2%) is an example of a keratoplastic agent. Stronger strengths of salicylic acid are keratolytic.

Keratolytics remove or soften the horny layer. Commonly used agents of this type include salicylic acid (4% to 10%), resorcinol (2% to 4%), urea (20% to 40%), and sulfur (4% to 10%). A strong destructive agent is trichloroacetic acid.

Urea in 5% to 10% concentration (Aquacare, Carmol) is moisturizing, while in 20% to 40% (Ultra Mide, Carmol) concentration, it is keratolytic.

Alpha hydroxy acids (lactic acid, glycolic acid) in 5% to 12% concentrations are moisturizers, while in higher concentrations up to 80%, they are keratolytic and can be used in the office for facial peeling, with caution.

Antieczematous agents remove oozing and vesicular excretions by various actions. The

SAUER NOTES

LOCAL THERAPY

1. The type of skin lesion (oozing, infected, or dry), more than the cause, should determine the local medication that is prescribed.
2. Do not harm. Begin local therapy for a particular case with mild drugs. The concentration of ingredients can be increased as the acuteness subsides.
3. Do not begin local corticosteroid therapy with the "biggest gun" available, particularly for chronic dermatoses.
4. Carefully instruct the patient or the nurse regarding the local application of salves, lotions, wet dressings, and baths. Many salves should be rubbed in for 5 to 10 seconds.
5. Prescribe the correct amount of medication for the area and the dermatosis to be treated. This knowledge comes with experience (see later in this chapter).
6. Change the therapy as the response indicates. If a new prescription is indicated and the patient has some of the first prescription left, instruct the patient to alternate using the old and the new prescriptions.
7. If a prescription is going to be relatively expensive, explain this fact to the patient.
8. For many diseases, "therapy plus" is indicated. Advise the patient to continue to treat the skin problem for a specified period after the dermatosis has apparently cleared. This may prevent or slow down recurrences.
9. Instruct the patient to telephone you if there are any questions or if the medicine appears to irritate the dermatosis.

common antieczematous agents include Burow's solution packs or soaks, coal tar solution (2% to 5%), and hydrocortisone (0.5% to 2%) and derivatives incorporated in lotions or salves.

Antiparasitic agents destroy or inhibit living infestations. Examples include Elimite cream for scabies, Kwell cream and lotion for scabies and pediculosis, and Nix for pediculosis.

Antiseptics destroy or inhibit bacteria, fungi, and viruses.

Antibacterial topical medications include gentamicin (Garamycin), mupirocin (Bactroban), bacitracin, and neomycin (Neomycin causes an appreciable incidence of allergic contact sensitivity).

Antifungal and **anticandidal topical agents** include miconazole (Micatin, Monistat-Derm), clotrimazole (Lotrimin, Mycelex), ciclopirox (Loprox), econazole (Spectazole), oxiconazole (Oxistat), naftifine (Naftin), ketoconazole (Nizoral), butenafine HCL (Mentax), and terbinafine (Lamisil). Sulfur (3% to 10%) is an older but effective antifungal and anticandidal agent (see Table 19-3).

Antiviral topical agents are acyclovir (Zovirax) ointment and penciclovir (Denavir).

Emollients soften the skin surface. Nivea oil, mineral oil, and white petrolatum are good examples. Newer emollients are more cosmetically elegant and effective.

SAUER NOTES

LOCALLY APPLIED GENERIC PRODUCTS

Advantages: Lower cost—you can prescribe a larger quantity at relatively less expense, and patients appreciate your sharing their concern regarding cost.

Disadvantages: With a proprietary product, you are quite sure of the correct potency and bioavailability of the agent, you know the delivery system, and you know the ingredients in the base.

If you prescribe a proprietary medication when a less expensive generic is available, explain to the patient your reason for doing this.

Types of Topical Dermatologic Medications

BATHS

1. Tar bath
   Coal tar solution (USP, LCD)   120.0
   Sig: Add 2 tbsp to a tub of lukewarm water, 6 to 8 inches deep.
   Actions: Antipruritic and antieczematous
2. Starch bath
   Limit or Argo starch, small box
   Sig: Add half box of starch to tub of cool water, 6 to 8 inches deep.
   Actions: Soothing and antipruritic
   Indications: Generalized itching and dryness of skin, winter itch, urticaria
3. Aveeno (regular and oilated) colloidal oatmeal bath
   Sig: Add 1 cup to the tub of water.
   Actions: Soothing and cleansing
   Indications: Generalized itching and dryness of skin, winter and senile itch
4. Oil baths (see section on oils and emulsions, below)

SOAPS AND SHAMPOOS

1. Oilatum soap unscented, Dove soaps, Neutrogena soaps, Cetaphil, Basis
   Action: Mild cleansing agent
   Indications: Dry skin, winter itch
2. Dial soap, Lever 2000
   Actions: Cleansing and antibacterial
   Indications: Acne, pyodermas
3. FS shampoo 120.0
   Sig: Shampoo as needed.
   Actions: Antiinflammatory, antipruritic, and cleansing
   Indications: Dandruff, psoriasis of scalp
   Comment: Contains fluocinolone acetonide, 0.01%
4. Selsun Suspension or Head and Shoulders Intensive Treatment shampoo 120.0
   Sig: Shampoo hair with three separate applications and rinses. You can leave the last application on the scalp for 5 minutes before rinsing off. Do not use another shampoo as a final cleanser.
   Actions: Cleansing and antiseborrheic
   Indications: Dandruff, itching scalp (not toxic if used as directed)
5. Tar shampoos: Polytar, T/Gel, X-Seb T, Pentrax, Ionil T, and so on
   Sig: Shampoo as necessary, even daily.
   Actions: Cleansing and antiseborrheic

Indications: Dandruff, psoriasis, atopic eczema of scalp
6. Nizoral shampoo 120.0
   Sig: Shampoo two or three times a week.
   Actions: Anticandidal and antiseborrheic
   Indication: Dandruff

WET DRESSINGS OR SOAKS

1. Burow's solution, 1:20
   Sig: Add 1 Domeboro tablet or packet to 1 pint of tap water. Cover affected area with sheeting wet with solution and tie on with gauze bandage or string. Do not allow any wet dressing to dry out. It can also be used as a solution for soaks.
   Actions: Acidifying, antieczematous, and antiseptic
   Indications: Oozing, vesicular skin conditions
   Comment: Do not use over a large area of the body.
2. Vinegar solution
   Sig: Add 1/2 cup of white vinegar to 1 quart of water for wet dressings or soaks, as above.
3. Salt solution
   Sig: Add 1 tbsp of salt to 1 quart of water for wet dressings or soaks, as above.

POWDERS

1. Purified talc (USP) or Zeasorb powder 60
   Sig: Dust on locally b.i.d. (Supply in a powder can)
   Actions: Absorbent, protective, and cooling
   Indications: Intertrigo, diaper dermatitis
2. Tinactin powder, Micatin powder, Zeasorb-AF powder, or Desenex powder
   Sig: Dust on feet in morning.
   Actions: Absorbent and antifungal
   Indications: Prevention and treatment of tinea pedis and tinea cruris
   Comment: The above powders are available over the counter.
3. Mycostatin powder 15.0
   Sig: Dust on locally b.i.d.
   Action: Anticandidal
   Indication: Candidal intertrigo

SHAKE LOTIONS

1. Calamine lotion (USP) 120
   Sig: Apply locally to affected area t.i.d. with fingers or brush.
   Actions: Antipruritic and antieczematous
   Indication: Widespread, mildly oozing, inflamed dermatoses
2. Nonalcoholic white shake lotion:

Zinc oxide	24.0
Talc	24.0
Glycerin	12.0
Distilled water q.s. ad	120.0

3. Alcoholic white shake lotion:

Zinc oxide	24.0
Talc	24.0
Glycerin	12.0
Distilled water q.s. ad	120.0

4. Colored alcoholic shake lotion:
   To alcoholic white shake lotion, add Sun Chemical pigments (brunette shade) 2.4
5. Proprietary lotions:
   Sarna lotion (with menthol and camphor), Cetaphil lotion

SAUER NOTES

1. Shake lotions 2, 3, and 4 are listed for physicians who desire specially compounded lotions, as I do. One or two pharmacists near your office will be glad to compound them and keep them on hand.
2. To these lotions you can add sulfur, resorcinol, menthol, phenol, and so on, as indicated.

OILS AND EMULSIONS

1. Zinc oxide, 40%
   Olive oil q.s. 120.0
   Sig: Apply locally to affected area by hand or brush t.i.d.
   Actions: Soothing, antipruritic, and astringent
   Indications: Acute and subacute eczematous eruptions
2. Bath oils:
   Nivea skin oil, Alpha-Keri
   Sig: Add 1 to 2 tbsp to the tub of water. Caution: Be careful to avoid slipping in tub.
   Actions: Emollient and lubricating
   Indications: Winter itch, dry skin, atopic eczema
3. Hand and body emulsions: A multitude of products are available over the counter. Some have phospholipids, some have urea or alpha hydroxy acids, and some are lanolin free.
   Sig: Apply locally as necessary.
   Actions: Emollient and lubricating
   Indications: Dry skin, winter itch, atopic eczema

4. Scalp oil:
Derma-Smoothe FS oil (fluocinolone acetonide 0.01%)   120.0
Sig: Moisten scalp hair and apply lotion overnight; wear a plastic cap.
Indications: Scalp psoriasis, lichen simplex chronicus, and severe seborrheic dermatitis

TINCTURES AND AQUEOUS SOLUTIONS

1. Povidone-iodine (Betadine) solution (also in skin cleanser, shampoo, and ointment)   15
Sig: Apply with swab t.i.d.
Actions: Antibacterial, antifungal, and antiviral
Indication: General antisepsis
2. Thimerosal tincture (N.F.)
Merthiolate tincture,   1:1000
Sig: Apply with swab t.i.d.
Actions: Antibacterial, antifungal, and drying
3. Gentian violet solution:
Gentian violet, 1%
Distilled water q.s.   30.0
Sig: Apply with swab b.i.d.
Actions: Antifungal and antibacterial
Indications: Candidiasis, leg ulcers
4. Antifungal solutions
   a. Lotrimin, Mycelex, Loprox, Tinactin, Micatin, Monistat-Derm, Lamisil spray among others   30.0
   Sig: Apply localy b.i.d.
   b. Fungi-Nail   30.0
   Sig: Apply locally b.i.d.
   Comment: Contains Resorcinol, salicylic acid, parachlorometaxylenol, and benzocaine in a base with acetic acid and alcohol.

PASTES

1. Zinc oxide paste (USP)
Sig: Apply locally b.i.d.
Actions: Protective, absorbent, and astringent
Indication: Localized crusted or scaly dermatoses

CREAMS AND OINTMENTS

A physician can write prescriptions for creams and ointments in two ways: (1) by prescribing proprietary creams and ointments already compounded by pharmaceutical companies, or (2) by formulating one's own prescriptions by adding medications to certain bases, as especially indicated for the particular patient being treated. For the physician who uses the second method, two different types of bases are used:

1. Water-washable cream bases: These bases are pleasant for the patient to use, are nongreasy, and are almost always indicated when treating intertriginous and hairy areas. Their disadvantage is that they can be too drying. A number of medications, as specifically indicated, can be added to these bases (*i.e.*, menthol, sulfur, tars, hydrocortisone, triamcinolone, antibiotics).
   a. Unibase
   b. Vanicream
   c. Acid Mantle Creme
   d. Dermovan
   e. Unscented cold cream (not water-washable)
2. Ointment bases: These Vaseline-type bases are, and should be, the most useful in dermatology. Although not as pleasant for the patient to use as the cream bases, their greasy quality alleviates dryness, removes scales, and enables the medicaments to penetrate the skin lesions. Any local medicine can be incorporated into these bases.
   a. White petrolatum (USP)
   b. Zinc oxide ointment (USP)
   c. Aquaphor (contains lanolin)
   d. Eucerin (contains lanolin)

For the physician who wishes to prescribe ready-made proprietary preparations, these are listed in groups:

3. Antifungal ointments and creams
Lotrimin cream, Mycelex cream, Spectazole cream, Loprox cream, Tinactin cream, Lamisil cream, Oxistat cream, Naftin cream, Nizoral cream, Mentax cream, and others (see Table 19-3).
Action: Antifungal
4. Antibiotic ointments and creams:
Bactroban ointment and cream, Garamycin ointment and cream, Neosporin ointment, Mycitracin ointment, Polysporin ointment. (Antibiotic solutions are discussed in Chapter 13 under Acne Therapy.)
5. Antiviral ointments
   a. Zovirax ointment (acyclovir)
   b. Denavir (penciclovir cream)
6. Corticosteroid ointments and creams (Table 5-1)
   a. Hydrocortisone preparations (.5% and 1% hydrocortisone creams and ointments are available over the counter and generically)
      • Hytone 1% and 2.5% cream and ointment

TABLE 5-1
POTENCY RANKING OF SOME COMMONLY USED TOPICAL CORTICOSTEROIDS*

Group I
Temovate cream 0.05%
Temovate ointment 0.05%
Temovate gel 0.05%
Diprolene AF cream 0.05%
Diprolene ointment 0.05%
Psorcon cream 0.05%
Psorcon ointment 0.05%
Ultravate cream 0.05%
Ultravate ointment 0.05%

Group II
Cyclocort ointment 0.1%
Diprosone ointment 0.05%
Elocon ointment 0.1%
Florone ointment 0.05%
Halog cream 0.1%
Lidex cream 0.05%
Lidex gel 0.05%
Lidex ointment 0.05%
Maxiflor ointment 0.05%
Maxivate cream 0.05%
Maxivate ointment 0.05%
Maxivate lotion 0.05%
Topicort cream 0.25%
Topicort gel 0.05%
Topicort ointment 0.25%

Group III
Aristocort cream HP 0.5%
Aristocort A ointment 0.1%
Cloderm cream
Cyclocort cream 0.1%
Cyclocort lotion 0.1%
Dermatop emollient cream 0.1%
Dermatop ointment
Diprosone cream 0.05%
Florone cream 0.05%
Halog ointment 0.1%
Halog solution 0.1%
Lidex E cream 0.05%
Maxiflor cream 0.05%
Pandel
Valisone ointment 0.1%

Group IV
Cordran ointment 0.05%
Elocon cream 0.1%
Elocon lotion 0.1%
Kenalog cream 0.1%
Kenalog ointment 0.1%
Synalar ointment 0.025%
Topicort LP cream 0.05%
Westcort ointment 0.2%

Group V
Cordran cream 0.05%
Diprosone lotion 0.05%
Kenalog lotion 0.1%
Kenalog ointment 0.025%
Locoid cream 0.1%
Locoid ointment 0.1%
Synalar cream 0.025%
Tridesilon ointment 0.05%
Valisone cream 0.1%
Westcort cream 0.2%

Group VI
Aclovate cream 0.05%
Aclovate ointment 0.05%
Aristocort cream 0.1%
DesOwen cream 0.05%
DesOwen ointment 0.05%
DesOwen lotion 0.05%
Kenalog cream 0.025%
Kenalog lotion 0.025%
Locoid solution 0.1%
Locorten cream 0.03%
Synalar cream 0.01%
Synalar solution 0.01%
Tridesilon cream 0.05%
Valisone lotion 0.1%

Group VII
Topicals with hydrocortisone, dexamethasone, flumethalone, prednisolone, and methylprednisolone

*Group I is the superpotency category. Potency descends with each group, to group VII, which is the least potent (groups II and III are potent corticosteroids; IV and V are mid-strength corticosteroids; VI and VII are mild corticosteroids). There is no significant difference between agents within groups II through VII. The compounds are arranged alphabetically within the groups. In group I, Temovate cream or ointment is most potent. (Courtesy of the late Richard B. Stoughton, MD, and Roger C. Cornell, MD)

b. Desonide preparations
- Tridesilon cream and ointment
- DesOwen cream and ointment

c. Triamcinolone preparations
- Kenalog ointment and cream
- Aristocort ointment and creams
- Also available generically

d. Other fluorinated corticosteroid preparations: See Table 5-1 for a listing of these preparations, which are ranked according to potency.

SAUER NOTES

1. Over-the-counter 0.5% or 1.0% Cortaid ointment (not the cream) has proved effective and well tolerated as an emergency nonprescription treatment.

2. Psorcon ointment is the only group I medication that has Food and Drug Administration approval to be used under occlusive dressing or for more than 2 consecutive weeks.

3. Do not use group I topical agents for longer than 2 weeks, or more than a 45-gram tube per week. A rest period must follow for 2 weeks.

---

7. Corticosteroid antibiotic ointments and creams
   Cortisporin ointment

8. Corticosteroid antifungal–antiyeast preparations
   a. Lotrisone cream
   b. Mycolog II cream and ointment

9. Antipruritic creams and lotions
   a. Eurax cream
   b. Sarna lotion
   c. Prax lotion
   d. PramaGel
   e. Doxepin (Zonalon) cream (may cause drowsiness)

10. Retinoic acid products:
    Retin-A cream (0.025%, 0.05%, 0.1%) and Retin-A gel (0.01% and 0.025%), Retin-A Micro (0.1%)
    Actions: Anti-acne comedones and small pustules (especially the gel) and antiphotoaging
    Indications: Acne of comedonal and small pustular type; aging wrinkles on face; removal of mild actinic keratoses, freckles, molluscum contagiosum, and flat warts
    Differin (adapalene gel 0.1%)
    Action: Retinoic acid receptor binder
    Indications: Acne of comedonal and small pustular type.
    Avita (tretinoin 0.025%) cream and gel
    Action: Anti-acne
    Indications: Acne of comedonal and small pustular type.

11. Miscellaneous creams, ointments, and gels
    a. MetroGel (metronidazole 0.75%)   15.0
       Noritate Cream (metronidazole 1%)   30.0
       Indications: Rosacea, perioral dermatitis
    b. Dovonex ointment (also comes as cream and scalp solution) 30.0 or 100.0
       Action: Antipsoriatic
       Comment: Moderately expensive
    c. Tazorac gel 0.05% and 0.1%
       Action: Antipsoriatic
       Comment: Very expensive, contraindicated in women with childbearing potential.

SAUER NOTES

COMPOUND PREPARATIONS

Compound proprietary preparations are frequently prescribed, particularly by family practice physicians and nondermatologic specialists. Physicians should know the ingredients in these compound preparations and should know the side effects. Here are some popular compounds:

Mycolog II cream: Contains mycostatin and triamcinolone. Beware: It is not beneficial for fungus (tinea) infections; the triamcinolone after long-term use can cause atrophy, striae and telangiectasia of the skin especially in intertriginous areas and on the face.

Lotrisone cream: Contains clotrimazole (Lotrimin) and betamethasone dipropionate. Beware: The betamethasone with long-term use can cause atrophy, striae and dilated vessels especially in intertriginous areas and on the face.

Vioform–hydrocortisone cream (Vytone): Contains Vioform plus 1% hydrocortisone. Beware: The Vioform causes a moderate yellow stain on the skin and clothing.

Cortisporin ointment: Contains 1% hydrocortisone with Neosporin, Polysporin, and bacitracin. Beware: Neomycin allergies occur infrequently.

12. Scabicidal and pediculicidal preparations
    a. Eurax cream and lotion
    Action: Scabicidal
    b. Kwell (lindane) lotion and cream
    Actions: Scabicidal and pediculicidal
    c. Elimite cream
    Action: Scabicidal
    d. Nix creme rinse
    Indications: Head lice, nits
13. Sunscreen creams and lotions:
    Aminobenzoic acid (and the esters of PABA) and octyl dimethyl paba (Padimate O), octocrylene, octyl salicylate, microfine zinc oxide, avobenzone (Parsol 1789), zinc oxide, cinnamates (octyl-methoxycinnamate), titanium dioxide, oxybenzone (benzophenone-3) are effective ultraviolet light blockers. There are many products on the market. Any sunscreen with a sun protective factor (SPF) of 15 or above offers effective sun-damage protection, if used correctly, frequently, early in age, and, for light-complexioned or sun-sensitive people, in the summer *and* winter. One sun-blocking agent is RVPaque cream.
    Sig: Apply to exposed areas before going outside.
    Action: Screening out ultraviolet rays
    Indications: Polymorphous light eruption, photoaging, systemic and chronic lupus erythematosus, possible prevention of skin precancers and skin cancers, especially in light-complexioned people

AEROSOLS AND FOAMS

1. Various local medications have been incorporated in aerosol and foam-producing containers. These include corticosteroids, antibiotics, antifungal agents, antipruritic medicines, and so on.
2. Kenalog spray (63-gram can), and Diprosone aerosol are effective corticosteroid preparations for scalp psoriasis and seborrhea.

CORTICOSTEROID MEDICATED TAPE

1. Cordran tape (also comes as a patch)
   Indications: Small areas of psoriasis, neurodermatitis, lichen planus

MEDICATED SKIN PATCHES

Several are available for transdermal delivery of such agents as nitroglycerin, EMLA patch for topical anesthesia, nicotine antismoking patches, and hormones.

FLUOROURACIL PREPARATIONS

See section on actinic keratosis therapy in Chapter 32.

LOCAL AGENTS FOR OFFICE USE

1. Podophyllum in cpd. tincture benzoin
   Podophyllum resin (USP) 25%
   Cpd. tct. benzoin q.s. ad 30.0
   Sig: Apply small amount to warts with cotton-tipped applicator every 4 or 5 days until warts are gone. Excess amount may be washed off in 3 to 6 hours after application, to prevent irritation.
   Action: Removal of venereal warts
   Comment: Other podophyllum proprietary preparations such as condylox are marketed.
2. Trichloroacetic acid solution (saturated)
   Sig: Apply with caution with cotton-tipped applicator. (Have water handy to neutralize.)
   Indications: Warts on children, seborrheic keratoses, xanthelasma
3. Modified Unna's boot
   a. Dome-Paste Bandage
   b. Gelocast
   c. Compression Gelatine bandage with zinc oxide and glycerine then wrapped with Coflex flexible wrap
   Indications: Stasis ulcers, localized neurodermatitis (lichen simplex)
4. Ace bandage, 3 or 4 inches wide
   Indications: Stasis dermatitis, leg edema

LOCAL THERAPY RULES OF THUMB

Students and general practitioners state that they are especially confused by dermatologists' reasons for using one chemical for one skin lesion and not another, or one chemical for unrelated skin diseases. The answer to this dilemma is not easily given. More often than not, the major reason for our preference is that experience has taught us, and those before us, that the particular drug works. Some drugs do have definite chemical actions, such as antiinflammatory, antipruritic, antifungal, or keratolytic actions, and these have been listed in the Formulary. But there is no definite scientific explanation for the beneficial effect of some of the other drugs, such as tar or sulfur on cases of psoriasis.

In an attempt to solve this apparent confusion, here are some generalizations summarizing our experience.

SAUER NOTES

1. I use compounded preparations with liquor carbonis detergens (LCD), sulfur, resorcinol, and salicylic acid every day in my practice.
2. These chemicals can be used to complement the corticosteroids in a mixture.
3. When prescribing one of these chemicals, always begin with the lower percentage of the drug. Increase the percentage only when a stronger action is desired.
4. I am quite aware of the arguments against the use of pharmacy-compounded prescriptions. They have worked exceptionally well for me and for my patients.

TARS (COAL TAR SOLUTION [LCD], 3% TO 10%; CRUDE COAL TAR, 1% TO 5%; ANTHRALIN, 0.1% TO 1%)

Consider for use in cases of:

Atopic eczema
Psoriasis
Seborrheic dermatitis
Lichen simplex chronicus

Avoid in intertriginous areas (can cause a folliculitis).

SULFUR (SULFUR, PRECIPITATED, 3% TO 10%)

Consider for use in cases of:

Tinea of any area of body
Acne vulgaris and rosacea
Seborrheic dermatitis
Pyodermas (combine with antibiotic salves)
Psoriasis

RESORCINOL (RESORCINOL MONOACETATE, 1% TO 5%)

Consider for use in cases of:

Acne vulgaris and rosacea (usually with sulfur)
Seborrheic dermatitis
Psoriasis

SALICYLIC ACID (1% TO 5%, HIGHER WITH CAUTION)

Consider for use in cases of:

Psoriasis
Lichen simplex chronicus, localized thick form

Tinea of feet or palms (when peeling is desired)
Seborrheic dermatitis
Avoid use in intertriginous areas.

MENTHOL (.25%); PHENOL (.5% TO 2%); CAMPHOR (1% TO 2%)

Consider for use in any pruritic dermatoses. Avoid use over large areas of body.

HYDROCORTISONE AND RELATED CORTICOSTEROIDS (HYDROCORTISONE POWDER, .5% TO 2%)

Consider for use in cases of:

Contact dermatitis of any area
Seborrheic dermatitis
Intertrigo of axillary, crural, or inframammary regions
Atopic eczema
Lichen simplex chronicus

Avoid use over large areas of body. New topical corticosteroids (such as fluticasone) with lower incidence of side effects and still with high potency may soon be available.

FLUORINATED CORTICOSTEROIDS LOCALLY

These chemicals are not readily available as powders for personal compounding, but triamcinolone, fluocinolone, and others are available as generic creams and ointments. Consider for use with or without occlusive dressings, in cases of:

Psoriasis, localized to small area (see Chap. 14)
Lichen simplex chronicus (see Chap. 11)
Lichen planus, especially hypertrophic type
Also anywhere that hydrocortisone is indicated
Avoid use over large areas of the body.

SAUER NOTES

LOCAL CORTICOSTEROID THERAPY

1. Avoid prescribing strong local corticosteroid preparations for generalized body use.
2. Do not prescribe the most potent ("biggest-gun") corticosteroid therapy on the initial visit.
3. The fluorinated corticosteroids should not be used on the face and intertriginous areas, where long-term use can result in atrophy and telangiectasia of the skin. There are exceptions.

4. The potent corticosteroids have a definite systemic effect.

5. Fluorinated corticosteroid prescriptions only rarely should be written for p.r.n. refills.

6. Continued long-term use of a local corticosteroid can result in a diminished effectiveness (tachyphylaxis).

7. The pros and cons of prescribing *generic* corticosteroids are discussed early in the chapter.

Quantity of Cream or Ointment to Prescribe

Several factors influence any general statements: severity of the dermatosis, acute or chronic dermatosis, base of the product (a petrolatum-based ointment spreads over the skin farther than a cream), whether dispensed in a tube or jar (patients use less from tubes), and the intelligence of the patient.

- 15 grams of a cream used b.i.d. will treat a mild hand dermatosis for 10 to 14 days.
- 30 grams of a cream used b.i.d. will treat an arm for 14 days.
- 60 grams of a cream used b.i.d. will treat a leg for 14 days.
- 480 to 960 grams or 1 to 2 lb of a cream used b.i.d. will treat the entire body for 14 days. This is seldom a practical prescription, but unmedicated white petrolatum or a cream base is economical to use over a large surface area. Other therapeutic agents should be used to make the dermatosis less extensive (*i.e.,* internal corticosteroids).

SPECIFIC INTERNAL DRUGS FOR SPECIFIC DISEASES

As in all fields of medicine, certain diseases can be treated best by certain specific systemic drugs. These drugs may not be curative, but they should be considered when beginning to outline a course of management for a particular patient. Many factors influence the decision to use or not use such a specific drug. Here follows a list of skin diseases and some systemic medicines considered specific (or as specific as possible) for the disease. *For proper dosage and contraindications,* check the appropriate sections in this book or in current books on therapy.

Acne vulgaris or rosacea in the scarring stage: antibiotics, spirinolactone, and in women birth control pills. For severe cases of cystic acne in men or women without indication of pregnancy, isotretinoin (Accutane) is indicated.

Acquired immunodeficiency syndrome (AIDS): Many systemic drugs are used, directed as specifically as possible against opportunistic organisms, tumors, and the human immunodeficiency virus.

Alopecia areata: corticosteroids in any of four forms—topical, intralesional or rarely parenteral, oral

Atrophie blanche vasculitis: pentoxifylline (Trental), corticosteroids

Creeping eruption: thiabendazole

Darier's disease: vitamin A, for controlled periods of time, and possibly isotretinoin, acitretin

Dermatitis herpetiformis: dapsone and sulfapyridine

Granuloma annulare: intralesional corticosteroids

Herpes simplex: acyclovir (Zovirax), famciclovir (Famvir), valacyclovir (Valtrex), foscarnet sodium (Foscavir).

Herpes zoster: acyclovir (Zovirax), famciclovir (Famvir), and valacyclovir (Valtrex)

Inflammation of the skin from many causes: antibiotics are indicated, in some cases, when local therapy is inadequate for control. Nonsteroidal antiinflammatory drugs are beneficial for some diseases.

Kawasaki's syndrome: intravenous gamma globulin and aspirin

Keloids: intralesional corticosteroids, 585-nm pulsed dye laser, 30 second liquid nitrogen cryosurgery and silicon gel sheets for 12 to 24 hours each day for at least 2 months.

Lichen simplex chronicus: intralesional corticosteroids

Lupus erythematosus: for systemic lupus erythematosus, use corticosteroids or immunosuppressive agents with care; for discoid form, use hydroxychloroquine and related antimalarials (beware of eye damage).

Mycosis fungoides: corticosteroids, antimetabolites, retinoids, and α_{2b}-interferon

Necrobiosis lipoidica diabeticorum: intralesional corticosteroids

Pemphigus: corticosteroids and antimetabolites

Pruritus from many causes: antihistamines and

tranquilizer-like drugs. Selected cases can be treated with oral corticosteroids.

Psoriasis, localized: intralesional corticosteroids

Psoriasis, severe: corticosteroids, psoralens and ultraviolet light (PUVA), methotrexate, cyclosporine (Neoral), and, in men or postmenopausal women, acitretin (Soriatane)

Pyodermas of skin: systemic antibiotics are valuable, when indicated.

Sarcoidosis: possibly corticosteroids, antimalarials

Sporotrichosis: saturated aqueous solution of potassium iodide and ketoconazole (Nizoral)

Syphilis: penicillin or other antibiotics

Tinea of scalp, body, crural area, nails: griseofulvin and, for selected cases, ketoconazole (Nizoral) and itraconazole (Sporanox), terbinafine hydrochloride (Lamisil)

Tuberculosis of the skin: dihydrostreptomycin, isoniazid, *p*-aminosalicylic acid, and rifampin

Urticaria: antihistamines and corticosteroids

SAUER NOTES

1. There are potential side effects from any systemic therapy. Be aware of these possible reactions by being knowledgeable concerning every drug you prescribe.

2. The risk/benefit ratio for your patient must always be considered.

3. Be aware of cross-reactions with a patient on multiple medications.

BIBLIOGRAPHY

Arndt KA. Manual of dermatologic therapeutics, ed 5. Philadelphia, Lippincott–Raven, 1995.

Barranco VP. Clinically significant drug interactions in dermatology. J Am Acad Dermatol 1998;38:4.

Drake LA, Dinehart SM, Farmer ER, et al. Guidelines of care for the use of topical glucocorticosteroids. J Am Acad Dermatol 1996;35:615.

Epstein E. Common skin disorders, ed 4. Philadelphia, WB Saunders, 1994.

Jackson EM. AHA-type products proliferate in 1993. Cosmetic Dermatol 1993;6:11.

Katz HI. Dermatologist's guide to adverse therapeutic interactions. Philadelphia, Lippincott–Raven, 1997.

Korting HC, Kerscher MJ. Glucocorticoids with improved benefit/risk ratio: do they exist? J Am Acad Dermatol 1992;27:87.

Lin AN, Reimer RJ, Carter DM. Sulfur revisited. J Am Acad Dermatol 1988;18:553.

Olsen EA. A double-blind controlled comparison of generic and trade-name topical steroids using the vasoconstriction assay. Arch Dermatol 1991;127:197.

Physician's Desk Reference. Oradell, NJ, Medical Economics, published yearly.

Wolverton SE. Monitoring for adverse effects from systemic drugs used in dermatology. J Am Acad Dermatol 1992;26:661.

6

Physical Dermatologic Therapy

The field of physical medicine embraces therapy with a variety of agents, which include massage, therapeutic exercise, water, air, radiation (heat, light, ultraviolet, x-rays, radium, and lasers), vibrations, refrigeration, and electricity of various forms. Many of these agents are used in the treatment of skin diseases.

HYDROTHERAPY

The physical agent most commonly used for dermatoses is hydrotherapy, in the form of medicated or nonmedicated wet compresses and baths. Distilled water and tap water are the vehicles and may contain any of the following chemicals in varying strengths: sodium chloride, aluminum acetate (Burow's solution), potassium permanganate, silver nitrate, tar, starch, and oatmeal (Aveeno). The instructions and the dilutions for Burow's solution compresses, starch baths, and tar baths are listed in the formulary in Chapter 5.

Wet Dressings

Wet dressings can be applied as open or closed dressings. The *open* compresses are used most frequently since excessive maceration of tissue occurs when the dressings are "closed" with plastic wrap or rubber sheeting. The compresses can be *hot*, *cold*, or *at room temperature*. Instructions to the patient or the nurse concerning correct application of the compresses should be explicit and detailed. For most conditions, the area to be treated should be wrapped with two or three layers of clean gauze sheeting or muslin. Additional gauze 3 inches wide should be wrapped around the sheeting to hold it firmly in place. After that, the dressing can be moistened with the solution by pouring it on or by squirting it under the dressing with a bulb syringe. In most instances, the dressing is wet with the solution before it is wrapped on the affected area. The compresses should never be allowed to dry out and should be left on only for the time specified by the physician. The solution used should be made fresh every day. For treating the face, hands, and genitalia, special masks, gloves, and slings can be improvised. The indications for wet compresses are any oozing, crusting, or pruritic dermatoses, regardless of cause.

SAUER NOTE

Over-the-telephone emergency therapy for an itching dermatitis should include the suggestion of cool wet packs or soaks applied for 20 minutes three times a day. Advantages: soothing, effective, and nothing to buy at the pharmacy.

Medicated Baths

Medicated baths should last from 15 to 30 minutes. Cool baths tend to lessen pruritus and are prescribed most frequently. Baths can be used for a multitude of skin diseases, except those conditions for which excessive dryness is to be avoided, such as for patients with atopic eczema, senile or winter pruritus, and ichthyosis.

ELECTROSURGERY

Electrosurgery is employed very commonly in treating or removing a multitude of skin lesions. One of several different types of available currents and instruments is employed to achieve a desired result. Five forms of electrosurgery are available.

SAUER NOTES

1. Use electrosurgery with caution on patients with cardiac pacemakers.
2. If alcohol has been used to prepare the surgery site, make sure that it has evaporated and that alcohol pledgets are removed from the area before performing electrosurgery.

Electrodesiccation or Fulguration

Electrodesiccation, or fulguration, is produced by an Oudin current of high voltage and low amperage, using a single or monoterminal electrode. The high-frequency current wave is damped. Such a current is produced by the Hyfrecator.

Electrocoagulation

Electrocoagulation is produced by a d'Arsonval current of relatively low voltage and high amperage, using biterminal electrodes. This current also is damped and can be obtained from the Hyfrecator using the spark-gap part of the machine. Electrocoagulation is more destructive than electrodesiccation, owing to the intense heat.

Electrosection

Electrosection, or cutting, is produced by a current that is undamped when delivered by a vacuum tube apparatus and moderately damped from a spark-gap apparatus. Biterminal electrodes are used. When the vacuum tube cutting current is used, the cut is clean, with practically no coagulation, whereas the current from a spark-gap machine produces some coagulation of the cut skin edge. Any coagulation can be minimized by making a rapid stroke. Tissue skillfully removed in this manner can be studied histologically, if necessary.

Electrocautery

Electrocautery is simply produced by applying heat to the skin. This can be supplied by many instruments. Some operators prefer this form of electrosurgery to electrodesiccation or electrocoagulation.

Electrolysis

Electrolysis uses a direct galvanic current to produce chemical cauterization of tissue due to the formation of sodium hydroxide in the tissues, with liberation of free hydrogen at the negative electrode. Battery machines or rectified direct-current instruments accomplish this. Electrolysis is used mainly to remove superfluous hair. A faster and less painful technique of hair epilation is to use the high-frequency current set at a very low intensity, at which it will deliver a small electrodesiccation spark.

The dermatoses most commonly treated by electrosurgery are warts of all kinds, actinic and seborrheic keratoses, leukoplakia, spider hemangiomas, hypertrichosis, and basal cell and squamous cell carcinomas. The skill and the experience of the therapists determine the scope of their use of the surgical diathermy machine. Disposable electrode tips are available.

CRYOSURGERY

Therapeutic refrigeration of the skin can be accomplished by the use of solid carbon dioxide or more commonly liquid nitrogen.

Solid carbon dioxide is readily available from a tank of carbon dioxide, as blocks from ice cream manufacturers. The temperature of solid carbon dioxide is $-78.5°$ C. The solid carbon dioxide, that used to be used commonly, was shaped into an appropriately sized "pencil" for treat-

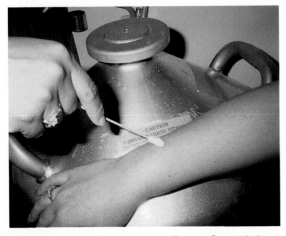

Figure 6-1. Liquid nitrogen applicator. One technique of applying liquid nitrogen to skin lesions is with a large or small cotton-tipped applicator.

ment of superficial skin growths, warts, or seborrheic keratoses.

Liquid nitrogen, which provides freezing at −195.8° C, has become more readily available for office use. Many dermatologists have a 25-liter, refillable container in their office. This amount lasts for 2 or 3 weeks with normal usage. A loosely wound cotton-tipped applicator is used to hold the smoking liquid (Fig. 6-1). The applicator is applied to the skin for only a few seconds. The pain varies from moderate to quite marked. A blister forms within 24 hours after the application, and it is hoped that the growth comes off entirely when the dead skin peels away in 10 to 14 days. Additional liquid nitrogen applications may be indicated. Liquid nitrogen can be sprayed on the skin. Several spray units are available that have varying degrees of sophistication and cost. Liquid nitrogen is used to remove warts, seborrheic keratosis, actinic keratoses, and other superficial skin growths. Therapeutically, liquid nitrogen can also be used to flatten excoriated folliculitis, prurigo nodularis, and Kaposi's sarcoma in patients with acquired immunodeficiency syndrome.

SAUER NOTES

1. The length of application of liquid nitrogen cryosurgery should err on the short side rather than on the long side.
2. Seldom does one need to treat a keratosis or wart for longer than 10 to 20 seconds.

3. Overzealous therapy is painful for the patient, is rarely necessary, and prompts phone calls to the physician at night with concern over a large blood blister.
4. Overtreatment can also cause unsightly hypopigmentation, scars, and rarely nerve damage.
5. Danger: Cryotherapy below the knee in elderly patients can result in slow-healing ulcers.

RADIATION

Radiation agents are important in the field of skin diseases.

Ultraviolet Therapy

Ultraviolet therapy is commonly used and available. There are several sources of artificial ultraviolet radiation.

The *hot quartz mercury vapor lamp* is used for dermatoses. This operates at a high vapor pressure and relatively high temperature, producing middle-wave ultraviolet radiation, in the 290- to 320-nm range, or UVB. These rays cause erythema and tanning of the skin.

Fluorescent sunlamps are low-pressure mercury vapor lamps in glass tubes internally coated with a white phosphor. They produce waves of moderate intensity, with the main emission in the 280- to 350-nm range. They cause erythema and tanning and are used in specially constructed, booth-like units.

The dermatoses most commonly treated with the UVB lamp are psoriasis, acne, pityriasis rosea, and seborrheic dermatitis, and less commonly parapsoriasis, pityriasis lichenoides chronica, eosinophilic pustular folliculitis, pruritus of HIV infection, and uremic pruritus. Narrowband UVB (311–313nm) is possibly more efficacious than standard UVB therapy and may be safer.

UVA lamps produce high-intensity long-wave ultraviolet radiation, in the 315- to 400-nm range. For decades, these wavelengths were believed to be biologically inactive. Newly developed intensified light sources of these wavelengths have been produced. When oral or topical psoralens are given to patients who are then exposed to this light source, the procedure is known as PUVA therapy. This routine is used to treat psoriasis and vitiligo.

The true risk of skin cancer from PUVA therapy may not be known for years. There is an increased incidence of squamous cell carcinoma of the skin. PUVA-induced lentigines, although so far benign, and malignant melanoma are another reason for concern. Tanning salons use UVA lamps of lower intensity, but some UVB is emitted. The safety of these units is variable, and regulation, unfortunately, is minimal. These should be avoided.

The *cold quartz lamp* operates at a low vapor pressure and low temperature, producing essentially a monochromatic source, at 254 nm, in the UVC range. These rays have insignificant tanning effect and mainly produce desquamation. The use of this lamp in dermatology is limited.

New types of narrowband or limited spectrum therapies are being developed.

Photophoresis is the extracorporeal exposure of blood to ultraviolet radiation. When the blood is returned to the body of a patient with a cutaneous T-cell lymphoma, there is in some cases a suppressive effect on the remaining untreated malignant cells. Efficacy in therapy with photophoresis has also been tried for progressive systemic sclerosis of scleroderma and for several other diseases.

X-Ray Therapy

Another of the physical therapeutic agents used for skin diseases is x-ray therapy. A detailed discussion of x-ray therapy is not within the scope of this book since it is a specialized subject of considerable magnitude. X-ray therapy should be administered only by an adequately trained dermatologist or radiologist. If correct shielding and dosage are observed, x-ray therapy is quite safe, as has been proved by many well-controlled studies.

X-ray therapy finds its greatest use in the treatment of skin cancers, various pruritic dermatoses, and cutaneous lymphomas (particularly mycosis fungoides).

SAUER NOTES

X-ray therapy, when first used, caused a large amount of skin cancer and disfigurement. As with any therapy, when used by an experienced physician, in an appropriate setting, it can have many valuable uses.

For most dermatoses, excluding malignancies, the physical factors of superficial x-ray therapy are 70 to 100 kV-peak, 2 to 5 mA, 20 to 30 cm focal skin distance, and no filter. The half-value layer with these factors varies with the machine from 0.6 to 1 mm of aluminum. The average superficial x-ray therapy dose for dermatoses is 75 rad per week. This weekly dose can be given up to a maximum total of 600 to 1200 rad, if absolutely indicated. The top maximum dose depends on many factors, such as seriousness of the lesion being treated, response of the dermatosis to therapy, and complexion and age of the patient. *Under no circumstances should such a maximum course of x-ray therapy ever be repeated.* Grenz ray therapy is an even more superficial form of x-ray therapy, and therefore it is potentially less harmful.

Laser

The laser (an acronym for *light amplification by stimulated emission of radiation*) is an instrument that generates an intensely strong beam of light that is capable of cauterizing, and thus destroying, various skin lesions. The carbon dioxide laser, which produces a beam of intense invisible infrared electromagnetic energy with a wavelength of 10,600 nm, is the laser that is most often used for treating dermatologic lesions.

The lesions treated include cutaneous vascular growths, inflammatory masses, tattoos, nevoid lesions, and other growths.

Many newer specialized lasers have specific indications.

Photodynamic Therapy

This unique therapy has been used to treat actinic keratosis and superficial squamous cell carcinoma. It can also be used to tell tumor extent to help guide more conventional surgical therapy.

A photosensitization (usually δ-aminolevulinic acid) is applied to the skin and then a light source (laser or inherent light) causes tissue necrosis by generating light reactive oxygen intermediates that oxidize essential cellular components.

BIBLIOGRAPHY

Council on Scientific Affairs. Harmful effects of ultraviolet radiation. JAMA 1989;262:380.

Coven TR, Burack LH, Gilleaudeau R, et al. Narrowband UV-B produces superior clinical and histopathological resolution of moderate-to-severe psoriasis in patients compared with broadband UV-B. Arch Dermatol 1997;133:1514.

Dierickx CC, Anderson RR. New horizons in phototherapy: Photodynamic therapy in dermatology. Dermatology Foundation 1998;32:1.

Dover JS, Arndt KA, et al. Guidelines of care for laser surgery. AAD/Dermatology World Supplement, Oct 1998.

Fritsch C, Goerz G, Ruzicka T. Photodynamic therapy in dermatology. Arch Dermatol 1998;134:207.

Goldschmidt H, Panizzon RG. Modern dermatologic radiation therapy. New York, Springer-Verlag, 1991.

Hruza GJ. Lasers for pigmented lesions. Fitzpatrick's J Clin Dermatol 1994;Jul/Aug:47.

Kuflik EG. Cryosurgery updated. J Am Acad Dermatol 1994;31:6.

Luftl M, Degitz K, Plewig G, Rocken M. Psoralen Bath Plus UV-A Therapy. Arch Dermatol 1997;133:1597.

Sebben JE. Cutaneous electrosurgery. Chicago, Year Book Medical Publishers, 1989.

Spicer MS, Goldberg DJ. Lasers in dermatology. J Am Acad Dermatol 1996;34:1.

Fundamentals of Cutaneous Surgery

Frank Custer Koranda, M.D.*

Attention to detail is the essence of surgical perfection. Disregard of or ignorance of any of the fundamentals of surgery is often the difference between the optimal and the merely acceptable healed wound.

INSTRUMENT SELECTION

If an instrument facilitates one's surgery, it is usually worth its cost. Quality instruments are expensive. For most types of cutaneous surgery, the Webster needle holder, the neurosurgery needle holder, and the Halsey needle holder are well designed (Fig. 7-1A). Because of the smaller size of suture and the finer, precise needles that are generally best suited for cutaneous surgery, the needle holders should have smooth jaws. Serrated jaws can cut fine sutures and damage precision needles. For very delicate surgery and for very fine sutures, the Castroviejo needle holder is preferred (Fig. 7-1B). The amount of motion necessary to lock and unlock the Castroviejo is less than that required for the standard type of needle holder.

To lessen tissue damage the skin should be handled in the least traumatic manner. Gentle handling requires the use of skin hooks such as the single-hook Frazier or the fine double-hook Tyrell. When using forceps, usually finer types such as the Bishop-Harmon ophthalmic forceps are advantageous (Fig. 7-1C).

The no. 3 scalpel handle is used with the nos. 10, 11, and 15 blades. For very precise incisions, the 15C blade should be used. This blade was originally designed for periodontal surgery. For scissors dissection, the Metzenbaum, Malis, or Ragnell scissors may be used (Fig. 7-1D). For finer work, a Stevens scissor is well suited (Fig. 7-1E). For cutting sutures precisely and for suture removal, the pointed, delicately curved Gradle scissor is ideal (Fig. 7-1F).

A basic cutaneous surgical pack may include the following:

1. Webster or neurosurgery smooth jawed needle holder
2. Adson delicate forceps with teeth or Micro-Adson forceps with teeth
3. Dissecting scissors
4. Utility scissors
5. Halsted mosquito hemostats
6. Backhaus towel clips, 3 1/2 inch
7. Round toothpicks for skin marking (toothpicks dipped in methylene blue make a finer line than the standard marking pen and are less expensive)
8. Gauze sponges
9. Cotton tipped applicators are an option for point control of bleeding.

*Associate Clinical Professor, Department of Otolaryngology-Head and Neck Surgery, Division of Dermatology, University of Kansas Medical Center, Kansas City, Kansas; Staff Surgeon, Department of Otolaryngology-Head and Neck Surgery, St. Luke's Shawnee Mission, Shawnee Mission, Kansas.

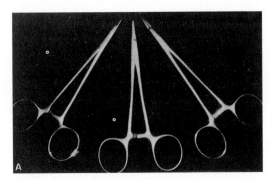

(A) Left to right: Webster needle holder, neuro-surgery needle holder, and Halsey needle holder.

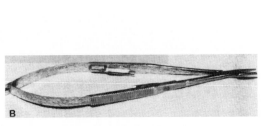

(B) Castroviejo needle holder.

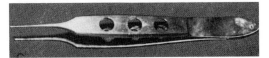

(C) Bishop-Harman ophthalmic forceps.

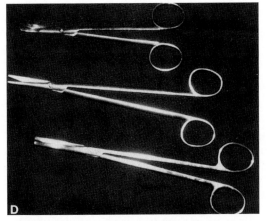

(D) Metzenbaum, Malis, and Ragnell scissors.

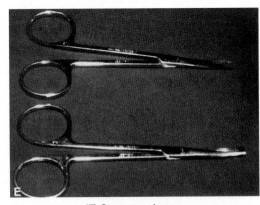

(E) Stevens scissors.

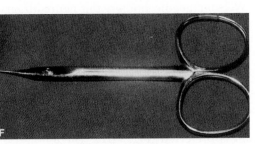

(F) Gradle scissors.

Figure 7-1. **Surgical instruments.**

SUTURE SELECTION

Sutures may be divided into two general groups, absorbable and nonabsorbable. The absorbable sutures are plain gut, chromic gut, polyglycolic acid (Dexon), polyglactin 910 (Vicryl), polydiox-anone (PDS), polyglyconate (Maxon), and poli-glecaprone (Monocryl).

Gut sutures that are made from the small intestine submucosal layer of sheep and the small intestine serosal layer of cattle undergo degradation by phagocytosis by eliciting a foreign body response. Plain gut gradually loses its tensile strength over 2 weeks. Chromic suture is gut suture that has been coated with chromic salts to delay its degradation. It has a slightly prolonged tensile strength over that of plain gut. Another modification of gut suture is the fast-absorbing plain gut. This is a suture that breaks down in 4 to 7 days and may be used for the skin stitch. After 4 to 7 days, the fast-absorbing suture may be wiped out of the wound with a moistened cotton-tipped applicator. In small children and for individuals who cannot return for suture removal, this is another option. The disadvantage is that there is more of an inflammatory response to this material than to nylon.

The synthetic absorbable sutures undergo degradation by hydrolysis. The synthetic sutures usually produce less of an inflammatory response in the subcutaneous tissue than do the gut sutures. Although Vicryl and Dexon are somewhat similar in their tensile strength properties, vicryl has a better tensile strength profile maintaining 65% at 2 weeks and 40% at 3 weeks. The hydrolysis and absorption of Vicryl is also significantly faster than that of Dexon. PDS and Maxon both maintain their tensile strength longer, 70% at 3 weeks, 50% at 4 weeks, and 25% at 6 weeks. Hydrolysis occurs at between 180 and 210 days.

The frequently used nonabsorbable sutures are silk, nylon, and polypropylene. Silk sutures are frequently used for eyelids and lips so that there are no sharp, irritating ends. The monofilament nylons such as Ethilon are general-purpose sutures. Prolene and Surgilene, a polypropylene type of monofilament suture, have the characteristics of increased memory and high tensile strength. They are good choices for a running intradermal stitch.

For subcutaneous sutures on the face usually a 4-0 or 5-0 size suture is used. For skin sutures on the face usually a 5-0 or 6-0 size suture is used. For delicate work a 7-0 size suture may be indicated. It is easier to handle the 7-0 size with a Castroviejo needle holder.

For skin and fascia one uses a reverse cutting needle. With the reverse cutting needle, the cutting edge is on the outside. For facial surgery and for other fine cutaneous surgery, precision-point needles should be used. There is reduced tissue drag and trauma with these super-smooth-finished, highly honed needles. In the Ethicon system, these needles have the code prefix P or PS (plastic or plastic surgery) and in the Davis and Geck systemic PR or PRE (plastic reconstructive). The P3 or PS 3 size needles have good utility for facial surgery. For general cutaneous surgery, an FS (for skin) reverse cutting needle may be used, but there is an appreciable drag as compared with the precision needles.

TYPES OF STITCHES

Buried Subcutaneous

The buried subcutaneous stitch (Fig. 7-2A) is used to close the dead space to prevent hematoma and a nidus for infection. It also reduces the tension on the incision line. Burying the knot decreases the amount of tissue reaction in the more superficial part of the wound so that the major part of the inflammatory response is away from the surface of the incision line and less apt to disrupt it.

To bury the knot, the needle is first inserted through the deeper tissue and exits more superficially on the same side as the wound and then enters superficially on the other side and exits through the deeper tissue on that side of the wound. An absorbable suture is usually used.

Simple Stitch

The simple stitch (Fig. 7-2B) is made through and through the epidermis and dermis from one side to the other. The entry and the exit points should be about 2 to 3 mm from the wound edge. With proper entry of the needle, a greater "bite" of tissue is taken more deeply than superficially. This helps to evert the wound edges.

The simple stitch is not only an approximating and everting stitch but is also used to adjust the height of wound edges so that they are even. If one side of the wound is lower than the other, a slightly deeper bite should be taken on the lower side for coarse adjustment of the wound edges. The knot is then placed on the lower side of the wound to further finely adjust the height of the wound edges.

Vertical Mattress Stitch

The vertical mattress stitch (Fig. 7-2C) tents up the skin edges. This eversion provides for good epidermal apposition and compensates for contracture that occurs in the wound and may cause a linear depression in the wound. If the edges of the wound are not everted sufficiently by the simple stitches, using a vertical mattress for every two or three simple sutures will usually provide good eversion.

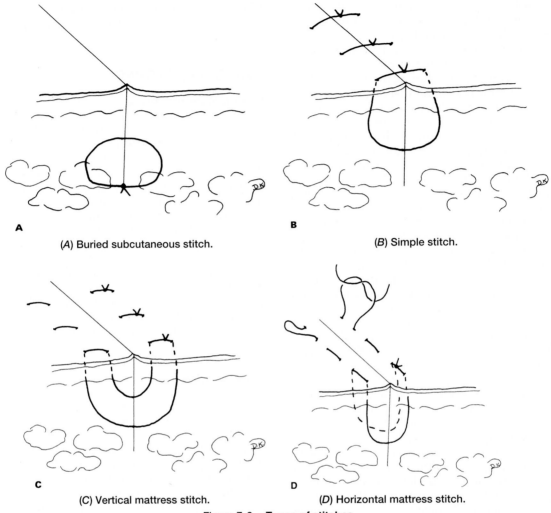

(A) Buried subcutaneous stitch.

(B) Simple stitch.

(C) Vertical mattress stitch.

(D) Horizontal mattress stitch.

Figure 7-2. **Types of stitches.**

Horizontal Mattress Stitch

The horizontal mattress stitch (Fig. 7-2D) is used for the closure of a wound under tension. It can cause strangulation of the skin. Because of this it is often used with a bolster such as a piece of a red Robinson catheter slipped over the part of the suture in contact with the skin to reduce pressure on the skin. In general it is not a suitable stitch for facial surgery.

Corner Stitch (Tip Stitch, Half-Buried Mattress)

The corner stitch (Fig. 7-3A) is used for V-shaped corners to prevent necrosis of the skin tip. It is inserted vertically down through the main seg-

ment of tissue and out through the dermis. It then enters horizontally through the dermal tissue in the tip of the flap and then back up through the main segment of tissue. The suture must enter and leave the flap tip in the same dermal plane that it exits and reenters the dermis of the main body of tissue.

Running Intradermal Stitch

The running intradermal stitch (Fig. 7-3B) is a dermally placed stitch that may be left in for an extended period without causing cross hatching. On some occasions, this stitch may be left in permanently. The stitch enters the skin at a point 4 to 5 mm beyond the end of the incision. From this point it is brought into the wound and then is

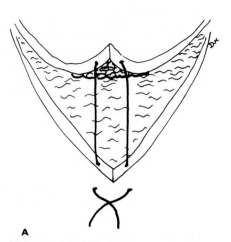

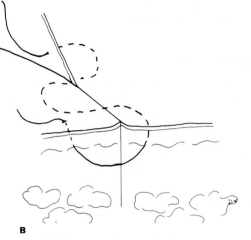

A

(*A*) Corner stitch (tip stitch, half-buried mattress stitch).

B

(*B*) Running intradermal stitch.

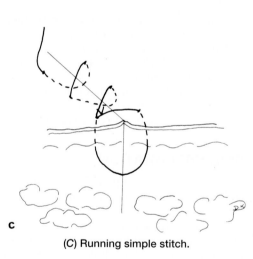

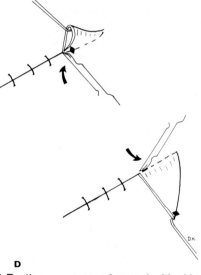

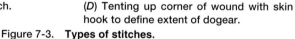

C

(*C*) Running simple stitch.

D

(*D*) Tenting up corner of wound with skin hook to define extent of dogear.

Figure 7-3. **Types of stitches.**

placed through the dermis on one side and crosses to the other side. The stitch is continued in a running "S" pattern, staying in the same plane of the dermis on both sides of the wound. In a long running intradermal stitch, it is wise to have it go out through the skin and then back down through the skin at the midpoint and then proceed intradermally. This will facilitate later removal, because this midpoint of the suture may be cut and only half the amount of suture needs to be pulled out from each end.

Although the intradermal stitch nicely coapts the wound, it is wise to also use a few sim-

ple stitches for the first 3 days for wound edge eversion and additional support.

Running Simple Stitch

The running simple stitch (Fig. 7-3C) is a repeated, continuous over-and-over simple stitch that is a rapid method of closure. This type of stitch can evenly distribute tension along the wound, and it is easier and less traumatic to remove than multiple interrupted stitches. By adjusting the depth of bite of tissue with each placement of the suture, the height of the wound edges may also be adjusted.

SUTURE TYING

Sutures should be tied so that they lie down as square knots. The sutures should be tied to coapt the wound edges but not to strangulate. Most individuals err by tying too tightly. One way of avoiding tight knots is to keep from snugging down the second throw of the suture. Leaving this throw slightly loose also compensates for the tissue edema that develops in wounds. Tying too tightly is a major cause of suture track marks on the skin. Leaving sutures in too long is another factor.

HEMOSTASIS

Meticulous hemostasis is essential to good wound healing. A rule of thumb on controlling bleeding vessels is that named vessels should be clamped and ligated and unnamed vessels may be electrocoagulated.

In tying vessels, use the smallest size suture that is practical. The suture should be cut on the knot to leave the least amount of foreign material in the wound that might cause foreign body reaction.

For electrocoagulation, a biterminal device may be used. With the biterminal unit, current enters the patient through an active or coagulating electrode. When tissue contact is made, heat is generated and coagulation occurs. The current passes through the patient and out via the dispersing electrode, the ground pad. The patient usually becomes part of the current circuit.

The grounding pad should be placed as close as possible to the surgical site. If possible, the heart should not be between the active electrode and the grounding pad, because it then becomes part of the current pathway.

The area of coagulation should be kept dry with sponging or with suction, because bleeding into the surrounding area disperses the current and diminishes the coagulation effect.

Biterminal coagulation is not bipolar coagulation. Bipolar coagulation refers to the system in which a single electrode has both terminals contained in it. With bipolar coagulation forceps, the current passes between the tines of the forceps, coagulating the tissue between the tines. Bipolar coagulation is more precise, produces less tissue damage, and does not involve current transmission through the patient.

Electrocautery is essentially a red-hot branding iron that seals blood vessels by the direct application of heat. Electrocautery systems use either low-frequency alternating current or direct current. The current remains in the electrode tip and does not pass into the patient. Electrocautery provides better hemostasis in a very wet field than does electrocoagulation. There are a variety of disposable, battery powered cautery pens.

PATIENT PREPARATION

Written instructions to the patient before extensive skin surgery help to prevent misunderstandings.

1. The patient should take no aspirin, aspirin-containing products, or nonsteroidal antiinflammatories for 2 weeks before surgery, because they interfere with platelet aggregation and prolong the bleeding time.
2. Shampoo the hair the night before or morning of surgery.
3. Apply no creams or make-up to face after washing the morning of surgery.
4. No smoking for 72 hours prior to surgery.
5. Take regularly prescribed medicines the morning of surgery.
6. Do not wear clothing that pulls over the head.
7. Wear loose, comfortable clothing.
8. Bring a companion to drive home.

SKIN PREPARATION

It is best to shave as little hair as possible. Do not shave the eyebrows, because they grow at a very slow rate.

Cleanse the skin with Betadine or Hibiclens, but do not use Hibiclens around the eye. Use Betadine or Shur-Clens (Poloxaner 188) about the eye. Prepare a large enough surgical area so that one may see not only the immediate surgical site but also the relationship to the surrounding anatomic landmarks to be sure that closure of the wound is not distorting some other structure such as the nose, lip, or eyelid.

The incision lines are marked out before any distortion by infiltrative anesthesia. Round toothpicks dipped in methylene blue or Bonney's blue make a more exact line than most skin marking pens.

ANESTHESIA

Most cutaneous surgery requires only local infiltrative or regional block anesthesia. The standard agent, 1% lidocaine, is an effective and safe anesthetic in which allergic reactions are exceedingly rare. By the addition of epinephrine, systemic absorption of lidocaine is lessened, the duration of action is markedly prolonged, and a local hemostatic effect is achieved. It usually takes 15 minutes to achieve optimal vasoconstriction. The available commercial preparations usually combine lidocaine with 1 : 100,000 epinephrine. Some patients react to epinephrine with apprehension, body tremors, diaphoresis, palpitations, tachycardia, and increased blood pressure. These side effects may be decreased or eliminated by increasing the dilution of epinephrine to 1 : 200,000 or even to 1 : 400,000 without significantly changing its efficacy.

The maximum recommended dosage of lidocaine is 500 mg, the equivalent of 50 ml of a 1% solution.

The injection of lidocaine, especially with epinephrine, is discomforting. This discomfort may be decreased by applying EMLA cream (lidocaine 2.5%, prilocaine 2.5%) to the skin under occlusion or in a patch form for 2 hours prior to a procedure to provide some dermal analgesia before lidocaine injection. This is particularly useful for young children and very apprehensive adults. Warming anesthetics to room temperature and buffering the anesthetic may decrease pain. One way of buffering 30 ml of lidocaine 1%, and epinephrine 1 : 100,000 is with 3 mL of 8.4% sodium bicarbonate injection. This shortens the shelf life of the lidocaine to 6 weeks or less.

PLACEMENT OF INCISIONS

Incisions should be planned so that they are parallel to or within wrinkle and smile lines. When there is lack of definite wrinkles, place incisions in the direction of relaxed skin tension lines. These lines run at right angles to the contraction vectors of the underlying muscle.

Another guide for camouflaging scars is to place incision lines at the boundaries of aesthetic and anatomic units. Examples are the vermilion junction, paranasal fold (the junction of the nose and the cheek), the submandibular area (the junction of the cheek and the neck), the submental area (the junction of the chin and neck), the preauricular area, and along the eyebrow or in the hair.

INCISIONS

Incisions should be made vertical to the skin surface. Obliquely angled incisions do not coapt as

well. An exception to the rule of vertical incisions is in the area adjacent to the eyebrows or in the hair. Incisions placed here should be at an angle that parallels the angle of the hair shaft as it emerges from the skin to avoid transection of the hair follicle.

Wounds, even small, should be undermined to reduce tension. Undermining may be done with a scissors or scalpel. On the face, the level or undermining is usually just under the dermal plexus. On the scalp, the level is between the aponeurosis and the periosteum, which is a relatively blood-free plane.

EXCISIONS

The standard excision is fusiform in shape. If the length-to-width ratio of the fusiform is less than 4:1 or if one side is longer than the other, redundant tissue will develop at the corners of the closure. These so-called dog ears or standing cones of tissue, if small, level out and flatten as the wound undergoes contracture. If large, they should be removed by tenting up the corner of the wound with a skin hook to define the extent of the dog ear. The dog ear is incised along its base on one side or the other. The final wound curves toward the side on which the incision is placed. After making the incision along one side of the base of the dog ear, the flap of tissue that is created is pulled across the incision. Where the base of the redundant tissue crosses the incision, it is transected. The dog ear is thus eliminated and the wound is closed (Fig. 7-3D).

WOUND DRESSINGS

In the first hours after the incision, a coagulum forms over the wound. Between 12 and 72 hours, there are two spurts of mitotic activity, and epidermal cells begin migrating across the wound. However, if a dried crust forms, it is a barrier to the epidermal migration. Rather than being able to migrate straight and level across the gap between the wound edges, the epidermal cells must find a plane of migration beneath the dried crust. This leads to a shallow linear depression in the healed incision.

To prevent wound crusting and the resultant linear trough in the healed wound, an occlusive dressing is used. For such a dressing, there is a variety of commercially available products such as Bioclusive or Tegaderm. However, another option is to use Dermicel tape. This is a hypoallergenic tape and the adhesive has some bacteriostatic properties. Benzoin or Mastisol is first applied to the skin. Dermicel tape is then applied directly down and over the wound. No ointment is used.

A moist environment develops under the dressing that inhibits formation of a crust and accelerates epidermal regeneration. Because of the abundant blood supply of the face, infection has not been a problem. The tape is left in place for 3 to 4 days.

SUTURE REMOVAL

There are no hard and fast rules for suture removal. If there is doubt about whether sutures should be removed, remove every other or every third one and observe for another day or so. Some guidelines for the time of suture removal are as follows:

Face	4 to 6 days
Neck	6 to 10 days
Back	10 to 14 days
Abdomen	7 to 10 days
Extremities	10 to 18 days

It is prudent to examine wounds 4 to 5 days after surgery, because this is when a wound infection is most likely to occur. If an infection occurs, antibiotics used topically or systemically should be effective against beta hemolytic streptococci and coagulase positive staphylococcus. If other organisms are suspected, a culture should be done before starting antibiotics.

In order not to disrupt the wound during suture removal, the sutures may be cut with fine scissors such as the Gradle or with a no. 11 blade. For correct suture removal, the suture is pulled toward the incision line. Pulling the incision away from the incision line might pull the wound apart.

The time at which sutures are removed from the face is the time at which the wound is the weakest, because fibroplasia is just beginning and only the epidermal bridging is holding the wound. The incision line may be reinforced with Steri-strips after suture removal.

WOUND DYNAMICS

Wound Healing

Wound healing is divided into four phases. However, these phases overlap and blend into each other.

During the beginning inflammatory phase, there is initial vasoconstriction with platelet aggregation. After 5 to 10 minutes of vasoconstriction, there is active venule dilatation and increased vascular permeability, lasting about 72 hours. Within a few hours of these vascular responses, a cellular response occurs. Polymorphonuclear leukocytes migrate into the area. There is a diapedesis of monocytes that transform into tissue macrophages. The macrophage is the dominant cell for the first 3 to 4 days. It initiates the fibroblastic phages.

While the inflammatory phase is still proceeding, the proliferative phase commences. Epidermal cells undergo changes and begin migrating into the wound. By the third day, migration of epidermal cells across an apposed incision is completed. Fibroblasts within the dermis begin to proliferate at 25 to 36 hours after the tissue injury.

By the fourth day, the fibroblastic phase is heralded by the synthesis of collagen and proteoglycans by the proliferating fibroblasts. Collagen fibers are laid down in a random pattern without orientation.

Overlapping and toward the latter part of fibroblastic phase the remodeling phase begins. This is a phase of differentiation, resorption, and maturation. Fibroblasts disappear from the wound, and collagen fibers are modeled into organized bundles and patterns.

Wound Contraction

In an open wound healing by second intention, there is an active drawing of the full thickness of the surrounding skin toward the center of the wound. Wound contraction begins during the proliferative phase of wound healing. There is a differentiation of fibroblasts or myofibroblasts, which are responsible for this dynamic process. Wound contraction usually proceeds until the wound is closed or until surrounding forces on the skin are greater than the contractile forces of the myofibroblasts.

Contracture

All scars undergo contracture with a resultant shortening along their axes. This process of contracture is due to collagen cross-linking, which occurs during the remodeling phase. Contracture is distinct and different from wound contraction.

Wound Strength

By 2 weeks, the wound gains 7% of its final strength; by 3 weeks, 20%; by 4 weeks, 50%. At full maturation, the healed wound regains only 80% of the strength of the original intact skin.

DOCUMENTATION AND ASSESSMENT

Although success or failure in cutaneous surgery may be readily apparent, it is important to document results with objective photography. Only by consistent, standardized photographs may one judge progress and analyze techniques and methods. Preoperative and postoperative photographs are essential, as are intraoperative photographs. Uniform clinic photography is a form of self-assessment and serves as a stimulus and a direction for improvement.

SAUER NOTES

1. One of the more common complaints after skin surgery, especially a more extensive procedure, is numbness or altered sensation in the area. This is not a complication, but an expected effect of cutting through the skin. It is best to warn patients of this possibility before the surgery and that this change in sensation may last for 6 to 12 months and in some cases may be permanent.

2. In areas of high sebaceous-gland concentration and activity such as the T area of the face and in patients with acne and rosacea, incisions often tend to spread and widen no matter how meticulous and precise the surgery. This is a phenomenon of wound healing. The patient should be preadvised that this is a potential problem. "What the patient is told before surgery is informed consent, what is told after surgery is an excuse."

3. Beware of the temporal branch of the facial nerve. As it exits from the parotid gland at the superior border it runs a superficial course over the zygomatic arch and into the temporal area. Transection of this branch causes paralysis of the frontalis muscle on that side and drooping of the eyebrow. With any excision in the temporal area this is a possibility. Forewarn the patient. A drooping eyebrow can be corrected with a browpexy.

4. Beware of the spinal accessory nerve in the posterior triangle of the neck. The spinal accessory nerve pierces through the posterior border of the sternocleidomastoid muscle a little above its midportion and enters the posterior triangle of the neck. The spinal accessory nerve then travels superficially just below the subcutaneous fat in the investing fascia covering the posterior triangle. There is also a chain of lymph nodes intimately associated with the spinal accessory nerve along its course in the posterior triangle. This nerve has been transected by those aware of its superficial location as well as by those unaware. "Good judgment is based on experience, which is often based on bad judgment."

5. No matter how careful and diligent the surgeon, the response of biologic systems is not always predictable and the outcome not always anticipated or desired. "If one wants to cut, one must be prepared to cry and to pray."

BIBLIOGRAPHY

Baker SR, Swanson NA. Local flaps in facial reconstruction. St. Louis, Mosby, 1995.

Coleman WP, Hanke CW, et al. Cosmetic surgery of the skin, ed 2. St. Louis, Mosby, 1997.

Lask GP. Principles and techniques of cutaneous surgery. New York, McGraw-Hill Publishing, 1996.

Lerner EV, et al. Topical anesthetic agents in dermatologic surgery. Dermatol Surg 1997;23:673.

Ratz JL, Geronemus RG, et al. Textbook of dermatologic surgery. Philadelphia, Lippincott–Raven, 1997.

Robinson JK. Atlas of cutaneous surgery. Philadelphia, WB Saunders, 1996.

Roenigk RK. Roenigk & Roenigk's dermatologic surgery, ed 2. New York, Marcel Dekker, 1996.

Seckel BR. Aesthetic laser surgery. Philadelphia, Lippincott-Raven, 1996.

Thomas JR, Roller J. Cutaneous facial surgery. New York, Thieme, 1992.

Usatine RP, Moy RL. Skin surgery, a practical guide. St. Louis, Mosby, 1998.

8

Cosmetics for the Physician

Marianne N. O'Donoghue, M.D.*

The complete physician is asked questions regarding skin care every day. People will always seek ways to enhance their appearance with cleansing products, moisturizing products, color cosmetics, and fragrance. These products are important for the care of skin, hair, and nails, and they contribute to a sense of well-being and self-esteem. It is important to know how cosmetics function, which products cause adverse reactions, and how we can recommend them for the better care of our patients.

To better understand the definition and labeling of cosmetics, it would be well to review their definition, labeling, and the regulations concerning them. The Food and Drug Administration (FDA) defines cosmetics as "(1) articles intended to be rubbed, poured, sprinkled, or sprayed on, introduced into, or otherwise applied to the human body or any part thereof for cleansing, beautifying, promoting attractiveness, or altering the appearance, and (2) articles intended for use as a component of any such article: except that such term shall not include soap." Cosmetics are not regulated as strictly as are drugs, but there is a voluntary registration by the cosmetic manufacturers. Cosmetic Ingredient Review is an independent panel of expert scientists and physicians established to examine all published and voluntarily submitted industry data and to summarize them in a safety monograph for each individual cosmetic ingredient or class of cosmetic ingredient.

In the United States the regulation for labeling cosmetics is that the manufacturer should label all ingredients in descending order of predominance for all ingredients greater than 1% of the product. Ingredients that compose less than 1% of the product may be listed in any order. The labels need only be on the outside wrapping.

Products intended for retail sale need a statement of identity, net quantity of content, name and place of business and the manufacturer or distributor, declaration of ingredient statement, any necessary warning statement, and directions for use. If not intended for retail sale (*e.g.*, cosmetics in a beauty salon) those specifications need not be met.

This means that the physician can trace the origin of any product to which a patient has an adverse reaction. The research and development departments of most cosmetic companies are helpful and knowledgeable. Industry has worked very hard to be helpful to the dermatologist.

CLASSIFICATION OF COSMETICS

Cosmetics can be classified into toiletries, skin care products, fragrance products, and make-up or color products.

---

*Associate Professor, Department of Dermatology, Rush Presbyterian—St. Luke Medical Center, Chicago, Illinois

1. Toiletries

These include soaps, shampoos, hair rinses and conditioners, hair dressings, sprays and setting lotions, hair color preparations, waving preparations, straightening (relaxing) agents, deodorants, antiperspirants, and sun protective agents. (These latter products may be considered drugs or cosmeceuticals and are addressed later.)

CLEANSERS

The purpose of cleansing is to remove sebum that attracts dirt, desquamate the skin, remove airborne pollutants, remove pathogenic organisms, and remove any existing makeup.

The classic cleanser, and the one that has been present for decades, is soap. This consists of a substance made up of fatty acid in oil or fat and an alkaline substance. Clear or transparent soap permits better control of the alkaline residue and rinses off more easily. Hard-milled soaps have been considered elegant for many years. Synthetic detergents (syndets) are shaped like soap in bars but consist of anionic surfactants, such as sodium lauryl sulfate, that can be adjusted as to the pH. This makes the syndet easier to rinse off in hard water, and the product can be adjusted to be less irritation to the skin. Special soaps can include medicaments, granules, emollients, or fragrance. Soaps and synthetic detergents have been tested as to irritancy, transepidermal water loss, pH, and many other qualities. All of these products have their advantages and disadvantages.

Shower gels have become popular especially in Europe. They may have potassium lauryl sulfate as their anionic surfactant or many other ingredients. These appear to rinse off well but may be a little more irritating in some individuals. Perfumed liquid gels using peppermint and pineapple scents have caused many cases of contact and irritant dermatitis in the late 1990s.

SHAMPOOS

Shampoos have three major components—water, detergent, and a fatty material. Like body cleansers, the soap shampoos contain alkali plus oil and fat. Because these may leave a precipitate on the hair shaft with hard water, soap shampoos are rarely used anymore.

Most shampoos are soapless and are made of sulfonated oil. They consist of (1) principal surfactants for detergent and foaming power, (2) secondary surfactants to improve and condition the hair, and (3) additives to complete the formulation and special effects. Because most of the damage to the hair shaft is from chemicals that have a high pH, such as color and permanent or straightening agents, many shampoos are formulated today with an acidic or neutral pH. Because shampoo contains a large component of water, preservatives (discussed later) must be added. Formaldehyde is the most common preservative in shampoo. Because shampoo is only left on the hair for a short period, contact dermatitis does not usually occur. Some of the other additives besides preservative, such as color and fragrance, occasionally can cause allergic reactions.

The major therapeutic agents added to shampoos are tar, salicylic acid, zinc pyrithione, and sulfur (ketoconazole and fluocinonide can be added as a drug by prescription only). It is important for physicians to know that these ingredients do not necessarily harm the hair. The formulation of these therapeutic shampoos can contain as many conditioners and beautifying ingredients as nontherapeutic shampoos. They can even be recommended for color-treated or permed hair. The formulation must simply be selected for the type of hair (*e.g.*, dry, oily, fine or coarse).

CONDITIONERS

Because of the trauma to the hair shaft from sun, wind, chemical treatment, and water, conditioners are a necessary hair-grooming product for both men and women. The original rinses to remove the soap shampoo film were lemon and vinegar. These substances are still helpful when a person is "roughing it" in the wild or simply not supplied with real conditioners. The other rinses coat the hair shaft so it does not become tangled with the hair shaft next to it. These products contain wax and paraffin, and they allow the hair to shine without static cling. Balsam is a product in that category.

The major conditioners for traumatized hair are cationic surfactant conditioners. Quaternary ammonium compounds, especially stearalkonium ammonium chloride, have been used for many years to make the hair manageable. It is possible to attach a polymer (such as polyvinylpyrrolidone) or other film formers to the quaternary ammonium compounds. These not only condition the hair, they add extra volume or body. There are even conditioners that contain sunscreens to protect the hair color. Occasionally, too frequent use of any of these conditioners can cause a build-up on the hair shaft so that the hair becomes too soft. This can be counteracted with an anionic shampoo to strip off the build-up, so that the hair is fresh and more easily managed.

Protein-based conditioners consist of amino acids and small polypeptide fragments of hydrolyzed protein. These can be incorporated into the cortex of the hair shaft when the hair has just been processed with color or permanent waving, or under a heat cap. This is advisable for hair that has been damaged through processing, wind, swimming, or sun.

Styling aids consist of lotions, gels, mousses, or hair spray. Most of these products contain water, copolymers, polyvinylpyrrolidone, quaternary salts, and fragrance. They waterproof the hair so that perspiration or mild rain does not upset the style.

PERMANENT WAVES AND RELAXERS

The three natural wave patterns of hair are straight, wavy, and kinky. To allow the hair to be curled differently, straightened, or become slightly wavy, a chemical reaction involving the disulfide bond is broken with heat, high pH, or with thioglycolates. For straightening, it is broken with sodium hydroxide, guanidine hydroxide, lithium hydroxide, heat, or thioglycolates. The hair is placed over rods or curlers, treated with the appropriate chemical until the shape of the hair shaft is changed, then neutralized with hydrogen peroxide with sodium perforate or potassium bromate. Some of the disulfide bonds are never repaired, so this process can be very hard on the hair shaft.

The mildest form of hair curling is the acid permanent—glycerol monothioglycolate. This is appropriate for fine or for color-treated hair. There are more cases of allergic contact dermatitis due to this chemical than to the other curling or straightening agents. This permanent wave must be administered in a professional salon.

The midstrength permanent wave is ammonium thioglycolate. This can be used on healthy hair for curling, or kinky hair for straightening. This may be performed at home because of its safety.

The strongest chemicals for these procedures are for resistant kinky hair and include lye (with the higher pH) or sodium, lithium, or calcium hydroxide. These products must be applied by professionals. If the chemicals are left on too long, the hair shaft may break.

HAIR COLORING

The five major types of hair coloring are temporary, gradual, natural, semipermanent, and permanent color.

The *temporary colors* are textile dyes. These dyes lie on the top of the cuticle and come off easily with perspiration or rain. Their advantage is to let the individual try a color and not cause any permanent change. These are safe and do not cause allergic reactions. The disadvantage is that the color can come off easily onto one's face or clothes.

The *gradual coloring* consists of metallic salts. The hair can go from gray to brown or black by the action of lead acetate and sulfur. These salts precipitate on the outside of the hair shaft and allow a gradual change in color.

Unfortunately, the hair looks very lusterless and can have a characteristic sulfur odor. The metal precipitate also precludes any other hair processing, such as permanent or other coloring procedures. The hair must grow out or have a stripping process before other cosmetic procedures may take place.

Natural coloring with henna from *Lawsonia inermis* is rarely used anymore. This is a vegetable dye that has no concern regarding carcinogenicity. It imparts red highlights to hair. This substance can precipitate asthma and allergies. Henna also stains gray hair an unpleasant orange color.

Semipermanent dyes are a nice first step for a person going from gray to a darker color. The active ingredients are low molecular-weight dyes specifically synthesized for hair coloring. Because the molecules are small, they can penetrate the cuticle and go into the cortex. These leave the hair shiny and attractive. Because those same molecules can slip out of the cuticle just as easily, the color only lasts for four to six shampoos. These dyes have low allergenicity, are easy to apply, and cause only minimal hair shaft damage. Because there is no peroxide used, the colors can only go darker, not lighter.

By far the most common products for hair color in men and women today are the *permanent hair color dyes*. In permanent or oxidative hair coloring, the formation of colorless molecules from their precursors occurs inside the cortex as a result of oxidation by hydrogen peroxide. The reaction is p-phenylenediamine + $H_2O_2 \rightarrow$ amines: amines + couplers $\rightarrow$ indo dyes. The indo dye molecules are so large that they cannot slip out of the cortex of the hair shaft. This color lasts for 4 to 6 weeks, until the new growth of scalp hair at the base becomes visible. The correct procedure then is simply to color the 1 or 1.5 cm of new growth.

Frosting or *highlighting* of the hair consists of taking strands of the hair and selectively bleaching them with the same procedure using 30 or 40 volumes percent for hydrogen peroxide (instead of 20 volumes percent, as in normal color).

For a real brunette to become a platinum blond, two processes must be used: first, a removal of all the color with peroxide, and then a dying of the hair as outlined above. This is the most traumatic procedure that can be performed on the hair.

With all of these chemical processes, the hair can be broken off at any point on the shaft.

Table 8-1 provides a summary of these color techniques.

2. Skin Care Products

According to the North American Contact Dermatitis Group, skin care products cause the greatest number of adverse reactions in cosmetics. These can be irritant dermatitis, allergic dermatitis, acne cosmetica, or folliculitis. To understand these products more thoroughly, it is important to study the types of ingredients compounded for these products. These consist of emollients, humectants, surfactants, preservatives, and fragrance.

EMOLLIENTS

Emollients are film-forming materials that add substance to cosmetic preparations and function on the skin to retard water loss. Five categories of emollients are hydrocarbons, waxes, natural lipid polyesters, lightweight esters and ethers, and silicone.

The *hydrocarbons* that are most familiar are mineral oil and petrolatum. Because these products contain no water, there is no need to add preservatives to them. It has been shown by tagging C^+ atoms that petrolatum actually penetrates into the intercellular substance of the epithelium. These hydrocarbons are heavy and may not be as aesthetically pleasing as other moisturizers. In the temperate zones in the winter, however, they are ideal for hands, feet, and other very dry areas on the body. They probably are too occlusive for facial skin.

Waxes consist of beeswax, synthetic beeswax, cholesterol, and lanolin. These substances usually cause no adverse reaction themselves, but esters of lanolin can occasionally be comedogenic (cause comedonal acne).

The *natural lipid polyesters* retard water loss by integrating with the proteins of the stratum corneum. Short-chain acids such as coconut oil,

capric or caprylic triglycerides, esters of lanolin, and synthesized unsaturated fatty acid esters such as sorbitol oleate or lanolin linoleate can be comedogenic because of their interaction with the stratum corneum. Long-chain polyesters are less likely to be comedogenic because of their molecular size.

Lightweight esters and *ethers*, such as isopropyl myristate and isopropyl stearate, also can be comedogenic. They are acceptable if they comprise less than 2% of the formulation. Some of these products act as preservatives at lower concentrations.

By far the most helpful emollient today is *silicone*. This inert product has been pulverized into tiny particles and then added to many products for "slip." It has replaced many of the acnegenic ingredients in facial cosmetics and has performed excellently. Silicone is lubricating, protective, and water repellant. There is no absorption of silicone topically, so concerns of safety with this product are absent. It has no adverse reaction regarding allergenicity or comedogenicity.

HUMECTANTS

Humectants are used to preserve moisture content of materials and attract and absorb water from their environment. Most of these products are cosmetically more pleasing to use. They are especially valuable in climates in which there is more humidity. Examples of humectants are glycerin, sodium pyroglutamic acid , sorbitol, urea, lactic acid, and propylene glycol.

Urea and lactic acid are very helpful ingredients for conditions of hyperkeratosis, such as ichthyosis, keratosis pilaris, Darier's disease, and severe dry skin. They can occasionally cause irritation or stinging but are not sensitizing. Propylene glycol is one of the favorite solvents for topical steroids. It is present in at least two thirds of the topical steroid cream products and in many of the ointments. It can be an irritant and occasionally cause contact dermatitis.

SURFACTANTS

Surfactants are surface-active ingredients that make it easier to mix the oil phase and water phase in an emulsion and effect a smoother contact between two surfaces. These substances can cause the skin to be more penetrable by lowering the barrier properties of the skin and allowing itself or other ingredients to penetrate the surface and cause irritation or sensitization.

TABLE 8-1
COLORING PRODUCTS AND THEIR KEY CHARACTERISTICS*

Type of Coloring Product	Recognition	Skill Involved	Type of Dye	Color Change Range	Site of Action	Lasting Quality	Overall Performance	Degree of Abuse of Hair Structure	Potential for Dermatologic Complaints
Temporary color rinses	Multiple-use package	Minimal Apply and dry	High-molecular-weight acid dyes as used in textiles, and certified food colors in a hydro-alcoholic suspension	Covers gray	Surface of shaft	Poor Removed by shampooing	Poor	Negligible	Negligible
Semi-permanent	Single- or multiple-use package; more viscous than no. 1 to prevent dripping off hair	Moderate Applied to freshly shampooed hair and left in place for 15–40 minutes; skin patch test required	Low-molecular-weight dyes: nitrophenylene-diamines, nitroamino-phenols, aminoanthro-quinones in shampoo vehicle or a solvent system	Covers gray; one to three shades on dark side of normal hair color	Penetrates to cortex	Gradually lost through three to five shampoos	Fair	Negligible	Negligible

	Packaging	Professional attention	Composition	Color range	Penetration	Permanence	Resistance to shampoo	Resistance to light	Hazards
Permanent oxidation type									
Single process	Two-unit system for mixing just before use	Moderate; skin patch test required	Several classes of dyes including PPD† intermediates in an alkaline peroxide "shampoo"	Covers gray; two or three shades on each side of normal	Cortex	Permanent; new growth touch-up every 4–8 weeks	Excellent	Moderate	Modest
Double process	Same as above	Professional attention necessary	As above, but hair must be previously decolorized (stripped)	Unlimited	Cortex	As above	Excellent	Significant	Moderate; hair breakage; local and systemic peroxide reactions
Progressive	Multiple-use package	None	Metallic salts particularly lead, in solution, cream, or pomade form	Discolors hair only	Surface and some beneath cuticle	As long as product is used regularly	Poor	Minimal	Negligible; a public health problem; incompatible with other chemical hair services
Vegetable	For all practical purposes, this does not exist and is not available.								
Henna	Although true henna is a vegetable dye, its color properties and lasting abilities make it unacceptable. Products are being marketed currently with this name but are actually henna coloring in the second and third categories above.								

*The late Dr. Earl Brauer compiled this chart for previous editions of this book.

†p-Phenylenediamine.

The four major types of surfactants are anionic, nonionic, cationic, and amphoteric.

The *anionic surfactants* are the principle ingredients in shampoos and synthetic detergent soaps. Sodium lauryl sulfate is an excellent cleanser, and it is the major workhorse for liquid facial cleansers as well as shampoos. Other anionics are alpha olefin sulfonates, NA/K stearate, triethanolamine (TEA-lauryl sulfate), and sulfosuccinates.

The *nonionic surfactants* are more gentle than the anionics. They allow for the removal of minerals from hard water, increase the viscosity and solubility of shampoos. and behave as emulsifiers. These include sorbitan fatty acids, polysorbates, polyethylene glycol (PEG) lipids, and lauramine oxide.

The *cationic surfactants* function largely as conditioners for hair, thickeners for shampoo, and hair grooming aids. These include stearalkonium chloride, quaternary ammonium salts, quaternary fatty acids, and amino acids.

The *amphoteric surfactants* contain a balance of positive and negative charges. These are not as aggressive products as the anionic surfactants and are the chief ingredients in baby shampoo.

PRESERVATIVES

Preservatives are second only to fragrance in causing contact dermatitis. They are absolutely necessary, however, to keep the products fresh and safe. The more water that there is in a product, the more important is the content of preservatives.

Preservatives are classified into three categories: antimicrobials, ultraviolet light absorbers, and antioxidants. The allergenicity of preservatives is variable. The variables include:

- Inherent sensitizing potential
- Concentration in the final product
- Whether it is a wash-off versus leave-on product
- The duration of the skin contact
- The state of the epidermal surface when applied
- The body region

Of all these variables, the first two are the most important. Preservatives are mixed and matched depending on whether there is a concern from gram-positive or gram-negative organisms, *Candida* sp, *Pityrosporum ovale*, or fungus.

The following is a review of five of the most commonly used groups of preservatives, their efficacy, and their disadvantages.

Formaldehyde and Formaldehyde Releasers. Free formaldehyde is present, especially in shampoos, because of its efficacy against *Pseudomonas aeruginosa*. Because it is left on for such a short time, patients usually have no reaction to it. However, hair dressers who shampoo their clients all day are likely to experience a contact or an irritant dermatitis from it. Formaldehyde treatment of corn starch in surgeons' gloves has been implicated as a potential source of sensitization. Formaldehyde-allergic people must avoid permanent-press or wrinkle-resistant garments. They should wash all new clothing items before wearing and wear protective undergarments when able.

Of the formaldehyde releasers, *quaternium 15* is number one, and *imidazolidinyl urea* is number two in causing contact dermatitis. Other formaldehyde releasers include *BNPD (Bronopol)*, *diazolidinyl urea (Germal II)*, and *DMDM hydantoin (Glydant)*. All of these products are very effective against *Pseudomonas*.

Parabens. Parabens are the least allergenic and most popular of all the preservatives. They are very effective against fungi and gram-positive bacteria. They are relatively water insoluble, so are not effective against *Pseudomonas* sp. Efficacy is enhanced by combining two parabens in the same formulation. Cross-reaction between individual parabens is the rule. As with the formaldehyde releasers, parabens are more likely to react with dermatitic skin, but sensitization is not common with these preservatives.

Antioxidants. Antioxidants are less frequently used. These include butylated hydroxyanisole (BHA), butylated hydroxytoluene (BHT), Triclosan, and sorbic acid. BHA and BHT are important for the prevention of spoilage. These are present in lipstick and sunscreens. Their widest use is in foods. Triclosan is a disinfectant and preservative in deodorants, shampoo, and soap. Sorbic acid is used often in creams and lotions. It is fungistatic but has poor bacterial inhibition.

Kathon CG (Methylchloroisothiazoline and Methylisothiazolinone). This organic preservative was considered the most complete and safest preservative until the past decade. It is an odorless and colorless biocide that exhibits microbicidal activity against a wide spectrum of fungi and gram-positive and gram-negative bacteria.

More than 80 publications in the past decade have reported allergic contact dermatitis to cleansing cream, hair tonics, hair balsam, wash softeners, cosmetics, and moist toilet paper. When these reports came in, a more serious study of Kathon CG took place. According to the North American Contact Dermatitis Group, the incidence of allergy is 1.9%. As long as the concentration is below 15 ppm in rinse-off products and less than 7.5 ppm in leave-on products, this substance is acceptable.

3. Fragrance and Fragrance Products

Fragrance as an ingredient in skin care products is the highest allergen. In one study, it accounted for 149 of 536 reactions. Together, fragrance and preservatives accounted for half of all the reactions to cosmetics.

Fragrance products include perfume, cologne, toilet water, bath-water additives, bath powder, and aftershave lotions.

The most common reaction to fragrance is allergic contact dermatitis; following are photodermatitis, contact urticaria, irritation, and depigmentation.

The common fragrance allergens are:

- Cinnamic alcohol
- Cinnamic aldehyde
- Hydroxycitronellal
- Isoeugenol
- Oak moss absolute

The most common photoallergen is musk ambrette.

Balsam of Peru as a patch test is a good screening agent for fragrance. In the past, oil of bergamot found in Shalimar perfume was the most common photoallergen. Now, those perfumes that contain oil of bergamot contain the bergapten-free variety, so there are fewer photodermatitis reactions.

4. Make-up (Color) Products

Color cosmetics include foundation, eye make-up (shadow, liner, mascara), lipstick, rouge, blush, and nail enamel.

The use of color cosmetics is likened to an artist painting a picture on a canvas. Foundation is used to give a simple flawless complexion on which other color cosmetics can be applied.

Spot coverage can be achieved with several products before foundation is applied. For patients with defects after surgery, telangiectasias, or lentigines, an erase stick or a heavier concealer product is applied before foundation. For patients with rosacea, scar tissue, laser resurfacing, or face peeling, a green-tint prefoundation may be used. These products are readily available.

The types of foundation vary with coverage and cream or moisture content. The concealing or covering quality varies with the amount of titanium dioxide and not the density of the product. Foundation can be transparent, imparting only color; translucent, offering more cover; or opaque, offering total coverage. This increasing amount of coverage does not affect the comedogenicity of the product.

Dermatologists are interested in the amount of cream or moisturizer in the foundation. For teenagers, a shake lotion–type foundation is less likely to contribute to acne. For 20- to 50-year-old women, a heavier make-up that is labeled noncomedogenic or oil-free may be appropriate. For most women 50 years old or older, any kind of moisturizing foundation is acceptable as long as they are not prone to adult acne.

The ingredients that are more likely to be comedogenic (this term is totally relative) are:

- Isopropyl myristate
- Isopropyl ester
- Oleic acid
- Stearic acid
- Petrolatum
- Lanolin (especially acetylated lanolin alcohols and lanolin fatty acids)

The products that have been substituted for the above ingredients, and that are less likely to be comedogenic, are low-dose mineral oil, octyl palmitate, isosteryl neopentanoate, cottonseed oil, corn oil, safflower oil, propylene glycol, spermaceti, beeswax, and sodium lauryl sulfate.

The final product, however, must be tested to decide if the compound is truly comedogenic or not. This is best tested on the face or back of patients who are acne prone. A good screening is with the rabbit ear.

With the clever use of highlighting with foundation or concealer, asymmetry, scleroderma, heavy cheeks, or an unclear jaw line can be concealed. It is not necessarily a physician's place to demonstrate this to the patient, but the physician should know where to send a patient who needs help to normalize his or her appearance. Even the medical tattooing of burned or scarred skin can be of assistance.

Blush adds color and the look of good health to the patient's appearance. Cream blush can be comedogenic and hard to apply. It may be best used by older patients who have dry skin. Powder blush seems to be the best choice. It should be applied in the same areas that children flush in when exercising. Usually, these products do not cause adverse reactions.

Lipsticks are made of waxes that are usually nonallergenic and noncomedogenic. When eosin dyes were used for long-lasting lipsticks there were cases of photodermatitis, so they are used less frequently now.

For women who have vertical lines above and below the vermilion border, the use of a lead lipstick pencil or liner can be helpful. This stops the waxy lipstick from "bleeding" into the vertical furrows when the patient eats or drinks. Lip liner is also recommended for women with asymmetry of their lips owing to removal of tumor or other lip surgery or too thin lips. The desired outline of the lips can be drawn with the pencil or line, and then the color can be filled in.

Eye make-up—shadow, liner, mascara—can be used to enlarge, brighten, or accentuate the eyes. Because of the need to prevent infection, most eye make-up contains preservatives. These preservatives are listed on the outside of the package and patients can check to see if they have had an adverse reaction to them. Generally, the preservatives are EDTA, BAL, thimerosal, parabens, quaternium 15, or phenylmercuric acetate/nitrate. Usually, each cosmetic company formulates its products with its specific preservatives. Therefore, a patient who cannot use one company's eye product may be able to use another company's product. Most American eye cosmetics are formulated without fragrance and with the simplest hypoallergic formula.

Eye shadow can function to conceal flaws or enlarge the eye. Usually, if the patient has an allergic reaction to cream eye shadow, a powder eye shadow is a good substitute.

Eye liner may help to change the shape of the eye as well as accentuate it. These products usually are waxes and therefore have no adverse reaction.

Mascara can be water-based or water-proof. The water-based products are healthier for the eyelashes because they can be removed easily with soap and water. Products with lengtheners, however, may add lacquer and may require special solvents to remove the old mascara. Water-proof mascara may have a lower concentration of preservatives and may therefore be less aller-

genic for some patients. It is necessary to use an eye make-up remover product to take mascara off. The use of the special remover may be more traumatic to the eyelashes. Because of this, patients with fragile lashes (*e.g.*, patients with alopecia areata) should wear water-washable mascara.

Eyelash curlers can be used to give the illusion of longer lashes and conceal blepharochalasia. The patient who is allergic to nickel or rubber should not use this instrument. If the eyelash curler is to be used, it must be used before the mascara is applied.

Nail enamels, including base coats and top coats, have similar composition:

Film former: nitrocellulose
Resin: toluene sulfonamide/formaldehyde resin, alkyl resins, acrylates, vinyls, or polyesters
Plasticizers: camphor, dibutyl phthalate, dioctyl phthalate, and tricresyl phosphate
Solvents: alcohol, toluene, ethyl acetate, and butyl acetate
Colorants: (optional)
Pearlizers: guanine and bismuth oxychloride (optional)

The major ingredient that causes allergic contact dermatitis is toluene sulfonamide. Butyl and ethyl methacrylate, which are in the glue used for sculptured nails, press-on nails, and nail mending, can also cause contact dermatitis. Cuticle remover (sodium or potassium hydroxide) is left on the cuticle to dissolve dead skin. If left on too long, this product becomes an irritant. The entire nail can be separated from the nail bed by too vigorous use of cuticle remover.

Cosmeceuticals

This term in an unofficial way is used to describe cosmetic-type products that are promoted with aggressive claims to have a favorable impact on the condition of the skin. These products include antioxidants (vitamins), tretinoin, α-hydroxy acids, β-hydroxy acids, antiperspirants, sunscreens, and self-tanners.

ANTIOXIDANTS

Antioxidants, such as alpha-tocopherol (vitamin E), prevent both formation of erythema and epidermal cytotoxicity to ultraviolet light exposure. It was suggested that sunburn cell formation can be prevented in skin by scavenging reactive oxygen species (Emerit et al, 1990). Formation of ultraviolet light-induced lipid peroxidates is also inhibited by alpha-tocopherol. The finding in several studies demonstrated that if a topical preparation of vitamin E can penetrate into the epidermis, there is less damage to the epidermal cells after sun or ozone exposure.

Researchers at Duke University have been working with vitamins C and E for photoprotection (Darr et al, 1992). When combining these vitamins with UVA or UVB sunblock, they appear to get better protection than with either product alone. Vitamin C appears to be more protective against UVA and vitamin E more protective against UVB. These researchers have succeeded in formulating vitamin C products that penetrate into the skin. Double-blind studies to prove that vitamin C is antiinflammatory and has antiaging qualities are still not available.

β-Carotene (vitamin A) taken by mouth is an antioxidant and a single oxygen quencher that helps the cells protect themselves against reactive oxygen species associated with environmental pollutants such as smog and ultraviolet light.

TRETINOIN

Tretinoin, a derivative of vitamin A, has been established clinically and histologically to reduce aging and photoaging of the skin (Olsen et al, 1997; Kligman et al, 1993). The actions of tretinoin are to normalize epidermal atypia, deposit new collagen, induce new blood formation (this enhances color and nutrition to the skin surface), increase epidermal thickness, and increase granular cell layer thickness. This compound may be irritating to the skin. Over the past few years newer formulations of tretinoin with improved delivery systems (Renova, Retin-A Micro, Avita) and adapalene gel have helped with this irritation. The use of daily sunscreen is advised with all of these products.

α-HYDROXY ACIDS

Lactic acid has been used by dermatologists for many years. The research by Van Scott has ushered into widespread use the rest of the α-hydroxy acids. These natural fruit acids exert their influence by diminishing corneocyte cohesion. The most commonly used ingredients are:

Glycolic acid: sugar cane
Lactic acid: sour milk
Malic acid: apples
Citric acid: citrus fruits
Tartaric acid: grapes

Leyden (1994) outlines the functions of these α-hydroxy acids clearly:

1. They bind water in the skin; therefore, the stratum corneum becomes more flexible.
2. They normalize desquamation of corneocytes from the stratum corneum. This may occur by interaction with stratum corneum lipids.
3. They release cytokines locally.
4. They cause a thickening of the epidermis.
5. They increase production of hyaluronic acid within the dermis. This may be due to the increased production of transforming growth factor-β.
6. In both ichthyosis and thickening stratum corneum of dry skin, the α-hydroxy acids make the skin thin down toward normal.

The α-hydroxy acids have been incorporated into cosmetic formulation for shampoos, soap, face creams, and body creams. The difficulty in formulating these products is the need to be buffered. A 5% concentration in one product may not be as effective as a 5% concentration in another.

Glycolic acid peels have also been unpredictable because of this lack of standardization. The FDA is looking into these products.

β-HYDROXY ACIDS

In the search for a less irritating and stinging compound for creams and peels, β-hydroxy acids have become very popular. There is only one ingredient in this category, salicylic acid. This keratolytic has been known to dermatologists for years chiefly as an exfoliant for acne at a concentration of 2–3%, and a therapy for warts at concentrations of 10–15% in creams, and 40% in pastes. Salicylic acid appears to have an anti-inflammatory component and may have less stinging and irritancy than glycolic acid (Draelos, 1998).

β-Hydroxy acid face peels have also become popular for patients who cannot tolerate α-hydroxy or trichloracetic acid peels.

ANTIPERSPIRANTS

Antiperspirants are considered a drug (cosmeceutical) because of their physical interaction in the sweat duct. These products, which contain aluminum salts, act by causing a precipitation in the duct itself to block the secretion of sweat. They must have a specific amount of aluminum salts and in laboratory tests must reduce sweat by at least 20% in half of the people tested.

Deodorants contain bacteria-killing agents such as Triclosan, bacteria-retarding ingredients, and fragrance. They are a cosmetic because they do not change the function of the skin but just mask body odor.

For efficacy, roll-on products are best, then the sticks, and then the spray products.

SUNSCREENS

Sunscreens are the most important cosmetics men and women can use. Because these prevent skin cancer, they are considered a drug or cosmeceutical. These products are usually calibrated according to the sun-protective factor (SPF). The SPF value is the ration of UVB dose required to produce the minimal erythema reaction through the applied sunscreen product (2 mg/cm^2) compared with the UVB dose required to produce the same degree of minimal erythema reaction without the sunscreen.

The three major *physical* blocks are zinc oxide, talc, and titanium dioxide.

Zinc oxide has been used for lifeguards and children for many years on noses, ear tips, upper cheeks, and shoulders. Occasionally, bright neon colors have been added to this substance in sunblocks for children. The advantage of this substance is that it is inert and therefore not allergenic. The disadvantage is that it is messy. Newer products with pulverized zinc oxide are more cosmetically acceptable for people who are allergic to chemical sunscreens.

Talc has been added to other products to increase the opaque block of that substance.

With the perfecting of pulverization, *titanium dioxide* has become one of the most important ingredients. This ingredient is the chief one in hypoallergenic or "chemical free" sunblocks. Whereas this was unattractive and unnatural looking in the past, it has become cosmetically very elegant. These are the sunscreens selected when a patient has a photoallergic reaction to the benzophenones. It is one of the most popular additions in all the products formulated against UVB and UVA. All these products have been formulated in a waterproof formulation.

The *chemical* absorbers have been formulated against UVB and UVA.

UVA absorbers are active against the sunburn spectrum from 290 to 320 nm. This is especially important for the prevention of nonmelanoma skin cancer.

p-Aminobenzoic acid (PABA) and PABA esters (Padimate O, Padimate A, glycerol PABA) were the major sunblocks in the United States until the mid-1980s. Their advantages were that they protect against the 290- to 320-nm wavelength, they are easy to work with cosmetically, the esters are nonstaining, and they bind to the horny layer. If a patient applied these 3 days in a row, he or she might still have protection on the fourth day. The disadvantages were the lack of protection for UVA, cross-sensitivity with benzoin and p-phenylenediamine, and that PABA itself may stain. Today, only Padimate O is readily available.

Cinnamates (octyl methoxycinnamate and cinoxate) have largely replaced PABA in many products. These are incorporated into many face make-ups in which an SPF of 6 to 12 may be desired. These are easy to work with and rarely sensitizing. These are the most common ingredients in cosmetic products for sun protection.

Salicylates (homomenthyl, octyl, triethanolamine) only have an SPF of 3.5 but are excellent additions to formulations to increase the SPF protection. Rarely they may cause photodermatitis.

There are many other UVB products, but these are the most commonly used.

As our knowledge of the damage from UVA (320 to 400 nm) grows, the need for better protectors grows. UVA can penetrate window glass and is responsible for a lot of the hyperpigmentation of melasma, photodamage in lupus erythematosus, actinic reticuloid, and photo-drug reactions. It may even be responsible for immune changes and for malignant melanoma.

Benzophenones were the chief UVA blockers until recently. Oxybenzone and dioxybenzone have a broad absorption spectrum of 200 to 350 nm, with peak absorption at about 290 to 325 nm. These ingredients are incorporated into compounds easily and are less allergenic than the PABA derivatives. There are many reports of photocontact dermatitis from oxybenzone and occasional reports of contact dermatitis and contact urticaria from dioxybenzone. The most common occurrence of the photocontact dermatitis from these products occurs with intense and very warm sun exposure such as is found near the equator. Many patients can use these products in temperate zones but react while on vacation. Physical sunblocks should then be substituted.

Parsol 1789 has been available since about 1989 in the United States. It has a spectrum of 310 to 400 nm, with a peak at 358 nm. Because of this spectrum, it is the sunblock of choice for all with special UVA needs. Of course it must be combined with a UVB block for total protection. The combinations for a few years did not work out, so new products with this ingredient were not released by the FDA until early 1998. This is now available in many excellent sunscreens from SPF 15–30.

As mentioned previously, vitamins C and E may be incorporated into some of the sunblocks in the future.

TANNING PRODUCT CATEGORIES

Self-tanning lotions consist primarily of dihydroxyacetone (DHA). These have a protein-staining effect from the DHA in the stratum corneum of the skin. These products used to be orange and streaky but have been perfected to an even-colored tone by the addition of silicone to the vehicle. Although these are nontoxic, they may accentuate freckles and seborrheic keratoses and may therefore not be desirable.

Bronzing gels consist of henna, walnut, juglone, and lawsone. These are water-soluble dyes to stain the skin. They can be messy to clothes and have the stickiness of a gel. They are usually noncomedogenic.

Tanning promoters, such as 5-methoxypsoralen, have been well documented to be highly phototoxic and carcinogenic. 5-Methoxypsoralen is not available over the counter in the United States.

Tanning pills consist of Canthaxanthin and are toxic to both skin and eyes. These are not available over the counter in the United States.

HOW TO TEST FOR COSMETIC ALLERGY

The items on the standard tray and the TRUE test that apply to cosmetics include imidazolidinyl urea, wool (lanolin) alcohols, p-phenylenediamine, thimerosal, formaldehyde, colophony, quaternium 15, balsam of Peru, and cinnamic aldehyde.

The cosmetics that can be tested without dilution are antiperspirants, blushes, eye liners, eye shadow, foundations, lipstick, moisturizers, perfumes, and sunscreens.

The cosmetics that are volatile and need to be allowed to dry on the patch or chamber before 48-hour occlusion are liquid eyeliner, mascara, and nail enamel.

The cosmetics that need to be diluted for testing are soaps, shampoos, shaving preparations, hair dyes, and permanent solutions, These may need open patch testing or usage testing.

SAUER NOTE

In conclusion, cosmetics are an important part of dermatology. The physician should know how they are used, what their components are , and how best to explain them to the patient.

BIBLIOGRAPHY

Adams RM, Maibach HI. A five-year study of cosmetic reactions. J Am Acad Dermatol 1985;12:1062.

Darr D, Combs S, Dunston S, Manning T, Pinnell S. Topical vitamin C protects porcine skin from ultraviolet radiation-induced damage. Br J Dermatol 1992;127:247.

Draelos ZD. Hydroxy acid update. Cosmetic Dermatol 1998;11:27.

Emerit I, Packer L, Auclair C. Antioxidants in therapy and preventive medicine. New York, Plenum Press, 1990:594.

FDC Act, 21 U.S. C.R. 321 (I).

Jackson EM. Tanning without sun: accelerators, promoters, pills, bronzing gels, and self-tanning lotions. Am J Contact Dermatitis 1994;5:38.

Kligman AM, Dogadkina D, Lavker RM. Effects of topical tretinoin on non-sun-exposed protected skin of the elderly. J Am Acad Dermatol 1993;29:25.

Larsen WG. Perfume dermatitis. J Am Acad Dermatol 1985;12:1.

Leyden J. Alphahydroxy acids. Dialog Dermatol 1994;34:3.

Maibach HI, Engasser PG. Dermatitis due to cosmetics. In: Fischer AA, ed. Contact dermatitis, ed 3. Philadelphia, Lea & Febiger, 2986:383.

McNamara SH. Cosmeceuticals: when is a cosmetic also regulated as a drug by FDA? Presented at the Symposium of Cosmetics, AAD Annual Meeting, Washington, DC, December 8, 1993.

Olsen EA, Katz HI, Levin N, et al. Tretinoin emollient cream for photodamaged skin: Results of 48-week, multicenter, double-blind studies. J Am Acad Dermatol 1997;37:217.

Pathak MA. Sunscreens and their use in the preventative treatment of sunlight-induced skin damage. J Dermatol Surg Oncol 1987;13:739.

9

Dermatologic Allergy

Contact dermatitis, industrial dermatoses, atopic eczema, and *drug eruptions* are included in this chapter because of their obvious allergenic factors. (However, some cases of contact dermatitis and industrial dermatitis are due to irritants.) *Nummular eczema* is also included because it resembles some forms of atopic eczema and may even be a variant of atopic eczema.

CONTACT DERMATITIS
(Figs. 9-1–9-4)

Contact dermatitis, or dermatitis venenata, is a very common inflammation of the skin caused by the exposure of the skin either to *primary irritant substances*, such as soaps, or to *allergenic substances*, such as poison ivy resin. Industrial dermatoses are considered at the end of this section.

PRIMARY LESIONS. Any of the stages, from mild redness, edema, or vesicles to large bullae with a marked amount of oozing, are seen.

SECONDARY LESIONS. Crusting from secondary bacterial infection, excoriations, and lichenification occurs.

DISTRIBUTION AND CAUSES. Any agent can affect any area of the body. However, certain agents commonly affect certain skin areas.

Face and Neck. See Fig. 9-5. Cosmetics, soaps, insect sprays, ragweed, perfumes or hair sprays (sides of neck), fingernail polish (eyelids), hat bands (forehead), mouthwashes, toothpaste, or lipstick (perioral), nickel metal (earlobes), industrial oil (facial chloracne).

Hands and Forearms. Soaps, hand lotions, wrist bands, industrial chemicals, poison ivy, and a multitude of other agents. Irritation from soap often begins under rings. Latex can cause a contact dermatitis and contact urticaria. It can be associated with life-threatening anaphylaxis and is becoming an increasing danger due to increased use of latex gloves and latex contraceptives.

Axillae. Deodorants, dress shields, or dry cleaning solutions.

Trunk. Clothing (new, not previously cleaned), rubber or metal attached to, or in, clothing, and transdermal drug patches.

Anogenital Region. Douches, dusting powder, contraceptives, colored toilet paper, poison ivy, or too strong salves for treatment of pruritus ani and fungal infections.

Feet. Shoes, foot powders, too strong salves for "athlete's foot" infection.

Generalized Eruption. Volatile airborne chemicals (paint, spray, ragweed), medicaments locally applied to large areas, bath powder, or clothing.

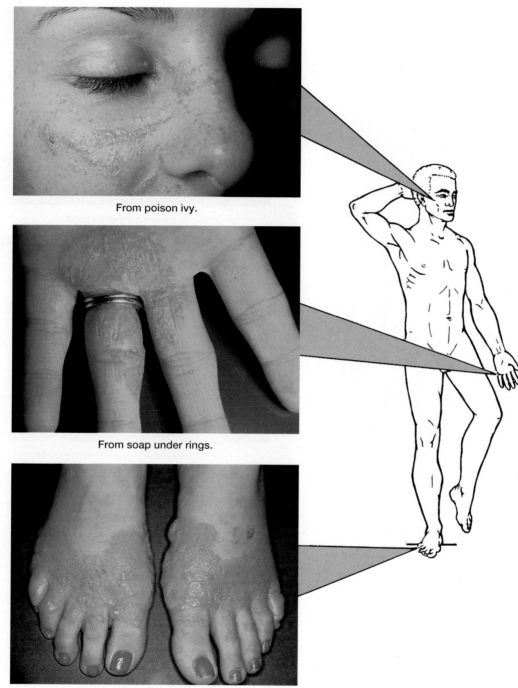

From poison ivy.

From soap under rings.

From shoe material.

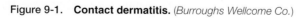

Figure 9-1. **Contact dermatitis.** (*Burroughs Wellcome Co.*)

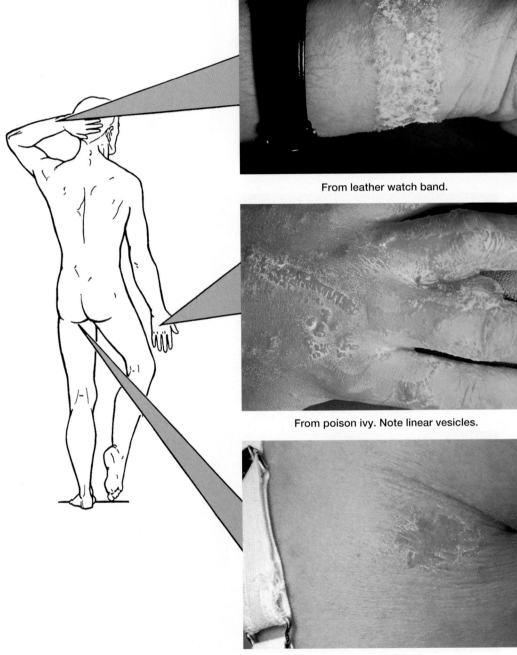

From leather watch band.

From poison ivy. Note linear vesicles.

From nickel metal in garter strap.

Figure 9-2. **Contact dermatitis.** (*Burroughs Wellcome Co.*)

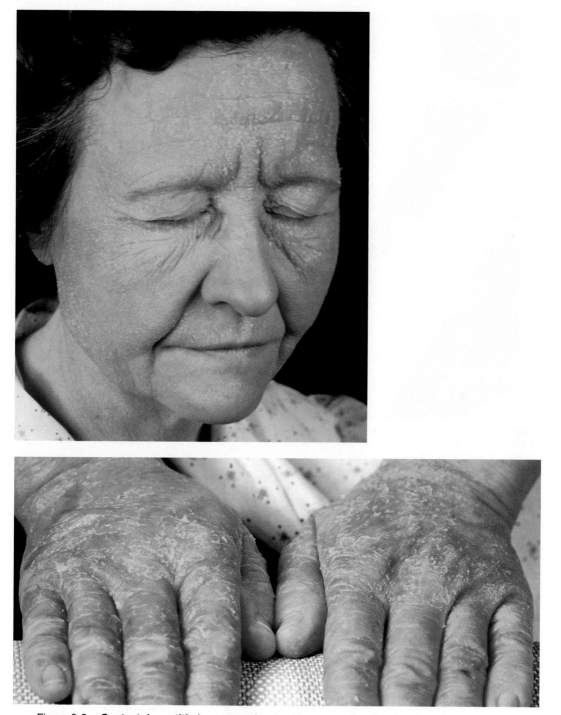

Figure 9-3. **Contact dermatitis in a nurse due to chlorpromazine.** The hands and face were involved most severely. This eruption was aggravated following exposure to sunlight. (*K.U.M.C.; Burroughs Wellcome Co.*)

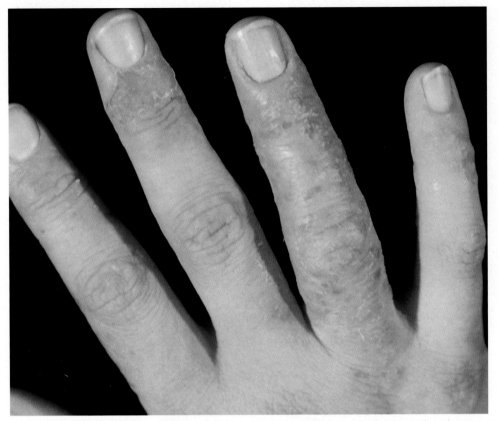

Figure 9-4. Contact dermatitis of the hand. This common dermatitis is usually due to continued exposure to soap and water. (*K.U.M.C.; Burroughs Wellcome Co.*)

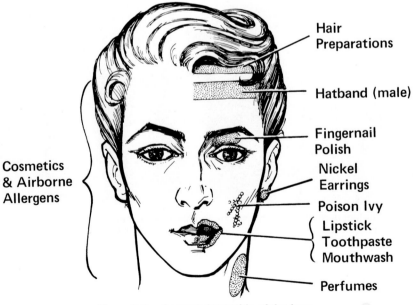

Hair Preparations

Hatband (male)

Fingernail Polish

Nickel Earrings

Poison Ivy

Lipstick
Toothpaste
Mouthwash

Perfumes

Cosmetics & Airborne Allergens

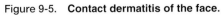

Figure 9-5. **Contact dermatitis of the face.**

COURSE. Duration can be very short to very chronic. As a general rule, successive recurrences become more chronic (*e.g.*, seasonal ragweed dermatitis can become a year-round dermatitis). An established hypersensitivity reaction is probably never lost. Also, certain people are more susceptible to allergic and irritant contact dermatitis than others.

SEASON. A very careful seasonal history of the onset, in chronic cases, may lead to discovery of an unsuspected causative agent, such as ragweed.

FAMILY INCIDENCE. This is not evident.

CONTAGIOUSNESS. The eczematous reaction (*e.g.*, the blister fluid of poison ivy) contains no allergen that can cause the dermatitis in another person. However, if the poison ivy oil or other allergen remains on the clothes of the affected person, contact of the allergen with a susceptible person could cause a dermatitis.

LABORATORY FINDINGS. Patch tests (see Chap. 2) are of value in eliciting the cause in a problem case. Careful interpretation is required.

Differential Diagnosis

A contactant reaction must be considered and ruled in or out in any case of eczematous or oozing dermatitis on any body area.

Treatment

Two of the most common contact dermatoses seen in the physician's office are *poison ivy* (or poi-son oak or *sumac*) *dermatitis* and *hand dermatitis*. The treatments for these two conditions are discussed next.

TREATMENT OF CONTACT DERMATITIS DUE TO POISON IVY

A patient comes to the office with a linear, vesicular dermatitis of the feet, the hands, and the face. He states that he spent the weekend fishing and that the rash broke out the next day. The itching is rather severe but not enough to keep him awake at night. He had "poison ivy" 5 years ago (Fig. 9-6).

FIRST VISIT

1. There are several mistaken notions about poison ivy dermatitis. Assure the patient that he cannot give the dermatitis to his family, or spread it on himself, from the blister fluid.
2. Suggest that the clothes worn while fishing be washed or cleaned to remove the allergenic resin.
3. Perform debridement. The blisters should be opened with manicure scissors, not by sticking with a needle. Cutting the top open with the scissors prevents the blister from reforming.
4. Prescribe Burow's solution wet packs.
   Sig: Add one packet of powder (Domeboro or Bluboro) to 1 quart of cool water. Apply sheeting or toweling, wet with the solution, to the blistered areas for 20 minutes twice a day. The wet packs need not be removed during the 20-minute period.
   (For a more widespread case of poison ivy dermatitis, take cool baths with half box of

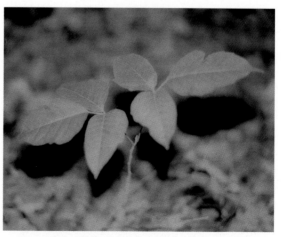

Figure 9-6.   **Large leaves of the poison ivy plant.**

Aveeno [colloidal oatmeal] or soluble starch to the tub, which gives considerable relief from the itching.)

5. 1% Hydrocortisone lotion q.s. 60.0 (1% Hytone lotion, 1% HC Pramosone lotion, etc.)
   Sig: Apply t.i.d. to the affected areas.

6. Chlorpheniramine maleate tablets, 4 mg **#60**
   Sig: 1 tablet t.i.d. (for relief of itching).
   Comment: Warn patient about side effect of drowsiness. This drug is available over the counter and is less expensive than if a generic prescription is written.

7. Use cortisone-type injection. Short- but rapid-acting corticosteroids are moderately beneficial, such as Celestone Phosphate (3 mg/mL in a dose of 1 to 2 mL subcutaneously), or Decadron LA (8 mg/mL) in a dose of 1 to 1.5 mL intramuscularly.

SUBSEQUENT VISITS

1. Continue the wet packs only as long as there are blisters and oozing. Extended use is too drying for the skin.

2. After 3 or 4 days of use, the lotion may be too drying. Substitute fluorinated corticosteroid emollient cream q.s.   60.0
   Sig: Apply small amount locally t.i.d., or more often if itching is present.

SEVERE CASES OF POISON IVY DERMATITIS

1. An oral corticosteroid is indicated in severe cases of poison ivy dermatitis: Prednisone, 10 mg   **#30**
   Sig: 5 tablets each morning for 2 days, 4 tablets each morning for 2 days, 3 tablets each morning for 2 days, 2 tablets each morning for 2 days, and 1 tablet each morning for 2 days.

SAUER NOTES

1. Most failures in the therapy for severe poison ivy or oak dermatitis result from the failure to continue the oral corticosteroid for 10 to 14 days or longer.

2. Medrol Dosepak therapy does not provide enough days of treatment for most cases of poison ivy dermatitis.

3. Explain to the patient that it is common for new lesions, even blisters, to continue to pop out during the entire duration of the eruption.

The use of poison ivy vaccine orally or intramuscularly is contraindicated during an acute episode. Desensitization may occur after a long course of oral ingestion of graduated doses of the allergen but pruritus ani, generalized pruritus, and urticaria probably make the treatment worse than the disease. Desensitization does not occur after a short course of intramuscular injections of the vaccine, and this form of prophylactic therapy is worthless. Barrier creams may decrease dermatitis if applied before exposure. Examples: Hydropel and Ivy-Block.

TREATMENT OF CONTACT DERMATITIS OF THE HAND DUE TO SOAP

A young housewife states that she has had a breakout on her hands for 5 weeks. The dermatitis developed about 4 weeks after the birth of her last child. She states that she had a similar eruption after her previous two pregnancies. She has used a lot of local medication of her own, and the rash is getting worse instead of better. The patient and her immediate family never had any asthma, hay fever, or eczema.

Examination of the patient's hands reveals small vesicles on the sides of all of her fingers, with a 5-cm area of oozing and crusting around her left ring finger.

FIRST VISIT

1. Assure the patient that the hand eczema is not contagious to her family.

2. Inform the patient that soap irritates the dermatitis and that it must be avoided as much as possible. A housewife will find this avoidance very difficult. One of the best remedies is to wear protective gloves when extended soap-and-water contact is unavoidable. Rubber gloves alone produce a considerable amount of irritating perspiration, but this is absorbed when thin white cotton gloves are worn under the rubber gloves. Lined rubber gloves are not as satisfactory because the lining eventually becomes dirty and soggy and cannot be cleaned easily.

3. For body cleanliness, a mild soap, such as Dove, can be used, or any of the following: Oilatum soap, Basis soap, Neutrogena soaps.

4. Tell the patient that the above prophylactic measures must be adhered to for several weeks *after* the eruption has apparently cleared, or there will be a recurrence. Injured skin is sensitive and needs to be pampered for an extended time.

5. Burow's solution soaks
   Sig: Add 1 packet of powder (Domeboro or Bluboro) to 1 quart of cool water. Soak hands for 15 minutes twice a day.
6. Fluorinated corticosteroid ointment (see Formulary in Chap. 5) 15.0
   Sig: Apply sparingly, locally, q.i.d.

SAUER NOTES

1. "Housewives' eczema" cannot usually be cured with a corticosteroid salve alone without observing the other protective measures.

2. After the dermatitis is clear, it is very important to advise the patient to treat the area for at least another week to prevent a recurrence. I call this "therapy plus."

RESISTANT, CHRONIC CASES

1. To the corticosteroid ointment add, as indicated, sulfur (3% to 5%), coal tar solution (3% to 10%), or an antipruritic agent such as menthol (0.25%) or camphor (2%).
2. Oral corticosteroid therapy. A short course of such therapy will rapidly improve or cure a chronic dermatitis.
3. Prevention of flares of contact dermatitis can be accomplished by frequent use of emollient preparations.

OCCUPATIONAL DERMATOSES

Sixty-five percent of all the industrial diseases are dermatoses. The patient with an average case of occupational dermatitis is compensated for 10 weeks, resulting in a total cost of over $100 million a year in the United States. The most common cause of these skin problems is contact irritants, of which cutting oils are the worst offenders. Lack of adequate cleansing is a big contributing factor to cutting oil dermatitis; on the other hand, harsh or abrasive cleansers can aggravate the dermatitis.

It is not possible to list the thousands of different chemicals used in the hundreds of varied industrial operations that have the potential of causing a primary irritant reaction or an allergic reaction on the skin surface. Excellent books on the subject of occupational dermatitis are listed in the bibliography at the end of this chapter.

Management of Industrial Dermatitis

A cutting-tool laborer presents with a pruritic, red, vesicular dermatitis on his hands, forearms, and face of 2 months' duration.

1. Obtain a careful, detailed history of his type of work and any recent change, such as use of new chemicals or new cleansing agents or exposure at home with hobbies, painting, and so on. Question him concerning remission of the dermatitis on weekends or while on vacation.
2. Question the patient concerning the first-aid care given at the plant. Too often this care aggravates the dermatitis. Bland protective remedies should be substituted for potential sensitizers, such as sulfonamide and penicillin salves, antihistamine creams, benzocaine ointments, nitrofuran preparations, and strong antipruritic lotions and salves.
3. Treatment of the dermatitis with wet compresses, bland lotions, or salves is the same as for any contact dermatitis (see previous discussion). Unfortunately, many of the occupational dermatoses respond slowly to therapy. This is due in part to the fact that most patients continue to work and are reexposed, repeatedly, to small amounts of the irritating chemicals, even though precautions are taken. Also, certain industrial chemicals, such as chromates, beryllium salts, and cutting oils, injure the skin in such a way as to prevent healing for months and years.
4. The legal complications with compensation boards, insurance companies, the industry, and the injured patient can be discouraging, frustrating, and time-consuming. However, most patients are not malingerers, and they do expect and deserve proper care and compensation for their injuries.

A comprehensive paper by Gordan C. Sauer on the percentages of skin impairment is entitled "A Guide to the Evaluation of Permanent Impairment of the Skin" (Arch Dermatol 1968; 97:566). A rather similar guide published by the American Medical Association (1990) is listed in the bibliography at the conclusion of this chapter.

ATOPIC ECZEMA
(Figs. 9-7–9-11)

Atopic eczema, or atopic dermatitis, is a rather common, markedly pruritic, chronic skin condition that occurs in two clinical forms: *infantile* and *adult*.

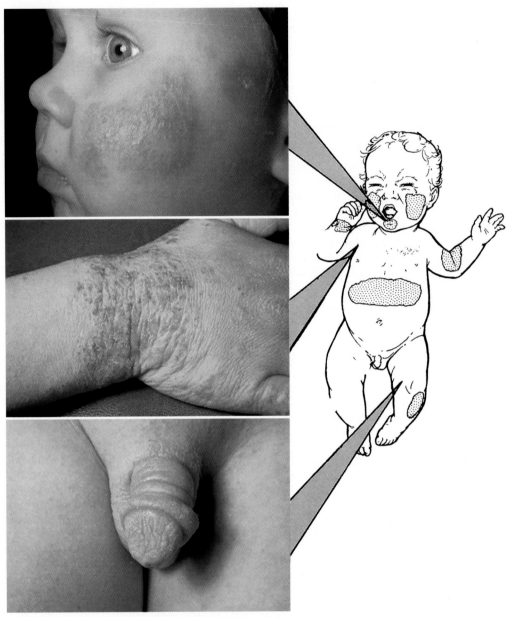

Figure 9-7. **Atopic eczema (infant).** (*Dome Chemicals*)

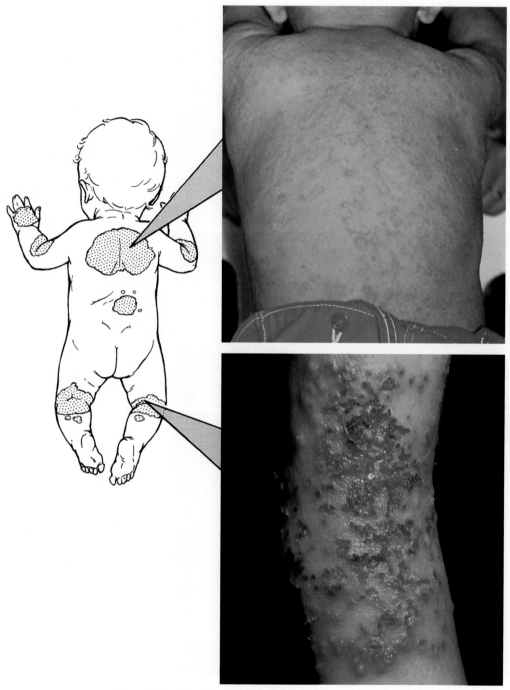

Figure 9-8. **Atopic eczema (infant).** (*Roche Laboratories*)

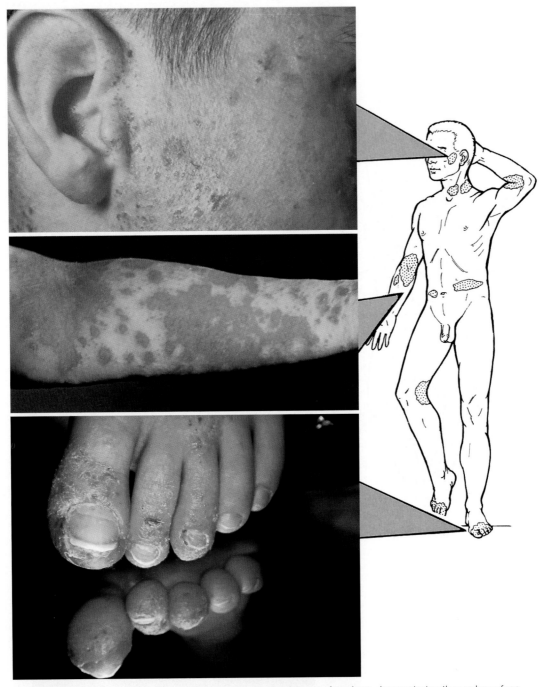

Figure 9-9. Atopic eczema. The bottom photograph, by the use of a mirror, demonstrates the undersurface of the toes. (*Sandoz Pharmaceuticals*)

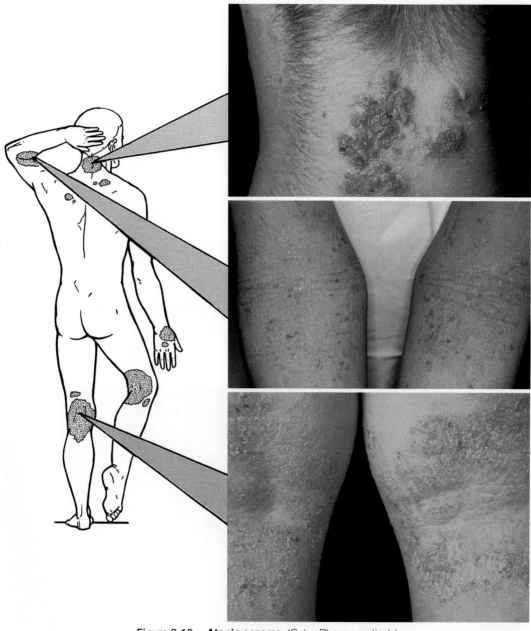

Figure 9-10. **Atopic eczema.** (Geigy Pharmaceuticals)

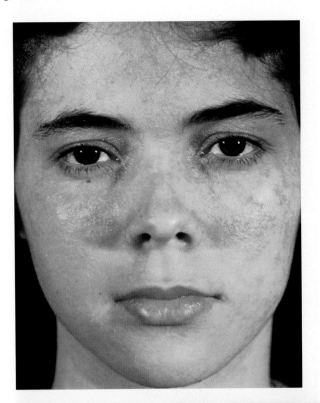

Figure 9-11. Atopic eczema. This case of facial atopic eczema (*top*) resembled acute lupus erythematosus. The arm eruption (*bottom*) is on another patient and exemplifies the chronic lichenified form of atopic eczema. (*K.U.M.C.; Dome Chemicals*)

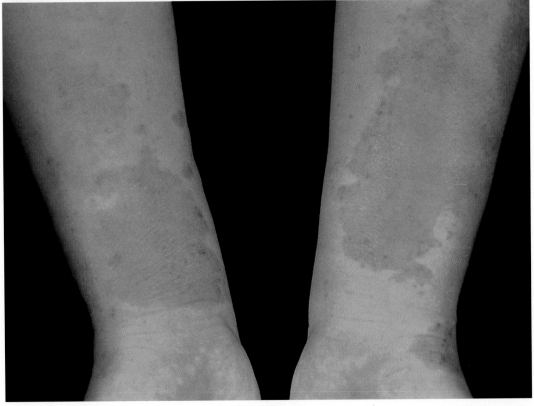

CLINICAL LESIONS. *Infantile form*: blisters, oozing, and crusting, with excoriation. *Adolescent and adult forms*: marked dryness, thickening (lichenification), excoriation, and even scarring.

DISTRIBUTION. *Infantile form*: on face, scalp, arms, and legs, or generalized. The diaper area is usually clear. *Adolescent and adult forms*: on cubital and popliteal fossae and, less commonly, on dorsa of hands and feet, ears, or generalized. Atopic eczema of the soles of the feet is quite common in adolescents.

COURSE. The course varies from a mild single episode to severe chronic, recurrent episodes resulting in the "psychoitchical" person. The infantile form usually becomes milder or even disappears after the age 3 or 4 years and approximately 70% of cases clear by puberty. During puberty and the late teenage years, flare-ups or new outbreaks can occur. Young housewives or househusbands may have their first recurrence of atopic eczema since childhood due to their new job of dishwashing and child care. Thirty percent of patients with atopic dermatitis eventually develop allergic asthma or hay fever.

CAUSES. The following factors are important:

- Heredity is the most important single factor. The family history is usually positive for one or more of the triad of allergic diseases: asthma, hay fever, or atopic eczema. Determination of this history in cases of hand dermatitis is important because often it enables the physician, on the patient's first visit, to prognosticate a more drawn-out recovery than if the patient had a simple contact dermatitis.
- Dryness of the skin is important. Most often, atopic eczema is worse in the winter owing to the decrease in home or office humidity. For this reason, the use of soap and water should be reduced. Emollients (lanolin free) can be applied after bathing.
- Wool and lanolin (wool fat) commonly irritate the skin of these patients. Wearing wool clothes may be another reason for an increased incidence of atopic eczema in the winter.
- Allergy to foods is a factor that is often overstressed, particularly with the infantile form. The mother's history of certain foods causing trouble should be a guide for eliminating foods. This can be tested by adding the incriminated foods to the diet, one new food every 48 hours, when the dermatitis is stable. Scratch tests and intracutaneous tests uncover very few dermatologic allergens.
- Emotional stress and nervousness aggravate any existing condition such as itching, duodenal ulcers, or migraine headaches. Therefore, this "nervous" factor is important but not causative enough to label this disease *disseminated neurodermatitis*.
- Concomitant bacterial infection of the skin, particularly with *Staphylococcus aureus*, is common.

Differential Diagnosis

Dermatitis venenata (contact dermatitis to plants): Positive history, usually, of contactants; no family allergic history; distribution rather characteristic (see Chap. 9).
Psoriasis: Patches localized to extensor surfaces, mainly knees and elbows with characteristic thick silvery-white scale (see Chap. 14).
Seborrheic dermatitis in infants: Absence of family allergy history; lesions scaling and greasy and often seen in the diaper area (see Chap. 13).
Lichen simplex chronicus: Single patches, mainly; no family allergy history (see Chap. 11).

General Management for Atopic Eczema

Inform the patient or family that this is usually a chronic problem; that this is an inherited allergy; that skin tests usually are not helpful; and that relief can occur from the dermatitis and the itch, but there is no "cure" except time.

Treatment of Infantile Form

A child, aged 6 months, presents with mild oozing, red, excoriated dermatitis on face, arms, and legs.

FIRST VISIT

1. Follow regular diet except for the avoidance of any foods that the mother believes aggravate the eruption.
2. Avoid exposure of infant to excessive bathing with soaps and to contact with wool and products containing lanolin.

3. Coal tar solution (LCD) or Balnetar bath oil
                                            120.0
   Sig: Add $1/2$ tbsp to the lukewarm bath water. Be sure to lubricate skin after each bath.
4. Hydrocortisone ointment, 1%   30.0
   Sig: Apply sparingly b.i.d. to affected areas.
   Comment: 1% Hytone ointment is in a petrolatum base without lanolin; I use it frequently. Other proprietary corticosteroid preparations are listed in the Formulary in Chapter 5.
5. Benadryl elixir   90.0
   Sig: 1 tsp b.i.d.
   Comment: Warn parent that this drug may paradoxically stimulate the child.
6. If infection is present, treat with appropriate systemic antibiotic, such as erythromycin or cloxacillin.

SUBSEQUENT VISITS

Add coal tar solution such as LCD (3% to 10%) to the above ointment.

SEVERE OR RESISTANT CASES

1. Restrict diet to milk only, and after 3 days, add one different food every 24 hours. An offending food will cause a flare-up of the eczema in several hours.
2. Hydrocortisone liquid: Cortef   90.0
   Sig: 1 tsp (10 mg) q.i.d. for 3 days, then 1 tsp t.i.d. for 1 week.
   Comment: Decrease the dose or discontinue as improvement warrants. Vary the dosage according to the weight of the child.
3. Hospitalization with change of environment may be necessary for a severe case. This may be necessary in a case of parental negligence.

Treatment of Adult Form

A young adult presents with dry, scaly, lichenified patches in cubital and popliteal fossae.

FIRST VISIT

1. Stress avoidance of excess soap for bathing, of lanolin preparations locally, and of contact with wool.
2. Coal tar solution (LCD)   5%
   Fluorinated corticosteroid ointment or emollient cream (see Chap. 5) q.s.   30.0
3. Chlor-trimeton, 8 or 12 mg   #60
   Sig: 1 tablet b.i.d.
   Comment: Available generically. Warn patient about side effect of drowsiness.

> **SAUER NOTE**
>
> Do not initiate local corticosteroid therapy with the strongest "big guns." Save these stronger corticosteroids for later use, if necessary.

SUBSEQUENT VISITS

1. Gradually increase the concentration of the coal tar solution in the previously mentioned salve up to 10%.
2. Increase the potency of the corticosteroid ointment or emollient cream.
3. For patients with infected crusted lesions (all patients have an element of infection), an antibiotic such as erythromycin, 250 mg, may be prescribed b.i.d. or t.i.d. for several weeks.
4. Systemic corticosteroid therapy may be indicated for severe and resistant cases.
5. Topical doxepin hydrochloride cream (Zonalon)
   Sig: Thin coat q.i.d. on pruritic areas.
   Comment: Can cause drowsiness with overuse and may sting or burn when therapy is first initiated.
6. Leukotriene inhibitors have shown to be of benefit recently by some authors. An example is zafirlukast (Accolate).
   Sig: 20 mg/tab 1 tab by mouth b.i.d.
7. Recombinant human interferon-γ has shown some benefit in some studies. 50 $\mu g/m^2$ is given subcutaneously daily.

> **SAUER NOTES**
>
> 1. With every visit, reemphasize the fact of the chronicity of atopic eczema and the ups and downs that occur, particularly with seasons and stress.
> 2. Emollient (lanolin-free) lotions are helpful in aborting recurrences.

NUMMULAR ECZEMA
(Fig. 9-12)

Nummular eczema is a moderately common, distinctive eczematous eruption characterized by coin-shaped (nummular), papulovesicular patches, mainly on the arms and the legs of young adults and elderly patients.

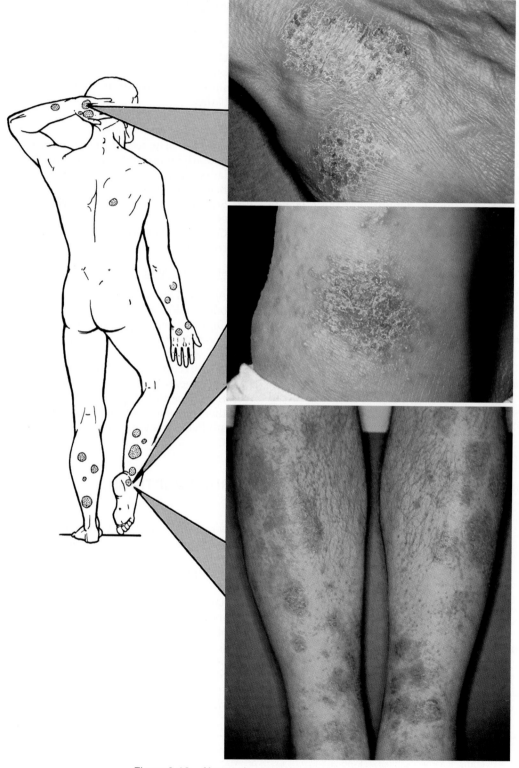

Figure 9-12. **Nummular eczema.** (*Schering Corp.*)

PRIMARY LESIONS. Coin-shaped patches of vesicles and papules are usually seen on the extremities, occasionally on the trunk.

SECONDARY LESIONS. Lichenification and bacterial infection occur.

COURSE. This is very chronic, particularly in older people. Recurrences are common, especially in fall and winter.

SUBJECTIVE COMPLAINTS. Itching is usually quite severe.

CAUSES. Nothing is definite, but these factors are important:

- History is usually positive for asthma, hay fever, or atopic eczema, particularly in the young adult.
- Bacterial infection of the lesions may occur.
- The low indoor humidity of winter causes dry skin, which intensifies the itching, particularly in elderly patients.

Differential Diagnosis

Atopic eczema: Mainly in cubital and popliteal fossae, not coin-sized lesions (see preceding section).
Psoriasis: Not vesicular; see scalp and fingernail lesions (see Chap. 14).
Contact dermatitis: Will not see coin-sized lesions on both arms and legs (see beginning of this chapter).
"Id" reaction, from stasis dermatitis of legs or a localized contact dermatitis: Impossible to differentiate this clinically from nummular eczema, but patient will have history of previous primary dermatitis that suddenly became aggravated.

Treatment

An elderly man presents in the winter with five to eight distinct, coin-shaped, excoriated, vesicular, crusted lesions on the arms and the legs.

FIRST VISIT

1. Instruct the patient to avoid excess use of soaps.
2. Use superfatted soaps such as Dove and lubricate the skin immediately after every bath or shower. Use water as cool as is tolerable to bathe.
3. Corticosteroid ointment   60.0
   Sig: Apply t.i.d. locally.
   Comment: The use of the *ointment* base is particularly important in the therapy for nummular eczema.
4. Benadryl, 50 mg   #15
   Sig: 1 capsule h.s. for antipruritic and sedative effect.
   Comment: Available generically and over the counter

RESISTANT CASES

1. Add coal tar solution, 3% to 10%, to the previously mentioned salve.
2. Oral antibiotic therapy may be beneficial. Prescribe erythromycin, 250 mg, t.i.d. for several weeks.
3. A short course of oral corticosteroid therapy is effective, but relapses are common.
4. Experimental topical immunosuppressive therapies such as tacrolimus (FK506) are being studied for severe recalcitrant atopic dermatitis.

DRUG ERUPTIONS
(Fig. 9-13)

It can be stated almost without exception that any drug systemically administered is capable of causing a skin eruption.

   To jog the memory of patients I often ask, "Do you take any medicine for any condition? What about medicated toothpaste, laxatives, vitamins, aspirin, and tonics? Have you received any shots in the past month?" As stated in Chapter 4, this questioning also gives the physician some general information regarding other ills of the patient that might influence the skin problem. (An eruption due to allergy or primary irritation from *locally* applied drugs is a contact dermatitis.)

Figure 9-13.   Drug eruptions. (*A*) Erosions of tongue and lips from sulfonamides. (*B*) Bismuth line of gums. (*C*) Phenolphthalein fixed eruption of lips of an African-American boy. (*D*) Whitening of scalp hair from chloroquine therapy for lupus erythematosus. (*E*) Erythema multiforme-like eruption of palm from oral antibiotic therapy. (*F*) Striae of buttocks of 30-year-old man following 9 months of corticosteroid therapy. (*G*) Papulosquamous eruption of chest from phenolphthalein. (*E.R. Squibb*)

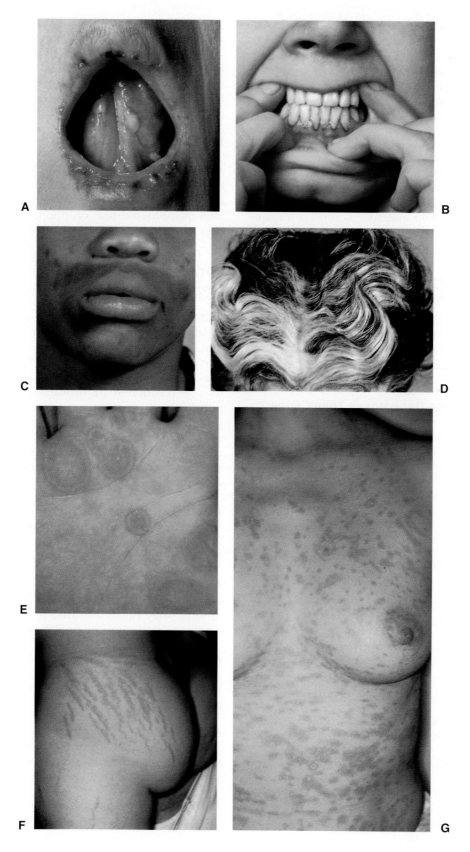

Any of the larger dermatologic texts have extensive lists of common and uncommon drugs, with their common and uncommon skin reactions. These books must be consulted for the rare reactions, but the following paragraphs cover 95% of these idiosyncrasies.

Photosensitivity reactions from drugs are also covered in Chapter 30. Hepatic drug metabolism pathway involving cytochrome P-450 enzymes defines the most significant and largest group of drug–drug interactions. These complex drug–drug interactions are summarized by Singer et al. (See bibliography at end of chapter.)

Adverse drug interactions must always be considered.

> ### SAUER NOTE
>
> Any patient with a generalized skin eruption should be *carefully* questioned concerning the use of oral or parenteral medicinal drugs.

Drugs and the Dermatoses They Cause

Drug eruptions are usually not characteristic for any certain drug or group of drugs. However, the following drugs most commonly cause the associated listed skin lesions. Drug reactions affecting organs other than the skin are not stressed in this chapter.

ACCUTANE. See *Isotretinoin*.

ACETAMINOPHEN (TYLENOL). This drug is an infrequent cause of drug eruption.

ACETOPHENETIDIN (PHENACETIN). Urticaria and erythematous eruptions are noted.

ADRENOCORTICOTROPIC HORMONE (ACTH). Cushing's syndrome, hyperpigmentation, acneiform eruptions, seborrheic dermatitis-like eruptions, and hirsutism have been seen.

ALLOPURINOL (ZYLOPRIM). Erythema, maculopapular rash, and severe bullae are noted.

AMANTADINE. Livedo reticularis is seen.

AMINOSALICYLIC ACID. Scarlatiniform or morbilliform rash, fixed drug eruption, and nummular eczema-like rash are seen.

AMIODARONE. Causes photosensitivity reaction and blue-gray discoloration of skin.

AMPHETAMINE (BENZEDRINE). Coldness of extremities and redness of neck and shoulders occur; it increases itching in lichen simplex chronicus.

AMPICILLIN. See *Antibiotics*.

ANGIOTENSIN-CONVERTING ENZYME (ACE) INHIBITORS. These can cause maculopapular eruption with eosinophilia, pemphigus, a bullous pemphigoid-like eruption, angioedema, rosacea, urticaria, and possibly can flare psoriasis.

ANTABUSE. Redness of face and acne may be noted.

ANTIBIOTICS. Various agents have different reactions, but in general, candidal overgrowth in oral, genital, and anal orifices results in pruritus ani, pruritus vulvae, and generalized pruritus. Candidal skin lesions may spread out from these foci. Also common are urticaria and erythema multiforme-like eruptions, particularly from penicillin. Ampicillin not infrequently causes a generalized maculopapular rash. This is very common in patients with infectious mononucleosis. See *Streptomycin* and later section on photosensitivity reactions.

ANTICOAGULANTS. Bishydroxycoumarin (Dicumarol), sodium warfarin (Coumadin), and heparin can cause severe hemorrhagic skin infarction and necrosis.

ANTIHISTAMINES. These drugs are found in Coricidin, Super-Anahist, and many other preparations. They cause urticaria, eczematous dermatitis, and pityriasis rosea-like rash.

ANTINEOPLASTIC AGENTS. These can cause many skin and mucocutaneous reactions, including alopecia, stomatitis, radiation recall reaction, and erythema.

ANTITOXIN. Immediate reaction occurs with skin manifestations of pruritus, urticaria, and sweating; delayed serum sickness reaction is evidenced by urticaria, redness, and purpura.

APRESOLINE. Systemic lupus erythematosus-like reaction occurs.

ARSENIC. Inorganic arsenic (Fowler's solution, Asiatic pills) causes erythematous, scarlatiniform, vesicular, or urticarial rashes. Delayed reactions include palmar and plantar keratoses and eventual carcinomatous changes. Organic arsenic (Mapharsen, Neoarsphenamine, Tryparsamide) causes similar skin changes plus a severe form of exfoliative dermatitis. A mild erythema on the 9th day of therapy is not unusual. British Anti-Lewisite (BAL) is effective therapy if given early for the skin reactions due to organic arsenicals.

ASPIRIN AND SALICYLATES. Aspirin is found as an ingredient in a multitude of cold and antipain remedies. Pepto-Bismol contains salicylates. Urticaria, purpura, and bullous lesions result.

ATABRINE. Universal yellow pigmentation, blue macules on face and mucosa, and lichen planus–like eruption are found.

ATROPINE. Scarlet fever–like rash occurs.

BARBITURATES. This class of drugs can cause urticarial, erythematous, bullous, or purpuric eruptions and fixed drug eruptions.

β-BLOCKERS. These can cause alopecia and can flare psoriasis.

BISMUTH. Bluish pigmentation of gums and erythematous, papulosquamous, and urticarial skin eruptions have been reported.

BLEOMYCIN. An antitumor antibiotic can cause gangrene, erythema, sclerosis, nail changes, and characteristic striate lesions.

BORIC ACID. Accidental oral ingestion can cause exfoliative dermatitis and severe systemic reaction.

BROMIDES. See *Iodides.* Bromides are found in neurosin, Bromo Quinine, Bromo-Seltzer, Shut-Eye, and other drugs. Acne-like pustular lesions that can spread to form deep granulomatous pyodermas that heal with marked scarring are mainly seen. These must be differentiated from other granulomas.

CAPTOPRIL. Pemphigus-like eruption may occur. See *Angiotensin-converting Enzyme Inhibitors.*

CHEMOTHERAPY AGENTS. See *Antineoplastic Agents.*

CHLORAL HYDRATE. Urticarial, papular, erythematous, and purpuric eruptions occur.

CHLOROQUINE. Erythematous or lichenoid eruptions with pruritus and urticaria have been noted. (Ocular retinal damage from long-term use of chloroquine and other antimalarials can be irreversible.)

CHLOROTHIAZIDE DIURETICS. Petechial and purpuric eruptions, especially of legs. See later section on photosensitivity reactions.

CHLORPROMAZINE (THORAZINE). Maculopapular rash, increased sun sensitivity, purpura with agranulocytosis, and icterus from hepatitis may occur. With long-term therapy, a slate-gray to violet discoloration of the skin can develop.

CIMETIDINE. Dry, scaly skin may result.

CLOFIBRATE. Alopecia may occur.

CODEINE AND MORPHINE. Erythematous, urticarial, or vesicular eruption has been noted.

COLLAGEN, BOVINE, INJECTED. Skin edema, erythema, induration, and urticaria may be seen at implantation sites.

CONTRACEPTIVE DRUGS. Chloasma-like eruption, erythema nodosum, and hives occur, and some cases of acne are aggravated.

CORTISONE AND DERIVATIVES. Cutaneous allergy is rare.

COUMADIN. See *Anticoagulants.*

DAPSONE. Red, maculopapular, vesicular eruption with agranulocytosis occurs, occasionally resembling erythema nodosum.

DICUMAROL. See *Anticoagulants.*

DIETHYLPROPION HYDROCHLORIDE (TENUATE, TEPANIL). Measles-like eruption has been reported.

DIGITALIS. An erythematous, papular eruption is seen rarely.

DILANTIN. See *Phenytoin.*

ESTROGENIC SUBSTANCES AND STILBESTROL. Edema of legs with cutaneous redness progressing to exfoliative dermatitis is seen.

FELDENE. See *Piroxicam* in later section on photosensitivity reactions.

FLAGYL. See *Metronidazole*.

FUROSEMIDE. Bullous hemorrhagic eruption occurs.

GLUTETHIMIDE. Erythema, urticaria, purpura, or (rarely) exfoliative dermatitis has been reported.

GOLD. There is eczematous dermatitis of hands, arms, and legs or a pityriasis rosea-like eruption. Seborrheic-like eruption, urticaria, and purpura have also been found.

HEPARIN. See *Anticoagulants*.

HYDROXYUREA. Dermopathy mimicking cutaneous findings of dermatomyositis. Atrophic, erythematous dermatitis over the back of the hands that may be photoinduced and leg ulcers may develop.

IBUPROFEN (MOTRIN, NAPRIN, ADVIL). Bullous eruptions, including erythema multiforme, Stevens-Johnson syndrome, toxic epidermal necrolysis, urticaria, photosensitivity and fixed drug reactions.

IMIPRAMINE. Can cause slate-gray discoloration of skin.

INSULIN. Urticaria with serum sickness symptoms and fat atrophy at injection site can result.

IODIDES. See *Bromides*. Papular, pustular, ulcerative, or granulomatous lesions occur mainly on acne areas or legs. Administration of chloride hastens recovery.

ISONIAZID. Eruptions may be erythematous and maculopapular, generalized, purpuric, bullous, and nummular eczema-like. Acne may be aggravated.

ISOTRETINOIN. Dry red skin and lips are common; alopecia is rare.

LASIX. See *Furosemide*.

LAMOTRIGINE. At least 10% with cutaneous drug reactions. May be similar to phenytoin cutaneous drug reactions.

LITHIUM. Acne-like lesions occur on the body. Lithium can exacerbate psoriasis.

LIVER EXTRACT. Urticaria, diffuse redness, and itching occur.

MECLIZINE HCL (ANTIVERT). Urticaria may be present.

MEPHENYTOIN (MESANTOIN). Macular rash and severe bullous eruption occur.

MEPROBAMATE. Small purpuric lesions and erythema multiforme-like eruption are found.

MERCURY. Erythema, pruritus, scarlatiniform eruption, and stomatitis have been noted.

MESANTOIN. See *Mephenytoin*.

METHANDROSTENOLONE (DIANABOL). An acne-like eruption is seen.

METRONIDAZOLE (FLAGYL). Urticaria and pruritus occur.

MINOCYCLINE. This can discolor skin (muddy skin syndrome), teeth, and scars. Rarely hypersensitivity, sickness-like reaction and drug-induced lupus erythematosus. Rare syndrome of hepatitis, exfoliative dermatitis, fever, lymphadenopathy, eosinophilia and lymphocytosis. Rarely a systemic lupus-like syndrome may occur.

MORPHINE. See *Codeine*.

NAPROXEN. A lichen planus-like eruption is found.

NONSTEROIDAL ANTIINFLAMMATORY DRUGS. Urticaria, erythema multiforme-like eruption, and toxic epidermal necrolysis occur. There are many drugs in this grouping, including ibuprofen (Motrin), naproxen (Naprosyn), indomethacin (Indocin), fenoprofen (Nalfon), piroxicam (Feldene), diclofenac (Voltaren), and so on.

PENICILLIN. See *Antibiotics*.

PENICILLAMINE. Lupus-like rash, lichen planus-like rash, and pemphigus foliaceous are noted.

PHENACETIN. See *Acetophenetidin*.

PHENOLPHTHALEIN. This product is found in 4-Way Cold tablets, Ex-Lax, Bromo Quinine,

Phenolax, Agoral, Bile Salts, and pink icing on cakes. A fixed drug eruption, which consists of hyperpigmented or purplish, flat or slightly elevated, discrete, single or multiple patches occurs.

PHENOTHIAZINE GROUP. See later section on photosensitivity reactions.

PHENYLBUTAZONE. Widespread erythematous bullous eruptions have been seen.

PHENYTOIN (DILANTIN). Hypertrophy of gums and an erythema multiforme-like eruption occurs. This drug can cause a pseudolymphoma syndrome. The fetal hydantoin syndrome manifests with many organ defects plus nail hypoplasia.

PROCAINAMIDE. This drug can cause systemic lupus erythematosus-like reaction.

PROPRANOLOL (INDERAL). Drug eruption is rare. See β-*Blockers*.

PSORALENS. See later section on photosensitivity reactions.

QUINIDINE. There may be edema, purpura, or a scarlatiniform eruption that may progress to exfoliative dermatitis.

QUININE. Any kind of diffuse eruption may occur.

***RAUWOLFIA* ALKALOIDS (RESERPINE).** Urticaria, photosensitivity reactions, and petechial eruptions have been reported.

RIFAMPIN.
Pruritus, urticaria, acne, bullous pemphigoid, mucositis, exfoliative erythroderma, red urine and red soft contact lenses.

SALICYLATES. See *Aspirin*.

SILVER. A diffuse bluish or grayish pigmentation of skin and gum margins is found owing to a deposit of silver salts.

STILBESTROL. See *Estrogenic Substances and Stilbestrol*.

STREPTOMYCIN. Urticaria and erythematous, morbilliform, and purpuric eruptions are noted.

SULFONAMIDES. There may be urticaria, scarlatiniform eruption, erythema nodosum, eczema-tous flare of exudative dermatitis, erythema multiforme-like bullous eruption, or fixed eruption. See later section on photosensitivity reactions. AIDS patients develop allergic drug eruptions quite often.

SULFONYLUREA HYPOGLYCEMICS. See *Sulfonamides* and later section on photosensitivity reactions.

SURAMIN. 80% have cutaneous reaction especially morbilliform, ultraviolet light recall (skin eruptions at site of previous ultraviolet exposure), urticaria and "suramin keratoses."

TESTOSTERONE AND RELATED DRUGS. Acne-like lesions and hypertrichosis have been reported.

TETRACYCLINE. Teeth staining under 8 years of age. See *Antibiotics*. Fixed drug eruption, photosensitivity, and serum sickness-like reaction.

THIAZIDES. See later section on photosensitivity reactions.

TRIETHYLENEMELAMINE (TEM). Pruritic maculopapular eruption results.

TRIMETHADIONE (TRIDIONE). Acneiform eruption of face occurs.

TRIMETHOPRIM (TRIMPEX). This drug is rarely incriminated in drug eruptions.

TRYPTOPHAN. This drug can cause eosinophilic myalgia syndrome.

VITAMINS

> *Vitamin A.* Long-term therapy with large doses causes scaly, rough, itchy skin with coarse, dry, scant hair growth, and systemic changes.

> *Vitamin D.* Skin lesions are rare, but headache, nausea, diarrhea, increased urination, and sore gums and joints are found.

> *Vitamin B Group.* Urticaria, pruritic redness, and even anaphylactic reactions occur after intramuscular or intravenous administration. Nicotinic acid quite regularly causes a red flush, pruritus and, less often, hives, within 15 to 30 minutes after oral ingestion of 50 to 100 mg. The patient should be warned concerning this flush to eliminate unnecessary alarm.

WARFARIN, SODIUM. See *Anticoagulants*.

Dermatoses and the Drugs That Cause Them

As stated previously, drug eruptions are usually not characteristic for any particular chemical, but experience has shown that certain *clinical pictures* commonly follow absorption of certain drugs. (For a description of these eruptions see the disease mentioned.)

ACNE-LIKE OR PUSTULAR LESIONS. Bromides, iodides, lithium, trimethadione, testosterone, methandrostenolone (Dianabol), and corticosteroids.

ACRAL ERYTHEMA. Redness, pain, and swelling of the hands and feet associated with various chemotherapeutic agents including cyclophosphamide, cytosine arabinoside, docetaxel, doxorubicin, fluorouracil, hydroxyurea, mercaptopurine, methotrexate, and mitotane.

ALOPECIA. Amethopterin (methotrexate) and other antineoplastic agents, also colchicine, clofibrate, testosterone, β-blockers, heparin, dicumarol, and coumarin derivatives.

ANGIOEDEMA. Aspirin, nonsteroidal antiinflammatory drugs, and ACE inhibitors.

DIDMOS. (Drug-induced delayed [3–6 weeks] multiorgan hypersensitivity syndrome of Sontheimer and Houpt, also called DRESS [drug rash with eosinophil and systemic symptoms of Bocquet and Roujeau].) An exanthematous or papulopustular febrile eruption with hepatitis (also possible lung, renal, hypothyroid involvement), lymphadenopathy, and eosinophilia. Dapsone, carbamazepine, phenobarbital, minocycline, trimethoprim, sulfamethoxazole, procarbazine, allopurinol, terbinafine.

ECZEMATOUS ERUPTION. Quinine, procaine, antihistamines, gold, mercury, sulfonamides, penicillin, and organic arsenic.

ERYTHEMA MULTIFORME-LIKE ERUPTION. Penicillin and other antibiotics, sulfonamides, phenolphthalein, barbiturates, phenytoin, and meprobamate.

ERYTHEMA NODOSUM-LIKE ERUPTION. Sulfonamides, iodides, bromides, salicylates, contraceptive drugs, and dapsone.

EXFOLIATIVE DERMATITIS. In the course of any severe generalized drug eruption, particularly due to arsenic, penicillin, sulfonamides, allopurinol, and barbiturates.

FIXED DRUG ERUPTION. (See *Phenolphthalein* in preceding list for description.) Phenolphthalein, acetaminophen, barbiturates, organic arsenic, gold, salicylates, sulfonamides, tetracycline, and many others.

KERATOSES AND EPITHELIOMAS. Arsenic, mercury, PUVA therapy, and immunosuppressive agents.

LICHEN PLANUS-LIKE ERUPTION. Atabrine, arsenic, naproxen, gold, and others.

LUPUS ERYTHEMATOSUS. Minocycline, hydralazine, procainamide, isoniazid, methyldopa, chlorpromazine, and quinidine.

LINEAR IgA BULLOUS DERMATOSIS. Rare, vancomycin most common.

MEASLES-LIKE ERUPTION. Barbiturates, arsenic, sulfonamides, quinine, and many others.

MUCOUS MEMBRANE LESIONS. Many drugs can cause various types of lesions, including pigmentation of gums from bismuth, hypertrophy of gums from phenytoin, and erosive lesions from sulfonamides, antineoplastic agents, and many other drugs.

NAIL CHANGES. Demethylchlortetracycline (Declomycin) and tetracycline can cause distal detachment of nails (onycholysis), apparently due to a phototoxic reaction.

NUMMULAR ECZEMA-LIKE ERUPTION. From combination of isoniazid and *p*-amino-salicylic acid.

NECROSIS OF THE SKIN. Coumarin and heparin (both localized and distant site) derivatives. Recombinant α interferon at localized site.

PEMPHIGUS-LIKE LESIONS. Rifampin, phenylbutazone, penicillamine, and captopril aminopyrine, captopril, phenylbutazone, and pyrazolone derivatives.

PHOTOSENSITIVITY REACTION. Several of the newer drugs and some of the older ones cause a dermatitis on exposure to sunlight. These skin reactions can be urticarial, erythematous, vesicular, or plaque-like. The mechanism can be either phototoxic or photoallergic, but this distinction can be difficult to ascertain. Here is a rather complete list of *photosensitizing drugs*, but also consult Chapter 31.

Sulfonamides: Sulfonylurea Hypoglycemics
Tolbutamide (Orinase)
Chlorpropamide (Diabinese)
Acetohexamide (Dymelor)

Antibiotics
Demethylchlortetracycline (Declomycin)
Doxycycline (Doryx, Monodox, Vibramycin)
Griseofulvin (Fulvicin, Grifulvin, Gris-PEG)
Lomefloxacin (Maxaquin)
Nalidixic Acid (NegGram and others)
Tetracycline

Benzofurans
Amiodarone (Cordarone)

Chlorothiazide diuretics
Chlorothiazide (Diuril)
Hydrochlorothiazide (HydroDIURIL, Esidrix, Oretic)
Methyclothiazide (Enduron)

Phenothiazines
Chlorpromazine (Thorazine)
Promazine (Sparine)
Prochlorperazine (Compazine)
Promethazine (Phenergan)

Psoralens
8-Methoxypsoralen (Oxsoralen)
Trioxsalen (Trisoralen)

Oxicams
Piroxicam (Feldene)

PIGMENTARY CHANGES. Contraceptive drugs, atabrine, chloroquine, chlorpromazine, minocycline, amiodarone, bismuth, gold, and silver salts.

PITYRIASIS ROSEA-LIKE ERUPTION. Bismuth, gold, barbiturates, and antihistamines.

PSEUDOLYMPHOMA. Antidepressants, diphenylhydantoin, alpha-agonists, angiotensin-converting enzyme inhibitors, anticonvulsants, antihistamines, benzodiaze-pine, β-blockers, calcium-channel blockers, lipid-lowering agents, lithium, nonsteroidal antiinflammatory drugs, phenothiazines, procain- amide, estrogen, and progesterone.

PSORIASIS EXACERBATION. Lithium, β-blockers, ACE inhibitors, antimalarials, nonster-oidal antiinflammatory drugs and terbinafine.

PURPURIC ERUPTIONS. Barbiturates, salicylates, meprobamate, organic arsenic, sulfonamides, chlorothiazide diuretics, dicumarol, and long-term use of corticosteroids.

SCARLET FEVER-LIKE ERUPTION OR "TOXIC ERYTHEMA." Arsenic, barbiturates, codeine, morphine, mercury, quinidine, salicylates, sulfonamides, and others.

SEBORRHEIC DERMATITIS-LIKE ERUPTION. Gold and ACTH.

URTICARIA. Penicillin, salicylates, serums, sulfonamides, barbiturates, opium group, contraceptive drugs, *Rauwolfia* alkaloids, and ACE inhibitors.

VESICULAR OR BULLOUS ERUPTIONS. Sulfonamides, penicillin, phenylbutazone, and mephenytoin.

WHITENING OF HAIR. Chloroquine and hydroxychloroquine can cause this in blond or red-haired people.

Course of Drug Eruptions

The course of drug eruptions depends on many factors, including the type of drug, severity of the cutaneous reaction, systemic involvement, general health of the patient, and efficacy of corrective therapy. Most cases with bullae, purpura, or exfoliative dermatitis have a serious prognosis and a protracted course.

Treatment

1. Eliminate the drug. This simple procedure is often delayed, with resulting serious consequences, because a careful history is not taken. If the eruption is mild and the drug necessary, discontinuation of the drug may not be mandatory.
2. Further therapy depends on the seriousness of the eruption. Most barbiturate measles-like eruptions subside with no therapy. An itching drug eruption should be treated to relieve the itch. Cases of exfoliative dermatitis or severe erythema multiforme-like lesions require corticosteroid and other supportive therapy.

SAUER NOTES

1. When confronted with any diffuse or puzzling eruption, routinely question the patient regarding *any* medication taken by *any* route.

2. Ask: "Are you taking any vitamins, laxatives, nerve pills, and so forth?" This jogs the patient's memory.

3. Remember, any chemical ingested can cause an eruption, such as toothpaste, mouthwash, breath-freshener, and chewing gum.

BIBLIOGRAPHY

Adams RM. Occupational skin disease, ed 2. Orlando, FL, Harcourt Brace Jovanovich, 1990.

American Academy of Dermatology. Guidelines of care for atopic dermatitis. J Am Acad Dermatol 1992;26:485.

American Medical Association. Guides to the evaluation of permanent impairment, ed 3. Chicago, AMA, 1990.

Brehler R, Hildebrand A, Luger TA. Recent developments in the treatment of atopic eczema. J Am Acad Dermatol 1997;36:1.

DeShazo RD, Smith DL. Primer on allergic and immunologic diseases. JAMA 1992;268:2785. This entire issue is devoted to allergic diseases.

Drake LA, Dorner W, Goltz RW, et al. Guidelines of care for contact dermatitis. J Am Acad Dermatol 1995;32:109.

Drake LA, Dinehart SM, Farmer ER, et al. Guidelines of care for cutaneous adverse drug reactions. J Am Acad Dermatol 1996;35:458.

Drugs that cause photosensitivity. Med Lett Drugs Ther 1995;37:35.

Fisher AA. Contact dermatitis, ed 4. Philadelphia, Lea & Febiger, 1995.

Fisher AA. The diagnosis and management of health personnel allergic to natural rubber latex gloves: Part II. Cutis 1997;59:168.

Goh CL, Wong JS, Giam YC. Skin colonization of Staphylococcus aureus in atopic dermatitis patients seen at the National Skin Centre, Singapore. Int J Dermatol 1997;36:653.

Goldstein SM. Adverse cutaneous reactions to medication. Baltimore, Williams & Wilkins, 1996.

Guin JD. Practical contact dermatitis: A handbook for the practitioner. McGraw-Hill, 1995.

Hanifin IM. Atopic dermatitis: new therapeutic considerations. J Am Acad Dermatol 1991;24:1097.

Lepoittevin JP, Basketter DA, et al. Allergic contact dermatitis. Springer, 1998.

Leung DY. Atopic dermatitis: From pathogenesis to treatment. Chapman & Hall, 1996.

Maibach HI. Occupational and industrial dermatology, ed 2. Boca Raton, FL, CRC Press, 1986.

Menne T, Maibach HI. Hand eczema. CRC Press, 1994.

Physicians' desk reference to pharmaceutical specialties and biologicals. Oradell, NJ, Medical Economics, published yearly. Toxic reactions to specific drugs are listed.

Plotnick H. Analysis of 250 consecutively evaluated cases of workers' disability claims for dermatitis. Arch Dermatol 1990;126:782.

Rietschel RL. Fisher's contact dermatitis, ed 4. Williams & Wilkins, 1995.

Roujeau JC, Stern RS. Severe adverse cutaneous reactions to drugs. N Engl J Med 1994;331:1272.

Warshaw EM. Latex allergy. J Am Acad Dermatol 1998;39:1.

10

Dermatologic Immunology

Richard S. Kalish, M.D., Ph.D.*

The purpose of this chapter is to give an overall view of the skin diseases in which immunologic reactions play a significant role.

BASIC IMMUNOLOGY

Historically, the immune system was divided into two basic branches: *humoral immunity* and *cellular immunity*. In fact, the immune response is an active interplay of both humoral and cellular immunity, along with cytokines (Table 10-1) made by a multitude of cells including lymphocytes, Langerhans' cells, macrophages, and keratinocytes.

Humoral Immunity

Humoral immunity is mediated by antibodies produced by B lymphocytes. When activated by antigen, antigen-presenting cells, and helper T lymphocytes, the B lymphocytes differentiate into plasma cells, which produce antibodies. Antibodies can specifically bind their appropriate antigen with high affinity. These antibodies can be divided into five classes: immunoglobulin G (IgG), immunoglobulin A (IgA), immunoglob-

ulin M (IgM), immunoglobulin D (IgD), and immunoglobulin E (IgE, reagin). IgA is the principal antibody secreted at mucosal surfaces. These antibodies, with varying degrees of efficiency, can fix (activate) complement (IgG, IgM), aid macrophages in cytotoxicity or cell killing and phagocytosis (IgG), and trigger release of immunoreactive substances from mast cells (IgE).

Complement System

The complement system is a complex set of proteins that, when activated, can lyse cells and aid in phagocytosis by macrophages, cause mast cells to release histamines, and be chemotactic for neutrophils. Activation of complement occurs as a cascade of factors, resulting in amplification. Complement can be activated by antibodies and immune complexes through the classic pathway. The sequence of activation of factors in the classic complement pathway is C1qrs, C2, C4, C3, C5, C6, C7, C8, C9. Complement can also be activated by bacteria, fungi, and endotoxins through the alternate pathway by activation of properdin. This results in cleavage and activation of C3. C5a is produced by cleavage of C5 during activation and is an "anaphylatoxin" that induces histamine release, vascular permeability, and chemotaxis of inflammatory cells. The final components of complement form a complex (C5b6789) that can lyse cells.

*Associate Professor, Department of Dermatology, Health Sciences Center, State University of New York at Stony Brook, Stony Brook, New York

TABLE 10-1
T-CELL CYTOKINES

IL1	Costimulatory signal for T-lymphocyte activation by antigen, chemotactic, induces acute phase reactants, induces and synergizes with other cytokines; produced by macrophages, Langerhans' cells, keratinocytes, and many additional cells; only released by keratinocytes following cell damage
IL2	T-lymphocyte growth factor: required for growth of most T cells. Immune response does not happen without IL-2. Most IL-2 is made by CD4$^+$ cells. CD8$^+$ cells can make IL-2, but CD8$^+$ cells are a minor source. IL-2 receptor (Tac, CD25) expression is essential for T-cell proliferation and is tightly regulated.
IL3	Growth factor for mast cells
IL4	Induces IgE production growth factor for subset of T cells (TH2), produced by TH2 CD4$^+$ T cells
IL5	B-cell differentiation factor, TH2 cytokine
IL6	Induces acute phase reactants, synergizes with other cytokines
IL8	Chemotactic for neutrophils
IL10	Produced by TH2 cells; inhibits production of γ-interferon by TH1 cells
GM-CSF	Activates monocytes and neutrophils, colony-stimulating factor for growth of monocyte and neutrophil precursors in bone marrow
γ-INF	Gamma-interferon; induces DR, ICAM-1 on keratinocytes and endothelial cells, inhibits IgE production, antiviral major effector of delayed hypersensitivity (TH1), produced by TH1 cells
TNF-α	Tumor necrosis factor; TNF-α produced by keratinocytes, macrophages, etc.; TNF-β produced by T lymphocytes; direct cytotoxic effects, induces ICAM-1 mediator of inflammation

Cellular Immunity

Cellular immunity involves T lymphocytes (T cells), antigen-presenting cells, and natural killer (NK) cells. T cells are subdivided into CD4+ and CD8+ cells. The CD4+ T cells act as helper cells both in the production of antibodies and CD8+ T-cell responses. CD8+ T cells can kill target cells with specific antigens (cytotoxicity). CD8+ T cells may also suppress immune responses (suppressor cells). Both CD4+ and CD8+ T-cells produce hormones termed *interleukins*, which mediate many of their effects. CD4+ cells generally produce greater amounts of those interleukins that promote T-cell proliferation, and B-cell antibody production, hence providing help. Production of antibodies by B cells is generally dependent upon such help from T cells. Therefore, the separation of immune responses into humoral and cellular is artificial.

Antigen Presentation

T cells cannot see antigen without the aid of antigen-presenting cells. Antigen-presenting cells include macrophages and dendritic antigen-presenting cells, such as the Langerhans' cells of the skin. Langerhans' cells are the primary antigen-presenting cell of the epidermis and are central to epidermal T cell-mediated reactions such as allergic contact dermatitis. Presentation of antigens to T cells generally requires that protein antigens are first degraded to peptides and presented by special antigen-presenting molecules. Antigens that derive from inside the cells are generally presented on major histocompatibility complex (MHC) class I molecules (*e.g.*, HLA-A, B, C), to CD8+ T cells. Examples of internal antigens are viral antigens, tumor-associated antigens, and transplantation antigens. CD8+ cytotoxic cells are thus positioned to recognize and kill these cells.

Extracellular antigens are phagocytosed by the antigen presenting cells and presented on MHC class II molecules (*e.g.* HLA-DR, DP, DQ) to CD4+ T cells. Examples of extracellular antigens are bacteria, toxins, and vaccines. The CD4+ cells are thus positioned to help in the production of antibodies to these proteins.

Interleukins, Interferons, and Cytokines

Many of the effects of T cells are mediated by hormones that go by the names of cytokines (Table 10-1), interleukins, or interferons. Interleukin 2 (IL-2) is the principal growth factor of T cells. Production of IL-2 by CD4+ cells is closely regulated and is one of the major controls in the immune response. Cytokines are divided into TH1 cytokines, which promote cellular immunity, and TH2 cytokines, which promote antibody production, especially IgE. Both TH1 and TH2 cytokines are made by CD4+ cells, which may differentiate into TH1 and TH2 CD4+ cells. Classic TH1 cytokines are interferon-γ, interleukin 2 (IL-2), and tumor necrosis factor-α. TH2 cytokines include IL-4, IL-5, and IL-10.

Immunity and Skin Disease

Response to an antigen (either foreign or self) is divided into four types according to the Gel and Coombs classification. Type I is anaphylaxis or immediate hypersensitivity, which is an IgE-mediated response. Type II involves binding antibodies to cell membranes. Type III is mediated by circulating immune complexes that fix complement to induce inflammation. Type IV is cell-mediated or delayed hypersensitivity. Although this classification is useful, many conditions are a combination of these types.

IMMUNE-MEDIATED SKIN CONDITIONS

ATOPIC DISEASE AND ATOPIC ECZEMA. Atopic conditions include asthma, allergic rhinitis, urticaria, and atopic dermatitis. These conditions are generally associated with elevated serum IgE levels and serum IgE responses to allergens. The role of IgE and exogenous antigens in atopic dermatitis is extremely controversial (see Chap. 9). Candidate antigens include food, animal dander, inhalants, *Staphylococcus aureus,* and house dust mite. Atopic diseases are believed to result from a predominance of TH2 CD4+ immune responses. TH2 T cells produce cytokines (*e.g.*, IL-4, IL-5) which favor the production of IgE.

ALLERGIC CONTACT DERMATITIS. Poison ivy is the prototypic allergic contact dermatitis. It is mediated by T-cell recognition of a small chemical (hapten) or allergen that is bound to protein and presented by epidermal Langerhans' cells. Both CD4+ and CD8+ T cells can have a role in the inflammation. Allergic contact dermatitis often presents with a linear or asymmetric distribution, matching exposure to the inciting hapten. Patch tests are used clinically to discover the cause of allergic contact dermatitis.

DRUG ERUPTIONS. Recognition of drugs by the immune system generally requires that the small chemical entities bind to protein and act as a hapten, or directly to MHC molecules. Drug eruptions take many forms, some of which are immune-mediated. Urticarial or anaphylactic reactions can be medicated by IgE degranulation of mast cells. Vasculitic reactions (*e.g.*, palpable purpura) and serum sickness result from deposition of immune complexes and complement in vessels. There is evidence suggesting that morbilliform and bullous (blistering) drug reactions may be mediated by T lymphocytes.

ERYTHEMA MULTIFORME AND TOXIC EPIDERMAL NECROLYSIS. Erythema multiforme is a severe bullous eruption, marked by necrosis of the full thickness of the epidermis. When involving more than 30% of body surface, it is called *toxic epidermal necrolysis.* Toxic epidermal necrolysis has a significant mortality rate. Erythema multiforme involving mucous membranes and systemic toxicity is also called Stevens Johnson syndrome. These conditions may be a continuous spectrum. It is proposed that they are mediated by T lymphocytes. Mild, recurrent erythema multiforme may result from recurrent herpes simplex infection. Severe forms are generally drug reactions.

URTICARIA. The classic type I or immediate hypersensitivity reaction can cause urticaria and also the true systemic anaphylactoid reactions, which can include bronchospasm with asthma-like reactions, laryngeal edema, convulsions, nausea, diarrhea, hypotension, and in its most exaggerated state, shock. Allergic urticaria results from IgE-mediated degranulation of mast cells.

CUTANEOUS AUTOIMMUNE CONDITIONS

AUTOIMMUNE BULLOUS ERUPTIONS. Autoantibodies against epidermal adhesion molecules can induce blisters that correspond histologically to the site of the autoantigen. Pemphigus vulgaris results from IgG directed against desmoglein III, which is associated with desmosomes. The IgG is deposited between epidermal cells and stains in an intercellular pattern on immunofluorescence. Blisters form within the epidermis of skin and mucosa. Pemphigus is a classic Gel and Coombs type II reaction, and transfer of pemphigus IgG to neonatal mice induces similar blisters and immunofluorescent findings. In contrast, bullous pemphigoid is associated with IgG against proteins associated with hemidesmosomes. Immunofluorescence shows a linear band of IgG at the dermal–epidermal junction. The blisters are below the epidermis, through the lamina lucida of the basement membrane. Autoantibodies in epidermolysis bullosa acquisita are directed against type VII collagen, which is present in the anchoring filaments below the basement membrane. Blisters are below the basement membrane, which results in scarring. Dermatitis herpetiformis differs in that immune complexes containing IgA are deposited in the dermal papillae. This is associated with micropustules of neutrophils and clefts below the epidermis, resulting in extremely pruritic grouped vesicles. Table 10-2 contains a partial list of autoimmune blistering diseases, which are also discussed in Chapter 22.

ALOPECIA AREATA. This condition results in loss of hair in circular patches. It may extend to the entire scalp or all body hair. Histology demonstrates an infiltrate of T cells around affected hair follicles. Both autoantibodies and autoreactive T cells have been demonstrated. It is possible to transfer alopecia areata to human scalp on immunosuppressed mice by injection of T cells.

VITILIGO. The primary defect in vitiligo is the absence of melanocytes from affected skin. This

TABLE 10-2
BULLOUS SKIN DISEASES ASSOCIATED WITH AUTOIMMUNITY*

Disease	Immune Reaction	Clinical Cutaneous Response
Bullous pemphigoid	IgG and C3† direct IF at BMZ; IgG and C3 by IE in lamina lucida and hemidesmosomes; IgG indirect IF on sodium chloride split skin on either epidermal or epidermal and dermal sides at BMZ	Large tense bullae; urticarial or circinate lesions; may have underlying cancer
Cicatricial pemphigoid (benign mucous membrane pemphigoid)	Direct IF same as bullous pemphigoid; indirect IF may be positive depending on substrate; IgG by IE positive at lamina lucida and lamina densa	Bullae healing with scars; oral mucous membrane erosions; severe ocular disease with scars
Pemphigus	IgG and C3 direct IF at intercellular substance; IgG indirect IF at intercellular substance; IgG and C3 by IE localized to the cell membrane	Large flaccid bullae arising on skin and mucous membranes
Dermatitis herpetiformis	IgA direct IF in uninvolved skin; IgA indirect IF antiendomysial antibodies in 70%.	Grouped papulovesicular and pustular eruption, especially elbows, knees, and buttocks; very pruritic; heals with marked hyperpigmentation
Epidermolysis bullosa acquisita	IgG and C3 direct IF at BMZ; IgG indirect IF on sodium split skin on dermal side of BMZ	Trauma-induced acral blisters with scars
Linear IgA dermatosis	IgA direct IF at BMZ; IgA rare indirect IF at BMZ; IgA by IE at lamina lucida, sublamina densa, or both	Similar to dermatitis herpetiformis or bullous pemphigoid
Herpes gestationis	C3 direct IF at BMZ; indirect IF rarely shows Hg factor (complement-fixing IgG anti-BMZ antibody); C3 by IE at lamina densa	Mimicks bullous pemphigoid, intense pruritus; occurs during pregnancy
Chronic bullous disease of childhood	IgA direct IF at BMZ; IgA indirect IF may be present at BMZ	Annular arrays of blisters in preschool children, especially perianal and perioral
Paraneoplastic pemphigus	IgG and C3 direct IF at BMZ and intraepidermal; indirect IF on rat bladder transitional epithelium	Painful oral and eye lesions; polymorphous skin lesions (bullae, vesicles, lichenoid papules, erythematous macules); underlying cancer present; poor prognosis

IF, immunofluorescence; BMZ, basement membrane zone; IE, immunoelectron microscopy.
* Considered to be type II immune response, except dermatitis herpetiformis, which is type III immune response.
† Third component of complement

is associated with autoantibodies against melanocyte antigens.

PSORIASIS. This condition is marked by increased proliferation of epidermal keratinocytes, associated with an infiltrate of neutrophils and lymphocytes. T-lymphocyte functions are necessary to induce and maintain psoriasis lesions. Psoriasis responds to a variety of immunosuppressive treatments, including fusion toxins that specifically target only T cells. It is also possible to induce psoriasis in human skin grafted onto immunodeficient mice by transferring T cells. Bacterial superantigens, which activate T cells, may have a role in flaring psoriasis.

CONNECTIVE TISSUE DISEASE. A final division of autoimmune disease is the connective tissue or *collagen vascular diseases* (Table 10-3). These include lupus erythematosus, scleroderma, and dermatomyositis. Most of these diseases are associated with autoantibodies, including antinuclear antibodies. Clinical presentation, serology, and histology are used to classify the disorders. Overlap syndromes combining one or more of these illnesses are common.

VASCULITIS. The types of vasculitis are listed in Table 10-4. The immune response in vasculitis is thought to be type III or immune complex disease, and this can be demonstrated by comple-

TABLE 10-4
TYPES OF VASCULITIS: IMMUNE AND CLINICAL RESPONSES

Immune Response

Type III immune complex; complement and immunoglobulin found in vessel walls

Circulating immune complexes found in serum

Clinical Response

Urticarial lesions that are not evanescent; palpable purpura (most common and characteristic); gangrene; cutaneous infarcts

Types of Vasculitis

Hypersensitivity angiitis (leukocytoclastic vasculitis)

Henoch-Schönlein purpura (usually IgA)

Urticarial vasculitis (may have low complement)

Cryoglobulinemia (cryoglobulins precipitated in vessels)

Vasculitis associated with collagen vascular disease (rheumatoid arthritis, systemic lupus erythematosus, dermatomyositis, acute rheumatic fever, Sjögren's syndrome)

Polyarteritis nodosa (may be associated with hepatitis B associated surface antigen)

Wegner's granulomatosis (positive for anti-neutrophil cytoplasmic antibody with cytoplasmic accentuation)

Lymphatoid granulomatosis (behavior may mimic lymphoma)

Giant cell arteritis (temporal artery is only skin distribution of vasculitis)

TABLE 10-3
AUTOIMMUNE CONNECTIVE TISSUE DISEASES IN THE SKIN

Disease	Evidence of Immune Response	Clinical Cutaneous Response
Dermatomyositis	Associated with other collagen vascular diseases (overlap syndrome); auto-antibodies usually absent	Periorbital heliotrope, erythema over joints
SLE, DLE disease localized to skin	IgG direct IF at DEJ, ANA (especially homogeneous) positive 5% in DLE and 99% in SLE, anti-DNA positive 70% of SLE, low complement; low white blood count; immune complexes in serum	Wide range (scaling, scarring, erythema, vasculitis, bullae, alopecia)
Rheumatoid arthritis	IgM rheumatoid factor	Vasculitis; subcutaneous nodules
Scleroderma	ANA-positive (especially nucleolar, speckled) in systemic form and may have increased interleukin-8, ANA usually negative in localized form (morphea)	Sclerosis of skin
Sjögren's syndrome	Anti-SS-A, anti-SS-B	Dry skin; decreased sweating, pruritus; dry mouth; dry eyes (keratoconjunctivitis sicca)
Still's disease (chronic juvenile polyarthritis)	Autoantibodies negative	Evanescent evening morbilliform eruption

DEJ, dermoepidermal junction; ANA, antinuclear antibody; DLE, discoid lupus erythmatosus; SLE, systemic lupus erythematosus; IF, immunofluorescence.

ment and immunoglobulins in vessel walls as circulating serum immune complexes. The most common clinical manifestation of all these diseases is palpable purpura, but other manifestations can include urticarial lesions, gangrene, and ischemic ulcers.

GRAFT-VERSUS-HOST DISEASE (GVH). This condition results from transplanted T cells attacking the recipient. Target organs are skin, gut, and liver. It is manifested as a sunburn type rash, diarrhea, and elevated liver enzymes. The requirements for GVH are transferred T cells capable of attacking the host as foreign and an inability of the host to eliminate the hostile T cells. The most common setting for GVH is bone marrow transplantation, but transfusion of immunosuppressed patients with blood that has not been irradiated can have the same result. The rash of GVH can vary from macular erythema to epidermal necrosis and death.

SKIN DISEASE ASSOCIATED WITH IMMUNODEFICIENCY

Immunodeficiency can be acquired, as in AIDS (see Chap. 18) or other viral infections, or genetic. Genetic immune defects can selectively target antibody production (*e.g.*, agammaglobulinemias), or T-lymphocyte function (*e.g.*, ataxia telangiectasia). Other immunodeficiencies can alter neutrophil chemotaxis, lysosomal function, or oxidative burst. Genetic deficiencies of complement components can inhibit resistance to encapsulated bacteria (*e.g.*, C3 deficiency) or predispose to autoimmune disease (*e.g.*, C4). Deficiency of antibody production is correlated with infection with encapsulated bacteria, whereas deficiency of T-cell function results in viral infections. Severe combined immunodeficiency results in defects in both antibody and T-cell mediated immunity. (See Table 10-5 for a list of skin diseases associated with immunodeficiency.)

TABLE 10-5
SKIN DISEASES ASSOCIATED WITH IMMUNODEFICIENCY

Disease	Immune Defect	Cutaneous Manifestations
Acquired immunodeficiency (AIDS; human immunodeficiency virus infection)	CD4 (helper-inducer cells) depleted, polyclonal increase in immunoglobulins due to B-cell activation	Acute viral exanthem, candidiasis, herpes simplex, Kaposi's sarcoma, seborrhea, dry skin, malignancies (see Chap. 18)
Agammaglobulinemia (three types: transient, congenital X-linked recessive, acquired)	Associated with pernicious anemia, vitiligo, drug eruptions, decreased IgG	Staphylococcal pyodermas, granulomas, dermatomyositis-like syndrome, eczema, angiodema, lymphoma, aphthous ulcers
Ataxia-telangiectasia (autosomal recessive)	Type IV immunodeficiency, IgA absent	Telangiectasias
Chédiak-Higashi syndrome	Defect of lysosomes	Oculocutaneous albinism, streptococcal and staphylococcal infections
Chronic granulomatous disease (X-linked recessive)	Increase of all immunoglobulins, polymorphonuclear lymphocytes are defective	Chronic abscesses
Chronic mucocutaneous candidiasis	Absent delayed skin test for candidiasis, may have T-cell defect; may have autoimmune abnormality; endocrine abnormalities may be present	Chronic candidiasis infection of mucous membranes and skin
Job's syndrome (hyperimmunoglobulin E recurrent infection syndrome)	IgE greater than 1000, decreased suppressor-T cells, decreased neutrophil chemotaxis	Eczema, chronic recurrent abscesses
Severe combined immunodeficiency	Autosomal recessive—absence of T-lymphocytes; X-linked—absence of T-lymphocytes and decreased B-lymphocytes	Pyoderma, morbilliform rash, candidiasis
Wiskott-Aldrich syndrome	Decreased serum IgM, increased serum IgA	Eczema, purpura, pyoderma

IMMUNOMODULATION OF SKIN DISEASE

Most inflammatory skin disease responds to topical or systemic corticosteroids. However, long-term use of corticosteroids has significant toxicity and there are multiple nonsteroidal immunosuppressive agents used in dermatology. "Steroid sparing" agents used in the treatment of autoimmune bullous diseases include azathioprine, cyclophosphamide, dapsone, gold, and methotrexate. Immunosuppressive agents useful for psoriasis include cyclosporine A, hydroxyurea, mycophenolate mofetil, and methotrexate. Phototherapy with UVB, or psoralen plus UVA, has immunosuppressive effects. Antimalarials (*e.g.*, hydroxychloroquine) are useful for connective tissue disease. Additional immunomodulatory therapies used in dermatology include extracoporeal photophoresis, interferons, interferon inducers, and topical nitrogen mustard. Nonsteroidal antiinflammatory agents under investigation for skin conditions include FK506 and related compounds that can have topical activity. With the use of molecular biology it has been possible to create molecules that specifically target T cells, cytokines, or antigen-presentation molecules. Several such designer molecules have show efficacy in phase I trails for psoriasis. The future promises increasingly sophisticated nonsteroidal antiinflammatory therapies.

BIBLIOGRAPHY

Belsito DV. The rise and fall of allergic contact dermatitis. Am J Contact Dermatitis 1997;8:193.

Bos JD, Wierenga EA, Smitt JHS, et al. Immune dysregulation in atopic eczema. Arch Dermatol 1992;128:1509.

Castellino F, Zhong G, Germain RN. Antigen presentation by MHC class II molecules: Invariant chain function, protein trafficking, and the molecular basis of diverse determinant capture. Hum Immunol 1997;54:159.

Del Prete G. The concept of type-1 and type-2 helper T-cells and their cytokines in humans. Int Rev Immunol 1998;16 : 427.

Dahl MV. Clinical immunodermatology, ed 3. New York, Mosby, 1996.

Fine JD. Management of acquired bullous skin diseases. N Engl J Med 1995;333 : 22.

Jennette CJ, Milling DM, Falk RJ. Vasculitis affecting the skin: A review [editorial]. Arch Dermatol 1994;130:899.

Johnson ML, Farmer ER. Graft-versus-host reactions in dermatology. J Am Acad Dermatol 1998;38:3.

Jordon RE. Immunologic diseases of the skin. East Norwalk, CT, Appleton & Lange, 1990.

Kalish RS. Drug eruptions: A review of clinical and immunologic features. Adv Dermatol 1991;6:221.

Kalish RS. Antigen processing: The gateway to the immune response [review]. J Am Acad Dermatol 1995;32:640.

Kondo S, Sauder DN. Epidermal cytokines in allergic contact dermatitis. J Am Acad Dermatol 1995;33:786.

Kuhn CA, Hanke CW. Current status of melanoma vaccines. Dermatol Surg 1997;23:649.

Leung DY. Atopic dermatitis: immunobiology and treatment with immune modulators. Clin Exp Immunol 1997;107(Suppl 1):25.

11

Pruritic Dermatoses

Pruritus, or itching, brings more patients to the physician's office than any other skin disease symptom. Itchy skin is not easily cured or even alleviated. Many hundreds of proprietary over-the-counter and prescription drugs are touted as effective antiitch remedies, but none is 100% effective. However, many are partially effective, but it is unfortunate that the most effective locally applied chemicals frequently irritate or sensitize the skin.

Pruritus is a symptom of many of the common skin diseases, such as contact dermatitis, atopic eczema, seborrheic dermatitis, hives, some drug eruptions, and many other dermatoses. Relief of itching is of prime importance in treating these diseases.

In addition to the pruritus that occurs as a symptom of many skin diseases, there are other clinical forms of pruritus that deserve special consideration. These special types include *generalized pruritus* of the winter, senile, and essential varieties and *localized pruritus* of the lichen simplex type, of the ears, anal area, lower legs in men, back of the neck in women, and genitalia.

GENERALIZED PRURITIS

Diffuse itching of the body without perceptible skin disease usually is due to winter dry skin, senile skin, underlying illness (especially Hodgkin's disease), or unknown causes.

Winter Pruritis

Winter pruritus, or pruritus hiemalis, is a common form of generalized pruritus, although most patients complain of itching confined mainly to their legs. Every autumn, a certain number of elderly patients, and occasionally young ones, walk into the physician's office complaining bitterly of the rather sudden onset of itching of their legs. These patients have dry skin due to the low humidity in their furnace-heated homes, or occasionally from the low humidity resulting from cooling air conditioning. Clinically, the skin shows excoriations and dry, curled, scaling plaques resembling a sun-baked, muddy beach at low tide. The dry skin associated with winter itch is to be differentiated from *ichthyosis*, a congenital dermatosis of varying severity, which is also worse in the winter.

Treatment of winter pruritus consists of the following:

1. Bathing should involve as cool water as possible and as little soap as possible.
2. A bland soap, such as Dove, Oilatum, Cetaphil, or Basis, is used sparingly.
3. An oil is added to the bath water, such as Lubath, RoBathol, Nivea, or Alpha-Keri. (The patient should be warned to avoid slipping in the tub.)
4. Emollient lotions are beneficial, such as Complex 15, Pen-Kera or Moisturel. α-Hydroxy acid preparations include LactiCare,

Lac-Hydrin, and Eucerin Plus. Urea products that are beneficial include Aquacare HP, Carmol, and Eucerin Plus. These lubricants should be applied immediately after bathing.

5. A low-potency corticosteroid ointment applied twice daily is effective.

6. Oral antihistamines are sometimes effective, such as chlorpheniramine (Chlor-Trimeton), 4 mg h.s. or q.i.d, or diphenhydramine (Benadryl), 50 mg h.s.

SAUER NOTE

When the presenting complaint is generalized itching of the skin, always stroke the skin on the forearm with your nail or a tongue depressor. After 5 minutes or so, if there is a wheal reaction at the stroking site, you have a diagnosis of dermographism. This is a common problem that is easily overlooked.

Senile Pruritis

Senile pruritus is a resistant form of generalized pruritus in the elderly patient. It can occur at any time of the year and may or may not be associated with dry skin. There is some evidence that these patients have a disorder of keratinization. This form of itch occurs most commonly on the scalp, the shoulders, the sacral areas, and the legs. Clinically, some patients have no cutaneous signs of the itch, but others may have linear excoriations. *Scabies* should be ruled out, as well as the diseases mentioned under the next form of pruritus to be considered, essential pruritus.

Treatment is usually not very satisfactory. In addition to the agents mentioned previously in connection with winter pruritus, the injection of 30 mg triamcinolone acetonide suspension (Kenalog-40) intramuscularly every 4 to 6 weeks for two or three injections is quite beneficial.

Essential Pruritus

Essential pruritus is the rarest form of the generalized itching diseases. No person of any age is exempt, but it occurs most frequently in the elderly patient. The itching is usually quite diffuse, with occasional "bites" in certain localized areas. All diffuse itching is worse at night, and no exception is made for this form of pruritus. Before a diagnosis of essential pruritus is made, the fol-

lowing diseases must be ruled out by appropriate studies: *drug reaction, diabetes mellitus, uremia, lymphoma* (mycosis fungoides, leukemia, or Hodgkin's disease), *liver disease, bullous pemphigoid, AIDS,* and *intestinal parasites.* Treatment is the same as for senile and winter pruritus.

LOCALIZED PRURITIC DERMATOSES

Lichen Simplex Chronicus

Other common terms for lichen simplex chronicus include *localized neurodermatitis* and *lichenified dermatitis.* There are pros and cons for all the terms.

Lichen simplex chronicus (Figs. 11-1 and 11-2) is a common skin condition characterized by the occurrence of single or, less frequently, multiple patches of chronic, itching, thickened,

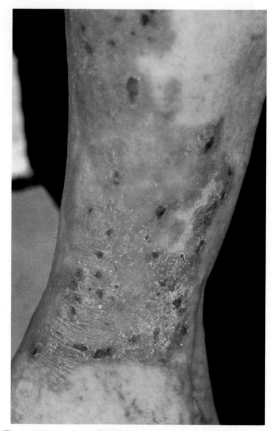

Figure 11-1. Localized lichen simplex chronicus of the leg. This is a common location. Note the lichenification and the excoriations due to the marked pruritus. *(K.U.M.C.; Duke Labs, Inc.)*

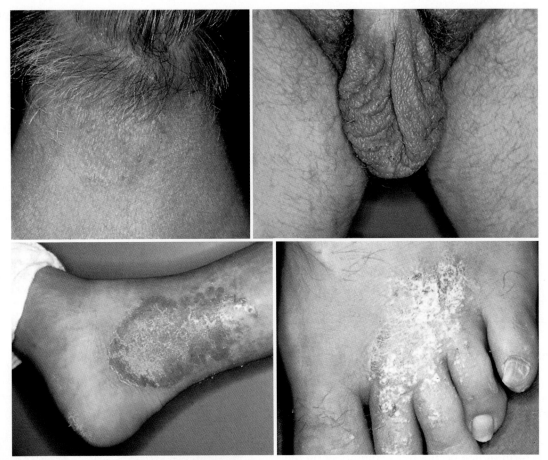

Figure 11-2. Localized lichen simplex chronicus. (*Top left*) In occipital area of scalp. (*Top right*) Of scrotum, with marked lichenification and thickening of the skin. (*Bottom left*) Of medial aspect of ankle, following lichen planus of the area. (*Bottom right*) On dorsum of foot. (*Duke Labs, Inc.*)

scaly, dry skin in one or more of several classic locations. It is unrelated to atopic eczema.

PRIMARY LESIONS. This disease begins as a small, localized, pruritic patch of dermatitis that might have been an insect bite, a chigger bite, contact dermatitis, or other minor irritation, which may or may not be remembered by the patient. Because of various etiologic factors mentioned, a cycle of itching, scratching, more itching, and more scratching supervenes, and the chronic dermatosis develops.

SECONDARY LESIONS. These include excoriations, lichenification, and, in severe cases, marked verrucous thickening of the skin, with pigmentary changes. In these severe cases, healing is bound to be followed by some scarring.

DISTRIBUTION. This condition is seen most commonly at the hairline of the nape of the neck and on the wrists, the ankles, the ears (see external otitis), anal area (see pruritus ani), and so on.

COURSE. The disease is quite chronic and recurrent. Most cases respond quickly to correct treatment, but some can last for years and defy all forms of therapy.

SUBJECTIVE COMPLAINTS. Intense itching, often paroxysmal, usually worse at night, occurs even during sleep.

CAUSES. The initial cause (a bite, stasis dermatitis, contact dermatitis, seborrheic dermatitis, tinea cruris, psoriasis) may be very evanescent, but it is generally agreed that the chronicity of the lesion is due to the nervous habit of scratching. It is a rare patient who will not volunteer the information or admit, if questioned, that the itching is worse when he or she is upset, nervous, or tired. Why some people with a minor skin injury respond with the development of a lichenified patch of skin and others do not is possibly due to the personality of the patient.

AGE GROUP. It is very common to see localized neurodermatitis of the posterior neck in menopausal women. Other clinical types of neurodermatitis are seen in any age.

FAMILY INCIDENCE. This disorder is unrelated to allergies in patient or family, thus differing from atopic eczema. Atopic people are more "itchy," however.

RELATED TO EMPLOYMENT. Recurrent exposure and contact to irritating agents at work can lead to lichen simplex chronicus.

DIFFERENTIAL DIAGNOSIS

Psoriasis: Several patches on the body in classic areas of distribution; family history of disease; classic silvery whitish scales; sharply circumscribed patch (see Chap. 14).

Atopic eczema: Allergic history in patient or family; multiple lesions; classically seen in cubital and popliteal areas and face (see Chap. 9).

Contact dermatitis: Acute onset; contact history positive; usually red, vesicular, and oozing; distribution matches site of exposure of contactant; may be acute contact dermatitis overlying lichen simplex chronicus due to overzealous therapy (see Chap. 9).

Lichen planus, hypertrophic form on anterior tibial area: Lichen planus in mouth and on other body areas; biopsy specimen usually characteristic (see Chap. 14).

Seborrheic dermatitis of scalp: Does not itch as much; is better in summer; a diffuse, scaly, greasy eruption (see Chap. 13).

TREATMENT

A 45-year-old woman presents with a severely itching, scaly, red, lichenified patch on back of the neck at the hairline.

FIRST VISIT

1. Explain the condition to the patient and tell her that your medicine will be directed toward stopping the itching. If this can be done, and if she will cooperate by keeping her hands off the area, the disease will disappear. Emphasize the effect of scratching by stating that if both arms were broken, the eruption would

be gone when the casts were removed. However, this is not a recommended form of therapy.

2. For severe bouts of intractable itching, prescribe ice cold Burow's solution packs.
   Sig: Add 1 packet of Domeboro powder to 1 quart of ice cold water. Apply cloth wet with this solution for 15 minutes p.r.n.

3. A moderate-potency corticosteroid ointment or emollient cream   15.0
   Sig: Apply q.i.d., or more often, as itching requires.

   The moderate-potency fluorinated corticosteroid creams (Synalar, Cordran, Lidex, Diprosone, Cutivate) can be used under an occlusive dressing of plastic wrap on lesions on an extremity. The dressing can be left on overnight.

   Warning: Long-continued occlusive dressing therapy with corticosteroids can cause atrophy of the skin.

SUBSEQUENT VISITS

1. Add menthol (0.25%) or coal tar solution (3% to 10%) to above ointment or cream for greater antipruritic effect.

2. Intralesional corticosteroid therapy. This is a very effective and safe treatment. The technique is as follows. Use a 1-inch long No. 26 needle or 30-1/2 needle and a Luer-Lok type syringe. Inject 5 or 10 mg of triamcinolone parenteral solution (Kenalog-10 or Aristocort Intralesional Suspension) intradermally or subcutaneously, directly under the skin lesion. An equal amount of saline should be mixed with the solution in the syringe. Do not inject all the solution in one area, but spread it around as you advance the needle. The injection can be repeated every 2 or 3 weeks as necessary to eliminate the patch of dermatitis.
   Warning: A complication of an atrophic depression at the injection site can occur. This usually can be avoided if the concentration of triamcinolone in one area is kept low, and when it occurs, it usually disappears after months.

RESISTANT CASES

1. A tranquilizer
2. Prednisone 10 mg
   Sig: 1 tablet q.i.d. for 3 days, then 2 tablets every morning for 7 days.
3. Dome-Paste boot or Coban wrap. Apply in office for cases of neurodermatitis localized to

arms and legs. This is a physical deterrent to scratching. Leave on for a week at a time.
4. Psychotherapy is of questionable value.

External Otitis

External otitis is a descriptive term for a common and persistent dermatitis of the ears due to several causes. The agent most frequently blamed for this condition is "fungus," but pathogenic fungi are rarely found in the external ear. The true causes of external otitis, in order of frequency, are as follows: seborrheic dermatitis, lichen simplex chronicus, contact dermatitis, atopic eczema, psoriasis, pseudomonas bacterial infection (which is usually secondary to other causes) and, lastly, fungal infection, which also can be primary or secondary to other factors. For further information on the specific processes, refer to each of the diseases mentioned.

TREATMENT

Treatment should be directed primarily toward the specific cause, such as care of the scalp for seborrheic cases or avoidance of jewelry for contact cases. When this is done, however, certain special techniques and medicines must be used in addition to clear up this troublesome area.

An elderly woman presents with an oozing, red, crusted, swollen left external ear, with a wet canal but an intact drum. A considerable amount of seborrheic dermatitis of the scalp is confluent with the acutely inflamed ear area. The patient has had itching ear trouble off and on for 10 years, but in the past month, it has become most severe.

First Visit

1. Always inspect the canal and the drum with an otoscope. If excessive wax and debris are present in the canal, or if the drum is involved in the process, the patient should be treated for these problems or referred to an ear specialist. An effective liquid to dry up the oozing canal is as follows:
   Hydrocortisone powder   1%
   Burow's solution, 1:10 strength q.s.   15.0
   Sig: Place 2 drops in ear t.i.d.
2. Burow's solution wet packs
   Sig: Add 1 packet of Domeboro powder to 1 quart of cool water. Apply wet cloths to external ear for 15 minutes t.i.d.

3. Corticosteroid ointment   15.0
   Sig: Apply locally to external ear t.i.d., not in canal.

Subsequent Visits

Several days later, after decreased swelling, cessation of oozing, and lessening of itching, institute the following changes in therapy:

1. Decrease the soaks to once a day.
2. Sulfur, ppt.   5%
   Corticosteroid ointment q.s.   15.0
   Sig: Apply locally t.i.d. to ear with the little finger, *not* down in the canal with a cotton-tipped applicator.

For persistent cases, a short course of oral corticosteroid or antibiotic therapy often removes the "fire" so that local remedies will be effective.

Pruritus Ani

Itching of the anal area is a common malady that can vary in severity from mild to marked. The patient with this very annoying symptom is apt to resort to self-treatment and therefore delay the visit to the physician. Usually, the patient has overtreated the sensitive area, and the immediate problem of the physician is to quiet the acute contact dermatitis. The original cause of the pruritus ani is often difficult to ascertain.

PRIMARY LESIONS. These can range from slight redness confined to a very small area to an extensive contact dermatitis with redness, vesicles, and oozing of the entire buttock.

SECONDARY LESIONS. Excoriations from the intense itching are very common, and after a prolonged time, they progress toward lichenification. A generalized papulovesicular id eruption can develop from an acute flare-up of this entity.

COURSE. Most cases of pruritus ani respond rapidly and completely to proper management, especially if the cause can be ascertained and eliminated. Every physician, however, will have a patient who will continue to scratch and defy all therapy.

CAUSES. The proper management of this socially unacceptable form of pruritus consists in searching for and eliminating the several factors that contribute to the persistence of this symptom complex. These factors can be divided into general and specific etiologic factors.

GENERAL FACTORS

Diet: The following irritating foods should be removed from the diet: chocolate, nuts, cheese, and spicy foods. Coffee, because of its stimulating effect on any form of itching, should be limited to 1 cup a day. Rarely, certain other foods are noted by the patient to aggravate the pruritus.

Bathing: Many patients have the misconception that the itching is due to uncleanliness. Therefore, they resort to excessive bathing and scrubbing of the anal area. This is harmful and irritating and must be stopped.

Toilet care: Harsh toilet paper contributes greatly to the continuance of this condition. Cotton or a proprietary cleansing cloth (Tucks) must be used for wiping. Mineral oil or Balneol lotion can be added to the cotton if necessary. Rarely, an allergy to the pastel tint in colored toilet tissues is a factor causing the pruritus.

Scratching: As with all the diseases of this group, chronic scratching leads to a vicious cycle. The chief aim of the physician is to give relief from this itching, but a gentle admonishment to the patient to keep hands off is indicated. With the physician's help, the itch-and-scratch habit can be broken. The emotional and mental personality of the patient regulates the effectiveness of this suggestion.

SPECIFIC ETIOLOGIC FACTORS

Oral antibiotics: Pruritus ani from oral antibiotic therapy is seen frequently. It may or may not be due to an overgrowth of candidal organisms. The physician who automatically questions patients about recent drug ingestion will not miss this diagnosis.

Lichen simplex chronicus: It is always a problem to know which comes first, the itching or the "nervousness." In most instances, the itching comes first, but there is no denying that once pruritus ani has developed, it is aggravated by emotional tensions and "nerves." However, only the rare patient has a "deep-seated" psychological problem.

Psoriasis: In this area, psoriasis is common. Usually, other skin surfaces are also involved.

Atopic eczema: Atopic eczema of this site in adults is rather unusual. A history of atopy in the patient or family is helpful in establishing this cause.

Fungal infection: Contrary to old beliefs, this cause is quite rare. Clinically, a raised, sharp, papulovesicular border is seen that commonly is confluent with tinea of the crural area. If a scraping or a culture reveals fungi, then local or systemic antifungal therapy is indicated for cure.

Worm infestation: In children, pinworms can usually be implicated. A diagnosis is made by finding eggs on morning anal smears or by seeing the small white worms when the child is sleeping. Worms are a rare cause of adult pruritus ani.

Hemorrhoids: In the lay person's mind, this is undoubtedly the most common cause. Actually, it is an unimportant primary factor but may be a contributing factor. Hemorrhoidectomy alone is rarely successful as a cure for pruritus ani.

Cancer: This is a very rare cause of anal itching, but a rectal or proctoscopic examination may be indicated.

TREATMENT

A patient states that he has had anal itching for 4 months. It followed a 5-day course of an antibiotic for the "flu." Many local remedies have been used; the latest, a supposed remedy for athlete's foot, aggravated the condition. Examination reveals an oozing, macerated, red area around the anus.

FIRST VISIT

1. Initial therapy should include removal of the general factors listed under Causes and giving instructions as to diet, bathing, toilet care, and scratching.
2. Burow's solution wet packs

Sig: Add 1 packet of Domeboro to 1 quart of cool water. Apply wet cloths to the area b.i.d. while lying in bed for 20 minutes, or more often if necessary for severe itching. Ice cubes may be added to the solution for more anti-itching effect.

3. Low-potency corticosteroid cream or ointment q.s.   15.0
   Sig: Apply to area b.i.d.

4. Benadryl, 50 mg
   Sig: 1 capsule h.s. (for itching and sedation).
   Comment: Available over the counter

SAUER NOTES

1. Do not prescribe a fluorinated corticosteroid salve for the anogenital area. It can cause telangiectasia and atrophy of the skin after long-term use.

2. One of my favorite medications for pruritus ani or genital pruritus is 1% Hytone ointment applied sparingly locally two or three times a day. The petrolatum base is well tolerated.

3. If the anogenital pruritus is resistant to therapy and especially if the involvement is unilateral, a biopsy should be performed to rule out Bowen's disease or extramammary Paget's disease.

SUBSEQUENT VISITS

1. As tolerated, add increasing strengths of sulfur, coal tar solution, or menthol (0.25%) or phenol (0.5%) to the above cream, or Vytone cream with hydrocortisone 1%.

2. Intralesional corticosteroid injection therapy. This is very effective. Usually, the minor discomfort of the injection is quite well tolerated because of the patient's desire to be cured. The technique is given in the section on lichen simplex chronicus.

Genital Pruritus

Itching of the female vulva or the male scrotum can be treated in much the same way as pruritus ani if these special considerations are borne in mind.

VULVAR PRURITUS. Etiologically, vulvar pruritus is due to candida or trichomonas infection; contact dermatitis from underwear, douche chemicals, contraceptive jellies, and diaphragms; chronic cervicitis; neurodermatitis; menopausal or senile atrophic changes; lichen sclerosus et atrophicus; or leukoplakia. Pruritus vulvae is frequently seen in patients with diabetes mellitus and during pregnancy.

Treatment can be adapted from that for pruritus ani (see preceding section) with the addition of a daily douche, such as vinegar, 2 tablespoons to 1 quart of warm water.

Vulvodynia is a difficult problem to manage. The sensation of burning and pain in the vulvar area is not uncommon and requires careful etiologic evaluation. Most cases can be managed as a contact dermatitis, but there is a strong psychological element. A minimal dose of haloperidol (Haldol), 1 mg, b.i.d., or amitriptyline (Elavil), 10 mg h.s., is occasionally indicated and effective. Larger doses may be necessary. Scrotodynia is a similar variant in males.

SCROTAL PRURITUS. Etiologically, scrotal pruritus is due to tinea infection; contact dermatitis from soaps, powders, or clothing; or lichen simplex chronicus (see Fig. 11-2).

Treatment is similar to that given for pruritus ani in the preceding section.

Notalgia Paresthetica

Notalgia paresthetica is a moderately common localized pruritic dermatosis that is usually confined to the middle upper back or scapular area. A pigmented patch is formed by the chronic rubbing. Some evidence exists for a hereditary factor. EMLA anesthetic cream and capsaicin (Zostrix) cream may be beneficial.

BIBLIOGRAPHY

Denman ST. A review of pruritus. J Am Acad Dermatol 1986;14:375.

Leibsohm E. Treatment of notalgia paresthetica with capsaicin. Cutis 1992;49:335.

Long CC, Marks R. Stratum corneum changes in patients with senile pruritus. J Am Acad Dermatol 1992;27:560.

12

Vascular Dermatoses

Urticaria, erythema multiforme and its variants, and erythema nodosum are included under the heading of vascular dermatoses because of their vascular reaction patterns. Stasis dermatitis is included because it is a dermatosis due to venous insufficiency in the legs.

URTICARIA
(Fig. 12-1)

The commonly seen entity of urticaria, or hives, can be acute or chronic and due to known or unknown causes. Numerous factors, both *immunologic* and *nonimmunologic*, can be involved in its pathogenesis. The urticarial wheal results from liberation of histamine from tissue mast cells and from circulating basophils.

Nonimmunologic factors that can release histamine from these cells include chemicals, various drugs (including morphine and codeine), ingestion of lobster, crayfish, and other foods, bacterial toxins, and physical agents. Examples of the type caused by physical agents are the linear wheals that are produced by light stroking of the skin, known as *dermographism*. (Consult the Dictionary–Index for the triple response of Lewis reaction.)

Immunologic mechanisms are probably involved more often in acute than in chronic urticaria. The most commonly considered of these mechanisms is the type I hypersensitivity state that is triggered by polyvalent antigen bridging two specific immunoglobulin E molecules that are bound to the mast cell or basophil surface (see Chap. 10).

LESIONS. Pea-sized red papules to large circinate patterns with red borders and white centers that can cover an entire side of the trunk or the thigh may be noted. Vesicles and bullae are seen in severe cases, along with hemorrhagic effusions. A severe form of urticaria is labeled *angioedema*. It can involve an entire body part, such as the lip or the hand. Edema of the glottis and bronchospasm are serious complications.

COURSE. Acute cases may be mild or explosive but usually disappear with or without treatment in a few hours or days. The chronic form has remissions and exacerbations for months or years.

CAUSES. After careful questioning and investigation, many cases of hives, particularly of the chronic type, are concluded to result from no apparent causative agent. Other cases, mainly the acute ones, have been found to result from the following factors or agents:

> *Drugs or Chemicals.* Penicillin and derivatives are probably the most common causes of acute hives, but any other drug, whether ingested, injected, inhaled, or, rarely, applied on the skin, can cause the reaction (see Chap. 9).

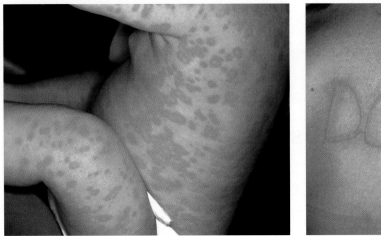

(*A*) Acute urticaria from penicillin in 6-month old child.　　　　(*B*) Dermographism on back.

Figure 12-1.　**Vascular dermatoses.** *(Dermik Laboratories, Inc.)*

Foods. Foods are a common cause of acute hives. The main offenders are seafood, strawberries, chocolate, nuts, cheeses, pork, eggs, wheat, and milk. Chronic hives can be caused by traces of penicillin in milk products.

Insect Bites and Stings. Insect bites, stings from mosquitoes, fleas, or spiders, and contact with certain moths, leeches, and jellyfish cause hives.

Physical Agents. Hives result from heat, cold, radiant energy, and physical injury. *Dermo-graphism* is a term applied to a localized urticarial wheal produced by scratching the skin in certain people (see Fig. 12-1) .

Inhalants. Nasal sprays, insect sprays, dust, feathers, pollens, and animal danders are some offenders.

Infections. A focus of infection is always considered, sooner or later, in chronic cases of hives, and in unusual instances it is causative. The sinuses, the teeth, the tonsils, the gallbladder, and the genitourinary tract should be checked.

Internal disease. Urticaria has been seen with liver disease, intestinal parasites, cancer, rheumatic fever, and others.

"Nerves." After all other causes of chronic urticaria have been ruled out, there remain a substantial number of cases that appear to be related to nervous stress, worry, or fatigue. These cases benefit most from the establishment of good rapport between the patient and the physician.

Contact Urticaria Syndrome. This uncommon response can be incited from the local contact on the skin of drugs and chemicals, foods, insects, animal dander, and plants.

Cholinergic Urticaria. Clinically, small papular welts are seen that are caused by heat (hot bath), stress, or strenuous exercise.

Differential Diagnosis

Hebra's erythema multiforme: Systemic fever, malaise, and mouth lesions are noted in children and young adults (see the next section of this chapter).

Dermographism: A common finding in young adults, especially those who present complaining of welts on their skin or vague itching of the skin with no residual lesions. To make the diagnosis, stroke the skin firmly to see if an urticarial response develops. The course can be chronic, but hydroxyzine, 10 mg b.i.d. or t.i.d., is quite helpful.

(Warn the patient about the possibility of drowsiness.)

Urticarial vasculitis: Lesions may last more than 24 hours, be painful, leave a bruise, and be associated with hypocomplementemia.

Treatment

For a case of *acute* hives due to penicillin injection 1 week previously for a "cold":

1. Colloidal bath
   Sig: Add 1 cup of starch or oatmeal (Aveeno) to 6 to 8 inches of lukewarm water in the tub. Bathe for 15 minutes once or twice a day.
2. Sarna Lotion or PrameGel OTC
   Sig: Apply p.r.n. locally for itching.
3. Hydroxyzine (Atarax), 10 mg   #30
   Sig: Take 1 tablet t.i.d., a.c. (drowsiness warning).
4. Diphenhydramine (Benadryl), 50 mg
   Comment: Available over the counter
5. Betamethasone sodium phosphate (Celestone), 3 mg/mL
   Sig: Inject 1 to 1.5 mL subcutaneously.

For a more severe case of acute hives:

1. Benadryl injection
   Sig: Inject 2 mL (20 mg) subcutaneously, *or*
2. Epinephrine hydrochloride
   Sig: Inject 0.3 to 0.5 mL of 1:1000 solution subcutaneously, *or*
3. Prednisone tablets, 10 mg   #30
   Sig: Take 1 tablet q.i.d. for 3 days, then 1 tablet in morning as necessary.

For treatment of patient with *chronic* hives of 6 months' duration when cause is undetermined after careful history and examination:

1. Hydroxyzine (Atarax), 10 to 25 mg   #60
   Sig: Take 1 tablet t.i.d. depending on drowsiness and effectiveness. Continue for weeks or months.
   Clemastine (Tavist) 1.34 or 2.68 mg   #30
   Sig: Take 1 tablet b.i.d.
   Cyproheptadine (Periactin) 4 mg   #60
   Sig: One by mouth t.i.d.
2. Loratadine (Claritin) 10 mg   #30
   Sig: Take 1 tablet once a day
   Cetirizine (Zyrtec) 5 mg or 10 mg   #30
   Sig: Take 1 tablet once a day
   Fexofenadine (Allegra), 60 mg   #30
   Sig: Take 1 tablet once a day
3. Cimetidine (Tagamet), 300 mg   #60
   Sig: Take 1 tablet t.i.d.
   Comment: This H2 blocker is of benefit in some cases, and can be added to HI blockers.

4. Suggest avoidance of chocolate, nuts, cheese and other milk products, seafood, strawberries, pork, excess spicy foods, and excess of coffee or tea.
5. Keep a diet diary of everything ingested (including all foods, all medicines, even over-the-counter, candy, menthol cigarettes, chewing gum, chewing tobacco, mouthwash, breath fresheners, etc.) and then see what items were used 12 to 24 hours before the episode of hives occurred.
6. A mild sedative or tranquilizer such as meprobamate, 400 mg t.i.d., or chlordiazepoxide (Librium), 5 mg t.i.d., may help.
7. Doxepin (Sinequan) 10 mg   #60
   Sig: 1 tablet t.i.d.
   Comment: This is a tricyclic antidepressant with potent antihistaminic properties. It can cause drowsiness, dry mouth, and other side effects of this classification of drugs.
8. Immunosuppressive drugs such as Prednisone are unfortunately necessary in severe cases.
9. Ketotifen fumarate is a mast cell stabilizer not yet approved in the United States but found in other countries with benefit in severe cases.

ERYTHEMA MULTIFORME
(*Fig. 12-2*)

The term *erythema multiforme* introduces a flurry of confusion in the mind of any student of medicine. It is our purpose in this section to attempt to dispel that confusion. Erythema multiforme, as originally described by Hebra, is an uncommon, distinct disease of unknown cause characterized by red iris-shaped or bull's eye-like macules, papules, or bullae confined mainly to the extremities, the face, and the lips. It is accompanied by

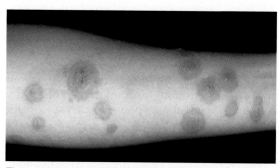

Figure 12-2. **Vascular dermatoses.** Erythema multiforme-like eruption on arm during pregnancy. (*Dermik Laboratories, Inc.*)

mild fever, malaise, and arthralgia. It occurs usually in children and young adults in the spring and the fall, has a duration of 2 to 4 weeks, and frequently is recurrent for several years.

The only relation between Hebra's erythema multiforme and the following diseases or syndromes is the clinical appearance of the eruption.

Stevens-Johnson syndrome is a severe and rarely fatal variant of erythema multiforme. It is characterized by high fever, extensive purpura, bullae, ulcers of the mucous membranes, and, after 2 to 3 days, ulcers of the skin. Eye involvement can result in blindness. It can be related to drugs and it's severest form is considered by some to be the same as toxic epidermal necrolysis (see Chapter 22).

Erythema multiforme bullosum is a severe, chronic, bullous disease of adults (see Chap. 22). There is an opinion that this syndrome is completely separate from erythema multiforme. More macular, truncal lesions and more epidermal necrosis and less infiltrate may be seen in Stevens-Johnson syndrome (toxic epidermal necrolysis). Sulfonamides, anticonvulsant agents, allopurinol, chlormezanone and nonsteroidal antiinflammatory drugs.

Erythema multiforme-like drug eruption is frequently due to phenacetin, quinine, penicillin, mercury, arsenic, phenylbutazone, barbiturates, trimethadione, phenytoin, sulfonamides, and antitoxins (see Chap. 9).

Erythema multiforme-like eruption is seen rather commonly as part of a herpes simplex outbreak and also in conjunction with rheumatic fever, pneumonia, meningitis, measles, Coxsackievirus infection, pregnancy, and cancer, as well as after deep x-ray therapy, and as an allergic reaction to foods.

The *erythema perstans* group or figurate erythemas of diseases includes over a dozen clinical entities with impossible-to-remember names. (See Dictionary–Index under *erythema perstans*.) All have various sized erythematous patches, papules, or plaques with a definite red border and a less active center, forming circles, half circles, groups of circles, and linear bands. Multiple causes have been ascribed, including tick bites; allergic reactions; fungal, bacterial, viral, and spirochetal infections; and internal cancer. The duration of and the response to therapy varies with each individual case.

Erythema chronicum migrans is the distinctive cutaneous eruption of the multisystem tick-borne spirochetosis Lyme disease. The deer tick, *Ixodes dammini*, is the vector for the spirochete.

Early therapy with doxycycline or ampicillin may prevent late manifestations of the disease (see Chap. 16).

Reiter's syndrome is a triad of conjunctivitis, urethritis, and, most important, arthritis, that occurs predominantly in males and lasts about 6 months. The skin manifestations consist of psoriasiform dermatitis that is called balanitis circinata on the penis and keratoderma blenorrhagica on the palms and soles.

Behçet's syndrome consists of a triad of genital, oral, and ophthalmic ulcerations seen most commonly in males; it can last for years, with recurrences. Other manifestations include cutaneous pustular vasculitis, synovitis, and meningoencephalitis. It is more prevalent in eastern Mediterranean countries and Japan.

Differential Diagnosis

Urticaria: Clinically, urticaria may resemble erythema multiforme, but hives are associated with only mild systemic symptoms; it can occur in any age group; iris lesions are unusual; usually, it can be attributed to penicillin or other drug therapy; and it responds rapidly but often not completely to antihistamine therapy (see first part of this chapter). It is evanescent and dissipates or moves to a new area in less than 24 hours.

Treatment

A 12-year-old boy presents with bull's eye-like lesions on his hands, arms, and feet; erosions of the lips and mucous membranes of the mouth; malaise; and a temperature of 101° F (38.3° C) orally. He had a similar eruption last spring.

1. Order bed rest and increased oral fluid intake.
2. Acetaminophen (Tylenol), 325 mg OTC
   Sig: Take 1 to 2 tablets q.i.d, *or*
   Prednisone, 10 mg   #16
   Sig: Take 2 tablets stat and then 2 tablets every morning for 7 days.
3. For severe cases, such as the Stevens-Johnson form, hospitalization is indicated, where intravenous corticosteroid therapy (debatable), intravenous infusions, immune globulin, and other supportive measures can be administered.

ERYTHEMA NODOSUM
(Fig. 12-3)

Erythema nodosum is an uncommon reaction pattern seen mainly on the anterior tibial areas of the legs. It appears as erythematous nodules in successive crops and is preceded by fever, malaise, and arthralgia.

PRIMARY LESIONS. Bilateral red, tender, rather well-circumscribed nodules are seen mainly on the pretibial surface of the legs but also on the arms and the body. Later, the flat lesions may become raised, confluent, and purpuric. Only a few lesions develop at one time.

SECONDARY LESIONS. The lesions never suppurate or form ulcers.

COURSE. The lesions last several weeks, but the duration can be affected by therapy directed to the cause, if it is known. Relapses are related to the cause. It can be idiopathic and have a chronic course.

CAUSES. Careful clinical and laboratory examination is necessary to determine the cause of this toxic reaction pattern. The following tests should be performed: complete blood cell count, erythrocyte sedimentation rate, urinalysis, serologic test for syphilis, chest roentgenogram, and specific skin tests, as indicated. The causes of erythema nodosum are streptococcal infection (rheumatic fever, pharyngitis, scarlet fever, arthritis), fungal infection (coccidioidomycosis, trichophyton infection), pregnancy, sarcoidosis, lymphogranuloma venereum, syphilis, chancroid, drugs (contraceptive pills, sulfonamides, iodides, bromides), and, rarely, tuberculosis.

AGE AND SEX INCIDENCE. The disorder occurs predominantly in adolescent girls and young women.

LABORATORY FINDINGS. Histopathologic examination reveals a nonspecific but characteristically localized inflammatory infiltrate in the subcutaneous tissue and in and around the veins.

Differential Diagnosis

Erythema induratum: Chronic vasculitis of young women that occurs on the posterior calf area and often suppurates; biopsy shows a tuberculoid-type infiltrate, usually with caseation. A tuberculous causation has been suggested, again.

Necrobiosis lipoidica diabeticorum: An uncommon cutaneous manifestation of diabetes mellitus, characterized by well-defined patches of reddish-yellow atrophic skin, primarily on anterior areas of legs; the lesions can ulcerate; biopsy results are characteristic, but biopsy is usually not necessary or indicated because of the possibility of poor healing (see Chap. 26).

Periarteritis nodosa: A rare, usually fatal arteritis that most often occurs in males; 25% of patients show painful subcutaneous nodules and purpura, mainly of the lower extremities. There is a cutaneous variety.

Nodular vasculitis: Chronic, painful nodules of the calves of middle-aged women, which rarely ulcerate and recur commonly; biopsy is of value; this disorder may be a chronic variant of erythema nodosum.

Superficial thrombophlebitis migrans of Buerger's disease: An early venous change of Buerger's disease commonly seen in male patients, with painful nodules of the anterior tibial area; biopsy is of value.

Nodular panniculitis or Weber-Christian disease: Occurs mainly in obese middle-aged women; tender, indurated, subcutaneous nodules and plaques are seen, usually on the thighs and the buttocks; each crop is preceded by fever and malaise; residual atrophy and hyperpigmentation occur.

Leukocytoclastic vasculitis: Includes a constellation of diseases, such as allergic angiitis, allergic vasculitis, necrotizing vasculitis, and

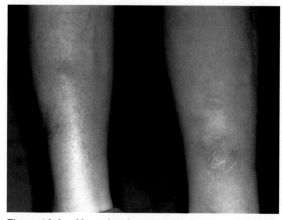

Figure 12-3.   Vascular dermatoses. Erythema nodosum on legs. *(Dermik Laboratories, Inc.)*

cutaneous systemic vasculitis. Clinically, palpable purpuric lesions are seen, most commonly on the lower part of the legs. In later stages, the lesions may become nodular, bullous, infarctive, and ulcerative. Various etiologic agents have been implicated, such as infection, drugs, and foreign proteins. Treatment includes bed rest, pentoxifylline (Trental), and corticosteroids (see Chap. 10).

For completeness, the following five very rare syndromes with *inflammatory nodules of the legs* are defined in the Dictionary–Index: (1) subcutaneous fat necrosis with pancreatic disease, (2) migratory panniculitis, (3) allergic granulomatosis, (4) necrobiotic granulomatosis, and (5) embolic nodules from several sources.

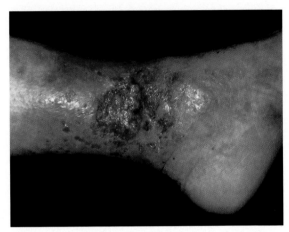

Figure 12-4. Vascular dermatosis. Stasis dermatitis. *(Dermik Laboratories, Inc.)*

Treatment

1. Treat the cause, if possible.
2. Rest, local heat, and aspirin are valuable. The eruption is self-limited if the cause can be eliminated.
3. Chronic cases can be disabling enough to warrant a short course of corticosteroid therapy. Some cases have benefited from naproxen (Naprosyn), 250 mg b.i.d. (or other nonsteroidal antiinflammatory drugs), for 2 to 4 weeks.

STASIS (VENOUS) DERMATITIS AND ULCERS
(Fig. 12-4; see also Fig. 34-12)

Stasis dermatitis is a common condition due to impaired venous circulation in the legs of older patients. Almost all cases are associated with varicose veins, and because the tendency to develop varicosities is a familial characteristic, stasis dermatitis is also familial. The medial malleolus area of the ankle is the most common location. Stasis ulcers can develop in the impaired skin.

PRIMARY LESIONS. Early cases of stasis dermatitis begin as a red, scaly, pruritic patch that rapidly becomes vesicular and crusted, owing to scratching and subsequent secondary infection. The bacterial infection may be responsible for the spread of the patch and the chronicity of the eruption. Edema of the affected ankle area results in a further decrease in circulation and, conse-

quently, more infection. The lesions may be unilateral or bilateral.

SECONDARY LESIONS. Three secondary conditions can arise from untreated stasis dermatitis:

Hyperpigmentation: This is inevitable following the healing of either simple or severe stasis dermatitis of the legs. This reddish-brown increase in pigmentation is slow to disappear, and in many elderly patients it never does.
Stasis ulcers: These can occur as the result of edema, trauma, deeper bacterial infection, or improper care of the primary dermatitis.
Infectious eczematoid dermatitis: This can develop on the legs, the arms, and even the entire body, either slowly, or as an explosive, rapidly spreading autoeczematous or "id" eruption (see Chap. 15).

COURSE. The rapidity of healing of stasis dermatitis depends on the age of the patient and on other factors listed under Causes. In elderly patients who have untreated varicose veins, stasis dermatitis can persist for years with remissions and exacerbations. If stasis dermatitis develops in a patient in the 40- to 50-year-old age group, the prognosis is particularly bad for future recurrences and possible ulcers. Once stasis ulcers develop, they can rapidly expand in size and depth. Healing of the ulcer, if possible for a given patient, depends on many factors.

CAUSES. Poor venous circulation due to the sluggish blood flow in tortuous, dilated varicose veins is the primary cause. If the factors of obe-

STASIS (VENOUS) DERMATITIS AND ULCERS **111**

sity, lack of proper rest or care of the legs, pruritus, secondary infection, low-protein diet, and old age are added to the circulation problem, the result can be a chronic, disabling disease.

Differential Diagnosis

Contact dermatitis: History is important, especially regarding nylon hose, new socks, contact with ragweed, high-top shoes, and so on; no venous insufficiency is noted (see Chap. 9).

Lichen simplex chronicus: Thickened, dry, pruritic patch; no venous insufficiency is found (see Chap. 11).

Atrophie blanche: Characterized by small ulcers that heal with irregular white scars; seen mainly over the ankles and legs. Telangiectasis and hyperpigmentation surround the scars. This arterial vasculitis can respond to pentoxifylline (Trental).

Differential diagnosis for stasis ulcers includes *pyodermic ulcers*, *arterial ulcers* (such as mal perforans of diabetes), *necrobiosis lipoidica* ulcers, *pyoderma gangrenosum malignancies*, and ulcers from hematologic and other internal problems. Blood tests, cultures, and biopsies help to establish the type of ulcer.

Treatment of Stasis Dermatitis

A 55-year-old laborer presents with scaly, reddish, slightly edematous, excoriated dermatitis on the medial aspect of the left ankle and leg of 6 weeks' duration.

1. Prescribe rest and elevation of the leg as much as possible by lying in bed. The foot of the bed should be elevated 4 inches by placing two bricks under the legs. Attempt to elevate the leg when sitting. Avoid prolonged standing or sitting with the legs bent. Taking time to walk on long train, car, or plane trips is a good idea.
2. Burow's solution wet packs
   Sig: Add 1 packet of powder to 1 quart of warm water. Apply cloths wet with this solution for 30 minutes, b.i.d.
3. An antibiotic and corticosteroid ointment mixture q.s. 30.0
   Sig: Apply to leg t.i.d.

For *more severe cases* of stasis dermatitis with oozing, cellulitis, and 3-pitting edema, the following treatment should be ordered, in addition:

1. Hospitalization or enforced bed rest at home for the purpose of (1) applying the wet packs for longer periods of time and (2) strict rest and elevation of the leg
2. A course of an oral antibiotic
3. Prednisone, 10 mg   #36
   Sig: Take 2 tablets b.i.d. for 4 days, then 2 tablets in the morning for 10 days
4. Ace elastic bandage, 4 inches wide, no. 8

After the patient is dismissed from the hospital and is ambulatory, give instructions for the correct application of this bandage to the leg before arising in the morning. This helps to reduce the edema that could cause a recrudescence of the dermatitis.

Treatment of Stasis Ulcer

As for any chronic difficult medical problem, there are many methods touted for successful management.

Consider a 75-year-old obese woman on a low income who has a 4-cm ulcer on her medial right ankle area with surrounding dermatitis, edema, and pigmentation.

1. Manage the primary problem or problems. Attempt to remedy the obesity, make sure there is adequate nutrition, and treat systemic or other causes of the ulcer.
2. Correct the physiologic alterations. Control the edema with adhesive flexible bandages of adequate width (4 inches wide usually) and with correct application from foot up to knee. A Jobst-type support stocking or pump may be indicated in resistant cases.
3. Treat contributing factors. Control the dermatitis, itching, and infection.
4. Promote healing. Occlusion of the ulcer has been proved to accelerate healing. Unna boots, adhesive flexible bandage dressings, and polyurethane-type films have been used with success. Enzymatic granules have their proponents as well as newer collagen granules.
5. Skin grafting may be indicated in deep, stubborn ulcers. Artificial skin substitutes such as Apligraft may be used.

Here is the technique we would use for this case. The diagnosis is stasis or venous ulcer.

1. Advise a multiple vitamin and mineral supplement tablet once a day, including zinc and magnesium.
2. Elevate leg as much as possible lying down prone.

3. Erythromycin, 250 mg #100
   Sig: Take 2 to 3 tablets a day until ulcer is healed.
   Comment: Infection is common.

4. Prednisone, 10 mg #60
   Sig: Take 1 tablet every morning.
   Actions: Antipruritic, antiinflammatory

5. Occlusive dressing. This is to be applied in the office. If there is a lot of drainage and debris, the frequency of dressing should be every 3 to 4 days at first, then weekly. Use a foot-rest stand for the leg. Keep a record on the size of the ulcer.
   a. Apply Bactroban ointment to a Telfa dressing.
   b. Place gauze squares in four layers over the Telfa dressing.
   c. Apply adhesive flexible bandage wrap over the gauze, down to the foot arch and up to below the knee. Do not apply too tightly at first.
   d. Wrap an adhesive flexible bandage, 4 inches wide, over the Coban.
   e. Leave the dressing on for 3 to 7 days, and then reapply.

   Another variant of occlusive dressing is as follows:
   a. Zeasorb powder on ulcer
   b. Mid-strength cortisone cream around the ulcer
   c. Zinc oxide wrap around the entire leg with a tighter wrap distally.
   d. Flexible adhesive bandage as a second wrap. Change every week, and keep dry.

No management of a venous stasis ulcer is 100% effective, but this routine with modifications is the one we use.

After the ulcer has healed, which will take many weeks, advise the patient to wear an elastic bandage or support hose *constantly* during the day, primarily as *protection* against injury of the damaged and scarred skin and to decrease recurrent edema.

PURPURIC DERMATOSES
(Fig. 12-5)

Purpuric lesions are caused by an extravasation of red blood cells into the skin or mucous membranes. The lesions can be distinguished from erythema and telangiectasia by the fact that purpuric lesions do not blanch under pressure applied by the finger or by diascopy.

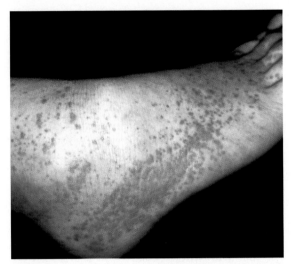

Figure 12-5. Vascular dermatoses Acute purpura, of unknown etiology, in 12-year-old boy. *(Dermik Laboratories, Inc.)*

Petechiae are small, superficial purpuric lesions. *Ecchymoses*, or bruises, are more extensive, round or irregularly shaped purpuric lesions. *Hematomas* are large, deep, fluctuant, tumor-like hemorrhages into the skin.

The purpuras can be divided into the *thrombocytopenic* forms and the *nonthrombocytopenic* forms.

Thrombocytopenic purpura may be idiopathic or secondary to various chronic diseases or to a drug sensitivity. The platelet count is below normal, the bleeding time is prolonged, and the clotting time is normal, but the clot does not retract normally. This form of purpura is rare.

Nonthrombocytopenic purpura is more commonly seen. *Henoch-Schönlein purpura* is a form of nonthrombocytopenic purpura most commonly seen in children that is characterized by recurrent attacks of purpura accompanied by arthritis, hematuria, IgA glomerulonephritis, and gastrointestinal disorders.

The ecchymoses, or *senile purpura*, seen in elderly patients after minor injury are very common. Ecchymoses are also seen in patients who have been on long-term systemic corticosteroid therapy and also occur after prolonged use of the high-potency corticosteroids *locally* and from corticosteroid nasal inhalers.

Another common purpuric eruption is that known as *stasis purpura*. These lesions are associated with vascular insufficiency of the legs and occur as the early sign of this change, or they are seen around areas of stasis dermatitis or stasis ulcers.

Frequently seen is a petechial *drug eruption* due to the chlorothiazide diuretics.

Pigmented Purpuric Eruptions

A less common group of cases are those seen in middle-aged adults, classified under the name *pigmented purpuric eruptions*. Some cases of pigmented purpuric eruptions itch severely. The cause is unknown; most cases have a positive tourniquet test, but other bleeding tests are normal. Clinically, these patients have grouped petechial lesions that begin on the legs and extend up to the thighs, and occasionally up to the waist and onto the arms.

Some clinicians are able to separate these pigmented purpuric eruptions into *purpura annularis telangiectodes (Majocchi's disease), progressive pigmentary dermatosis (Schamberg's disease)*, and *pigmented purpuric lichenoid dermatitis (Gougerot and Blum disease)*. Majocchi's disease commonly begins on the legs but slowly spreads, to become generalized. Telangiectatic capillaries become confluent and produce annular or serpiginous lesions. The capillaries break down, causing purpuric lesions. Schamberg's disease is a slowly progressive pigmentary condition of the lower part of the legs that fades after a period of months. The Gougerot-Blum form is accompanied by severe itching and eczematous changes; otherwise it resembles Schamberg's disease.

Treatment

For these pigmented purpuric eruptions, therapy may not be necessary. Occlusive dressing therapy with a corticosteroid cream can be beneficial.

For resistant cases, prednisone, 10 mg, 1 to 2 tablets in the morning for 3 to 6 weeks, is indicated.

Telangiectases

Telangiectases are abnormal dilated small blood vessels. Telangiectases are divided into *primary forms*, in which the causes are unknown, and *secondary forms*, which are related to some known disturbance.

The primary telangiectases include the simple and compound hemangiomas of infants, essential telangiectasias, and spider hemangiomas (see Chap. 32).

Diseases with numerous telangiectasias include cirrhosis of the liver, Osler-Weber-Rendu disease, lupus erythematosus, scleroderma, dermatomyositis and rosacea.

Secondary telangiectasia is very commonly seen on the fair-skinned person as a result of aging and chronic sun exposure. X-ray therapy and burns can also cause dilated vessels.

Treatment for the secondary telangiectasias can be accomplished quite adequately with very light electrosurgery to the vessels, which is usually tolerated without anesthesia or for many extensive lesions use of laser therapy. Injectable sclerosing agents are available for therapy on the lower legs.

BIBLIOGRAPHY

Centers for Disease Control. Henoch-Schönlein purpura: Connecticut. Arch Dermatol 1988;124:639.

Cooper KD. Urticaria and angioedema. J Am Acad Dermatol 1991;25:166.

Eaglstein WH. Experiences with biosynthetic dressings. J Am Acad Dermatol 1985;12:434.

Falanga V, Eaglstein WH. A therapeutic approach to venous ulcers. J Am Acad Dermatol 1986;14:777.

Ghersetich I, Panconesi E. The purpuras. Int J Dermatol 1994;33:1.

Henz BM, Zuberbier T, Monroe E. Urticaria: Clinical, diagnostic and therapeutic aspects. 1998.

Heymann WR. Acquired angioedema. J Am Acad Dermatol 1997;36:4.

Jacobson KW, Branch LB, Nelson HS. Laboratory tests in chronic urticaria. JAMA 1980;243:1644.

Jennette JC. Small-vessel vasculitis. N Engl J Med 1997;337:21.

Mangelsdorf HC, White WL, Jorizzo JL. Behcet's disease. J Am Acad Dermatol 1996;34:5.

Ollert MW, Thomas P, Korting HC, et al. Erythema induratum of Bazin. Arch Dermatol 1993;129:469.

Sabroe RA, Greaves MW. The pathogenesis of chronic idiopathic urticaria. Arch Dermatol 1997;133.

13

Seborrheic Dermatitis, Acne, and Rosacea

SEBORRHEIC DERMATITIS

(Figs. 13-1–13-3; see also Fig. 33-27)

Seborrheic dermatitis, in our opinion, is a synonym for dandruff. The former is the more severe manifestation of this dermatosis.

Seborrheic dermatitis is exceedingly common on the scalp but less common on the other areas of predilection: ears, face, sternal area, axillae, intergluteal area, and pubic area. It is well to consider seborrheic dermatitis as a *condition* of the skin and not as a *disease*. It occurs as part of the *acne seborrhea complex*, most commonly seen in brown-eyed brunettes who have a family history of these conditions. Dandruff is spoken of as oily or dry, but it is all basically oily. If dandruff scales are pressed between two pieces of tissue paper, an oily residue is expressed, leaving its mark on the tissue.

Certain misconceptions that have arisen concerning this common dermatosis need to be corrected. Seborrheic dermatitis cannot be cured, but remissions for varying amounts of time do occur naturally or as the result of treatment. Seborrheic dermatitis does not cause permanent hair loss or baldness unless it becomes grossly infected. Seborrheic dermatitis is not contagious. The cause is unknown, but an important etiologic factor is the yeast *Pityrosporum ovale*.

Seborrheic dermatitis in AIDS patients can be widespread and recalcitrant to therapy.

PRIMARY LESIONS. Redness and scaling appear in varying degrees. The scale is of the greasy type (see Fig. 13-1).

SECONDARY LESIONS. Rarely seen are excoriations from severe itching and secondary bacterial infection. Lichen simplex chronicus can follow a chronic itching and scratching habit.

COURSE. Exacerbations and remissions are common, depending on the season, treatment, and age and general health of the patient. Because this is a condition of the skin, and not a disease, a true cure is impossible.

SEASONAL INCIDENCE. This condition is worse in colder weather, presumably due to lack of summer sunlight.

AGE INCIDENCE. Seborrhea occurs in infants (called *cradle cap*) but usually disappears by age of 6 months. It may recur again at puberty.

Differential Diagnosis

SCALP LESIONS

Psoriasis: Sharply defined, silvery-white, dry, scaly patches; typical psoriasis lesions on elbows, knees, nails, or elsewhere (see Chap. 14)

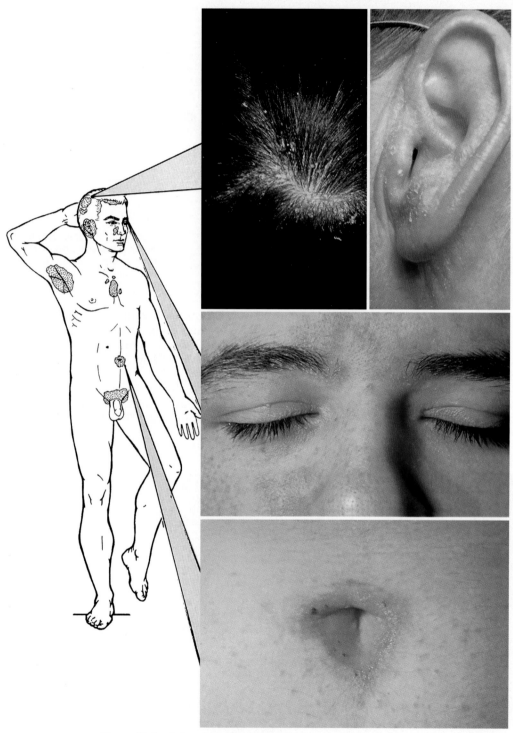

Figure 31-1. **Seborrheic dermatitis.** (*Owen Laboratories, Inc.*)

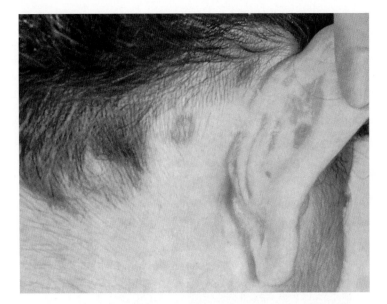

Figure 13-2. **Seborrheic dermatitis behind the ear and at the border of the scalp.** (*Smith Kline & French Laboratories*)

Lichen simplex chronicus: Usually a single patch on the posterior scalp area or around the ears; intense itching; excoriation; thickening of the skin (see Chap. 11)

Tinea capitis: Usually occurs in a child; broken-off hairs, with or without pustular reaction; some types fluoresce under Wood's light; positive culture (see Chap. 19)

Atopic eczema: Usually occurs in infants (where it spares diaper area) or children; diffuse dry scaliness; eczema also on face, arms, and legs (see Chap. 9)

FACE LESIONS

Systemic lupus erythematosus: Faint, reddish, slightly scaly, "butterfly" eruption, aggra-

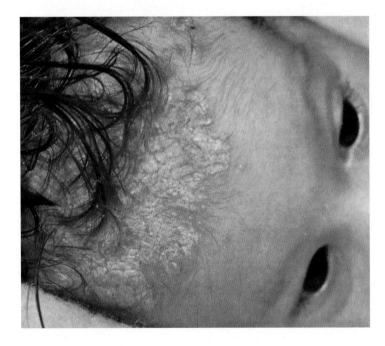

Figure 13-3. **Seborrheic dermatitis of infancy.** This is one of the causes of "cradle cap." (*Smith Kline & French Laboratories*)

vated by sunlight, with fever, malaise, and positive antinuclear antibody test (see Chap. 25)

Chronic discoid lupus erythematosus: Sharply defined, red, scaly, atrophic areas with large follicular openings with keratotic plugs, resistant to local therapy, often leaves scars (see Chap. 25)

BODY LESIONS

Tinea corporis (see Chap. 19)
Psoriasis (see Chap. 14)
Pityriasis rosea (see Chap. 14)
Tinea versicolor (see Chap. 14)

Treatment

A young man presents with recurrent red, scaly lesions at the border of the scalp and forehead and diffuse, mild, whitish scaling throughout the scalp

1. Management of cases of dandruff must include explaining the disease and stating that it is not contagious, that there is no true cure, that it will not cause baldness, and that there are seasonal variations. Therapy can be very effective, but only for keeping the dandruff under control.
2. With the above information in mind, tell the patient that shampooing offers the best management. There are several shampoos available, and the patient may have to experiment to find the one most suitable. The following types can be suggested:
   a. Selenium sulfide $2^1/_2$% suspension (Selsun, Head and Shoulders Intensive Treatment which is OTC)   120.0
   Sig: Shampoo as frequently as necessary to alleviate itching and scaling. Use no other soap. Refill prescription p.r.n.
   b. Additional shampoos:
      • Tar shampoos, such as Ionil T, Tarsum, Reme-T, Pentrax, X Seb T, and T-Gel
      • Zinc pyrithione shampoos, such as Zincon, Head & Shoulders, and DHS Zinc
      • Ketoconazole (Nizoral) shampoo (OTC) or FS shampoo (contains triamcinolone, by prescription)
   Sig: Shampoo as frequently as necessary to keep scaling and itching to a minimum.

3. Triamcinolone (Kenalog) spray, 63 mL
   Sig: Apply sparingly to scalp at night. Squirt the spray through a plastic tube that is supplied.
   Comment: A spray is less messy on the scalp than a corticosteroid solution, but solutions are available.
4. A low-potency corticosteroid cream 15.0
   Sig: Apply b.i.d. locally to body lesions.
5. Ketoconazole (Nizoral) 2% cream 15.0 (OTC)
   Sig: Apply b.i.d. on scalp or body lesions.
   Comment: This is a corticosteroid-sparing agent.

SAUER NOTES

1. Do not prescribe a fluorinated corticosteroid cream for long-term use on the face or in intertriginous areas.
2. Reiterate that there is no cure for seborrheic dermatitis; long-term management is necessary.
3. Reassure the patient that seborrheic dermatitis does not cause permanent hair loss.

ACNE
(Figs. 13-4–13-6)

Acne vulgaris is a common skin condition of adolescents and young adults. It is characterized by any combination of comedones (blackheads), pustules, cysts, and scarring of varying severity.

Severe cystic acne is called acne conglobata. When accompanied by systemic symptoms such as arthralgia, leukocytosis, and fever, the term acne fulminans can be used.

Hidradenitis suppurativa, also termed acne inversa, is a debilitating disease of deep undermining cysts and fistulas in the axillary, inguinal, and perirectal areas. Treatment is difficult and includes surgery, antibiotics, and isotretinoin (Accutane).

Dissecting cellulitis of the scalp (perifolliculitis capitis abscedens et suffodiens) is an inflammatory disease of the scalp with undermining cysts and fistulas of the scalp resulting in scarring alopecia. Treatment is difficult but an-

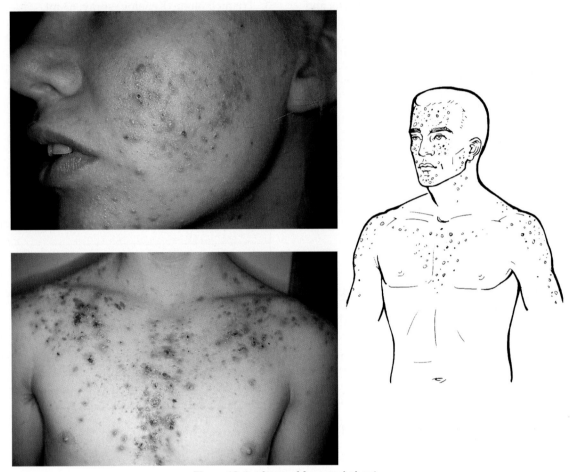

Figure 13-4. **Acne of face and chest.**

tibiotics, surgery, and intralesional corticosteroids may be helpful.

Acne conglobata, hidradenitis suppurativa, and dissecting cellulitis of the scalp have been referred to as the *follicular occlusion triad*. Pilonidal sinus is added by some authors to make this a tetrad.

PRIMARY LESIONS. Comedones, papules, pustules, and, in severe cases, cysts occur.

SECONDARY LESIONS. Pits and scars are evident in severe cases. Excoriations of the papules are seen in some adolescents, but most often they appear as part of the acne of women in their 20s and 30s, and when severe it is called acne excoriae des jeunes filles.

DISTRIBUTION. Acne occurs on the face and neck and, less commonly, on the back, chest, and arms.

COURSE. The condition begins at ages 9 to 12 years, or later, and lasts, with new outbreaks, for months or years. It subsides in most cases by the age of 18 or 19 years, but occasional flare-ups may occur for years. The residual scarring varies with severity of the case and response to treatment.

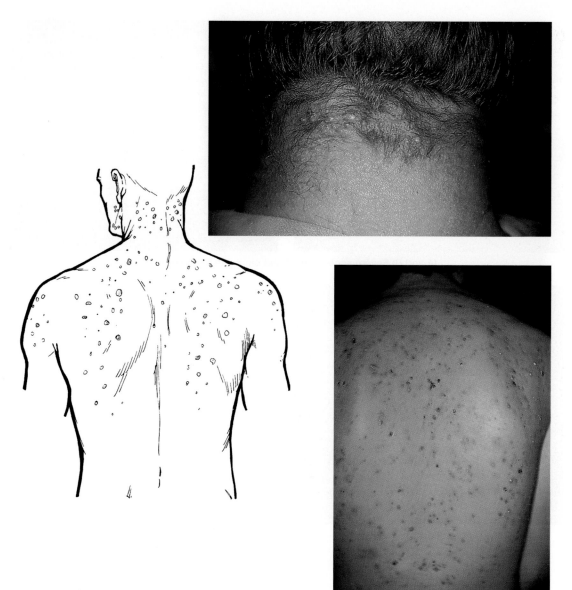

Figure 13-5. **Acne of neck and back.**

SUBJECTIVE COMPLAINT. Tenderness of the large pustules and itching may be reported (rarely). Emotional upset is common as a result of the unattractive appearance.

CAUSES. These factors are important: heredity, hormonal balance, diet, cleanliness, and general health.

In a case of severe adult acne, one should rule out an endocrine disorder. Hirsutism or abnormal menstrual periods in women are clues.

SEASON. Most cases are better during the summer.

CONTAGIOUSNESS. Acne is not contagious.

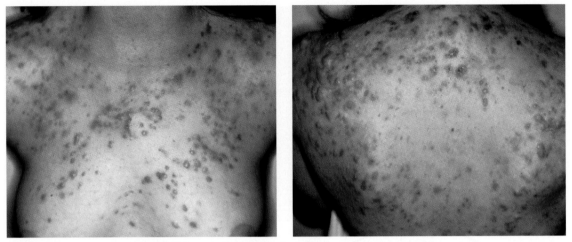

(*A* and *B*) Severe acne of chest and back of a 15-year-old girl.

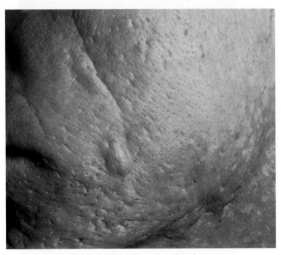

(*C*) Acne scars on cheek.

Figure 13-6. Severe acne vulgaris. (*Hoechst-Roussel Pharmaceuticals, Inc.*)

Differential Diagnosis

Drug eruption: Note history of ingestion of lithium, corticosteroids, iodides, bromides, trimethadione, or testosterone (including anabolic steroids used by athletes and body builders), and adrenocorticotropic hormone by injection (see Chap. 9).

Contact dermatitis from industrial oils (see Chap. 9)

Perioral dermatitis (see Fig. 13-7): Red papules, small pustules, and some scaling on chin, upper lip, and nasolabial fold. The cause is unknown, but formaldehyde in Kleenex-type tissues, toothpastes, and new clothes may be a factor; acne and seborrhea may also be factors. *Corticosteroid creams, locally, eventually aggravate the eruption and usually should not be prescribed.* Tetracycline, orally, as for acne, is the therapy of choice. Metronidazole gel (MetroGel) is an alternative local therapy for children under 12 years of age. Some authors think this should be called periorificial dermatitis as it can occur around the eyes and in the diaper area often associated with topical corticosteroid abuse.

Adenoma sebaceum: Rare; associated with epilepsy and mental deficiency

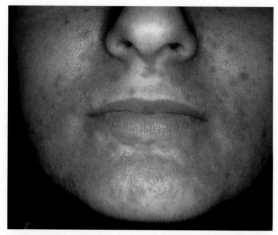

Figure 13-7. Perioral dermatitis. (*Hoechst-Roussel Pharmaceuticals, Inc.*)

Treatment

An 11-year-old patient presents with a moderate amount of facial blackheads and pustules.

FIRST VISIT

1. Give instructions regarding skin care (see sheet that can be given to patient, "What You Should Know About Acne"). Stress to the patient and the parent that not one factor but several factors (heredity, hormones, diet, stress, season of the year, greasy cosmetics, cleanliness, and general health) influence acne breakouts. Some of these factors cannot be altered.
2. Bar soap. The affected areas should be washed twice a day with a washcloth and a noncreamy soap, such as Dial, Neutrogena for Acne-Prone Skin, and Purpose.

3. Sulfur, ppt., 6%
   Resorcinol, 4%
   Colored alcoholic shake lotion (see Formulary in Chap. 5) q.s.   60.0
   Sig: Apply locally at bedtime with fingers.
   Comment: Proprietary products for the above lotion include Sulfacet-R, Novacet lotion, Klaron lotion, and Seba-Nil liquid and cleanser.
4. Benzoyl peroxide preparations:
   Benzoyl peroxide gel (5% or 10%) as in Benzagel, Desquam-X, Benzac-W, Panoxyl, Persa-Gel, Brevoxyl, and others. Some of these are also available as emollient gels. Benzamycin lotion is a combination of benzoyl peroxide and erythromycin.
   Sig: Apply locally once a day.
   Comment: Some dryness of skin is to be expected. Fabric can be bleached by the benzoyl peroxide.
5. Tretinoin (Retin A) gel (0.01% or 0.025%) or cream (0.025%, 0.05% or 0.1%): tretinoin (Retin A Micro), tretinoin (Avita)
   Sig: Apply locally once a day at night. Patient toleration varies considerably.
   Comment: Especially valuable for comedo acne.
6. Local antibiotic solutions, pledgets, and gels:
   Clindamycin 1% or erythromycin 2% lotion q.s.   30.0
   Sig: Apply locally once or twice a day.
7. Adapalene (Differin) 0.1% q.s. 15 gm
   Sig: Thin coat each night
   Comment: May be less irritating and more effective than Retin A.
8. Remove the blackheads with a comedone extractor (Fig. 13-8) in the office.

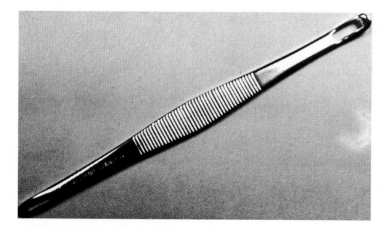

Figure 13-8. Comedone extractor. The most frequently used instrument in my office. Firm but gentle pressure with the smaller end over a comedone will force the comedone out of the sebaceous gland opening.

TREATMENT FOR A CASE OF SCARRING ACNE

1. Tetracycline, or similar antibiotic, 250 mg #100
Sig: Take 1 capsule q.i.d. for 3 days, then 1 capsule b.i.d. This dose can be continued for weeks, months, or years, or the dose can be lowered to 1 capsule a day for maintenance, depending, of course, on the extent of the involvement. Severe cases respond to 3 to 6 capsules a day.

    Tetracycline should be taken 30 minutes before meals or 2 hours after a meal, and not concurrently with iron or calcium for optimal absorption.
Comment: Other effective antibiotics include erythromycin, 250 mg b.i.d. or t.i.d., minocycline, 100 mg/day, and doxycycline (Monodox) 100 mg b.i.d. Retin A Micro (tretinoin), Avita (tretinoin) and Differin (adapalene) may be substituted as less irritating.

2. Other treatments:
    a. Vitamin A (water-soluble synthetic A), 50,000 U #100

Sig: Take 1 capsule b.i.d. for 5 months, then off 2 months to prevent liver toxicity.

    b. Abrasive cleansers are somewhat effective in removing comedones but if too irritating may actually aggravate acne.

    c. Large papules or early cysts. Intralesional corticosteroid can be injected with care. Dilute Kenalog suspension (4 mg/mL) with equal part of saline, and inject about 0.1 mL into the lesion. Atrophy can result if too large a quantity is injected.

    d. Incision of fluctuant acne cysts. *Never* incise these widely, but if you believe the pus must be drained, do it through a very small incision.

    e. Short-term prednisone systemic therapy is effective for severe cystic acne, especially for *acne fulminans*, an acute, disabling form of acne.

    f. Isotretinoin (Accutane). For severe, scarring, cystic acne this therapy has proved very beneficial. The usual dosage is 1 mg/kg/day given for 4 to 5 months. There are many minor and major side effects with this therapy (notably *teratogenic effects on pregnant women*), so isotretinoin should *only* be prescribed by those knowledgeable in its use.

3. The residual scarring of severe acne (see Fig. 13-6) can be lessened by surgical dermabrasion, using a rapidly rotating wire brush or diamond fraise or laser resurfacing. Microdermabrasion is a newer alternative. These procedures are being done by many dermatologists and plastic surgeons.

ROSACEA
(Fig. 13-9)

A common pustular eruption with flushing and telangiectasias of the butterfly area of the face may occur in adults in the 40- to 60-year-old age group.

PRIMARY LESIONS. Diffuse redness, papules, pustules, and, later, dilated venules, mainly of the nose, the cheeks, and the forehead, are seen.

SECONDARY LESIONS. Severe, longstanding cases eventuate in the bulbous, greasy, hypertrophic nose characteristic of *rhinophyma*.

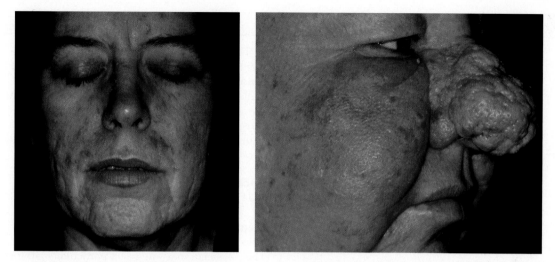

(*A*) Rosacea of a 47-year-old woman.   (*B*) Rosacea, chronic, with rhinophyma.

Figure 13-9. **Rosacea.** (*Hoechst-Roussel Pharmaceuticals, Inc.*)

COURSE. The pustules are recurrent and difficult to heal. Rosacea keratitis of the eye may occur.

CAUSES. Several factors influence the disease: (1) hereditary factor of oily skin; (2) excess ingestion of alcoholic beverages, hot drinks, and spicy foods; (3) *Demodex* mites have been implicated as causative for some cases of rosacea. Excess sun exposure and emotional stress can aggravate some cases of rosacea.

Differential Diagnosis

Systemic lupus erythematosus: No papules or pustules; positive ANA blood test (see Chap. 25)

Boils: Usually only one large lesion; can be recurrent but may occur sporadically; an early case of rosacea may look like small boils (see Chap. 15).

Iodide or bromide drug eruption: Clinically similar, but drug eruption usually is more widespread; history positive for drug (see Chap. 9)

Seborrheic dermatitis: Pustules uncommon; red and scaly; also in scalp (see earlier)

Rosacea-like tuberculid of Lewandowsky: rare; biopsy helpful

Treatment

A 44-year-old man presents with redness and pustules on the butterfly area of the face.

1. Prescribe avoidance of these foods: chocolate, nuts, cheese, cola drinks, iodized salt, seafood, alcohol, spices, and very hot drinks.
2. Metronidazole gel (MetroGel, Metrocream or Noritate cream)
   Sig: Apply thin coat b.i.d. Response to therapy is slow, taking 4 to 6 weeks to benefit.
3. Sulfur, ppt.   6%
   Resorcinol   4%
   Colored alcoholic shake lotion q.s.   60.0
   Sig: Apply to face h.s.
   Similar proprietary lotions are Sulfacet-R lotion and Novacet lotion.
4. Tetracycline, 250-mg capsules
   Sig: Take 1 capsule q.i.d. for 3 days, then 1 capsule b.i.d. for weeks, as necessary for benefit.
5. Therapy for *Helicobacter pylori* in the same treatment regimen as for peptic ulcer disease has been tried with some benefit in severe cases.

WHAT YOU SHOULD KNOW ABOUT ACNE*

Acne is a disorder in which the oil glands of the skin are overactive and the duct of the oil gland is unable to drain the extra oil. It usually involves the face and frequently the chest and the back, since these areas are the richest in oil glands. When an oil gland opening becomes plugged, a blackhead is formed and irritates the skin in exactly the same way as any other foreign body, such as a sliver of wood. This irritation takes the form of red pimples or deep painful cysts. This inflammation may destroy tissues and, when healed, may result in permanent scars.

The tendency to develop acne runs in families, especially those in which one or both parents have oily skin. Acne is aggravated by certain foods, improper care of the skin, lack of adequate sleep, and nervous tension. In girls, acne is usually worse before a menstrual period. Even in boys, acne flares on a cyclic basis. Any or all of these factors can exaggerate the tendency of the oily skin to develop acne. Therefore, the prevention of acne depends on correcting not one but several of these factors.

Because acne is so common, is not contagious, and does not cause loss of time from school or work, many people tend to ignore it or regard it as a necessary part of growing up. Actually, the old statement, "You'll be all right when you're married," has little or no significance. Marriage itself has no relation to acne, except that ordinarily by the time a person is ready to get married, he or she is past the acne age and the acne would have cleared anyway.

REASONS FOR TREATING ACNE

There are at least two very important reasons for seeking medical care for acne. The first is to prevent the scarring mentioned previously. Once scarring has occurred, it is permanent. Then a patient must go through the rest of life being embarrassed and annoyed by the scars, even though active pimples are no longer present. This scarring may vary from tiny little pits, which are frequently mistaken for enlarged pores, to deep, large, disfiguring pockmarks.

*This information is from an instruction sheet that I give to my acne patients. I am well aware of differences of opinion regarding the role of diet in acne, but I am presenting my belief. (G.C.S.)

The second reason for starting active treatment for acne, even without scarring, is that the condition may become the source of much psychological disturbance to a patient. Even though the acne may appear to others to be mild and inconspicuous, it may seem very noticeable to the patient and lead to embarrassment, worry, and nervousness.

TREATMENT MEASURES TO BE CARRIED OUT BY THE PATIENT

Cleaning Measures. Your face is to be washed twice a day with soap. Do not scrub too roughly. The physician may suggest a particular soap for use. Do not use any face cream, cold cream, cleansing cream, nourishing cream, or any other kind of grease on the face. This includes the avoidance of so-called pancake-type makeup, which may contain oil, grease, or wax. Acne is caused by excessive oiliness. You may think your face is dry because of the flakes on it, but these are actually flakes of dried oil or the greasy scaling of seborrhea. Later, when the treatment begins to take effect, your skin will actually become dry, even to the point where it is chapped and tender, especially around the mouth and the sides of the chin. When this point is reached, you will be advised as to suitable corrective measures for this temporary dryness. If the skin becomes red and uncomfortable between office visits, the applied remedy may be discontinued for one or two nights.

Girls may use face powder, dry rouge or blush (not cream rouge), lipstick, but no face creams. Boys with acne should shave as regularly as necessary and should not use oils, greases, pomades, or hair tonics, except those that may be prescribed by the physician. Hair should be dressed only with water.

Many cases of acne are associated with oily hair and dandruff and, for these cases, suitable local scalp applications and shampoos will be prescribed by the physician.

Plenty of rest is important. You should have at least 8 hours of sleep each night. Exercise is usually accompanied by increased activity of the oil glands and an acne flare. Wiping the skin off with a cool damp cloth and showering as soon as possible may be helpful. Moderate suntanning is beneficial for acne, but a sunburn does more harm than good and all sun exposure adds to the cumulative risk of skin cancer. When you get out in the sun, do not use oily or greasy suntan preparations.

Diet. In Gordon Sauer's opinion, certain foods aggravate the acne condition. This is controversial, but I think for completeness and for the patient who wants to try diet therapy, it is important to list the diet. It is advisable to avoid or limit the following foods.

Chocolate: This includes chocolate candy, chocolate ice cream, chocolate cake, chocolate-covered nuts, chocolate sodas, cocoa, and cola drinks. Hard candy (not chocolate) and soft drinks, other than the cola drinks, are all right in small or moderate amounts. You can drink the diet-type colas.

Nuts: Especially avoid peanuts, peanut butter, Brazil nuts, and coconuts. Almonds, walnuts, and pecans *can* be eaten in moderation.

Milk products: Avoid whole milk (homogenized) and 2% butterfat milk. You can drink up to two glasses of *skim* milk a day. Avoid sour cream, whipped cream, butter, margarine (allowed in moderation), rich creamy cheeses, ice cream, and sharp cheeses. Cottage and cheddar cheese are permitted. Sherbet can be eaten.

Fatty meats: Avoid meats such as lamb, pork, hamburgers, and tender steaks. Fish, chicken, and turkey *can* be eaten unless fried in coconut oil or animal fat. Mazola oil or other corn oils should be used in cooking. French fried potatoes should be avoided.

Spicy foods: Reduce as much as possible the use of spicy sauces, Worcestershire sauce, chili, catsup, spicy smoked meats, delicatessen products, and pizzas.

Following this diet does not mean that you should starve yourself. Eat plenty of lean meats, fresh and cooked vegetables, fruits (and their juices), and all breads. Drink plenty of water (4 to 6 glasses) daily.

MEDICAL TREATMENT OF ACNE

In addition to the prescribed treatment you apply yourself, there are several aspects of the treatment of acne that must be carried out by the physician or the nurse.

One important method of treatment is the proper removal of blackheads. *This is often part of the physician's job.* Pimples that have pus in them and are ready to open should be opened by the physician or the nurse. This is done with surgical instruments that are designed for the purpose and do not damage tissue or cause scars. Picking of pimples by the patient can cause scarring and should be avoided. When the blackheads are removed and the pustules opened in the physician's office, the skin heals faster and scarring is minimized.

Tetracycline or other antibiotics are frequently prescribed for the acne patient who is developing scars or pits. This antibiotic therapy may be continued by the physician for many months or even years. Occasionally, one develops an upset stomach, diarrhea, or a genital itch from an overgrowth of yeast organisms. Oral fluconazole (Diflucan) has made control of vaginal yeast infection much easier. If these problems develop, stop the medication and call the physician.

Here are other important comments about oral tetracycline therapy:

1. Tetracycline may make the skin more sensitive to sunlight. Therefore, if you go skiing or to a sunny climate it may be necessary to lower the dosage or stop the tetracycline 4 days before the trip.

2. If a woman is on birth control pills and also on tetracycline, there is the remote possibility that the birth control pills may be less effective. Additional birth control measures are indicated at possible times of conception.

3. Do not take tetracycline or similar antibiotic if you become pregnant because, after the fifth month of pregnancy, it can permanently discolor the teeth of the child.

4. The effectiveness of the tetracycline medication is decreased if iron or milk products are ingested at the same time as the tetracycline capsules. The best rule is for you to take tetracycline 30 minutes before meals or 2 hours after a meal.

5. Serious side effects from long-term therapy are almost nonexistent, but if there is any question concerning an illness and the taking of the antibiotic, call your physician. Do not continue taking an antibiotic unless you are under the continued care of your physician. Stop the antibiotic for acne while taking an antibiotic for another condition.

Other internal medications may be prescribed by the physician for acne, such as vitamin A.

For very severe cases of cystic scarring acne, isotretinoin (Accutane) can be prescribed, with suitable precautions. *Women of childbearing age should be aware of the fact that Accutane can cause birth defects if the woman is or becomes pregnant during therapy.*

Ultraviolet light treatments are also beneficial for some cases, but the danger of photodamage must be considered.

Do not take any other medicines internally while under acne therapy without informing your physician.

FOLLOW-UP CARE FOR YOUR COMPLEXION PROBLEMS

When active therapy for your complexion problem by the physician is terminated, this does not mean that you also stop the home care. The routine that was outlined for you on the first visit to the physician should be adhered to so that your complexion can continue to remain as clear as possible.

First, it is important that you continue using the soap that was prescribed for you.

Second, it is important that you continue to observe the diet. As the months go by and your skin matures, however, you will find that it is less important to watch your diet strictly.

Third, any local preparation that was prescribed should be continued for several months, or even years, if you continue to have complex-ion problems. These have been prescribed especially for you and probably are stronger than any other product that can be bought over the counter.

Fourth, there are certain times when *your complexion can flare up again.* This especially happens in the fall. If this happens, it is imperative that you begin active medical therapy with your physician as soon as possible to prevent any scarring of the skin.

If you follow the above measures, you should continue to have a good complexion so that after you have passed through this stage of complexion problems you will not have any scars on your face. It is only rarely that we have complexion-problem cases so difficult that nothing can be done to prevent or minimize the scarring tendency.

CONCLUSION

Do not become discouraged! Treatment is effective in at least 95% of all cases. It may be 4 to 6 weeks before noticeable improvement appears. There may be occasional mild flare-ups, but eventually your skin will improve and you and your friends will notice the difference.

It is very important for you and your parents to realize that your physician cannot shorten the length of time it takes for your oil glands to work normally. This maturing process of your skin can take several years, even into the 20s, 30s, or, for a few persons, (especially females) longer.

BIBLIOGRAPHY

Abramowicz M. Adapalene for acne. Med Lett 1997;39:995.

American Academy of Dermatology guidelines: Acne vulgaris. J Am Acad Dermatol 1990;22:676.

Bergfeld WF, Odom RB. New perspectives on acne. J Am Acad Dermatol 1995;32:5.

Layton AM, Cunliffe WJ. Guidelines for optimal use of isotretinoin in acne. J Am Acad Dermatol 1992;27:52.

Leyden JJ. Therapy for acne vulgaris. N Engl J Med 1997;336:16.

Reingold SB, Rosenfield RL. The relationship of mild hir-sutism or acne in women to androgens. Arch Dermatol 1987;123:209.

Rosenberg EW. Acne diet reconsidered. Arch Dermatol 1981;117:193.

Sauer GC. Safety of long-term tetracycline therapy for acne. Arch Dermatol 1976;112:1603.

Stratigos JD, Antoniou C, Katsambas A, et al. Ketoconazole 2% cream versus hydrocortisone 1% cream in the treatment of seborrheic dermatitis. J Am Acad Dermatol 1988;19:850.

Weiss JS. Current options for the topical treatment of acne vulgaris. Pediatr Dermatol 1997;14:6.

14

Papulosquamous Dermatoses

The papulosquamous dermatoses include several specific entities that predominantly affect the chest and the back with clinically similar macular, papular, and scaly lesions. The most common diseases in the group are psoriasis, pityriasis rosea, tinea versicolor, lichen planus, seborrheic dermatitis, secondary syphilis, and drug eruptions. The last three conditions are considered elsewhere in this book. To be complete with regard to the differential diagnoses of this group, the following rarer diseases can also be included: parapsoriasis and its variants, lichen nitidus, and pityriasis rubra pilaris.

PSORIASIS
(Figs. 14-1–14-4; see also Fig. 33-23)

Psoriasis is a common, chronically recurring, papulosquamous disease, characterized by various sized silvery-white, scaly patches seen most commonly on the elbows, the knees, and the scalp.

    Generalized pustular psoriasis (pustular psoriasis of von Zambusch) and generalized erythrodermic psoriasis can be life-threatening, usually related to overwhelming sepsis and rarely seen in association with adult respiratory distress syndrome. A form of pustular psoriasis localized to the palms and soles (pustular psoriasis of Barber, acropustulosis) can be a difficult therapeutic problem. The pustules are sterile in both conditions.

PRIMARY LESIONS. Erythematous, papulosquamous lesions vary in shape and size from drop size to large circinate areas, which can become generalized. The scale is usually thick and silvery and bleeds from minute points when it is removed by the fingernail (Auspitz's sign).

    Pustular psoriasis is a severe type of psoriasis involving the palms and soles (acropustulosis or pustular psoriasis of the palms and soles of Barber), or it can be generalized on the body (von Zumbusch variant).

SECONDARY LESIONS. Although unusual, excoriations, thickening (lichenification), and oozing can be found.

DISTRIBUTION. Psoriasis most commonly occurs on the scalp, the elbows, and the knees, but it can involve any area of the body, including the nails.

COURSE. Psoriasis is notoriously chronic and recurrent. However, cases have been known to clear and not recur.

    Human immunodeficiency virus-positive patients can have recalcitrant psoriasis.

CAUSES. The cause of psoriasis is unknown. About 30% of patients with psoriasis have a family history of the disease.

    An acute form of psoriasis, called *guttate psoriasis*, frequently develops after a streptococcal

127

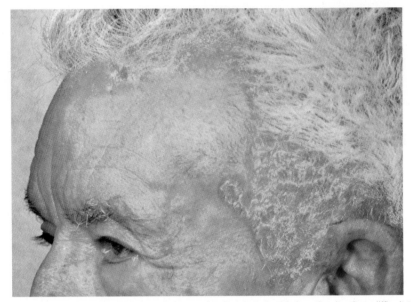

Figure 14-1. **Psoriasis of the border of the scalp.** Psoriasis in this location is often difficult to distinguish from seborrheic dermatitis. (*Smith Kline & French Laboratories*)

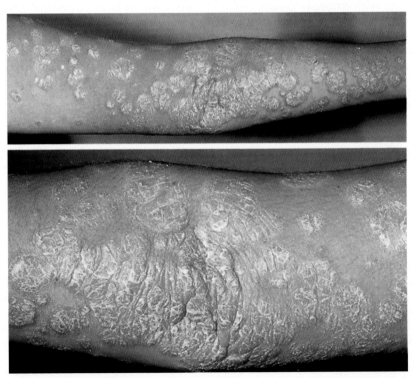

Figure 14-2. **Psoriasis on elbows of a 17-year-old girl.** Moderately extensive psoriasis in classic distribution on back and knees. (*K.U.M.C.; Roche Laboratories*) (continued)

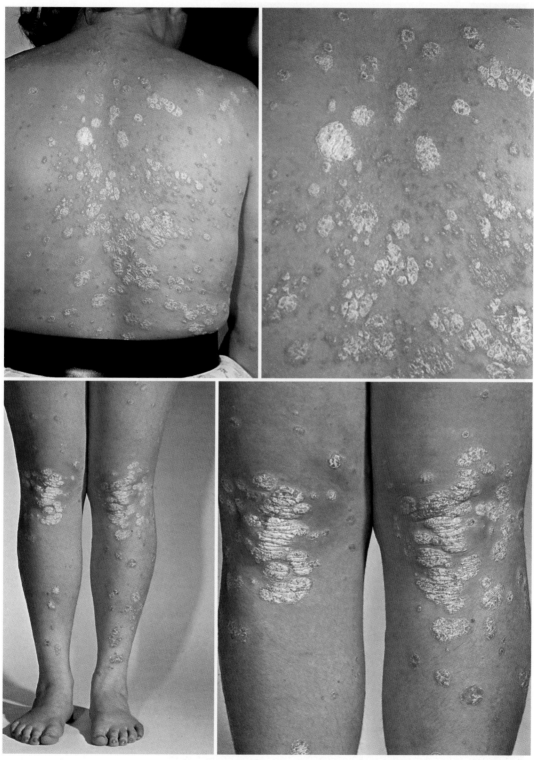

Figure 14-2. *(Continued)*

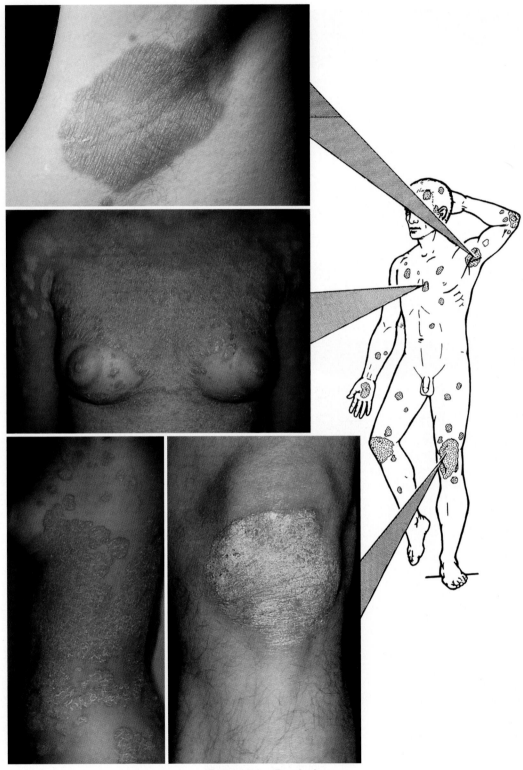

Figure 14-3. **Psoriasis.**

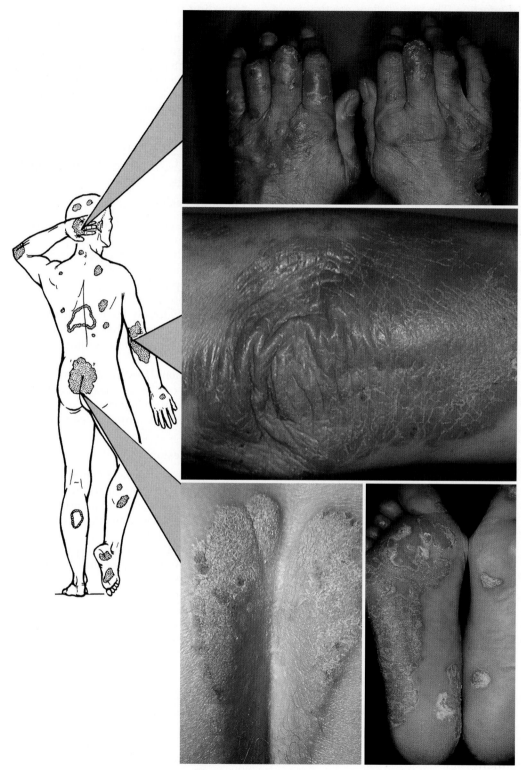

Figure 14-4. **Psoriasis.**

throat infection. The scaly lesions are the size of drops, hence guttate. This form of psoriasis is usually seen in children and young adults.

Medications such as Lithium, β-blockers, antimalarials, and possibly angiotensin-converting enzyme inhibitors can flare psoriasis. Discontinuance of alcohol and tobacco smoking (especially in pustular cases) may be beneficial.

SUBJECTIVE COMPLAINTS. Fortunately, only 30% of patients with psoriasis itch.

SEASON. Psoriasis is usually worse in winter, probably because of low indoor humidity and relative lack of sunlight.

AGE GROUP. The disease may affect a person of any age but is unusual in children.

CONTAGIOUSNESS. Psoriasis is not contagious.

RELATION TO EMPLOYMENT. Psoriatic lesions can develop or flare up in areas of skin injury (Koebner's phenomenon).

LABORATORY FINDINGS. Microscopic section is somewhat characteristic in typical cases.

Differential Diagnosis

Tinea corporis: Single lesion, usually round with healing in center; scraping and culture positive for fungi (see Chap. 19)
Seborrheic dermatitis: Lesions more greasy and occur in hairy areas; scalp lesions are often impossible to differentiate from psoriasis (see Chap. 13)
Pityriasis rosea: "Herald patch"; "Christmas tree" configuration; acute onset (see later in this chapter)
Atopic eczema: Patches on flexural surfaces; allergic history (see Chap. 9)
Secondary or tertiary syphilis: Can be psoriasiform; blood serology positive; local therapy of little value (see Chap. 16)
Lichen planus: Lesions violaceous; small papules; very little scaling (see later in this chapter)

A single lesion of psoriasis may resemble lichen simplex chronicus.

Psoriasis of nails (see Fig. 28-11) is similar in appearance to tinea of nails.

Treatment

It is most important in the management of patients with psoriasis that you be frank with them

regarding the prognosis and "cure." Reassure them that it is not contagious, that the disease disappears in rare cases, and that you can help them manage the disease. But be straightforward in saying that no physician at this moment knows a cure for psoriasis. It might help the patient (or it might not) for you to say that psoriasis should not be considered a disease but should be thought of as a hobby.

FIRST VISIT OF A PATIENT PRESENTING WITH RED SCALY LESIONS ON THE SCALP AND ELBOWS ONLY

For Body Lesions

1. Medium-potency fluorinated corticosteroid cream or ointment   30.0
   Sig: Apply q.s. to body lesions, *or*
2. Coal tar solution (LCD)   5%
   Sulfur, ppt.   5%
   White petrolatum q.s.   30.0
   Sig: Apply locally b.i.d. to body lesions.
        This treatment has the added value of being inexpensive and without corticosteroid side effects.
3. Calcipotriene (Dovonex) ointment 100, 30, or 15
   Sig: Thin coat on psoriasis b.i.d. It is expensive and may cause irritation. Combination with a corticosteroid ointment can decrease irritation.

For Scalp Lesions

1. Tar shampoo (see list in Formulary in Chap. 5).
2. FS shampoo (contains triamcinolone) 120.0
   Sig: Shampoo scalp frequently.
        Use without any other soap; also useful in relieving itching.
3. Triamcinolone (Kenalog) spray, 63 grams
   Sig: Apply to scalp at night with plastic tube applicator.
4. Derma-Smoothe FS with or without LCD, 5%, is effective when applied overnight under shower cap.
5. Calcipotriene (Dovonex Scalp Lotion) 0.0005% 60 ml
   Sig: Thin coat to scalp b.i.d.

SUBSEQUENT VISITS OF A PATIENT WITH LOCALIZED PSORIASIS

1. For body lesions, gradually increase the strength of the medicines in the previously listed salves.
2. Occlusive dressing with corticosteroid therapy. For localized areas of psoriasis, especially on the extremities, a low-potency fluorinated

corticosteroid cream can be applied at night and covered with an occlusive plastic dressing such as Saran Wrap. This wrapping should be left on overnight.

For greater therapeutic effectiveness, on subsequent visits, coal tar solution (3% to 6%) can be incorporated in the corticosteroid cream.

3. Intralesional corticosteroid therapy. For localized patches of psoriasis, parenteral triamcinolone can be injected under the lesions. This is an effective treatment for small lesions.
4. Anthralin U.S.P. (Drithocreme), 0.1%   60.0
Sig: Apply q.s. locally b.i.d. Avoid salve near the eyes.

There is also a technique of applying anthralin and removing it in 30 minutes, done once a day (short-contact therapy). The concentration of the anthralin can be increased cautiously, as necessary, up to 1%. Anthralin stains the skin and clothing and can irritate the skin.

5. Tazorac (Tazarotene Gel) 0.1% and 0.05%
Sig: Apply thin coat once a day. It is contraindicated in pregnancy and is expensive. Due to the irritation, it is often combined with a topical corticosteroid ointment.
6. Micanol (anthralin cream 1%)   50g
Sig: Thin coat 30 minutes before bathing. It has less staining and less irritations than other anthralin preparations.

FIRST VISIT OF A PATIENT WITH PSORIASIS ON 65% OR MORE OF THE BODY SURFACE.

1. Coal tar solution (LCD)   180.0
Sig: Add 2 tablespoons to the bathtub, with 6 to 8 inches of warm water. Soak for 15 minutes once a day. Soap may be used, unless there is much itching.

Later, the concentration can be slowly increased.

2. Mild body salve:
Coal tar solution (LCD)   3%
White petrolatum q.s.   120.0
Sig: Apply locally b.i.d.
3. Ultraviolet therapy (UVB), in increasing suberythema doses, once or twice a week can be used after a daily thin application of a tar salve, similar to the Goeckerman regimen.

The combination of oral psoralen and ultraviolet A therapy (PUVA) for extensive or persistent psoriasis is being used with definite benefit. This therapy requires special UVA light sources, equipment, timers, and trained personnel. Many precautions must be observed with PUVA therapy. There is an increased risk of skin cancer.

SAUER NOTES

MANAGEMENT OF PSORIASIS

1. Give written information to the patient on the diagnosis and whether it can be cured or not (there is no cure, but there is help available). Tell the patient that the cause of psoriasis is unknown, that it is cyclic and seasonal, and that it is aggravated by stress. Provide an outline of your proposed therapy.

2. I rarely prescribe a silver or plastic tube of *single* medication salve for psoriasis. My prescription is compounded with LCD, 3% to 10%, sulfur, ppt 3% to 10%, salicylic acid, 3% to 6%, singly or in combination, in a base of corticosteroid ointment, or in Unibase or white petrolatum. I am aware of the pros and cons of mixing locally applied salves, but this is what I do.

3. I begin with lower concentrations of any medication and increase or further modify the mixtures according to the patient's individual response.

4. There is evidence that β-blocking drugs, lithium, and antimalarials can aggravate psoriasis.

SUBSEQUENT VISITS OF A PATIENT WITH RATHER GENERALIZED PSORIASIS

1. Gradually increase the strength of the medicines in the above salves.
2. Methotrexate therapy. In cases of severe psoriasis, dermatologists occasionally use this oral or intramuscular injection method of therapy with good results. Because methotrexate is a potent and dangerous drug, those wishing to use it must consult recently published papers on the subject to become thoroughly familiar with the side effects.
3. Acitretin (Soriatane) therapy. For a severe case of psoriasis in a man (or in a woman not capable of conception), this therapy is effective, but there are many side effects. This drug has a

half-life of 50 hours and is not stored in adipose tissue. It has replaced etretinate (Tegison), which has a half-life of up to 6 months and is stored in adipose tissue. Ingestion of ethanol converts acitretin to etretinate. These drugs are teratogenic and have many other side effects. They are especially effective for pustular psoriasis.

4. Some other aggressive therapies are being used for severe cases of psoriasis. These include cyclosporine, mycophenolate mofetil, and Re-PUVA (combination retinoid and PUVA therapy).

PITYRIASIS ROSEA

(Figs. 14-5–14-7)

Pityriasis rosea is a moderately common papulosquamous eruption, mainly occurring on the trunk of young adults. It is mildly pruritic and occurs most often in the spring and fall.

PRIMARY LESIONS. Papulosquamous, oval erythematous discrete lesions are seen. A larger "herald patch" resembling a patch of "ringworm" may precede the general rash by 2 to 10 days. A collarette of fine scaling is seen around the edge of the lesions.

SECONDARY LESIONS. Excoriations are rare. The effects of overtreatment or contact dermatitis are commonly seen.

DISTRIBUTION. The lesions appear mainly on the chest and trunk along the lines of cleavage. Many cases have the oval lesions in a "Christmas tree branches" pattern over the back. In atypical cases, the lesions are seen in the axillae and the groin only. Face lesions are rare in Caucasian adults but are rather commonly seen in children and African-Americans.

COURSE. After the development of the "herald patch," new generalized lesions continue to appear for 2 to 3 weeks. The entire rash commonly disappears within 6 to 8 weeks. Recurrences are rare.

SUBJECTIVE COMPLAINTS. Itching varies from none to severe.

CAUSE. The cause is unknown.

SEASON. Spring and fall "epidemics" are common.

AGE GROUP. Young adults are most often affected.

CONTAGIOUSNESS. The disease is not contagious.

Differential Diagnosis

Tinea versicolor: Lesions tannish and irregularly shaped; fungi seen on scraping, fine dry adherent scale becomes apparent when the physician scratches the area with the fingernail.

Drug eruption: No "herald patch"; positive drug history for gold, bismuth, or sulfa (see Chap. 9).

Secondary syphilis: No itching (99% true); history or presence of genital lesions; positive blood serology (see Chap. 16).

Psoriasis: Also usually on elbows, knees, and scalp; lesions have silvery-white scale.

Seborrheic dermatitis: Greasy, irregular, scaly lesions on sternal and other hairy areas (see Chap. 13).

Lichen planus: Lesions more papular and violaceous; on mucous membranes of mouth and lip.

Parapsoriasis: Rare, chronic may have fine "cigarette paper" atrophy. Can develop into mycosis fungoides.

SAUER NOTE

If the pityriasis rosea-like rash does not itch, obtain blood serologic test for syphilis if you have any uncertainty about the diagnosis and especially if palm and sole lesions are present with adenopathy.

Treatment

FIRST VISIT

1. Reassure the patient that he or she does not have a "blood disease," that the eruption is not contagious, and that it would be rare to get it again.
2. Colloidal bath
   Sig: Use 1 packet of Aveeno oatmeal preparation to the tub containing 6 to 8 inches of lukewarm water. Bathe for 10 to 15 minutes every day or every other day.
   Comment: Avoid soap and hot water as much as possible to reduce any itching.
3. Nonalcoholic white shake lotion or Calamine lotion q.s.   120.0
   Sig: Apply b.i.d. locally to affected areas.

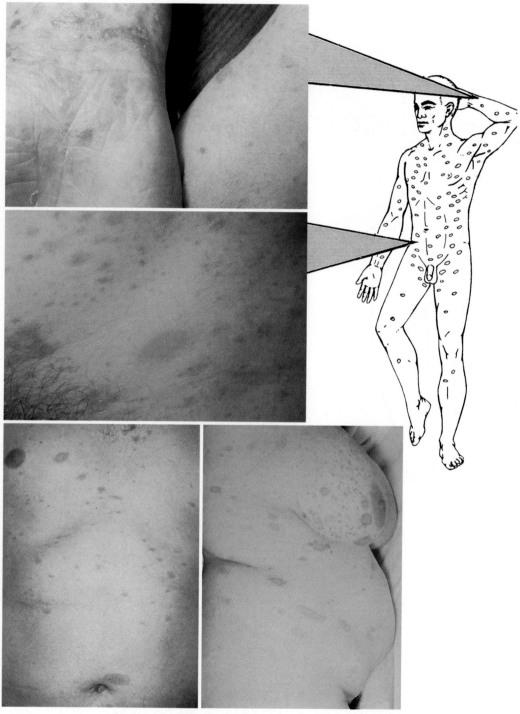

Figure 14-5.   **Pityriasis rosea.** (*Westwood Pharmaceuticals*)

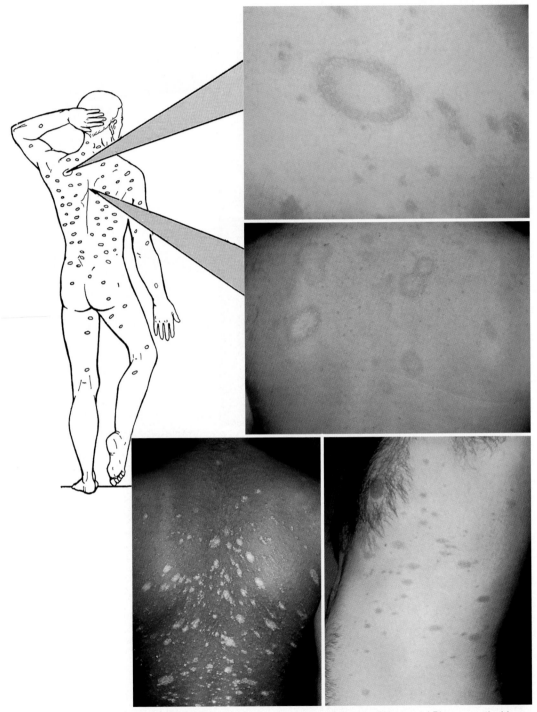

Figure 14-6.   **Pityriasis rosea.** Bottom left photograph is of a black man. (*Westwood Pharmaceuticals*)

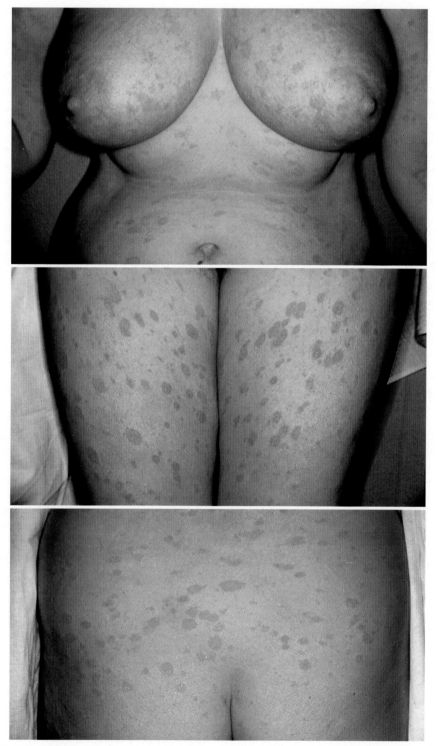

Figure 14-7.   **Pityriasis rosea of chest, thighs, and buttocks of one patient.** (*Syntex Laboratories, Inc.*)

4. If there is itching, prescribe an antihistamine drug, such as:

Cyproheptadine (Periactin), 4 mg   #60

Sig: Take 1 tablet a.c. and h.s.

5. UVB therapy in increasing suberythema doses once or twice a week may be given. The severity is decreased but itching and disease duration are probably not altered.

SUBSEQUENT VISITS

1. If the skin becomes too dry from the colloidal bath and the lotion, stop the lotion or alternate it with the following:

Hydrocortisone cream or ointment, 1% q.s.   60.0

Sig: Apply b.i.d. locally to dry areas.

2. Continue the ultraviolet treatments.

SEVERELY PRURITIC CASES

1. In addition to the above, add:

Prednisone, 5 mg   #40

Sig: Take 1 tablet q.i.d. for 3 days, then 1 tablet t.i.d. for 4 days, then 2 tablets every morning for 1 to 2 weeks, as symptom of itching demands.

TINEA VERSICOLOR
(Fig. 14-8)

Tinea versicolor is a moderately common skin eruption with characteristics of tannish-colored, irregularly shaped scaly patches causing no discomfort that are usually located on the upper chest and back. It is caused by a lipophilic yeast (see Chap. 19). Dry scaling can be revealed by stroking the skin with a fingernail (coup d'ongle).

PRIMARY LESIONS. Papulosquamous or maculosquamous, tan, and irregularly shaped lesions occur.

SECONDARY LESIONS. Relative depigmentation results because the involved skin does not tan when exposed to sunlight. This cosmetic defect, obvious in the summer, often brings the patient to the office.

DISTRIBUTION. The upper part of the chest and the back, neck, and arms are affected. Rarely are the lesions on the face or generalized.

COURSE. The eruption can persist for years unnoticed. Correct treatment is readily effective, but the tinea usually recurs.

CAUSE. The causative agent is a lipophilic yeast, *Pityrosporum orbiculare*, which has a hyphae form called *Pityrosporum* or *Malassezia furfur*.

CONTAGIOUSNESS. The disease is not contagious and is not related to poor hygiene.

LABORATORY FINDINGS. A scraping of the scale placed on a microscopic slide, covered with a 20% solution of potassium hydroxide and a coverslip, shows the hyphae. Under the low-power lens of the microscope, very thin, short, mycelial filaments are seen. Diagnostic grape-like clusters of spores are seen best with the high-power lens. The appearance of spores and hyphae is referred to as "spaghetti and meatballs." The dimorphic organism does not grow on routine culture media.

Differential Diagnosis

Pityriasis rosea: Acute onset; lesions oval with collarette of fine adherent dry scale (see earlier in this chapter)

Seborrheic dermatitis: Greasy scales in hairy areas, mainly (see Chap. 13)

Mild psoriasis: Thicker scaly lesions on trunk and elsewhere (see earlier in this chapter)

Vitiligo: Because tinea versicolor commonly manifests with depigmentation of the skin, many cases have been called vitiligo. This is indeed unfortunate because tinea versicolor is quite easy to treat and has a much better prognosis than vitiligo (see Chap. 24)

Secondary syphilis: Lesions are more widely distributed and present on palms and soles (see Chap. 16)

Treatment

Selenium (Selsun or Head and Shoulders Intensive Treatment) suspension   120.0

Sig: Bathe and dry completely. Then apply medicine as a lotion to all the involved areas, usually from neck down to pubic area. Let it dry. Bathe again in 24 hours and wash off the medicine. Repeat procedure again at weekly intervals for four treatments.

Comment: Recurrences are rather common and can be easily retreated. May be irritating.

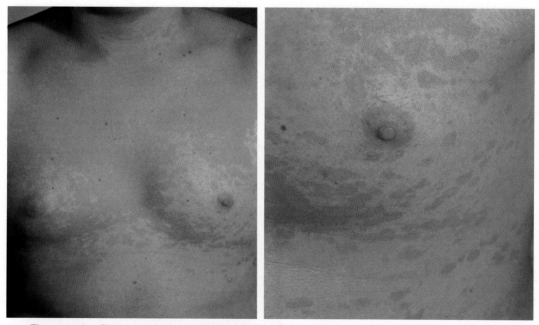

Figure 14-8.   Tinea versicolor on the chest. The dark areas of the skin are infected with the fungus. (*K.U.M.C.; Sandoz Pharmaceuticals*)

SAUER NOTES

1. It is important to tell the patient that depigmented spots may remain after the tinea versicolor is cured. These can be tanned by gradual exposure to sunlight or ultraviolet light.

2. A topical imidazole cream (clotrimazole, econazole, ketoconazole, miconazole) twice a day topically for 2 weeks with or without a sulfur soap can be used. Terbinafine spray (Lamisil) twice a day for 1 week.

3. Ketoconazole (Nizoral) orally in various short term regimens and itraconazole (Sporanox) 200 mg orally for 1 week have been used.

LICHEN PLANUS

(Figs. 14-9–14-12; see also Fig. 3-1B)

Lichen planus is an uncommon, chronic, pruritic disease characterized by violaceous flat-topped papules that are usually seen on the wrists and the legs. Mucous membrane lesions on the cheeks or lips are whitish.

PRIMARY LESIONS. Flat-topped, violaceous papules and papulosquamous lesions appear. On close examination of a papule, preferably after the lesion has been wet with an alcohol swipe, intersecting small white lines or papules (Wickham's striae) can be seen. These confirm the diagnosis. Uncommonly, the lesions may assume a ring-shaped configuration or may be hypertrophic, atrophic, or bullous. On the mucous membranes, the lesions appear as a whitish, lacy network.

SECONDARY LESIONS. Excoriations and, on the legs, thick, scaly, lichenified patches have been noted.

DISTRIBUTION. Most commonly the lesions appear on the flexural aspects of the wrists and the ankles, the penis, and the oral mucous membranes, but they can be anywhere on the body or become generalized.

COURSE. The outbreak is rather sudden, with the chronic course averaging 9 months' duration. Some cases last several years. There is no effect on the general health except for itching. Recurrences are moderately common.

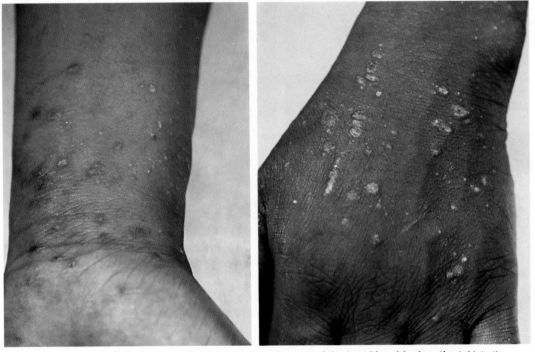

Figure 14-9. Lichen planus on the wrist and the dorsum of the hand in a black patient. Note the violaceous color of the papules and the linear Koebner phenomenon on the dorsum of the hand. (*E.R. Squibb*)

CAUSE. The cause is unknown. The disorder is rather frequently associated with nervous or emotional upsets. It may represent an autoimmune process, and some cases have a distinct pattern on direct immunofluorescence. Hepatitis C or hepatitis B is present in some cases (possibly up to 10%).

SUBJECTIVE COMPLAINTS. Itching varies from mild to severe.

CONTAGIOUSNESS. Lichen planus is not contagious.

RELATION TO EMPLOYMENT. As in psoriasis, the lichen planus lesions can develop in scratches or skin injuries (Koebner phenomenon).

LABORATORY FINDINGS. Microscopic section is quite characteristic.

Differential Diagnosis

Secondary syphilis: No itching; blood serology positive (see Chap. 16)
Drug eruption: History of taking atabrine, arsenic, or gold (see Chap. 9)

Psoriasis: Lesions more scaly, whitish on knees and elbows (see earlier in this chapter)
Pityriasis rosea: "Herald patch" mainly on trunk (see earlier in this chapter)

Lichen planus on leg may resemble *neurodermatitis* (usually one patch only; intensely pruritic; no mucous membrane lesions; see Chap. 11) or keloids (secondary to injury with no Wickham's striae).

Treatment

A patient presents with generalized papular eruption and moderate itching.

FIRST VISIT

1. Assure the patient that the disease is not contagious, is not a blood disease, and is chronic but not serious.
2. Avoid excess bathing with soap.
3. Low-potency corticosteroid cream   60.0
   Sig: Apply locally b.i.d.
4. Over-the-counter antihistamine such as chlorpheniramine, 4 mg   **#**60
   Sig: Take 1 tablet b.i.d. for itching.
   Comment: Warn the patient of drowsiness at onset of therapy.

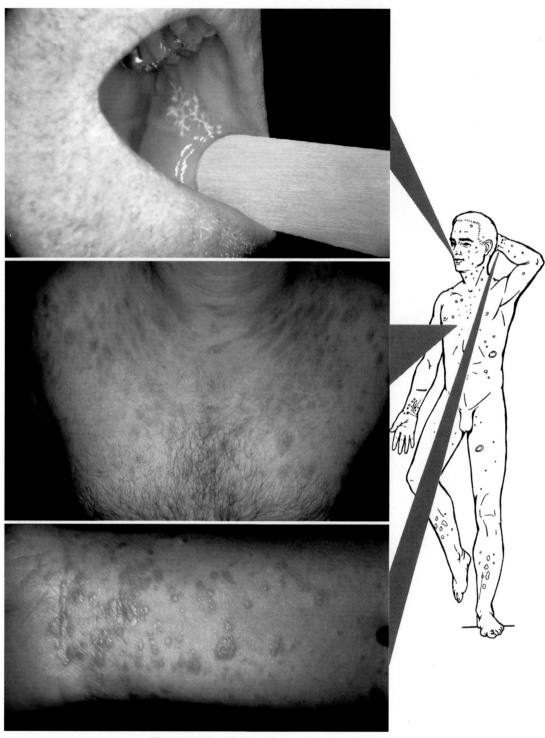

Figure 14-10.   **Lichen planus.** (*Johnson & Johnson*)

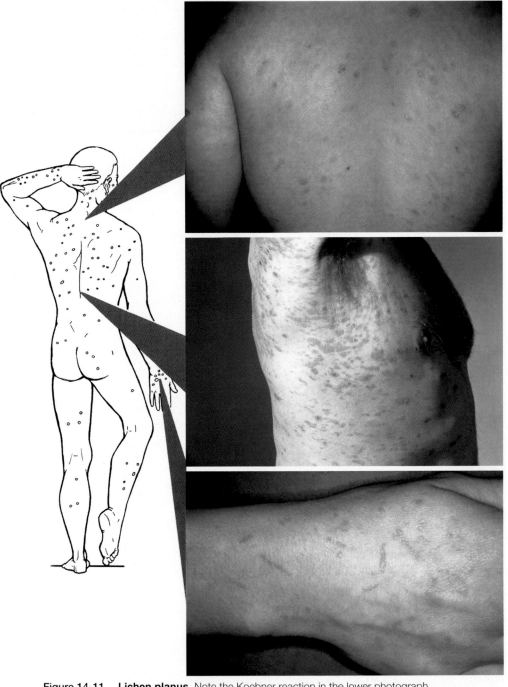

Figure 14-11. **Lichen planus.** Note the Koebner reaction in the lower photograph.

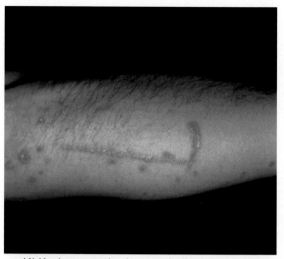

(*A*) Koebner reaction in scratched areas on arm.

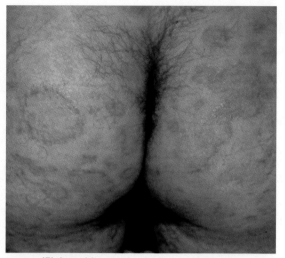

(*B*) Atrophic scarring lesions on buttocks.

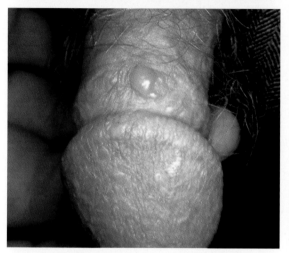

(*C*) Bullous and vesicular lesions on penis.

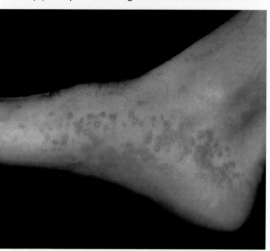

(*D*) Lichen planus on sole of foot.

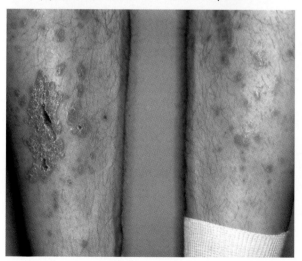

(*E*) Hypertrophic lesions on anterior tibial area of legs.

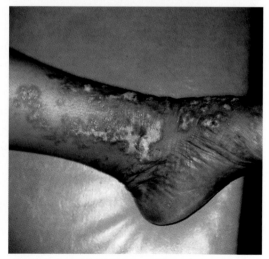

(*F*) Hypertrophic lesions on leg of an African-American woman.

Figure 14-12.   **Lichen planus, unusual variations.** (*Neutrogena Corp.*)

<u>Subsequent Visits</u>

1. Occlusive dressing with corticosteroid therapy. This is quite effective for localized cases. I have also found that if occlusive dressings are applied only to the lichen planus on the legs, the rest of the body lesions improve.
2. Meprobamate, 400 mg   #100
   Sig: Take 1 tablet t.i.d., *or*
   Chlordiazepoxide (Librium), 5 mg
   Sig: Take 1 tab t.i.d.
3. It is important in some resistant cases to rule out a focus of infection in teeth, tonsils, gallbladder, genitourinary system, and so on.
4. Corticosteroids orally or by injection are of definite value for temporarily relieving the acute cases that have severe itching or a generalized eruption.

BIBLIOGRAPHY

Abramowicz M. Two new retinoids for psoriasis. Med Lett 1997;39:1013.

American Academy of Dermatology guidelines: Psoriasis. J Am Acad Dermatol 1993;18:632.

Baughman RD. A 61-year-old man with psoriasis. JAMA 1996;276:17.

Boyd AS, Neldner KH. Lichen planus. J Am Acad Dermatol 1991;25:593.

Camisa C. Handbook of psoriasis. 1998.

Faegemann J, Fredriksson T. Tinea versicolor: some new aspects on etiology, pathogenesis, and treatment. Int J Dermatol 1982;21:8.

Fox BJ, Odum RB. Papulosquamous diseases: A review. J Am Acad Dermatol 1985;12:597.

Krueger GG, Drake LA, Elias PM, et al. The safety and efficacy of tazarotene gel, a topical acetylenic retinoid, in the treatment of psoriasis. Arch Dermatol 1998;134:57.

Lebwohl M, Abel E, et al. Topical therapy for psoriasis. Int J Dermatol 1995;34:10.

Liem WH, McCullough JL, Weinstein GD. Effectiveness of topical therapy for psoriasis. Cutis 1995;55:306.

Menter MA, See JA, et al. Proceedings of the Psoriasis Combination and Rotation Therapy Conference. J Am Acad Dermatol 1996;34:2.

O'Hagan ML. New horizons in the management of psoriasis. Cutis 1998;61:2S.

Roenigk HH, Auerbach R, et al. Methotrexate in psoriasis: Consensus conference. J Am Acad Dermatol 1998;38:3.

Sunenshine PJ, Schwartz RA, Janniger CK. Tinea versicolor. Int J Dermatol 1998;37:648.

Wolverton SE. Systemic drug therapy for psoriasis. Arch Dermatol 1991;127:565.

15

Dermatologic Bacteriology

Bacteria exist on the skin as normal nonpathogenic resident flora or as pathogenic organisms. The pathogenic bacteria cause primary, secondary, and systemic infections. For clinical purposes it is justifiable to divide the problem of bacterial infection into these three classifications.

PRIMARY BACTERIAL INFECTIONS

Impetigo
Ecthyma
Folliculitis
    Superficial folliculitis
    Folliculitis of the scalp
        Superficial—acne miliaris necrotica
        Deep scarring—folliculitis decalvans
    Folliculitis of the beard
    Stye
Furuncle
Carbuncle
Sweat gland inflammations
Erysipelas

SECONDARY BACTERIAL INFECTIONS

Cutaneous diseases with secondary infection
Infected ulcers
Infectious eczematoid dermatitis
Bacterial intertrigo

SYSTEMIC BACTERIAL INFECTIONS

Scarlet fever
Granuloma inguinale
Chancroid

Mycobacterial infections
    Tuberculosis of the skin
    Leprosy
Gonorrhea
Rickettsial diseases
Actinomycosis

With an alteration in immune capabilities in a person, bacteria and other infectious agents can have erratic behavior. Ordinary nonpathogens can act as pathogens, and pathogenic agents can act more aggressively.

PRIMARY BACTERIAL INFECTIONS (PYODERMAS)

The most common causative agents of the primary skin infections are the coagulase-positive micrococci (staphylococci) and the β-hemolytic streptococci. Superficial or deep bacterial lesions can be produced by these organisms.

In managing the pyodermas certain *general principles of treatment* must be initiated.

Improve the bathing habits: More frequent bathing and the use of bactericidal soap, such as Dial, is indicated. Any pustules or crusts should be removed during the bathing to facilitate penetration of the local medications.

General isolation procedures: Clothing and bedding should be changed frequently and

145

cleaned. The patient should have a separate towel and washcloth.

Systemic drugs: The patient should be questioned regarding ingestion of drugs that can cause lesions that mimic or cause pyodermas, such as iodides, bromides, testosterone, corticosteroids, and lithium.

Diabetes: In chronic skin infections, particularly recurrent boils, diabetes should be ruled out by history and laboratory examination.

Immunosuppressed patients: A good history of abnormal laboratory tests should alert the physician to the many patients now who are on chemotherapy for cancer or are post-transplant patients or have the acquired immunodeficiency syndrome (AIDS).

SAUER NOTE

Body piercing has been frequently associated with localized staphylococcal infection and pseudomonas infection and rarely bacteremia and endocarditis. Tuberculosis, hepatitis C and B, and even HIV may have been transmitted in this way. Noninfectious complications are keloids and allergic dermatitis. This fad should not be recommended, especially in tongue, lips, navels, nipples, and genitalia.

Impetigo

(Figs. 15-1 and 15-2; see also Fig. 3-1G)

Impetigo is a common superficial bacterial infection seen most often in children. This is the "infantigo" every mother respects.

PRIMARY LESIONS. The lesions vary from small vesicles to large bullae that rupture and discharge a honey-colored serous liquid. New lesions can develop in a matter of hours.

SECONDARY LESIONS. Crusts form from the discharge and appear to be lightly stuck on the skin surface. When removed, a superficial erosion remains, which may be the only evidence of the disease. In debilitated infants the bullae may coalesce to form an exfoliative type of infection called *Ritter's disease* or *pemphigus neonatorum*.

DISTRIBUTION. The lesions occur most commonly on the face but may be anywhere.

CONTAGIOUSNESS. It is not unusual to see brothers or sisters of the patient and, rarely, the parents similarly infected.

DIFFERENTIAL DIAGNOSIS

Contact dermatitis due to poison ivy or oak: Linear blisters; does not spread as rapidly; itches (see Chap. 9).

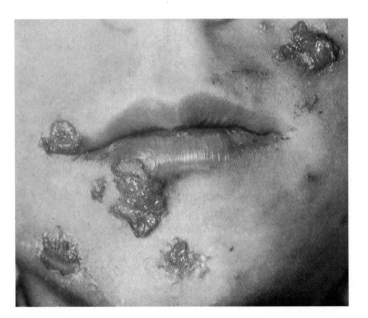

Figure 15-1. Impetigo of the face. The honey-colored crusts are typical. (*Abner Kurtin, Folia Dermatologica, No. 2. Geigy Pharmaceuticals*)

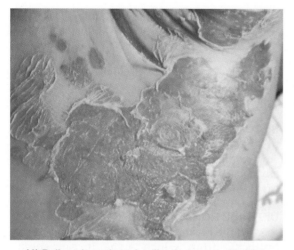

(*A*) Bullous impetigo of axillae in 1-year-old child.

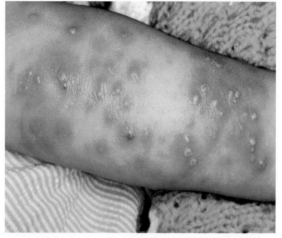

(*B*) Folliculitis of forearm in 7-month-old infant.

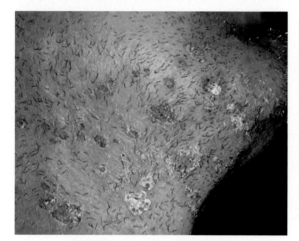

(*C*) Folliculitis of the beard area.

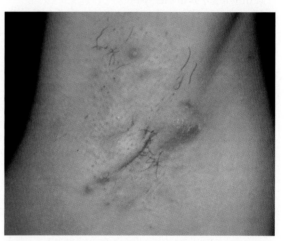

(*D*) Hidradenitis suppurativa of axilla of 6 years' duration.

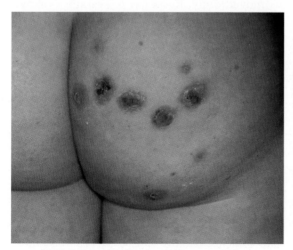

(*E*) Ecthyma of buttocks of 13-year-old boy.

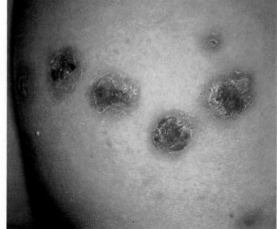

(*F*) Close-up of lesions.

Figure 15-2.　**Primary bacterial infections.** (*Burroughs Wellcome Co.*)

Tinea of smooth skin: Fewer lesions; spread slowly; small vesicles in annular configuration, which is an unusual form for impetigo; fungi found on scraping (see Chap. 19).

Bullous impetigo: In infants and rarely in adults, massive bullae (see Fig 15-4) can develop rapidly, particularly with staphylococcal infection. The severe form of this infection is known as the *staphylococcal scalded skin syndrome*, which is a type of toxic epidermal necrolysis (see Chap. 22).

TREATMENT

1. Outline the general principles of treatment. Emphasize the removal of the crusts once or twice a day during bathing with an antibacterial soap such as Lever 2000, or chlorhexidine (Hibiclens) skin cleanser.
2. Mupirocin (Bactroban) or gentamicin (Garamycin) ointment or Polysporin ointment q.s. 15.0
   Sig: Apply t.i.d. locally.

SAUER NOTES

1. I routinely add sulfur 5% and hydrocortisone 1% to 2% to the antibiotic cream or ointment for treatment of impetigo and other superficial pyodermas. Many patients with impetigo whom I see have been using a plain antibiotic salve with an oral antibiotic, and the impetigo persists. With this compound salve the impetigo heals.
2. Advise the patient that the local treatment should be continued for 5 days after the lesions apparently have disappeared to prevent recurrences—"therapy plus."
3. Systemic antibiotic therapy. Some physicians believe that every patient with impetigo should be treated with systemic antibiotic therapy to heal these lesions and also to prevent chronic glomerulonephritis. Erythromycin in appropriate dosages for 10 days would be effective in most cases. Resistance to erythromycin can occur, and then dicloxacillin or cephalexin is effective.

Ecthyma
(see Fig. 15-2)

Ecthyma is another superficial bacterial infection, but it is seen less commonly and is deeper than impetigo. It is usually caused by β-hemolytic streptococci and occurs on the buttocks and the thighs of children.

PRIMARY LESION. A vesicle or vesiculopustule appears and rapidly changes into the secondary lesion.

SECONDARY LESION. This is a piled-up crust, 1 to 3 cm in diameter, overlying a superficial erosion or ulcer. In neglected cases scarring can occur as a result of extension of the infection into the dermis.

DISTRIBUTION. Most commonly the disease is seen on the posterior aspect of the thighs and the buttocks, from which areas it can spread. Ecthyma commonly follows the scratching of chigger bites.

AGE GROUP. Children are affected mainly.

CONTAGIOUSNESS. Ecthyma is rarely found in other members of the family.

DIFFERENTIAL DIAGNOSIS

Psoriasis: Unusual in children; whitish, firmly attached scaly lesion, also in scalp, on knees, and elbows (see Chap. 14)
Impetigo: Much smaller crusted lesions, not as deep (see preceding section)

TREATMENT

1. The general principles of treatment are listed earlier in the chapter. The crusts must be removed daily. Response to therapy is slower than with impetigo, but the treatment is the same for both conditions.
2. Systemic antibiotics. Commonly with extensive ecthyma in children, but only rarely with impetigo, there is a low-grade fever and evidence of bacterial infection in other organs, such as the kidney. If so, one of the antibiotic syrups or tablets can be given orally q.i.d. for 10 days.

Folliculitis
(see Fig. 15-2)

Folliculitis is a common pyogenic infection of the hair follicles, usually caused by coagulase-positive staphylococci. Seldom does a patient consult the physician for a single outbreak of folliculitis. The physician is consulted because of recurrent and chronic pustular lesions. The patient realizes that the present acute episode will clear with the help of nature but seeks the medicine and the advice that will prevent recurrences. For this reason the *general principles of treatment* listed earlier, particularly the drug history and the diabetes investigation, are important. Some physicians believe that a focus of infection in the teeth, tonsils, gallbladder, or genitourinary tract should be ruled out when pyodermas are recurrent.

The folliculitis may invade only the superficial part of the hair follicle, or it may extend down to the hair bulb. Many variously named clinical entities based on the location and the chronicity of the lesions have been carried down through the years. A few of these entities bear presentation here, but most are defined in the Dictionary–Index.

Superficial Folliculitis

The physician is rarely consulted for this minor problem, which is most commonly seen on the arms, the scalp, the face, and the buttocks of children and adults with the "acne–seborrhea complex." A history of excessive use of hair oils, bath oils, or suntan oils can often be obtained. The use of these oily agents should be avoided.

Folliculitis of the Scalp (Superficial Form)

A *superficial form* has the appellation *acne necrotica miliaris*. This is an annoying, pruritic, chronic, recurrent folliculitis of the scalp in adults. The scratching of the crusted lesions occupies the patient's evening hours.

TREATMENT

1. Outline the general principles of treatment.
2. Selenium sulfide (Selsun, Head & Shoulders Intensive Treatment) suspension shampoo 120.0
   Sig: Shampoo twice a week as directed on the label.
3. Antibiotic and corticosteroid cream mixture q.s.   15.0
   Sig: Apply to scalp h.s.

Folliculitis of the Scalp (Deep Form)

The *deep form* of scalp folliculitis is called *folliculitis decalvans*. This is a chronic, slowly progressive folliculitis with an active border and scarred at-

rophic center. The end result, after years of progression, is patchy, scarred areas of alopecia, with eventual burning out of the inflammation. Cultures are negative.

SAUER NOTES

My routine for *chronic* folliculitis cases includes the following:

1. Sulfur ppt.   5%
   Hydrocortisone   1%
   Bactroban cream q.s.   15.0
   Sig: Apply b.i.d. locally.

2. Long-term low-dose antibiotic therapy can be used, such as erythromycin, 250 mg, q.i.d. for 3 days then two or three times a day for months.

3. Lichenified papules of excoriated folliculitis respond to superficial liquid nitrogen applications.

DIFFERENTIAL DIAGNOSIS

Chronic discoid lupus erythematosus: Redness; enlarged hair follicles (see Chap. 25).
Alopecia cicatrisata (pseudopelade of Brocq): Rare; no evidence of infection (see Chap. 27).
Tinea of the scalp: It is important to culture the hair for fungi in any chronic infection of the scalp; *Trichophyton tonsurans* group can cause a subtle noninflammatory clinical picture (black dot tinea in children) (see Chap. 19).
Excoriated folliculitis: Chronic thickened excoriated papules or nodules (can be called *prurigo nodularis*), usually seen on posterior scalp, posterior neck, anus, and legs. When allowed to heal, whitish scars remain. The infection can last for years. Liquid nitrogen applied to the papules is effective or intralesional corticosteroids.

TREATMENT

Results of treatment are disappointing. The routine for the superficial form of folliculitis should be followed and oral antibiotics prescribed.

Folliculitis of the Beard
(see Fig 15-2)

This is the familiar "barber's itch," which in the days before antibiotics was very resistant to therapy. This bacterial infection of the hair follicles is spread rather rapidly by shaving, but after treatment is begun, shaving should be continued.

DIFFERENTIAL DIAGNOSIS

Contact dermatitis due to shaving lotions: History of new lotion applied; general redness of the area with some vesicles (see Chap. 9).

Tinea of the beard: Very slowly spreading infection; hairs broken off; usually a deeper nodular type of inflammation; culture of hair produces fungi (see Chap. 19).

Ingrown beard hairs (pseudofolliculitis barbae): Hair circling back into the skin with resultant chronic infection; a hereditary trait, especially in African-Americans. Close shaving aggravates the condition. Local antibiotics rarely help, but locally applied depilatories may help. Other local therapy to consider is Retin-A gel, and Benzashave. Growing a beard or mustache eliminates the problem. Hairs may also become ingrown in axillae, pubic area, or legs, especially when closely shaved in places with curly hair.

TREATMENT

1. Outline the general principles of treatment, stressing the use of Dial or other antibacterial soap for washing of the face.
2. Shaving instructions:
   a. Change the razor blade daily or sterilize the head of the electric razor by placing it in 70% alcohol for 1 hour.
   b. Apply the following salve very lightly to the face before shaving and again after shaving. *Do not shave closely.*
3. Antibiotic and hydrocortisone cream mixture
   q.s.   15.0
   Sig: Apply to face before shaving, after shaving, and at bedtime.
   Comment: For stubborn cases, add sulfur 5% to the cream.
4. Oral therapy with erythromycin, 250 mg
   Sig: 1 capsule q.i.d. for 7 days, then 1 capsule b.i.d. for 7 days.

Stye (Hordeolum)

A stye is a deep folliculitis of the stiff eyelid hairs. A single lesion is treated with hotpacks of 1% boric acid solution and an ophthalmic antibiotic ointment. Recurrent lesions may be linked with the blepharitis of *seborrheic dermatitis* (dandruff). For this type, sulfacetamide ophthalmic ointment, or cleansing the eyelashes with Johnson's Baby Shampoo is indicated.

Furuncle
(Fig. 15-3)

A furuncle, or boil, is a more extensive infection of the hair follicle, usually due to *Staphylococcus*. A boil can occur in any person at any age, but certain predisposing factors account for most outbreaks. An important factor is the acne–seborrhea complex (oily skin, dark complexion, and history of acne and dandruff). Other factors include poor hygiene, diabetes, local skin trauma from friction of clothing, and maceration in obese persons. One boil usually does not bring the patient to the physician, but recurrent boils do.

DIFFERENTIAL DIAGNOSIS

SINGLE LESION

Primary chancre-type diseases: See list in Dictionary–Index.

MULTIPLE LESIONS

Drug eruption from iodides or bromides: See Chapter 9.

Hidradenitis suppurativa: See later in this chapter.

TREATMENT

A young man has had recurrent boils for 6 months. He does not have diabetes, is not obese, is taking no drugs, and bathes daily. He now has a large boil on his buttocks.

1. Burow's solution hot packs.
   Sig: 1 packet of Domeboro powder to 1 quart of hot water. Apply hot wet packs for 30 minutes twice a day.

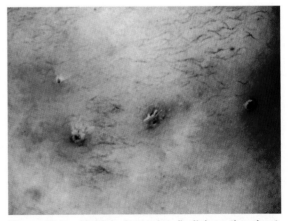

Figure 15-3. Multiple furuncles (boils) on the chest. *(Abner Kurtin, Folia Dermatologica, No. 2. Geigy Pharmaceuticals)*

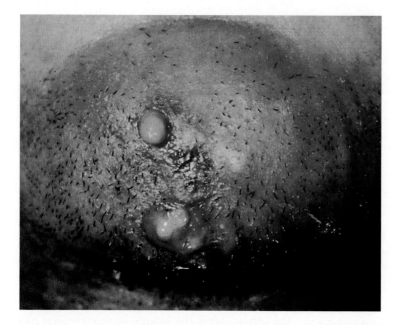

Figure 15-4.   Carbuncle on the chin. Notice the multiple openings. (*Abner Kurtin, Folia Dermatologica, No. 2. Geigy Pharmaceuticals*)

2. Incision and drainage. This should be done only on "ripe" lesions where a necrotic white area appears at the top of the nodule. Drains are not necessary unless the lesion has extended deep enough to form a fluctuant abscess.

3. Oral antistaphylococcal penicillin, such as dicloxacillin or cephalexin, should be prescribed for 5 to 10 days. (Bacteriologic culture and sensitivity studies are helpful in determining which antibiotic to use.)

4. For recurrent form:
   a. Outline general principles of treatment, use of an antibacterial soap.
   b. Rule out focus of infection in teeth, tonsils, genitourinary tract, and so on.
   c. Begin oral therapy with erythromycin, 250 mg, which is very effective in breaking the cycle of recurrent cases.
   Sig: 4 capsules a day for 4 days, then 1 capsule b.i.d. for weeks, until clear.

For *Staphylococcus aureus* resistant to erythromycin, penicillinase-resistant penicillins, cephalosporins, and azithromycin can be used.

Carbuncle

(Figs. 15-4 and 15-5)

A carbuncle is an extensive infection of several adjoining hair follicles that drains with multiple openings onto the skin surface. Fatal cases were not unusual in the preantibiotic days. A common location for a carbuncle is the posterior neck region. Large, ugly, criss-cross scars in this area in an older patient demonstrate the outdated treatment for this disease, namely, multiple bold incisions. Because a carbuncle is, in reality, a multiple furuncle, the same etiologic factors apply. Recurrences are uncommon.

TREATMENT

Treatment is the same as that for a boil (see preceding section) but with greater emphasis on systemic antibiotic therapy.

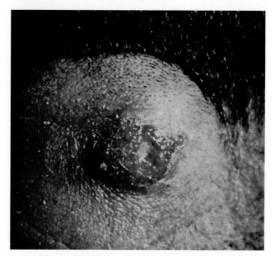

Figure 15-5.   Carbuncle on the back of the neck. (*J. Lamar Callaway, Folia Dermatologica, No. 4. Geigy Pharmaceuticals*)

Sweat Gland Inflammations
(Fig. 15-6)

Although not true infections, inflammations of the sweat gland are included here because of similar clinical appearance and similar treatment.

Primary *eccrine* sweat gland or duct infections are very rare. However, *prickly heat*, a sweat-retention disease, frequently develops secondary bacterial infection.

Primary *apocrine* gland inflammation is rather common. Two types of inflammation exist:

Apocrinitis denotes inflammation of a single apocrine gland, usually in the axilla, and is commonly associated with a change in deodorant. It responds to the therapy listed under furuncles. In addition, a lotion containing an antibiotic aids in keeping the area dry, such as an erythromycin solution (A/T/S, Erymax, EryDerm, Erycette, T-Stat, Staticin).

The second form of apocrine gland inflammation is *hidradenitis suppurativa* (Fig. 15-6). This chronic, recurring, inflammation is characterized by the development of multiple nodules, abscesses, draining sinuses, and eventual hypertrophic bands of scars. The most common location is in the axillae, but it can also occur in the groin, perianal, submammary, and suprapubic regions. It does not occur before puberty. Etiologically, there appears to be a hereditary tendency in these patients toward occlusion of the follicular orifice, and subsequent retention of the secretory products. Two other diseases are related to hidradenitis suppurativa and may be present in the same patient: (1) a severe form of acne called *acne conglobata* and (2) *dissecting cellulitis of the scalp*.

TREATMENT

The management of these cases is difficult. In addition to the general principles mentioned previously, one should use hot packs locally and an oral antibiotic for several weeks.

Plastic surgery or a marsupialization operation is indicated in severe cases. When draining canals or sinuses are present, the marsupialization operation is very curative and can be done in the office. After the bridge over the canal has been trimmed away, bleeding is controlled by electrosurgery. Etretinate (Accutane) can be tried for 5 to 10 months (see Chap 13).

Erysipelas
(Fig. 15-7)

Erysipelas is an uncommon β-hemolytic streptococcal infection of the subcutaneous tissue that produces a characteristic type of cellulitis, with fever and malaise. Recurrences are frequent.

PRIMARY LESION. A red, warm, raised, brawny, sharply bordered plaque enlarges peripherally. Vesicles and bullae may form on the surface of the plaque. Multiple lesions of erysipelas are rare.

DISTRIBUTION. Most commonly lesions occur on the face and around the ears (following ear piercing), but no area is exempt. Some authors now think the legs are the most common site.

COURSE. When treated with systemic antibiotics, the response is rapid. Recurrences are common in the same location and may lead to *lymphedema* of that area, which eventually can become irreversible. The lip, the cheek, and the legs are particularly prone to this chronic change, which is called *elephantiasis nostras*.

SUBJECTIVE COMPLAINTS. Fever and general malaise can precede the development of the skin

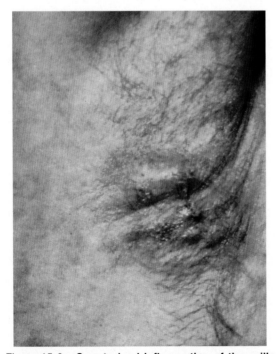

Figure 15-6. Sweat gland inflammation of the axilla (hidradenitis suppurativa). *(Abner Kurtin, Folia Dermatologica, No. 2. Geigy Pharmaceuticals)*

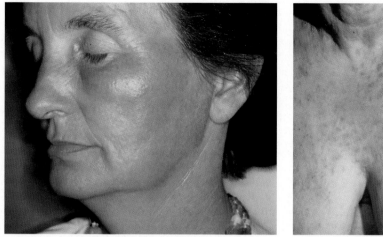

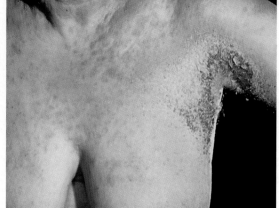

(*A*) **Erysipelas of cheek.**

(*B*) **Infectious eczematoid dermatitis from axilla.**

Figure 15-7.   **Bacterial infections of skin.** (*Burroughs Wellcome Co.*)

lesion and persist until therapy is instituted. Pain at the site of the infection can be severe.

DIFFERENTIAL DIAGNOSIS

Cellulitis: Lacks a sharp border; recurrences rare
Contact dermatitis: Sharp border absent; fever and malaise absent; eruption predominantly vesicular (see Chap. 9)

TREATMENT

1. Institute bed rest and direct therapy toward reducing the fever. If the patient is hospitalized, semiisolation procedures should be initiated.

2. Give an appropriate systemic antibiotic, such as erythromycin or a penicillin derivative, for 10 days.
3. Apply local, cool, wet dressing, as necessary for comfort.

Erythrasma
(*Fig. 15-8*)

Erythrasma is an uncommon bacterial infection of the skin that clinically resembles regular tinea or tinea versicolor. It affects the crural area, axillae, and webs of the toes with flat, hyperpigmented, fine, scaly patches. If the patient has not

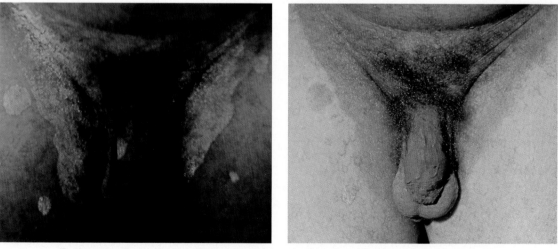

Erythrasma of crural area with fluorescence under Wood's light (*A*) and in natural light (*B*).

Figure 15-8.   **Bacterial infections of skin.** (*Burroughs Wellcome Co.*)

been using an antibacterial soap, these patches fluoresce a striking reddish orange under Wood's light. The causative agent is a diphtheroid organism called *Corynebacterium minutissimum.*

The most effective treatment is erythromycin, 250 mg, q.i.d. for 5 to 7 days. Locally the erythromycin lotions are quite effective (*e.g.,* Staticin, T-Stat, EryDerm, and A/T/S lotion). Apply twice daily for 10 days.

SECONDARY BACTERIAL INFECTIONS

Secondary infection develops as a complicating factor on a preexisting skin disease. The invasion of an injured skin surface with pathogenic streptococci or staphylococci is enhanced in skin conditions that are oozing and of long duration.

Cutaneous Diseases with Secondary Infection

Failure in the treatment of many common skin diseases can be attributed to the physician's not recognizing the presence of the secondary bacterial infection.

SAUER NOTE

Any type of skin lesion, such as hand dermatitis, poison weed dermatitis, atopic eczema, chigger bites, fungus infection, traumatic abrasion, and so on, can become secondarily infected.

The treatment is usually simple: An antibacterial agent is added to the local treatment one would ordinarily use for the dermatosis in question. For extensive secondary bacterial infection, the appropriate systemic antibiotic is indicated, based on bacterial culture and sensitivity studies.

Infected Ulcers
(see Fig 34-12)

Ulcers are deep skin infections due to injury or disease that invade the subcutaneous tissue and, on healing, leave scars. Ulcers can be divided into primary and secondary ulcers, but all become secondarily infected with bacteria.

PRIMARY ULCERS. Primary ulcers result from the following causes: gangrene due to pathogenic streptococci, staphylococci, and *Clostridium* species; syphilis; chancroid; tuberculosis; diphtheria; fungi; leprosy; anthrax; cancer; and lymphomas.

SECONDARY ULCERS. Secondary ulcers can be related to the following diseases: vascular disorders (arteriosclerosis, thromboangiitis obliterans, Raynaud's phenomenon, phlebitis, thrombosis); neurologic disorders (spinal cord injury with bedsores or decubiti, central nervous system syphilis, spina bifida, poliomyelitis, syringomyelia); diabetes; trauma; ulcerative colitis; immunosuppression; allergic local anaphylaxis; and other conditions. Finally, there is a group of secondary ulcers called *phagedenic ulcers,* variously described under many different names, that arise in diseased skin or on the apparently normal skin of debilitated persons. These ulcers undermine the skin in large areas, are notoriously chronic, and are resistant to therapy.

TREATMENT

1. For primary ulcers, specific therapy is indicated, if available. The response to therapy is usually quite rapid.
2. For secondary ulcers, appropriate therapy should be directed toward the primary disease. The response to therapy is usually quite slow. This is especially true for the *decubitus ulcer* of the immobile, incontinent person.
3. The basic rules of local therapy for ulcers can be illustrated best by outlining the management of a patient with a *stasis leg ulcer* (see Stasis Dermatitis and Stasis Ulcers in Chap. 12).
   a. Rest of the affected area. If rest in bed is not feasible, then an Ace elastic bandage, 4 inches wide, should be worn. This bandage is applied over the local medication and before getting out of bed in the morning. A more permanent support is a modification of Unna's boot (Dome-Paste bandage, Gelocast, or an easy to apply and effective adhesive flexible bandage). This boot can be applied for a week or more at a time if secondary infection is under control.
   b. Elevation of the affected extremity. This should be carried out in bed and can be accomplished by placing two bricks, flat surface down, under both feet of the bed. (Arteriosclerotic leg ulcers should not be elevated.)

c. Burow's solution wet packs
   Sig: 1 packet of Domeboro powder to 1 quart of warm water. Apply wet dressings of gauze or sheeting for 30 minutes t.i.d.
d. If debridement is necessary, this can be accomplished by enzymes, such as Debrisan, Santyl (collagenase) ointment, or Elase ointment, applied twice a day and covered with gauze.
e. Gentian violet   1%
   Distilled water q.s.   15.0
   Sig: Apply to ulcer b.i.d. with applicator.
   Comment: A liquid is usually better tolerated on ulcers than a salve. If the gentian violet solution becomes too drying, the following salve can be used alternately for short periods.
f. Bactroban or other antibiotic ointment q.s.
                                                          15.0
   Sig: Apply to ulcer and surrounding skin b.i.d.
g. Long-term erythromycin or cephalexin therapy: 250 mg, 1 capsule q.i.d. for 3 days, then 1 capsule b.i.d. for weeks, is helpful for chronic pyogenic ulcers. Other systemic antibiotics may be used.
h. Low-dose oral corticosteroid therapy: Prednisone,   10 mg
   Sig: 1 or 2 tablets every morning for 3 to 4 weeks, then 1 tablet every other morning for months. When this is added to the above routine many indolent ulcers will heal.
   Comment: The best treatment for one ulcer does not necessarily work for another ulcer. Many other local medications are available and valuable.

4. Surgical management, such as excision and grafting, may be indicated.
5. Various surgical dressings may be beneficial, such as OpSite, Duoderm, Tegaderm, or Polymem.

SAUER NOTE

The primary factor in the management of an ulcer is to not let it happen. This is especially appropriate for decubitus ulcers.

Infectious Eczematoid Dermatitis
(Fig. 15-9)

The term *infectious eczematoid dermatitis* or auto eczematous dermatitis is more often used incorrectly than correctly. Infectious eczematoid dermatitis is an uncommon disease characterized by the development of an acute eruption around an infected exudative primary site, such as a draining ear, mastitis, a boil, or a seeping ulcer. Widespread eczematous lesions can develop at a distant site from the primary infection, presumably due to an immune phenomenon.

PRIMARY LESIONS. Vesicles and pustules in circumscribed plaques spread peripherally from an infected central source. Central healing usually does not occur, as in ringworm infection.

SECONDARY LESIONS. Crusting, oozing, and scaling predominate in widespread cases.

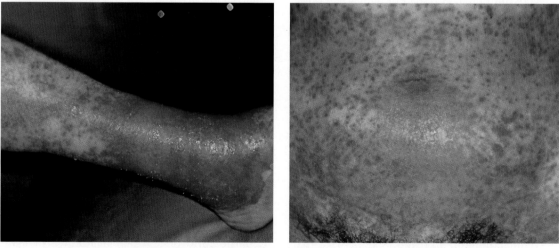

Infectious eczematoid dermatitis (*A*) from stasis dermatitis of legs with spread to body (*B*).

Figure 15-9. **Bacterial infections of skin**. *(Burroughs Wellcome Co.)*

DISTRIBUTION. Mild cases may be confined to a small area around the exudative primary infection, but widespread cases can cover the entire body, obscuring the initial cause.

COURSE. The course depends on the extent of the eruption. Chronic cases respond poorly to therapy. Recurrences are common even after the primary source is healed.

SUBJECTIVE COMPLAINTS. Itching is usually present.

CAUSE. Coagulase-positive staphylococci are frequently isolated.

CONTAGIOUSNESS. Despite the strong autoinoculation factor, passage of the infective material to another person rarely elicits a reaction.

DIFFERENTIAL DIAGNOSIS

Contact dermatitis with secondary infection: No history or finding of primary exudative infection; history of contact with poison ivy, new clothes, cosmetics, or dishwater; responds faster to therapy (see Chap. 9).
Nummular eczema: No primary infected source; coin-shaped lesions on extremities; clinical differentiation of some cases difficult (see Chap. 9).
Seborrheic dermatitis: No primary infected source; seborrhea–acne complex, with greasy, scaly eruption in hairy areas (see Chap. 13).
Eczematous Psoriasis: A recently described skin ailment with the appearance of diffuse severe nummular eczema but with a response to therapy mimicking that of psoriasis.

TREATMENT

An 8-year-old boy presents with draining otitis media and pustular, crusted dermatitis on the side of face, neck, and scalp.

1. Treat the primary source—the ear infection, in this case.
2. Apply Burow's solution wet packs
   Sig: 1 packet of Domeboro powder to 1 quart of warm water. Apply wet sheeting or gauze to area for 20 minutes t.i.d.
3. Apply antibiotic and corticosteroid cream, such as

Bactroban ointment	15.0
Triamcinolone 0.1% cream	15.0

   Sig: Apply t.i.d. locally, after the wet packs are removed.

A patient with a widespread case might require hospitalization, daily mild soap baths, oral antibiotics, and corticosteroid systemic therapy.

Bacterial Intertrigo

The presence of friction, heat, and moisture in areas where two opposing skin surfaces contact each other leads to a secondary bacterial, fungus, or yeast infection.

PRIMARY LESION. Redness from friction and heat of opposing forces and maceration from inability of the sweat to evaporate freely leads to an eroded patch of dermatitis.

SECONDARY LESION. The bacterial infection may become severe enough to result in fissures and cellulitis.

DISTRIBUTION. The inframammary region, axillae, umbilicus, pubic, crural, genital, and perianal areas, and area between the toes may be involved.

COURSE. In certain persons intertrigo tends to recur each summer.

CAUSES. The factors of obesity, diabetes, and prolonged contact with urine, feces, and menstrual discharges predispose to the development of intertrigo. AIDS may present with recurrent bullous groin impetigo.

DIFFERENTIAL DIAGNOSIS

Candidal intertrigo: Scaling at border of erosion; presence of surrounding small satellite lesions; scraping and culture reveals *Candida albicans* (see Chap. 19).
Tinea: Scaly or papulovesicular border; scraping and culture are positive for fungi (see Chap. 19).
Seborrheic dermatitis: Greasy red scaly areas, also seen in scalp; bacterial intertrigo may coexist with seborrheic dermatitis (see Chap. 13).

TREATMENT

A 6-month-old infant presents with red, fistular dermatitis in diaper area, axillae, and folds of neck.

1. Bathe child once a day in lukewarm water with antibacterial soap. Dry affected areas thoroughly.

2. Double rinse diapers to remove all soap, or use disposable diapers.

3. Change diapers as frequently as possible and apply a powder each time, such as

Talc, unscented   45.0

Sig: Place in powder can.

4. Hydrocortisone   1%

Bactroban ointment q.s.   15.0

Sig: Apply to affected areas t.i.d. Continue local therapy for at least 1 week after dermatitis is apparently clear—"therapy-plus." Allow only two refills of this salve to avoid atrophy of the skin.

SYSTEMIC BACTERIAL INFECTIONS

Scarlet Fever

Scarlet fever is a moderately common streptococcal infection characterized by a sore throat, high fever, and a scarlet rash. The eruption develops after a day of rapidly rising fever, headache, sore throat, and various other symptoms. The rash begins first on the neck and the chest but rapidly spreads over the entire body, except for the area around the mouth. Close examination of the pale scarlet eruption reveals it to be made up of diffuse pinhead-sized, or larger, macules. In untreated cases the rash reaches its peak on the 4th day, and scaling commences around the 7th day and continues for 1 or 2 weeks. The "strawberry tongue" is seen at the height of the eruption.

The presence of petechiae on the body is a grave prognostic sign. Complications are numerous and common in untreated cases. Nephritis, in mild or severe form, and rheumatic heart disease are serious complications.

DIFFERENTIAL DIAGNOSIS

Measles: Early rash on face and forehead; larger macular rash; running eyes; cough (see Chap. 17).

Drug eruption: Lack of high fever and other constitutional signs; atropine and quinine can cause eruption clinically similar to scarlet fever (see Chap. 9).

TREATMENT

Penicillin or a similar systemic antibiotic is the therapy of choice. Complications should be watched for and should be treated early.

Granuloma Inguinale
(Fig. 15-10)

Before the use of antibiotics, particularly streptomycin and tetracycline, this disease was one of the most chronic and resistant afflictions of humans. Formerly, it was a rather common disease. Granuloma inguinale should be considered a venereal disease, although other factors may have to be present to initiate infection.

PRIMARY LESION. An irregularly shaped, bright red, velvety appearing, flat ulcer with rolled border is seen.

SECONDARY LESIONS. Scarring may lead to complications similar to those seen with lymphogranuloma venereum. A *squamous cell carcinoma* can develop in old, chronic lesions.

DISTRIBUTION. Genital lesions are most common on the penis, the scrotum, the labia, the cervix, or the inguinal region.

COURSE. Without therapy, the granuloma grows slowly and persists for years, causing marked scarring and mutilation. Under modern therapy, healing is rapid, but recurrences are not unusual.

CAUSE. Granuloma inguinale is due to *Calymmatobacterium granulomatis*, which can be cultured on special media.

LABORATORY FINDINGS. Scrapings of the lesion reveal Donovan bodies, which are dark-staining, intracytoplasmic, cigar-shaped bacilli

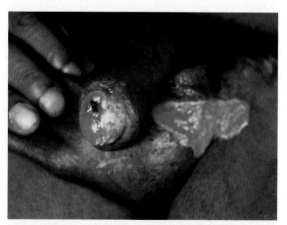

Figure 15-10. Systemic bacterial infections. Granuloma inguinale of penis and crural area. (*Derm-Arts Laboratories*)

found in large macrophages. The material for the smear can be obtained best by snipping off a piece of the lesion with a small scissors and rubbing the tissue on several slides. Wright or Giemsa stains can be used.

DIFFERENTIAL DIAGNOSIS

Granuloma pyogenicum: Small lesion; history of injury, usually; short duration; rarely on genitalia; no Donovan bodies.
Primary syphilis: Short duration; inguinal adenopathy; serology may be positive; spirochetes (see Chap. 16).
Chancroid: Short duration; lesion small, not red and velvety; no Donovan bodies (see next section).
Squamous cell carcinoma: More indurated lesion with nodule; may coexist with granuloma inguinale; biopsy specific.

TREATMENT

Tetracycline, 500 mg q.i.d., is continued until all the lesions are healed.

Chancroid
(Fig. 15-11)

Chancroid is a venereal disease with a very short incubation period of 1 to 5 days. It is caused by *Haemophilus ducreyi*.

PRIMARY LESION. A small, superficial or deep erosion occurs with surrounding redness and edema. Multiple genital or distant lesions can be produced by autoinoculation.

SECONDARY LESIONS. Deep, destructive ulcers form in chronic cases, which may lead to gangrene. Marked regional adenopathy, usually unilateral, is common and eventually suppurates in untreated cases.

COURSE. Without therapy most cases heal within 1 to 2 weeks. In rare cases, severe local destruction and draining lymph nodes (buboes) result. Early therapy is effective.

LABORATORY FINDINGS. The organisms arranged in "schools of fish" can often be demonstrated in smears of clean lesions.

DIFFERENTIAL DIAGNOSIS

> **SAUER NOTE**
>
> Syphilis must be considered in any patient with a penile lesion. It can be ruled out by darkfield examination or blood serology tests. The serology should be repeated in 6 weeks if clinical suspicion is high since the initial serology in primary syphilis may be negative.

Primary or secondary syphilis genital lesions: Longer incubation period; more induration; *Treponema pallidum* found on darkfield ex-

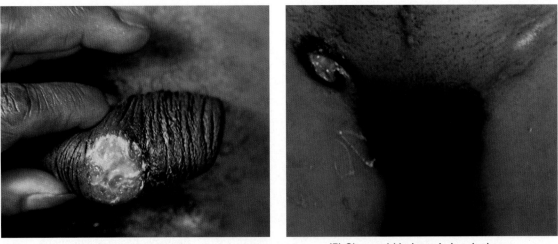

(*A*) Chancroid of penis.   (*B*) Chancroid buboes in inguinal area.

Figure 15-11.   Systemic bacterial infections. (*Derm-Arts Laboratories*)

amination; serology positive in late primary and secondary stage (see Chap. 16).

Herpes simplex progenitalis: Recurrent multiple painful blisters or erosions; mild inguinal adenopathy (see Chap. 17).

Lymphogranuloma venereum: Primary lesion rare; Frei test positive (see Chap. 17).

Granuloma inguinale: Chronic, red velvety plaque; Donovan bodies seen on tissue smear (see preceding section).

TREATMENT

The therapy for chancroid is a sulfonamide such as sulfisoxazole, 1 gram, q.i.d. for 2 weeks, or erythromycin, 2 grams/day for 10 to 15 days. Third-generation cephalosporins are effective also. A fluctuant bubo should never be incised but should be aspirated with a large needle.

Tuberculosis
(Fig. 15-12; see Fig. 3-2)

Skin tuberculosis is rare in the United States. However, a text on dermatology would not be complete without some consideration of this infection, and, although the incidence has been decreasing in the United States and leveled off worldwide since 1992, it is still a significant disease worldwide, and multidrug-resistant tuberculosis, especially in AIDS patients, is a particularly difficult problem. For this purpose the most common cutaneous tuberculosis infection, lupus vulgaris, is discussed. A classification of skin tuberculosis follows this section.

Lupus vulgaris is a chronic, granulomatous disease characterized by the development of

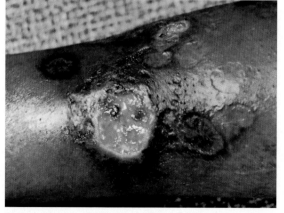

Figure 15-12. Systemic bacterial infections. Tuberculosis ulcer of leg. (*Derm-Arts Laboratories*)

nodules, ulcers, and plaques arranged in any conceivable configuration. Scarring in the center of active lesions or at the edge, in severe, untreated cases, leads to atrophy and contraction, resulting in mutilating changes.

DISTRIBUTION. Facial involvement is most common.

COURSE. The course is often slow and progressive, in spite of therapy.

LABORATORY FINDINGS. The histopathology shows typical tubercle formation with epithelioid cells, giant cells, and peripheral zone of lymphocytes. The causative organism, *Mycobacterium tuberculosis*, is not abundant in the lesions. The 48-hour tuberculin test is usually positive.

DIFFERENTIAL DIAGNOSIS

Other granulomas, such as those associated with *syphilis, leprosy, sarcoidosis, deep fungus disease,* and *neoplasm*, are to be ruled out by appropriate studies (see also Chap. 20).

TREATMENT

Early localized lesions can be treated by surgical excision. For more widespread cases, long-term systemic therapy offers high hopes for cure. Isoniazid is usually prescribed along with other antituberculous drugs, such as rifampin and ethambutol (Myambutol). Multidrug-resistant tuberculosis is an increasing problem in AIDS patients.

CLASSIFICATION OF CUTANEOUS TUBERCULOSIS

TRUE CUTANEOUS TUBERCULOSIS (LESIONS CONTAIN TUBERCLE BACILLI)

1. Primary tuberculosis (no previous infection; tuberculin-negative in initial stages)
   a. Primary inoculation tuberculosis Tuberculosis chancre (exogenous implantation into skin producing the primary complex)
   b. Miliary tuberculosis of the skin (hematogenous dispersion)
2. *Secondary tuberculosis* (lesions develop in person already sensitive to tuberculin as result of prior tuberculous lesion; tubercle bacilli difficult or impossible to demonstrate)
   a. Lupus vulgaris (inoculation of tubercle bacilli into the skin from external or internal sources)

b. Tuberculosis verrucosa cutis (inoculation of tubercle bacilli into the skin from external or internal sources)

c. Scrofuloderma (extension to skin from underlying focus in bones or glands)

d. Tuberculosis cutis orificialis (mucous membrane lesions and extension onto the skin near mucocutaneous junctions)

TUBERCULIDS (ALLERGIC ORIGIN; NO TUBERCLE BACILLI IN LESIONS)

1. *Papular forms*
   a. Lupus miliaris disseminatus faciei (purely papular)
   b. Papulonecrotic tuberculid (papules with necrosis)
   c. Lichen scrofulosorum (follicular papules or lichenoid papules)
2. *Granulomatous, ulceronodular forms*
   a. Erythema induratum (nodules or plaques subsequently ulcerating; may be a nonspecific vasculitis)

Leprosy
(Figs. 15-13 and 15-14)

Leprosy, or Hansen's disease, is to be considered in the differential diagnosis of any skin granulomas. It is endemic in the southern part of the United States and in semitropical and tropical areas the world over.

Two definite types of leprosy are recognized: lepromatous and tuberculoid. In addition, there are cases that cannot presently be classified in either of these two categories but eventually develop either lepromatous or tuberculoid leprosy.

Lepromatous leprosy is the malignant form, which represents minimal resistance to the disease, with a negative lepromin reaction, characteristic histology, infiltrated cutaneous lesions with ill-defined borders, and progression to death usually from secondary amyloidosis.

Tuberculoid leprosy is generally benign in its course because of considerable resistance to the disease on the part of the host. This is manifested by a positive lepromin test, histology that is not diagnostic, cutaneous lesions that are frequently erythematous with elevated borders, and minimal effect of the disease on the general health.

Early symptoms of the lepromatous type include reddish macules with an indefinite border, nasal obstruction, and nosebleeds. Erythema nodosum-like lesions occur commonly. The tuberculoid type of leprosy is diagnosed early by the presence of an area of skin with impaired sensation, polyneuritis, and skin lesions with a sharp border and central atrophy.

CAUSE. The causative organism is *Mycobacterium leprae*.

CONTAGIOUSNESS. The source of infection is believed to be from patients with the lepromatous form. Infectiousness is of a low order.

LABORATORY FINDINGS. The bacilli are usually discovered in the lepromatous type but seldom in the tuberculoid type. Smears should be obtained from the tissue exposed by a small incision made into the dermis through an infiltrated lesion.

The lepromin reaction, a delayed reaction test similar to the tuberculin test, is of value in differentiating the lepromatous form from the tuberculoid form of leprosy, as stated previously. False-positive reactions do occur.

Biologic false-positive tests for syphilis are common in patients with the lepromatous type of leprosy.

DIFFERENTIAL DIAGNOSIS

Consider any of the granulomatous diseases, such as *syphilis, tuberculosis, sarcoidosis*, and *deep fungal infections* (see also Chap. 20).

TREATMENT

Dapsone (diaminodiphenylsulfone), rifampin, and isoniazid are all effective.

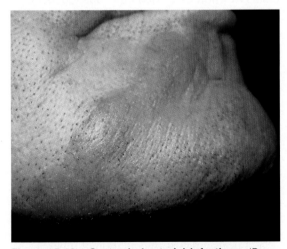

Figure 15-13. Systemic bacterial infections. *(Derm-Arts Laboratories)* Tuberculoid leprosy of the chin. *(Drs. W. Schorr and F. Kerdel-Vegas)*

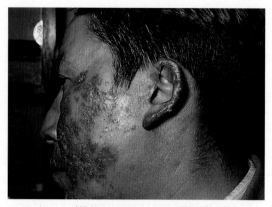

(A) Lepramatous leprosy.

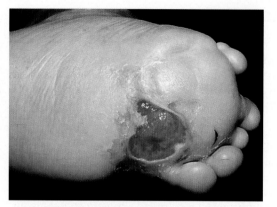

(B) Lepromatous leprosy on the foot.

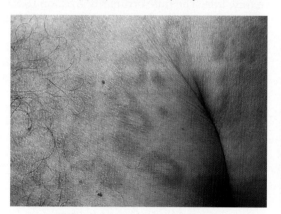

(C) Dimorphic leprosy on the chest.

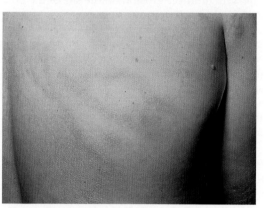

(D) Dimorphic leprosy on the back.

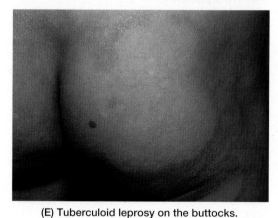

(E) Tuberculoid leprosy on the buttocks.

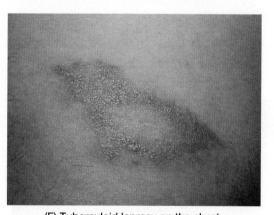

(F) Tuberculoid leprosy on the chest.

Figure 15-14. **Leprosy.** (*A and E, Dr. A. Gonzalez-Ochoa, Mexico; B and F, Dr. M. Rico, Durham, NC; C, Dr. R. Caputo, Atlanta, GA; D, Drs. W. Schorr, Wisconsin, and F. Kerdel-Vegas, Venezuela*).

Other Mycobacterial Dermatoses

Mycobacteria are pathogenic and saprophytic. *Mycobacterium marinum* can cause the *swimming pool granuloma* and also granulomas in fishermen and those involved with fish tanks. Minocycline, combinations of ethambutol and rifampin, clarithromycin, and levofloxacin have been used as treatments.

Mycobacterium avium-intracellulare is seen in patients with AIDS, but skin lesions are rare.

GONORRHEA
(Fig. 15-15)

Gonorrhea is considerably more prevalent than syphilis. Skin lesions with gonorrheal infection are rare. But a statement is due here on the therapy for uncomplicated gonorrhea.

The therapy suggested by the Centers for Disease Control is ceftriaxone, 250 mg, intramuscularly, one dose, or spectinomycin, 2 grams, intramuscularly, one dose.

Untreated or inadequately treated infection due to *Neisseria gonorrhoeae* can involve the skin through metastatic spread. *Primary cutaneous infection* with multiple erosions at the site of the purulent discharge is very rare.

Metastatic complications include a *bacteremia*, in which there is an intermittent high fever, arthralgia, and skin lesions. The skin lesions (see Fig. 15-15) are characteristic hemorrhagic vesiculopustules, most commonly seen on the fingers. Treatment with intravenous penicillin for 10 days at 5 to 10 million units per day is indicated.

The rarer *septicemic form*, with very high fever and meningitis or endocarditis, may have purpuric skin lesions similar to those seen in *meningococcemia*.

Rickettsial Diseases

The most common rickettsial disease in the United States is *Rocky Mountain spotted fever*, which is spread by ticks of various types. The skin eruption occurs after 3 to 7 days of fever and other toxic signs and is characterized by purpuric lesions on the extremities, mainly the wrists and the ankles, which then become generalized. The Weil-Felix test using *Proteus* OX19 and OX2 is positive. Tetracycline and chloramphenicol are effective.

The typhus group of rickettsial diseases includes *epidemic* or *louse-borne typhus, Brill's disease*, and *endemic murine* or *flea-borne typhus*. Less common forms include *scrub typhus* (tsutsugamushi disease), *trench fever*, and *rickettsialpox*. The last-named rickettsial disease is produced by a mite bite. The mite ordinarily lives on rodents. Approximately 10 days after the bite a primary lesion develops in the form of a papule that becomes vesicular. After a few days fever and other toxic signs are accompanied by a generalized eruption that resembles chickenpox. The disease subsides without therapy.

Ehrlichiosis is another rickettsial disease well known in dogs and now seen in humans. It is transmitted by tick bite. The nonspecific symptoms are similar to those of Rocky Mountain spotted fever, but only 20% of the patients have a rash.

Actinomycosis

Actinomycosis is a chronic, granulomatous, suppurative infection that characteristically causes the formation of a draining sinus. The most common location of the draining sinus is in the jaw region, but thoracic and abdominal sinuses do occur.

PRIMARY LESION. A red, firm, nontender tumor in the jaw area slowly extends locally to form a "lumpy jaw."

SECONDARY LESIONS. Discharging sinuses become infected with other bacteria and, if untreated, may develop into osteomyelitis.

COURSE. General health is usually unaffected unless extension occurs into bone or deeper neck tissues. Recurrence is unusual if treatment is continued long enough.

ETIOLOGY. *Actinomyces israelii*, which is an anaerobic bacterium that lives as a normal inhabitant of the mouth, particularly in persons who have poor dental hygiene, is the causative agent.

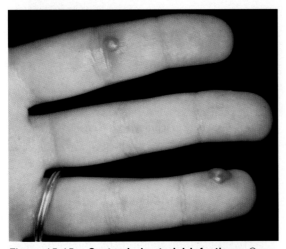

Figure 15-15. Systemic bacterial infections. Gonococcal septicemia with hemorrhagic vesicles. (*Derm-Arts Laboratories*)

Injury to the jaw or a tooth extraction usually precedes the development of the infection. Infected cattle are not the source of human infection. The disease is twice as frequent in men as in women.

LABORATORY FINDINGS. Pinpoint-sized "sulfur" granules, which are colonies of the organism, can be seen grossly and microscopically in the draining pus. A Gram stain of the pus will show masses of interlacing gram-positive fibers with or without club-shaped processes at the tips of these fibers. The organism can be cultured anaerobically on special media.

DIFFERENTIAL DIAGNOSIS

Consider *pyodermas, tuberculosis, draining dental abscess,* and *neoplasm.*

TREATMENT

1. Penicillin, 2.4 million units intramuscularly, is given daily, until definite improvement is noted. Then oral penicillin in the same dosage should be continued for 3 weeks after the infection apparently has been cured. In severe cases, 10 million or more units of penicillin given intravenously, daily, may be necessary.
2. Incision and drainage is performed of the lumps and the sinuses.
3. Good oral hygiene is required.
4. In resistant cases, broad-spectrum antibiotics can be used alone or in combination with the penicillin.

BIBLIOGRAPHY

Beck-Sague C, Dooley SW, Hutton MD, et al. Hospital outbreak of multidrug-resistant *Mycobacterium tuberculosis* infections. JAMA 1992;268:1280.

Bisno AL, Stevens DL. Streptococcal infections of skin and soft tissues. N Engl J Med 1996;334:4.

Boyd AS, Neldner KH. Typhus disease group. Int J Dermatol 1992;31:823.

Buntin DM, Rosen T, Lesher JL, et al. Sexually transmitted diseases: Bacterial infections. J Am Acad Dermatol 1991;25:287

Centers for Disease Control and Prevention. Estimates of future global tuberculosis morbidity and mortality. JAMA 1994;271:739.

Epstein ME, Amodio-Groton M, Sadick NS. Antimicrobial agents for the dermatologist: I. β-Lactam antibiotics and related compounds. J Am Acad Dermatol 1997;37:2.

Epstein ME, Amodio-Groton M, Sadick NS. Antimicrobial agents for the dermatologist: II. Macrolides, fluoroquinolones, rifamycins, tetracyclines, trimethoprim-sulfamethoxazole, and clindamycin. J Am Acad Dermatol 1997;37:3.

Johnson RA. Infectious folliculitis. Fitzpatrick's J Clin Dermatol 1995;3:38.

Modlin RL, Rea TH. Leprosy: New insight into an ancient disease. J Am Acad Dermatol 1987;17:1.

Parish LC. Color atlas of cutaneous infections. Blackwell Science 1995.

Parish LC, Witkowksi JA, Crissey JT. The decubitus ulcer in clinical practice. Springer, 1997.

Phillips TJ, Dover JS. Leg ulcers. J Am Acad Dermatol 1991;25:965.

Roth RR, James WD. Microbiology of the skin: Resident flora, ecology, infection. J Am Acad Dermatol 1989;20:367.

Sanders CV. Skin and Infection: A color atlas and text. Baltimore, Williams & Wilkins, 1995.

Sehgal VN, Sooneita AW. Cutaneous tuberculosis. Int J Dermatol 1990;23:237.

Spach DH, Liles WC, Campbell GL, et al. Tick-borne diseases in the United States: Review article. N Engl J Med 1993;329:936.

Tuberculosis morbidity—United States, 1996. JAMA 1997;278:16.

16

Spirochetal Infections

Two spirochetal diseases are discussed in this chapter: syphilis and Lyme disease.

SYPHILIS

When Gordon C. Sauer was stationed at the West Virginia State Rapid Treatment Center, from 1946 to 1948, the average admittance was 30 patients a day with venereal disease. Approximately one third of these patients had infectious syphilis. In 1949 the center was closed because of the low patient census. The incidence of reported syphilis has risen again to alarming heights. Many patients with acquired immunodeficiency syndrome (AIDS) also have syphilis. Because of this resurgence, it is imperative for all physicians to have a basic understanding of this polymorphous disease.

Cutaneous lesions of syphilis occur in all three stages of the disease.

Under what circumstances will the present-day physician be called on to diagnose, evaluate, or manage a patient with syphilis?

1. The cutaneous manifestations, such as a penile lesion or a rash that could be secondary syphilis, may bring a patient to the office.
2. A positive blood test found on a premarital examination or as part of a routine physical examination may be responsible for a patient's being seen by the physician.
3. Syphilis may be seen in conjunction with AIDS. The problem becomes complicated because the serologic test for syphilis may not be positive in patients with AIDS and routine antibiotic dosage regimens may be ineffective.
4. Cardiac, central nervous system, or other organ disease may be a reason for a patient to consult a physician.

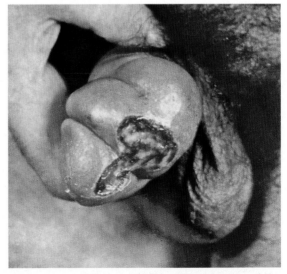

Figure 16-1. Primary syphilis with a chancre of the penis. This chancre is accompanied by marked edema of the penis. (*J.E. Moore and The Upjohn Company*)

To manage these patients properly a thorough knowledge of the natural *untreated* course of the disease is essential.

Primary Syphilis
(Figs. 16-1 and 16-2)

The first stage of acquired syphilis usually develops within 2 to 6 weeks (average 3 weeks) after exposure. The *primary chancre* most commonly occurs on the genitalia, but extragenital chancres are not rare and are often misdiagnosed. Without treatment the chancre heals within 1 to 4 weeks, depending on the location, the amount of secondary infection, and host resistance.

The blood serologic test for syphilis (STS) may be negative in the early days of the chancre

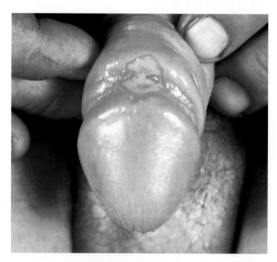

(*A*) Penile chancre.

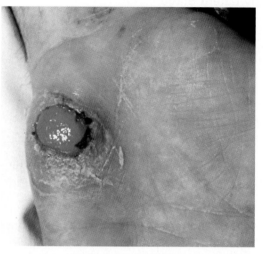

(*B*) Chancre of the palm.

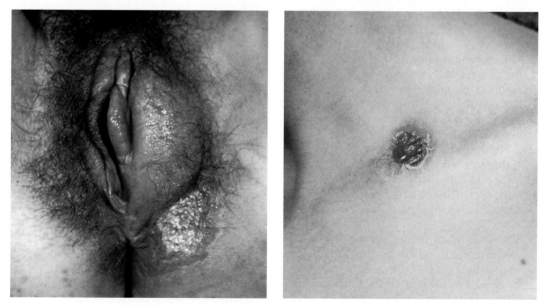

(*C*) Vulvar chancre with edema of the labia majora.

(*D*) Chancre over the clavicle.

Figure 16-2. **Primary syphilis.** (*The Upjohn Company*)

but eventually becomes positive. The spirochete, *Treponema pallidum*, is readily found with dark-field examination. A cerebrospinal fluid examination during the primary stage reveals invasion of the spirochete in approximately 25% of cases.

Clinically, the chancre may vary in appearance from a single small erosion to multiple indurated ulcers of the genitalia. Primary syphilis commonly goes unnoticed in the female patient. Bilateral or unilateral regional lymphadenopathy is common. Malaise and fever may be present.

Early Latent Stage

Latency, manifested by positive serologic findings and no other subjective or objective evidence of syphilis, may occur between the primary and the secondary stages.

Secondary Syphilis
(Figs. 16-3–16-5; see also Fig. 26-12)

Early secondary lesions may develop before the primary chancre has healed or after latency of a few weeks.

Late secondary lesions are more rare and usually are seen after the early secondary lesions have healed.

Both types of secondary lesions contain the spirochete *T. pallidum*, which can be easily seen with the darkfield microscope. The STS is positive (an exception is in a patient with AIDS), and approximately 30% of the cases have abnormal cerebrospinal fluid findings.

Clinically, the early secondary rash can consist of macular, papular, pustular, squamous, or eroded lesions or combinations of any of these lesions. The entire body may be involved or only the palms and the soles, the mouth, or the genitalia. A "moth-eaten" scalp alopecia may develop in the late secondary stage.

Condylomata lata is the name applied to the flat, moist, warty lesions teeming with spirochetes found in the groin and the axillae (see Figs. 16-4 and 16-5).

The late secondary lesions are nodular, squamous, and ulcerative and are distinguished from the tertiary lesions only by the time interval after the onset of the infection and by the finding of the spirochete in superficial smears of serum from the lesions. Annular and semiannular configurations of late secondary lesions are common.

Generalized lymphadenopathy, malaise, fever, and arthralgia occur in many patients with secondary syphilis.

Early Latent Stage

Following the secondary stage, many patients with untreated syphilis have only a positive STS. After 4 years of infection, the patient enters the late latent stage.

Late Latent Stage

This time span of 4 years arbitrarily divides the early infectious stages from the later noninfectious stages, which may or may not develop.

Tertiary Syphilis
(Fig. 16-6; see also Fig. 3-2)

This late stage is manifested by subjective or objective involvement of any of the organs of the body, including the skin. Tertiary changes may be precocious but most often develop 5 to 20 years after the onset of the primary stage. Clinically, the skin lesions are characterized by nodular and gummatous ulcerations (Fig. 16-7). Solitary multiple annular and nodular lesions are common. Subjective complaints are rare unless considerable secondary bacterial infection is present in a gumma. Scarring, on healing, is inevitable in the majority of the tertiary skin lesions. Larger texts should be consulted for the late changes seen in the central nervous system, the cardiovascular system, the bones, the eyes, and the viscera. Approximately 15% of the patients who acquire syphilis and receive no treatment die of the disease.

Late Latent Stage

Another latent period may occur after natural healing of some types of benign tertiary syphilis.

Congenital Syphilis

Congenital syphilis is acquired *in utero* from an infectious mother (Fig. 16-8; see also Fig. 33-4C). The STS required of pregnant women by most states has lowered the incidence of this unfortu-

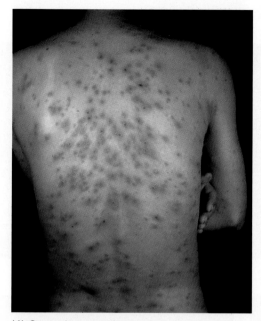

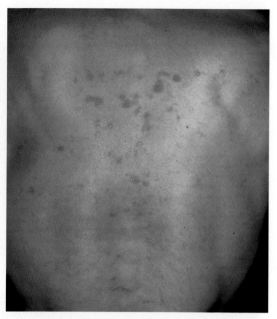

(*A*) Secondary papulosquamous lesions on the back.

(*B*) Papulosquamous lesions on the back.

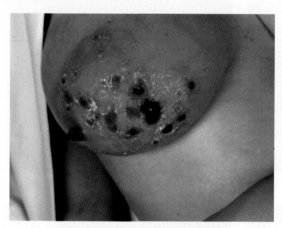

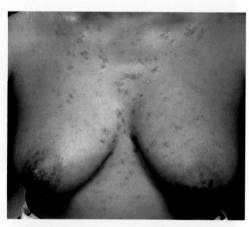

(*C*) Crusted lesions on the breast.

(*D*) Papular lesions on the chest. (*K.U.M.C.*)

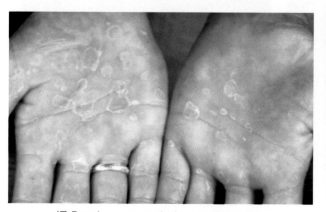

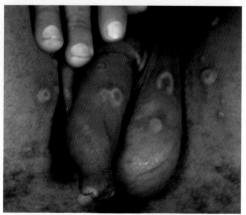

(*E*) Papulosquamous lesions on the palms.

(*F*) Late secondary annular lesions on penis and scrotum.

Figure 16-3. **Secondary syphilis.**

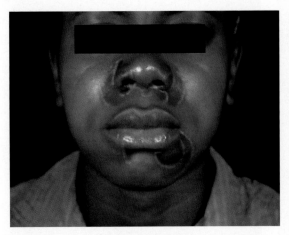

(*A*) Annular lesions.

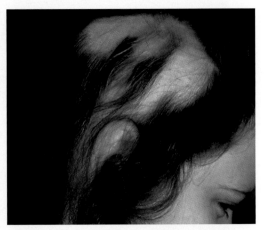

(*B*) Syphilitic alopecia.

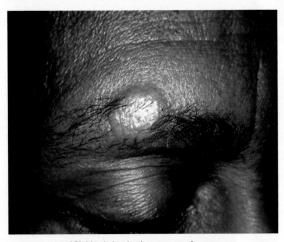

(*C*) Nodular lesion on eyebrow.

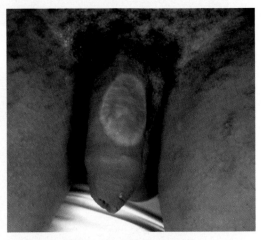

(*D*) Annular lesion on penis.

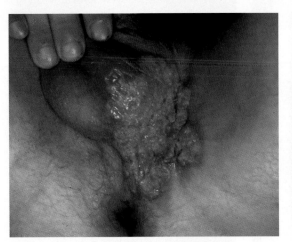

(*E*) Condylomata lata in groin area.

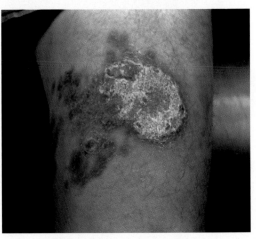

(*F*) Psoriatic-type lesion on leg.

Figure 16-4. **Late secondary syphilis.**

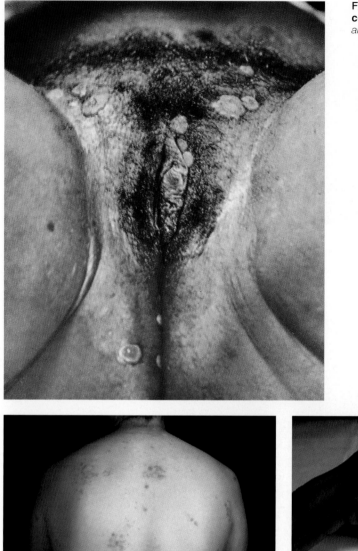

Figure 16-5. **Secondary syphilis with condylomata lata of the vulva.** (*J. E. Moore and The Upjohn Company*)

(*A*) Tertiary grouped papular lesions on the back.

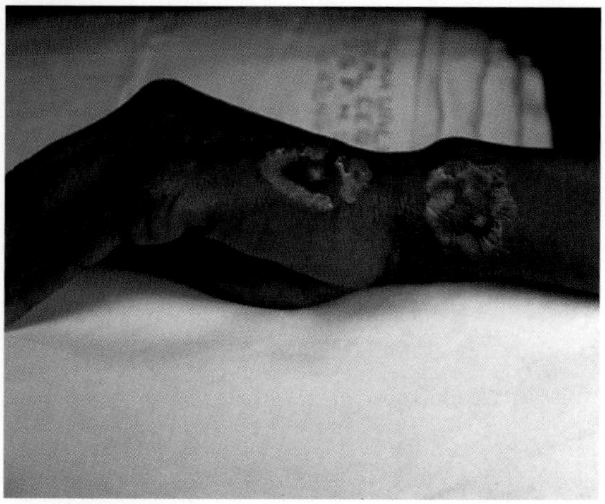

(*B*) Tertiary annula nodular lesions on hand.

Figure 16-6.   **Tertiary and congenital syphilis.**   *(continued)*

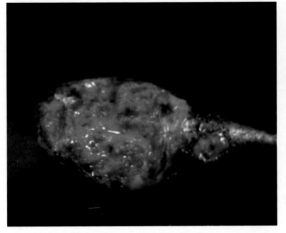

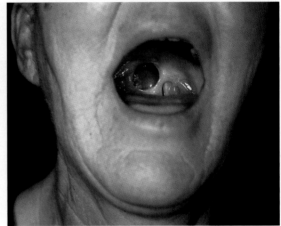

(C) Tertiary gumma on the leg.

(D) Tertiary perforation from old gumma of soft palate.

Figure 16-6. *(Continued)*

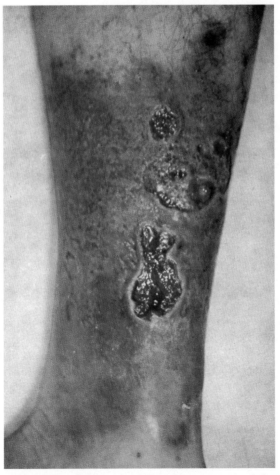

Figure 16-7. **Tertiary syphilis with a gumma of the leg.** This resembles a stasis ulcer. (*J.E. Moore and The Upjohn Company*)

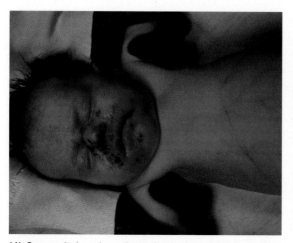

(*A*) Congenital scaly and erosive lesions with large liver (fatal).

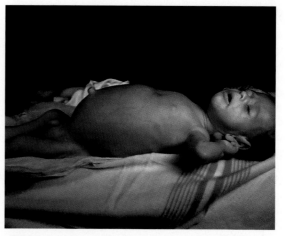

(*B*) Congenital syphilis with massively enlarged liver and spleen.

Figure 16-8. **Congenital syphilis.**

nate disease. Stillbirths are not uncommon from mothers who are untreated. After the birth of a live infected child, the mortality rate depends on the duration of the infection, the natural host resistance, and the rapidity of initiating correct treatment. Early and late lesions are seen in these children, similar to those found in the adult cases of acquired syphilis. Blistering can occur.

Laboratory Findings

DARKFIELD EXAMINATION

The etiologic agent, *T. pallidum*, can be found in the serum from the primary or secondary lesions. However, a darkfield microscope is necessary, and very few physician's offices or laboratories have this instrument. A considerable amount of experience is necessary to distinguish *T. pallidum* from other *Treponema* species.

SEROLOGIC TEST FOR SYPHILIS

The STS is simple and readily available and has several modifications. The rapid plasma reagin (RPR) test and the Venereal Disease Research Laboratories (VDRL) flocculation test are used most commonly. The fluorescent treponemal antibody absorption (FTA-ABS) test and modifications are more difficult to perform in the laboratory and therefore are used primarily when the RPR and VDRL tests are "reactive."

When a report is received from the laboratory that the STS is positive (RPR- or VDRL-reactive), a second blood specimen should be submitted to obtain a *quantitative* report. In many laboratories this repeat test is not necessary, because a quantitative test is run routinely on all positive blood specimens. A dilution of 1 : 2 is only weakly positive and might be a biologic false-positive reaction. A test positive in a dilution of 1 : 32 is strongly positive. In evaluating the response of the STS to treatment, one must remember that a change in titer from 1 : 2 to 1 : 4 to 1 : 16 to 1 : 32 to 1 : 64, or downward in the same gradations, is only a change in one tube, in each instance. Thus a change from 1 : 2 to 1 : 4 is of the same magnitude as a change from 1 : 32 to 1 : 64. Quantitative tests enable the physician to (1) evaluate the efficacy of the treatment, (2) discover a relapse before it becomes infectious, (3) differentiate between a relapse and a reinfection, (4) establish a reaction as a seroresistant type, and (5) differentiate between true and biologic false-positive serologic reactions.

In most laboratories it is now routine to do an FTA-ABS test on all patients with reactive RPR and VDRL tests. With rare exceptions, a positive FTA-ABS test means that the patient has or had syphilis and is not a biologic false-positive reactor.

The serologic test for syphilis may not be positive in patients with AIDS.

TISSUE EXAMINATION

A direct fluorescent antibody test for *T. pallidum* (DFA-TP) can be performed on lesion exudate or on biopsy tissue.

CEREBROSPINAL FLUID TEST

As has been stated, the cerebrospinal fluid is frequently positive in the primary and secondary stages of the disease. Invasion of the central nervous system is an early manifestation, even though the perceptible clinical effects are a late manifestation. The cerebrospinal fluid should be examined at least once during the course of the disease. Cerebrospinal fluid examination is appropriate for all patients with syphilis who are at a high risk for human immunodeficiency virus (HIV) infection. The best routine is to perform a cerebrospinal fluid test before treatment is initiated and repeat the test as indicated. If the cerebrospinal fluid is negative in a patient who has had syphilis for 4 years, central nervous system syphilis will not occur, and future cerebrospinal fluid tests are not necessary. If the test is positive, repeat tests should be done every 6 months for 4 years.

The following three tests are run on the cerebrospinal fluid:

1. *Cell count*: The finding of four or more lymphocytes or polymorphonuclear leukocytes per cubic millimeter is positive. The cell count is the most labile of the tests. It becomes increased early in the infection and responds fastest to therapy. Therefore, it is a good index of activity of the disease. The cell count must be done within an hour after the fluid is withdrawn.
2. *Total protein*: Measured in milligrams per deciliter, it normally should be below 40.
3. *Nontreponemal flocculation test*: Presently, the most common test performed is the qualitative and quantitative VDRL. This test is the last to turn positive and the slowest to return to negativity. In some cases, therapy causes a decrease in the titer, but slight positivity or "fastness" can remain for the lifetime of the patient.

Differential Diagnosis

Primary syphilis: From chancroid, herpes simplex, fusospirochetal balanitis, granuloma inguinale, and any of the *primary chancre-type diseases* (see Dictionary–Index).
Secondary syphilis: From any of the papulosquamous diseases (especially pityriasis rosea), fungal diseases, drug eruption, and alopecia areata.
Tertiary skin syphilis: From any of the granulomatous diseases, particularly tuberculosis, leprosy, sarcoidosis, deep mycoses, and lymphomas.
Congenital syphilis: From atopic eczema, diseases with lymphadenopathy, hepatomegaly, and splenomegaly.

A *true-positive syphilitic serology* is to be differentiated from a *biologic false-positive reaction*. This serologic differentiation is accomplished best by using the FTA-ABS test, or its modifications, along with a good history and a thorough examination of the patient. Many patients with biologic false-positive reactions develop one of the collagen diseases at a later date.

Treatment

A 22-year-old married man presents with a sore 1 cm in diameter on his glans penis of 5 days' duration. Three weeks previously he had extramarital intercourse, and 10 days before this office visit he had marital intercourse.

FIRST VISIT

1. Perform a darkfield examination of the penile lesion. Treatment can be started if *T. pallidum* is found. *If you cannot perform a darkfield examination, refer the patient to the local health department or another facility that can perform a darkfield examination.*
2. If a darkfield examination cannot be performed or is negative, obtain a blood specimen for an STS.
3. While waiting for the STS report, advise the patient to soak the site in saline solution for 15 minutes twice a day. The solution is made by placing 1/4 teaspoon of salt in a glass of water.
4. Advise the patient against sexual intercourse until the reports are completed.
5. Explain to the patient the seriousness of treating him for syphilis if he does not have it. The "syphilitic" label is one he should not want, if it is at all possible to avoid it.

SECOND VISIT

Three days later the lesion is larger and the STS report is "nonreactive."

1. Obtain blood specimen for a second STS.
2. Antibiotic ointment   15.0
   Sig: Apply t.i.d. locally after soaking in saline solution.
3. Explain again why you are delaying therapy until a definite diagnosis is made.

THIRD VISIT

Three days later the sore is smaller, but the STS report is "reactive." The diagnosis is now known to be "primary syphilis."

1. The patient is reassured that present-day therapy is highly successful but that he must follow your instructions closely.
2. His wife should be brought in for examination and a blood test. If the blood test is negative, it should be repeated weekly for 1 month. However, some syphilologists believe that therapy is indicated for the marital partner in the presence of a negative STS if the husband has infectious syphilis and is being treated. A single injection of 2.4 million units of a long-acting type of penicillin is used. This prevents "ping-pong" syphilis, which is a cycle of reinfection from one marital partner to another.
3. The patient's contact should be found. The patient knows her only as "Jane," and he cannot remember over which bar she presided. Report these findings to the local health department.
4. A cerebrospinal fluid specimen should be obtained. (The report was returned as normal for all three tests.)
5. Penicillin therapy should be begun. Here, two factors are important:
   a. The dose must be adequate.
   b. The duration of effective blood levels of medication must be maintained over 10 to 14 days.

DOSAGE

Primary and Secondary Syphilis
1. Administer 2.4 million units of benzathine penicillin G, half in each buttock, single session.
2. Consult larger texts or relevant literature for other treatment schedules.

Latent (Both Early and Late) Syphilis
1. If no cerebrospinal fluid examination, administer 7.2 million units benzathine penicillin G divided into three weekly injections.
2. If cerebrospinal fluid examination is nonreactive, give 2.4 million units in single dose.

Neurosyphilis or Cardiovascular Syphilis
1. Administer 9 to 12 million units of a long-acting penicillin.
2. For other routines or complicated cases, consult larger texts for therapy and care.

3. HIV-infected patients with neurosyphilis should be treated for 10 days at least with aqueous crystalline penicillin G in a dosage of 2 to 4 million units intravenously every 4 hours.

Benign Late Syphilis
Same as neurosyphilis.

Congenital Syphilis
1. Early congenital syphilis
   a. Younger than 6 months of age: Aqueous procaine penicillin G, 10 daily intramuscular doses totaling 100,000 to 200,000 units/kg.
   b. Six months to 2 years of age: As above, *or* benzathine penicillin G, 100,000 units/kg intramuscularly in one single dose.
2. Late congenital syphilis
   a. Ages 2 to 11 years, or weighing less than 70 pounds: Same as for 6 months to 2 years.
   b. Twelve years or older, but weighing more than 70 pounds: Same treatment as for adult-acquired syphilis, with comparable time and progression of infection.

LYME DISEASE

Originally described as Lyme arthritis, Lyme disease is caused by a spirochete that is transmitted by several species of *Ixodes* tick. Early removal of the tick (<24 hours) usually prevents disease transmission. The disease has been reported from most states and on every continent except Antarctica. Endemic areas include the northeastern United States and the upper midwestern states. Clinical manifestations include erythema chronicum migrans (ECM) skin lesions, flu-like symptoms, and possible neurologic, cardiac, and rheumatologic involvement.

Late manifestations of Lyme disease are *acrodermatitis chronica atrophicans* and, although controversial, possibly in some cases (especially in Europe) *morphea (localized scleroderma)*.

PRIMARY LESION. The erythematous circular rash appears at the site of the tick bite and enlarges with central clearing, but multiple ECM eruptions can occur. The rash typically develops from 2 to 30 days after the bite. The bite area can become necrotic.

SECONDARY LESION. Multiple ECM eruptions can develop.

DISTRIBUTION. Usually ECM begins at the site of the tick bite.

SEASON. The disease occurs from late May through early fall.

COURSE. In untreated patients the ECM lesions may last only 10 to 14 days, they may persist for months, or they may come and go over a year's time. The bite papule and ECM fade rapidly after therapy is begun. Late-stage cutaneous lesions include acrodermatitis chronic atrophicans and borrelia lymphocytoma (see Chap 26).

SUBJECTIVE COMPLAINTS. Flu-like symptoms, with fever, chills, myalgia, and headache, appear with the rash. Later other organs may be affected.

ETIOLOGY. The spirochete *Borrelia burgdorferi* is transmitted by *Ixodes* species of ticks and possibly by the hard-bodied ticks. The white-tailed deer and white-footed mouse are preferred hosts of the tick.

DIAGNOSIS. High index of suspicion, history of tick bite (patient is not always aware of bite), previous "ringworm-type" rash, and, later, positive Lyme disease antibody titer may be present (but these tests are not reliable).

The histology is not specific, and culture of the spirochete is often not practical. Polymerase chain reaction may be helpful on biopsy tissue in a qualified laboratory.

Differential Diagnosis

Cutaneously the ECM rash can resemble an allergic reaction or tinea.

Systemically many diseases can be considered, with fever, myalgia, cardiac, joint, or neurologic manifestations.

Treatment

Because diagnosis of Lyme disease is difficult, treatment may be indicated, especially in endemic areas, based on history and clinical findings.

Early therapy for this disease is doxycycline, 100 mg, b.i.d. for 21 days, or amoxicillin, 500 mg, t.i.d. for 21 days. Early tick removal in less than 24 hours probably prevents disease transmission. Removing deer and mice habitats such as brush, leaves, stonewalls, and woodpiles may be helpful.

For late stages of the disease with cardiac or neurologic manifestations, treatment is ceftriaxone, 2 to 4 grams/day IM or IV for 14 days. Since efficacy of therapy is difficult to evaluate, the literature is replete with other therapeutic regimens. Lyme vaccination is effective and should be considered in people at high risk in endemic areas. It takes 12 months to confer immunity.

Lymephobia is a common psychological problem due to the nonspecific nature of symptoms and the lack of specific tests. Permethrin 5% applied to clothing is a helpful tick repellant.

SAUER NOTES: SYPHILIS

1. Any patient treated for gonorrhea should have a serologic test for syphilis (STS) 4 to 6 weeks later.
2. Persons with HIV infection acquired through sexual contact or intravenous drug abuse should be tested for syphilis.
3. Seventy-five percent of the persons who acquire syphilis suffer no serious manifestations of the disease.
4. Syphilis does not cause vesicular or bullous skin lesions, except in infants with congenital infection.

PRIMARY STAGE

1. *Syphilis should be ruled in or out in the diagnosis of any penile or vulvar sores.*
2. Multiple primary chancres are moderately common.

SECONDARY STAGE

1. The rash of secondary syphilis, except for the rare follicular form, does not itch.
2. Secondary syphilis should be ruled in or out in any patient with a generalized, nonpruritic rash. A high index of suspicion is necessary.

LATENT STAGE

The diagnosis of "latent syphilis" cannot be made for a particular patient unless cerebrospinal fluid tests have been done and are negative for syphilis.

TERTIARY STAGE

1. Tertiary syphilis should be considered in any patient with a chronic granuloma of the skin, particularly if it has an annular or circular configuration.

2. Invasion of the central nervous system occurs in the primary and secondary stages of the disease. A cerebrospinal fluid test is indicated during these stages.

3. If the cerebrospinal fluid tests for syphilis are negative in a patient who has had syphilis for 4 years, central nervous system syphilis usually will not occur, and future spinal punctures are not necessary.

4. Twenty percent of patients with late asymptomatic neurosyphilis have a negative STS.

CONGENITAL SYPHILIS

An STS should be done on every pregnant woman to prevent congenital syphilis of the newborn. Congenital syphilis has been rapidly increasing in prevalence in the past decade.

SEROLOGY

1. The STS may be negative in the early days of the primary chancre. The STS is always positive in the secondary stage; an exception to this is in patients with AIDS.

2. A quantitative STS should be done on all syphilitic patients to evaluate the response to treatment or the development of relapse or reinfection.

3. The finding of a low-titer STS in a patient not previously treated for syphilis calls for a careful evaluation to rule out a *biologic false-positive reaction*.

BIBLIOGRAPHY

Syphilis

Baum EW, et al. Secondary syphilis, still the great imitator. JAMA 1983;249:3069.

Bennet ML, Lynn AW, Klein LE. Congenital syphilis: Subtle presentation of fulminant disease. J Am Acad Dermatol 1997;36:2.

Centers for Disease Control. Recommendations for diagnosing and treating syphilis in HIV-infected patients. Arch Dermatol 1989;125:15.

Centers for Disease Control. Treatment guidelines for sexually transmitted diseases. Fitzpatrick's J Clin Dermatol 1994;1:40.

Don PC, Rubenstein R, Christie S. Malignant syphilis (lues maligna) and concurrent infection with HIV. Int J Dermatol 1995;34:403.

Sexually Transmitted Diseases (STD) Bulletin. Monthly. F&M Projects, 152 Madison Avenue, New York, NY 10016.

Lyme Disease

Abele DC, Anders KH. The many faces and phases of borreliosis: I. Lyme disease. J Am Acad Dermatol 1990;23:167.

Abele DC, Anders KH. The many faces and phases of borreliosis: II. J Am Acad Dermatol 1990;23:401.

Burlington DB. FDA public health advisory: Assays for antibodies to Borrelia brugdorferi: Limitations, use, and interpretation for supporting a clinical diagnosis of lyme disease. FDA, July 7, 1997.

Golde WT. A vaccine for Lyme lisease: Current progress. Infections in Medicine 1998.

Lyme Disease-United States, 1996. Arch Dermatol 1997;133.

Stere AC, Taylor E, McHugh GL, et al. The overdiagnosis of Lyme disease. JAMA 1993;269:1812.

Treatment of Lyme disease. Med Lett 1997;39.

Trevisan G, Cinco M. Lyme disease. Int J Dermatol 1990;29:1.

17

Dermatologic Virology

Virus diseases of the skin are exceedingly common. The various clinical entities are distinct, and, because we have no specific antiviral drug, the treatment varies for each entity. The following list contains the virus diseases that are discussed here. The exanthems of children are covered in a cursory manner.

- Herpes simplex
- Kaposi's varicelliform eruption
- Zoster
- Chickenpox
- Smallpox, vaccinia, and cowpox
- Warts
- Molluscum contagiosum
- Lymphogranuloma venereum
- Exanthematous disease: measles, German measles, roseola, and erythema infectiosum

The human immunodeficiency virus (HIV) and the acquired immunodeficiency syndrome (AIDS) are discussed in Chapter 18.

HERPES VIRUSES
(Figs. 17-1 and 17-2)

Herpes simplex (fever blister) is an acute, moderately painful, viral eruption of a single group of vesicles that commonly occurs around the mouth or the genitalia. The most common type of herpes simplex is the *recurrent form* seen in adults.

An uncommon *primary form* of herpes simplex affects children and young adults. In this primary form, the vesicular lesions involve the mouth and the pharynx or vaginal and vulvar areas. High fever, regional lymphadenopathy, and general malaise accompany the painful sores that are often more severe than recurrent episodes. Most persons go through their primary infection with the herpesvirus without clinical manifestations and with only minimal lesions.

The following discussion refers to the common *recurrent form* of herpes simplex.

PRIMARY LESIONS. A group of vesicles appears.

SECONDARY LESIONS. Erosions and secondary bacterial infection are seen.

DISTRIBUTION. Lips, mouth, genital region of both males and females (herpes progenitalis), eye (marginal keratitis or corneal ulcer), distal finger (herpetic whitlow), or any body area may be involved.

COURSE. The vesicles last for 2 to 3 days before the tops come off. The residual erosions or crusted lesions last for another 5 to 7 days. Recurrences are common in the same area.

ETIOLOGY. The disease is caused by a relatively large DNA virus, the herpes simplex virus (HSV). There are two antigenically and biologi-

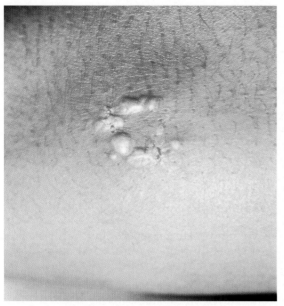

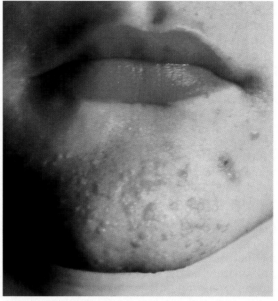

(*A*) Herpes simplex on arm.

(*B*) Herpes simplex on chin.

Figure 17-1.   **Dermatologic virology.**

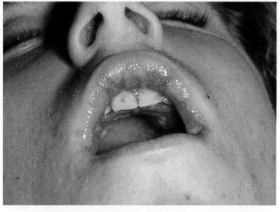

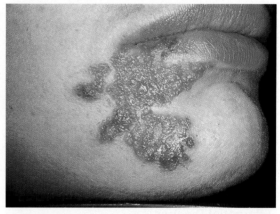

(*A*) Primary herpes simplex lips and interoral.

(*B*) Recurrent herpes simplex on chin with secondary bacterial infection.

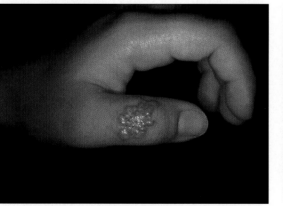

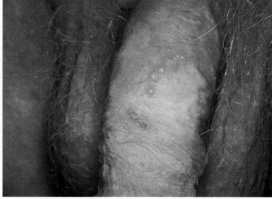

(*C*) Recurrent herpes simplex on a thumb.

(*D*) Recurrent herpes simplex on the penis.

Figure 17-2.   **Herpes simplex.** (*Dermik Laboratories, Inc.*)

cally different strains of the virus. Type 1 HSV is associated with most nongenital herpetic infections. Type 2 HSV occurs chiefly in association with genital infection and is venereally transmitted. However, herpetic pharyngitis in homosexual men is frequently caused by type 2 virus. Either viral type can "take" at any site on the body, if appropriately inoculated.

Certain precipitating factors are important in producing the recurrent eruptions. These factors, which include fever, common "cold," sunlight, immunodeficiency, psychic influences, stomach upsets, and trauma, apparently activate a dormant phase of the virus in the dorsal root ganglia.

CONTAGIOUSNESS. The disease is spread through intimate contact. On the average, recurrent herpes lesions "shed" infectious HSV for approximately 5 days after onset of the lesions. However, asymptomatic shedding of the HSV also occurs and is a major epidemiologic problem.

LABORATORY FINDINGS. The HSV may be isolated from the lesions by culture. If available, the polymerase chain reaction test is diagnostic. Cytodiagnosis slides (Tzanok preparation) (see Chap. 2) reveal large bizarre mononucleate and multinucleate giant cells and nuclear changes of "ballooning degeneration." The giant cells contain eight to ten nuclei, varying in size and shape. Occasionally, one may identify intranuclear inclusion bodies in these smears. Biopsy findings are also characteristic. Neutralizing antibodies in the blood show an increasing titer.

Differential Diagnosis

MOUTH LESIONS

Aphthous stomatitis: Only one or two painful, eroded lesions in the mouth not in a circumscribed area covered with grayish-white pseudomembrane, may be at sites of trauma; recurrent but at different sites; not caused by HSV (see Chap. 29).

BODY LESIONS

Zoster: More than one group of vesicles; nerve segment distribution; not recurrent at same site; different virus (see later section in this chapter).
Tinea of body: Early vesicular case can be clinically indistinguishable from herpes; later,

central healing in tinea; fungus grown from scraping by culture or seen from scraping with KOH preparation (see Chap. 19).

GENITAL LESIONS

Primary syphilis: Can be clinically similar to herpes simplex; history of sexual promiscuity; not recurrent, usually; darkfield examination is definitely indicated and would be positive, but this test is rarely available (see Chap. 16).

Treatment

A young woman presents with fever blisters on her lower lip that have recurred every 2 or 3 months for the past 2 years.

1. Acyclovir (Zovirax) therapy
   a. Acyclovir capsules, 400 mg #18
   Sig: 3 capsules a day for 5 days, in divided doses while awake.
   Comment: When therapy is begun at the early stages of the herpes simplex, acyclovir is more effective. The patient should be told to save 3 capsules to initiate early therapy if there is a future recurrence. There is evidence that this regimen shortens the course of the disease and also minimizes the discomfort. The current literature should be consulted for the dosage and side effects of an extended therapy regimen with acyclovir, which supposedly prevents recurrences. For instance, one routine is to prescribe acyclovir, 400 mg, b.i.d. for 6 months. (See following section).
   b. Acyclovir ointment, 5%   15.0
   Sig: Apply locally six times a day for 7 days. See directions on package insert.
   Comment: This therapy is indicated for the management of the *primary herpes simplex* eruption, along with a longer course of oral capsules. But there is some evidence that this local therapy favorably affects the course of *recurrent herpes simplex*, if it is used early.
   c. Penciclovir (Denavir) ointment, 1% 2 gram
   Sig: Apply locally 6 times a day for 7 days.
2. Valacyclovir (Valtrex) capsules, 500 mg, #10
   Sig: 1 p.o. b.i.d. for acute episodes or 1 p.o. q. day for prophylaxis
3. Famciclovir (Famvir) capsules 500 mg
   Sig: 125 mg capsule b.i.d. for 5 days for acute episodes, or 250 mg p.o. b.i.d. for prophylactic.
4. Antibiotic and corticosteroid ointment mixture q.s.   15.0
   Sig: Apply locally q.i.d.

Comment: This relieves the pain and the inflammation.

5. Burow's solution: Domeboro packet, one per quart of cold water.
   Sig: Apply as a cold wet compress for 20 minutes three times a day to relieve much of the pain and irritation.
6. Sunscreen preparations applied to the lips can prevent sun-induced herpes simplex.

RECURRENT GENITAL HERPES SIMPLEX

The management is the same as described previously. The long-term use of acyclovir capsules in a dosage of 400 mg b.i.d. for 5 to 6 months or famciclovir 250 mg b.i.d. or valacyclovin 500 mg a day is somewhat effective in preventing or decreasing the frequency of recurrence.

The difficult management problem with recurrent genital herpes simplex is that women and men are frightened of the disease and of the effect of herpes on a newborn. This serious problem of infecting the newborn is rare but has received a lot of lay publicity. The parents should be reassured that this is a rare complication of herpes simplex. If the mother, after careful examination, does not have the infection at the time of birth, the chance of infection of the infant is low. If the mother has herpes lesions before delivery, she can have cesarean section delivery and should the newborn get herpes simplex, therapy with acyclovir is beneficial; however, this is a serious problem.

Genital herpes simplex has been increasing since the 1970s, and its therapy and prevention are important because it can facilitate the transmission of the human immunodeficiency virus.

Human Herpesvirus 6 (HHV-6)

HHV-6 is the probable cause of roseola infantum (exanthem subitum, sixth disease). Ten percent of cases may be caused by human herpesvirus 8 (HHV-8).

Roseola is a common exanthem of children of 6 to 18 months of age. The incubation period is 10 days, but a contact history is rarely helpful. Characteristically, there is a temperature up to as high as 105°F (40.6°C) for 4 to 5 days. With the appearance of the rash the fever and the malaise subside. The rash is mainly on the trunk as a faint, red, macular eruption. It fades in a few days.

HHV-6 is rarely associated with fulminant hepatitis, hemophagocytosis, encephalitis, and pneumonia.

HHV-6 is associated with the acute rash of graft-versus-host disease and chronic fatigue syndrome.

Human Herpesvirus 7 (HHV-7)

HHV-7 may cause hepatitis and infectious mononucleosis-like syndrome.

Human Herpes Simplex 8 (HHS-8)

HHS-8 is associated with Kaposi's sarcoma in HIV-positive and -negative patients as well as angiosarcoma and angiolymphoid hyperplasia with eosinophilia.

KAPOSI'S VARICELLIFORM ERUPTION
(Fig. 17-3)

Kaposi's varicelliform eruption is an uncommon but severe complication in children who have atopic eczema. It is rarely associated with other widespread skin diseases. It results from self-inoculation by scratching, due to the virus of either herpes simplex (eczema herpeticum) or vaccinia. In the former type, a history of exposure to fever blisters may or may not be obtained. The vaccinia form (eczema vaccinatum) should be nonexistent now. With either type, the child is acutely ill, has a high fever, and has generalized, umbilicated, chickenpox-like skin lesions.

Acyclovir administered intravenously has proved beneficial in halting the progression of the disease and in promoting faster healing.

Supportive therapy consists of antibiotics systemically, intravenous infusions, and a calamine-like shake lotion, locally.

HERPESVIRUS INFECTION IN IMMUNOCOMPROMISED PATIENTS

Severe, ulcerative, life-threatening HSV infections can develop in immunocompromised children and adults who have undergone organ transplantation, have lymphomas or advanced metastatic carcinoma, have AIDS, or are receiving systemic corticosteroid or antimetabolite therapy.

Intravenous acyclovir or famciclovir therapy is helpful in controlling the viral proliferation.

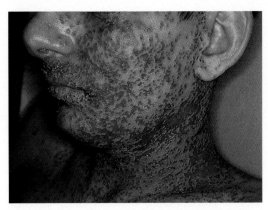

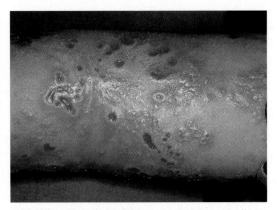

(*A*) Kaposi's varicelliform eruption: herpes simplex inoculated on atopic eczema.

(*B*) Kaposi's varicelliform eruption: smallpox vaccination inoculated on atopic eczema, age 4.

Figure 17-3.   **Kaposi's varicelliform eruption.** (*Glaxo Dermatology*)

ZOSTER
(Fig. 17-4; see also Figs. 18-2, 26-11A–C, and 34-7B)

Shingles is a common viral disease characterized by the appearance of several groups of vesicles distributed along a cutaneous nerve segment. Zoster and chickenpox are caused by the same virus. Susceptible children or rarely adults who are exposed to cases of zoster may develop chickenpox.

PRIMARY LESIONS. Multiple groups of vesicles or crusted lesions appear.

SECONDARY LESIONS. Bacterial infection with pustules occurs, rarely progressing to hemorrhagic gangrenous ulcers and scarring.

DISTRIBUTION. Unilateral eruption follows a nerve distribution, frequently in the thoracic region, the face, the neck, and, less frequently, the lumbosacral area and elsewhere. Eye involvement can be serious. Bilateral involvement of the body is rare but not fatal, contrary to the old wives' tale, and still predominates on one side of the body.

COURSE. New crops of vesicles can appear for 3 to 5 days. The vesicles then dry up and form crusts, which take 3 weeks, on the average, to disappear. The general health is seldom affected, except for low-grade fever and malaise. Recurrences are rare. The *post-herpetic pain* can persist for months or years in aged patients.

SUBJECTIVE COMPLAINTS. Pain of a neuritic type can precede the eruption and, if in the abdominal area, can lead to erroneous diagnoses and surgical procedures. The common simple pain of young persons with shingles is readily

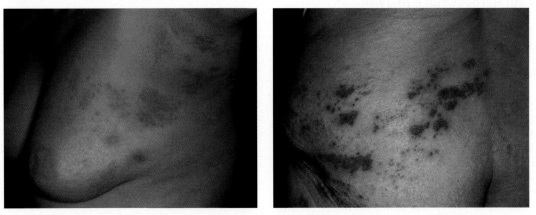

(*A*) Herpes zoster of left breast area.

(*B*) Hemorrhagic zoster of left hip area.

Figure 17-4.   **Zoster.** (*Dermik Laboratories, Inc.*)

treated and soon disappears. On the other hand, the severe, true post-herpetic pain of older patients can be very serious. To evaluate critically the therapeutic response to the many agents said to relieve this severe pain, *a nerve-distribution pain should not be labeled as the true post-herpetic type unless it has been present for over 30 days.* If this strict criterion is adhered to, many newly proclaimed treatments for such pain are found to be of limited value, but usage is common considering their low risk of side effects. For the best results use early in the course of disease.

ETIOLOGY. Zoster is caused by the same virus that causes chickenpox. Trauma of the nerve root is believed to play a role in development of some cases of shingles. "Nervousness" plays little if any role.

Severe cases of herpes zoster can develop in immunocompromised patients (see Chap. 18).

CONTAGIOUSNESS. The interrelationship between shingles and chickenpox has been referred to previously. You cannot catch shingles from someone with shingles.

LABORATORY FINDINGS. A cytodiagnostic test (Tzanck test) is positive for multinucleated giant cells. A culture or a polymerase chain reaction can be done.

Differential Diagnosis

Of the neuritic-type pain that precedes the skin lesions: Appendicitis, ureteral colic, sciatica, myocardial infarction, migraine, and so on.
Of the eruption: Herpes simplex (see single group of vesicles, recurrence history, refer to preceding section); blistered burn from hot application for neuritic pain (very commonly the patient really has shingles and erroneously attributes the blisters to the hot application for the preceding herpetic pain).

Treatment

CASE 1

A 40-year-old woman presents with multiple grouped vesicles on right cheek and forehead, causing moderately severe pain.

1. Reassure the patient that shingles, except in the elderly, is not a serious disease, and advise her not to believe what her well-meaning friends tell her about the disease.
2. Supply the name of an ophthalmologist to consult, to rule in or out eye complications if lesions are near the eye or on the end of the nose.
3. Hydrocortisone 1% lotion q.s.   60.0
   Sig: Apply locally to skin b.i.d.
4. Analgesic tablets   #50
   Sig: 1 to 2 tablets q.i.d. as needed for pain.
5. Acyclovir (Zovirax) capsules, 800 mg   #50
   Sig: 5 capsules a day in divided doses for 10 days.
   Comment: This therapy is not indicated for every case of zoster, but it is prescribed frequently. Valacyclovir (Valtrex) or famciclovir (Famvir) can be used and have the advantage of requiring less capsules per day. Early therapy is important to make disease less severe and decrease chance of postherpetic neuralgia.

CASE 2

A 70-year-old man presents with extensive zoster on the right side of the buttocks and down the thigh.

1. The therapy and admonitions in the previous case apply also.
2. Systemic therapy:
   a. Acyclovir (Zovirax) capsules, 800 mg #50
   Sig: 5 capsules a day in divided doses for 10 days.
   b. Famciclovir (Famvir) tablets, 500 mg   #21
   Sig: 1 tablet t.i.d. for 7 days.
   c. Valacyclovir (Valtrex) 1000 mg per tab #21
   Sig: 1 tablet t.i.d. for 7 days.

CASE 3

A 70-year-old man presents with severe post-herpetic pain of 5 weeks' duration.

1. Reassure him that most patients who have post-herpetic pain lose it gradually, day by day, week by week. It is extremely rare for the pain to remain persistent, but, when this does happen, it can be disabling. Be optimistic, however. The following treatment can alleviate the neuritis.
2. Capsaicin (Zostrix) cream, 45 g
   Sig: Apply three to four times a day locally. This treatment is of benefit for some patients.
3. Prednisone tablets, 10 mg   #40
   Sig: 2 tablets every morning for 6 days; then decrease dose slowly as symptoms subside.
4. Sedative capsule   #10

Sig: 1 capsule h.s. for sleep.
5. Doxepin (Zonalon) cream, 30 g and 45 g.
   Sig: Thin coat 4 to 5 times a day as needed for pain. This can cause drowsiness.
6. For resistant cases, consult larger texts for additional therapy or refer the patient to a pain clinic.

CASE 4

A 28-year-old man with AIDS has an extensive case of zoster on the right chest wall and also disseminated lesions.

Hospitalization is necessary for supportive therapy and for intravenous acyclovir therapy (see Chap. 18).

CHICKENPOX

Chickenpox is a common viral disease of childhood that is characterized by the development of tense vesicles, first on the trunk and then spreading, to a milder extent, to the face and the extremities. New crops of vesicles appear for 3 to 5 days, and healing of the individual lesions occurs in a week. The disease occurs 10 to 14 days after exposure to another child with chickenpox or to an adult with zoster. The clear vesicle becomes a pustule and then a crusted lesion before dropping off. Itching is more prominent during the healing stage.

Treatment

1. Usually nothing indicated, *or*
2. Menthol   0.25%
   Nonalcoholic white shake lotion (see Formulary in Chap. 5) or hydrocortisone, 1% lotion q.s.   120.0
   Sig: Apply locally t.i.d. for itching.
3. Benadryl hydrochloride elixir   60.0
   Sig: 1 teaspoon t.i.d. for moderately severe itching.
4. Oral acyclovir results in fewer lesions, more rapid healing, decreased symptoms, and less risk of complications.
5. Immunocompromised patients need to be treated with IV acyclovir, to avoid systemic complications such as pneumonitis, hepatitis, and encephalitis.
6. Immunization with live attenuated vaccine has recently been recommended, and the number of cases should be decreasing substantially.

SMALLPOX

Smallpox is an apparently eradicated viral disease. For historical interest here are some facts about smallpox and vaccination.

Smallpox is characterized by the development, after an incubation period of 1 to 3 weeks, of prodromal symptoms of high fever, chills, and various aches. After 3 to 4 days a rash develops, with lowering of the fever. The individual lesions are most extensive on the face and the extremities; they come out as a single shower and progress from papule to vesicle and, in 5 to 10 days, to pustule. With the occurrence of the pustule the fever goes up again, with a high white blood cell count. Hemorrhagic lesions usually indicate a severe form of the disease.

Alastrim is a mild form of smallpox resulting from a less virulent strain of the virus.

Varioloid is a mild form of smallpox that occurs in vaccinated persons. However, this strain of virus is very virulent, and when transmitted to a nonvaccinated person often causes a fulminating disease.

Severe systemic complications of smallpox include pneumonia, secondary bacterial skin infection, and encephalitis.

Treatment

Prophylactic treatment consists of vaccination. The best technique is by multiple puncture.

VACCINIA

Vaccinia is produced by the inoculation of the vaccinia virus into the skin of a person who has no immunity.

The *primary vaccination reaction* follows this timetable (the multiple puncture technique should be used): A red papule on a red base develops on the fourth day, becomes vesicular in 3 more days and pustular in 2 to 3 more days, and then gradually dries to form a crust, which drops off within 3 to 4 weeks after the vaccination. A mild systemic reaction may occur during the pustular stage. The vaccination site should be kept dry and uncovered.

Generalized vaccinia is rare but can occur from autoinoculation, by scratching, in atopic eczema patients (see *eczema vaccinatum*, earlier in this chapter). A biologic false-positive serologic test for syphilis develops in approximately 20% of vaccinated persons. The test becomes negative within 2 to 4 months.

A *vaccinoid reaction* develops in a partially immune person. A pustule with some surrounding redness occurs within 1 week.

An *immune reaction* consists of a papule that develops in 2 days, which may or may not persist for 1 week.

An *absent reaction* indicates that the vaccine was inactivated by the procedure (*e.g.*, alcohol used in cleaning the site) or that the vaccine was impotent.

A successful vaccination offers protection from smallpox within 3 weeks, and this immunity lasts for approximately 7 years or longer.

COWPOX

Jenner used the cowpox virus to vaccinate humans against smallpox. For that reason, the vaccinia virus and the cowpox virus have been believed to be the same. Evidence now exists that proves these viruses to be different, presumably as a result of a change in the vaccinia virus through years of passage. The term *cowpox* is now reserved for the viral disease of cows that occurs in Europe. Humans can get the disease from infected teats and udders. A solitary nodule appears, usually on the hand, which eventually suppurates and then heals in 4 to 8 weeks.

WARTS (VERRUCAE)
(Fig. 17-5; see Fig. 28-10)

Warts, or verrucae, are very common small tumors of the skin. It is doubtful if any human escapes this viral infection. Warts have been played with for centuries, and cures have been attributed to burying a dead black cat in the graveyard at midnight and other such feats. The interesting fact is that these examples of psychotherapy do work. Physicians attempt the same type of therapy under more professional guise and are pleased, but not surprised, when such therapy is effective. Children, fortunately, are most amenable to this suggestion therapy. On the other hand, however, every physician is also familiar with the stubborn wart that has been literally blasted from its mooring in the skin but keeps recurring.

ETIOLOGY. The human papillomavirus (HPV) is a DNA virus. Over 50 types of HPV have been identified by immunocytologic and molecular biologic techniques. Several of the types can cause clinically similar warts. HPV is associated with squamous cell carcinoma in epidermodysplasia verruciformis and immunosuppressed patients (especially renal, heart, and liver transplant patients). Oral squamous cell cancers, Bowen's disease, Buschke–Lowenstein tumors, juvenile laryngeal papillomas, and nail-bed cancer are all associated with HPV infection. Wart virus has been strongly associated with anogenital and cervical cancers (especially associated with HPV types 16, 18, 30, 31).

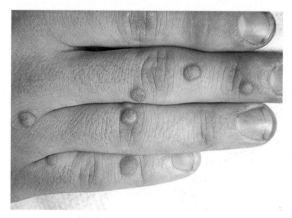

(*A*) Common warts on hand.

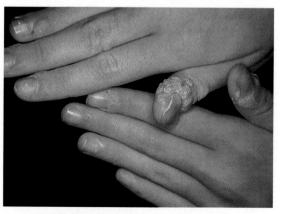

(*B*) Common and periungual warts.

Figure 17-5.   **Warts.** (*Reed & Carnrick Pharmaceuticals*)

DIAGNOSIS. The diagnosis is usually made by clinical examination. A skin biopsy is characteristic, and the polymerase chain reaction is diagnostic.

The various *clinical* types of warts relate to the appearance of the growth and to its location. The treatment varies somewhat for each clinical type of wart and is discussed separately for each type.

Common Wart
(see Fig. 17-5 A,B)

The appearance is a papillary growth, slightly raised above the skin surface, varying from pinhead size to large clusters of pea-sized tumors. These warts are seen most commonly on the hands. Rarely, they have to be differentiated from *seborrheic keratoses* (flatter, darker, velvety tumors of older adults; see Chap. 32) and *pigmented verrucous nevi* (projections are not dry and rough to touch; longer duration; often linear; biopsy may be indicated; see Chap. 33).

TREATMENT

1. Suggestion therapy can be attempted, particularly with children. One form of such therapy consists of the application by the physician of a colored solution, such as podophyllum in alcohol, 25% solution. This has the added benefit of being a cell-destroying chemical.
2. Single small (smaller than 6 mm) warts in adults or older children are removed best by electrosurgery. The recurrence rate is minimal, and one treatment usually suffices. The technique is to cleanse the area, anesthetize the site with 1% xylocaine or other local anesthetic, destroy the tumor with any form of electrosurgery (see Chap. 6), snip off or curette out the dead tissue, and desiccate the base. Recurrences can be attributed to failure to remove the dead tissue and to destroy the lesion adequately to its full depth. No dressing should be applied. The site will heal in 5 to 14 days with only minimal bacterial infection and scar formation. Warts around the nails have a high recurrence rate, and cure usually requires removal of part of the overlying nail. HPV type 16 has been associated with periungual squamous cell carcinoma.
3. If available, liquid nitrogen therapy is simple and effective, but moderately painful (see Chap. 6). The important admonition here is *freeze lightly* and not deeply.

> **SAUER NOTES**
>
> 1. A successful method of removing one or several warts, even in children, is the light application of liquid nitrogen to the wart followed by electrosurgery while the wart is thawing.
> 2. It is amazing how much electrosurgery some patients can tolerate before you need to stop. In those moments of toleration, many warts can be cured, or the procedure can be repeated every 3 weeks as necessary.

---

4. Salicylic acid   10%
   Flexible collodion q.s.   30.0
   Sig: Apply to warts cautiously every night for 5 to 7 nights. If irritation occurs, stop the application for three to four nights and resume again as necessary. The dead tissue can be removed with scissors, 10% lactic acid can be added to this formulation.

   Several prescription and proprietary medications of this therapy are available, such as DuoPlant (27% salicylic acid), DuoFilm (16.7% salicylic acid), Occlusal, and Compound W. Trans-plantar contains 21% salicylic acid in a dermal patch delivery system. A 40% salicylic acid plaster is available over the counter.

   This type of treatment is applicable for the patient with 20 or more warts on one hand or for larger warts to avoid scarring. The purpose is to remove as many warts as possible in this manner over a period of several weeks. Any remaining warts can be removed by electrosurgery or liquid nitrogen.

5. Another form of treatment for multiple warts or for warts in children is as follows:
   Mild corticosteroid cream   15.0
   Sig: Apply a very small quantity to each wart at night. Then cover the wart with Saran Wrap, and leave the occlusive dressing on all night or for 24 hours. Repeat nightly.
   Comment: This treatment has the advantage of being painless and quite effective. Salicylic acid (2% to 4%) can be added to the cream for further benefit.

6. Vitamin A, 50,000 units #50
   Sig: 1 tablet a day for no longer than 3 months.
   Comment: For the resistant case in an adult, and for the patient who says, "Doctor, aren't there any pills I can take for these warts," vit-

amin A is safe and warts have disappeared after such a course of treatment.

7. Intralesional interferon has been used with some success. It is expensive and painful.
8. Cimetidine in a dosage of 35 to 40 mg/kg per day for 3 to 4 months is safe and may be beneficial for recalcitrant warts.

Filiform Warts

Filiform warts have long, finger-like projections from the skin and most commonly appear on the eyelids, the face, and the neck. They are to be differentiated from *cutaneous horns* (which are seen in elderly patients with actinic keratosis or squamous cell carcinoma at the base and have a hard keratin horn; see Chap. 32), and from *pedunculated fibromas* (which occur on the neck and the axillae of middle-aged men and women; see Chap. 32).

TREATMENT

1. Without anesthesia, the wart is snipped off with a small scissors and trichloroacetic acid solution (saturated) is applied cautiously to the base. This is a fast and effective method, especially for children.
2. Electrosurgery can be performed as described previously for common warts.
3. Light application of liquid nitrogen is effective.

An annoying variant of this type of wart is the case with multiple small *filiform warts of the beard area.* Low-intensity electrosurgery without anesthesia is well tolerated and effective for these warts. However, to achieve a permanent cure, the patient should be seen every 3 to 4 weeks for as long a period as necessary to remove the young warts that are in the process of enlarging. The physician's job is to keep ahead of these warts and eliminate the reinfection that occurs from shaving.

Flat Warts

These small, flat tumors are often barely visible but can occur in clusters of 10 to 30 or more. They are commonly seen on the forehead and the dorsum of the hand and should be differentiated from small *seborrheic keratoses* or *nonpigmented nevi.* On women's legs, they are spread by shaving.

Flat warts can also occur on the penis and cervix. Acetic acid 3% to 5%, or vinegar solution, applied for 5 to 15 minutes to the area, with the use of a hand lens or colposcope, aids visualization. The flat warts appear whitish. Warts of HPV types 16 and 18 are believed to be related to the development of cervical, genital, and rectal cancer.

Squamous intraepithelial lesion (SIL) grade 1 involves the lower 1/3 of the epidermis. SIL grade 2 involves the lower 2/3 of the epidermis. Squamous cell carcinoma in situ (formerly Bowenoid papulosis) on the anogenital area and penis can clinically resemble flat warts and involves the full thickness of the epidermis. Histologically the flat papules exhibit changes of squamous cell carcinoma *in situ.* The course is usually benign. HPV has been found in these lesions.

TREATMENT

1. For flat warts on the face, cautious use of liquid nitrogen or light electrosurgery is done. *Care is taken so that scars do not form.* Retin-A gel (0.01%) applied locally once a day removes some flat warts. Suggestion therapy is effective for these warts in children.
2. For hand or leg flat warts, light electrosurgery is effective and tolerated quite well.
3. For genital flat warts, saturated solution of trichloroacetic acid, applied by the physician with great care, is beneficial. Light liquid nitrogen, electrosurgery, or both are effective. This is a tender area and local anesthesia is often necessary. Laser therapy is promoted by some but can scar and is expensive.

Some cases in adults can exhaust your therapeutic modalities, only to have the warts disappear with time.

Moist Warts (Condylomata Acuminata)
(Fig. 17-6; see Fig 18-5)

Moist warts are quite characteristic, single or multiple, soft, nonhorny masses that appear in the anogenital areas and, less commonly, between the toes and at the corners of the mouth. They are not always of a venereal nature. However, moist warts in the anal orifice or on the genitalia of a child can be a sign of sexual abuse.

Genital and anal warts are predominantly induced by HPV types 6, 11, 16, 18, and 31. Types 16 and 18 are associated with cervical cancer,

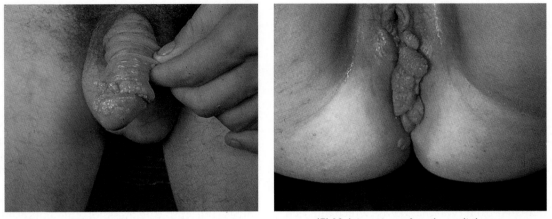

(A) Moist warts on penis.   (B) Moist warts on female genital area.

Figure 17-6. **Warts.** (*Reed & Carnrick Pharmaceuticals*)

squamous intraepithelial lesions, squamous cell carcinoma in situ, and anogenital cancer. Type 16 (especially cervical squamous carcinoma) and 18 (especially cervical adenocarcinoma) are associated with cervical and anogenital cancer and precancerous conditions.

TREATMENT

1. Podophyllum resin in alcohol (25% solution) is applied once to the warts, cautiously. Second or third treatments are usually necessary at weekly intervals. To prevent excessive irritation, the site should be bathed within 3 to 6 hours after the application.
2. Podofilox (Condylox) 0.5% is applied by the patient twice a day for 3 days, followed by 4 days of rest. This regimen is repeated for 2 to 4 weeks.
3. Occasionally, liquid nitrogen or electrosurgery or laser with local anesthesia is necessary.
4. Interferon α-2b (Intron A) is available for injection into the warts—*many* injections are needed.
5. Imiquimod (5%) cream (Aldara) applied three times a week overnight for 4 months is safe and may be effective. Its benefit may be due to inducing production of interferon α.

Plantar Warts
(*Fig. 17-7*)

(This is the layman's "planter's warts," which I am sure they believe are related to "Planter's Peanuts"). As the name signifies, this wart occurs

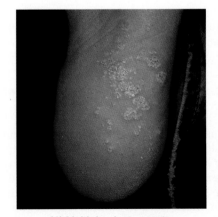 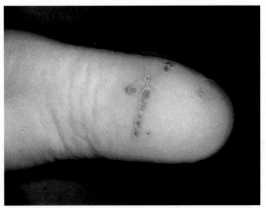

(A) Multiple plantar warts.   (B) Plantar warts that recurred in surgical excision site.

Figure 17-7. **Warts.** (*Reed & Carnrick Pharmaceuticals*)

on the sole of the foot, is flat, extends deep into the thick skin, and *on superficial trimming reveals small pinpoint-sized bleeding points*. Varying degrees of disability can be produced from the pressure type of pain. Single or multiple lesions can be present. The name *mosaic wart* is applied when the warts have coalesced into larger patches. One of the most vexing problems in dermatology is the patient with half of the sole of a foot covered with these warts.

Plantar warts are to be differentiated from a *callus* (no bleeding points visible on superficial trimming) and from *scar tissue from a previous treatment* (no bleeding points seen).

SAUER NOTE

Never treat a plantar lesion as a wart until you have proved your diagnosis by trimming to reveal the bleeding points of the wart. Too many *punctate keratoses, corns,* and *calluses* are mistaken for plantar warts. Rarely a verrucous carcinoma can be mistaken for a plantar wart.

TREATMENT

It would be impossible to list all of the forms of therapy that have proved to be curative for plantar warts or any other warts, but here are some favorite forms of therapy. We wager that if you start with number 1 and proceed to number 4, either the warts will have left or your patient will have gone to another physician.

1. Electrosurgery is the simplest and most successful form of therapy for a single small (smaller than 6 mm) plantar wart. The procedure is the same as for common warts except that the depth of the plantar wart is greater. Local anesthesia is usually necessary, and the injection is painful. Healing takes from 3 to 4 weeks to be complete. Some bleeding is to be expected a few days after the surgery. Most patients do not complain of much pain during the healing stage.
2. Liquid nitrogen therapy can be applied in two ways. When it is applied for 10 to 15 seconds, a blister forms in 24 hours and deep peeling of the wart ensues. This can be quite painful but is effective. When liquid nitrogen is applied lightly for 5 to 8 seconds, the larger warts or multiple warts can be removed gradually on

several visits with less pain and disability. Freezing, thawing, and refreezing greatly increases destruction of tissue in recalcitrant lesions.
3. Trichloroacetic acid–tape technique is useful for children and cases with multiple or large plantar warts. The procedure is as follows: Pare down the wart with a sharp knife, apply trichloroacetic acid solution (saturated) to the wart, then cover the area with plain tape. Leave the tape on for 5 to 7 days. Then remove the tape and curette out the dead wart tissue. Usually, more wart remains, and the procedure is repeated until the wart is destroyed. This course of treatment may take several weeks. After the first two visits the site may become tender and secondarily infected. If the disability and the infection are severe, therapy should be stopped temporarily and hot soaks instituted.
4. Fluorinated corticosteroid–occlusive dressing therapy. Have the patient apply a small amount of corticosteroid cream to the wart or warts at night and cover with Saran Wrap or Handi-Wrap. Leave on for 12 to 24 to 48 hours and reapply. This form of treatment is painless.

MOLLUSCUM CONTAGIOSUM
(Fig. 17-8; see Fig. 18-4)

Molluscum contagiosum is a common viral infection of the skin that is characterized by the occurrence, usually in children or sexually active young adults, of one or multiple small skin tumors. These growths occasionally develop in the scratched areas of patients with *atopic eczema*. The causative agent is a large DNA-containing poxvirus. Multiple facial lesions are common in HIV-positive patients.

PRIMARY LESION. An umbilicated, firm, waxy, skin-colored, raised papule varies in diameter from 2 to 5 mm and, rarely, is larger.

SECONDARY LESION. The skin is inflamed from bacterial infection or an eczematous reaction that may be immune in nature.

DISTRIBUTION. Most commonly the papules appear on the trunk, face, arms, and genital area, but they can occur anywhere.

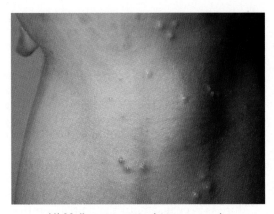

(A) Molluscum contagiosum on neck.

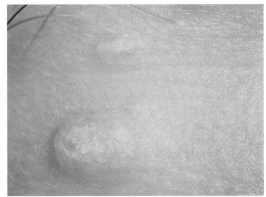

(B) Molluscum contagiosum close-up. (Drs. L. Calkins, A. Lemoine, and L. Hyde)

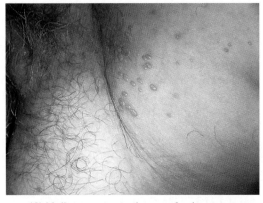

(C) Molluscum contagiosum of vulvar area.

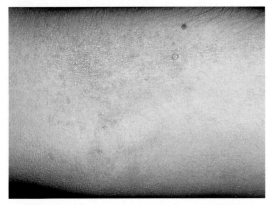

(D) Molluscum contagiosum with atopic eczema of cubital fossae.

Figure 17-8. **Molluscum contagiosum.** (*Glaxo Dermatology*)

COURSE. Onset of lesions is insidious, owing to lack of symptoms. Trauma or infection of a lesion causes it to disappear.

CONTAGIOUSNESS. This involves direct contact or autoinoculation.

Differential Diagnosis

Warts: No umbilication, not waxy (see earlier in this chapter)

Keratoacanthoma: Most commonly in older adults; larger lesion; rapid growth; biopsy findings characteristic (see Chap. 32)

Basal cell carcinoma: In older adults; slow growing; biopsy findings characteristic (see Chap. 32)

Treatment

A 6-year-old child presents with 10 small molluscum papules on his arms and upper trunk.

1. An excellent prescription (Verrusol) was removed from the market by the Food and Drug Administration because it contains more than one chemical. The pharmacy can mix up the following or some modification:

Cantharidin 1%
Salicylic acid 30%
Podophyllin 5%
Penederm 0.5%
Flexible collodion, 10 mL
Castor oil, 5 mL
Acetone 15 drops

Comment: A drop is *applied with care* by the physician on each lesion. A blister will form. This is an effective and painless therapy. Avoid on face, genital, or intetriginous areas.

2. Curettement. Each lesion is rapidly curetted, pressure is applied to stop bleeding, and then a bandage is applied. A small amount of trichloroacetic acid (saturated solution) on the broken pointed end of a swab stick helps to stop prolonged bleeding. Two or three visits may be necessary to treat recurrent lesions and new ones that have popped up.
3. Electrosurgery. Done lightly and rapidly, this is another effective method, especially for adults. It is not necessary to destroy the entire lesion, as for a wart, but only to induce some trauma and mild infection.
4. Cryosurgery is effective.
5. Topical and intravenous cidofovir has been shown to be beneficial in extensive molluscum seen in HIV-negative patients but is expensive and not yet available in a standardized topical form.

LYMPHOGRANULOMA VENEREUM

Lymphogranuloma venereum is an uncommon venereal disease characterized by a primary lesion on the genitals and secondary changes involving the draining lymph channels and glands.

The primary erosion or blister is rarely seen, especially on the female patient. Within 10 to 30 days after exposure, the inguinal nodes, particularly in the male patient, enlarge unilaterally. This inguinal mass may rupture if treatment is delayed. In the female patient the lymph drainage most commonly is toward the pelvic and the perirectal nodes, and their enlargement may be overlooked. Low-grade fever, malaise, and generalized lymphadenopathy frequently occur during the adenitis stage. Scarlatina-like rashes and erythema nodosum lesions also may develop. The later manifestations of lymphogranuloma venereum occur as the result of scarring of the lymph channels and fibrosis of the nodes. These changes result in rectal stricture, swelling of the penis or the vulva, and ulceration.

ETIOLOGY. Lymphogranuloma venereum is caused by the obligate intracellular parasite *Chlamydia trachomatis*, serotypes L_1, L_2, and L_3.

DIAGNOSIS. A complement fixation test (LGV-CFT) becomes positive 3 to 4 weeks after the onset of the disease in 80% to 90% of the patients.

TREATMENT. Tetracycline, 500 mg q.i.d., and minocycline, 100 mg b.i.d., are the drugs of choice. These are most effective in the early stages and should be continued for at least 3 weeks.

Fluctuant inguinal nodes should be aspirated to prevent rupture.

MEASLES (RUBEOLA)

Measles is a very common childhood disease. The characteristic points are as follows: the incubation period averages 14 days before the appearance of the rash. The prodromal stage appears around the ninth day after exposure and consists of fever, conjunctivitis, running nose, Koplik spots, and even a faint red rash. The Koplik spots measure from 1 to 3 mm in diameter, are bluish white on a red base, and occur bilaterally on the mucous membrane around the parotid duct and on the lower lip. With increasing fever and cough, the "morbilliform" rash appears first behind the ears and on the forehead and then spreads over face, neck, trunk, and extremities. The fever begins to fall as the rash comes out. The rash is a faint, reddish, patchy eruption, occasionally papular. Scaling occurs in the end stage.

Complications include secondary bacterial infection and encephalitis.

Differential Diagnosis

German measles: Postauricular nodes; milder fever and rash; no Koplik spots (see following section).
Scarlet fever: Circumoral pallor; rash brighter red and confluent (see Chap. 15).
Drug eruption: History of new drugs; usually no fever (see Chap. 9).
Infectious mononucleosis: Rash similar; characteristic blood picture; high titer of heterophile antibodies.

Treatment

PROPHYLACTIC. Measles virus vaccine, live, attenuated, can be administered.

ACTIVE. Supportive therapy for the cough, bed rest, and protection from bright light are measures for the active disease. The antibiotics have eliminated most of the bacterial complications.

Corticosteroids are of value for the rare but serious complication of encephalitis.

GERMAN MEASLES (RUBELLA)

Although German measles is a benign disease of children, it is serious if it develops in a pregnant woman during the first trimester, because it causes anomalies in a low percentage of newborns.

The incubation period is around 18 days, and, as in measles, there may be a short prodromal stage of fever and malaise. The rash also resembles measles, because it occurs first on the face and then spreads. However, the redness is less intense and the rash disappears within 2 to 3 days. Enlargement of the cervical and the postauricular nodes is a characteristic finding.

Serious complications are rare.

Differential Diagnosis

Measles: Koplik spots; the fever and the rash are more severe; no postauricular nodes (see previous section).
Scarlet fever: High fever; perioral pallor; rash may be similar (see Chap. 15).
Drug eruption: Get new drug history: usually no fever (see Chap. 9).

Treatment

PROPHYLACTIC. Rubella virus vaccine, live, attenuated, can be administered.

ACTIVE. Active treatment is usually unnecessary. Immune globulin given to an exposed pregnant woman in the first trimester of pregnancy may prevent the disease.

Congenital Rubella Syndrome

Infants born to mothers who had rubella in the first trimester of pregnancy can have multiple system abnormalities. The skin lesions include thrombocytopenic purpura; hyperpigmentation of the navel, forehead, and cheeks; acne; seborrhea; and reticulated erythema of the face and extremities.

ERYTHEMA INFECTIOSUM

Also known as "fifth disease," erythema infectiosum occurs in epidemics and is believed to be caused by parvovirus B19.

It affects children primarily, but in a large epidemic many cases are seen in adults.

The incubation period varies from 1 to 7 weeks. In children the prodromal stage lasts from 2 to 4 days and is manifested by low-grade fever and occasionally by joint pains. When the red macular rash develops, it begins on the arms and the face and then spreads to the body. The rash in children is measles-like on the body, but on the face it looks as though the cheeks had been slapped. On the arms and the legs the rash is more red and confluent on the extensor surfaces. A low-grade fever persists for a few days after the onset of the rash, which lasts for approximately 1 week.

In adults, the rash on the face (the "slap") is less conspicuous, joint complaints are more common, and itching is present.

ETIOLOGY. Parvovirus B19 is the causative agent.

Differential Diagnosis

Drug eruption: See Chap. 9.
Measles: Coryza; eruption begins on face and behind ears (see earlier in this chapter).
Other measles-like eruptions

Treatment

Treatment usually is not necessary.

COXSACKIEVIRUS INFECTIONS

Coxsackievirus infections are identified by type-specific antigens that appear in the blood 7 days or so after the onset of the disease.

Differential Diagnosis

Measles, German measles, scarlet fever, infectious mononucleosis, and drug eruption must be differentiated.

Treatment

No treatment is necessary except to reduce the high fever.

Herpangina

Herpangina is an acute febrile disease that occurs mainly in children in the summer months. The first complaints are fever, headache, sore throat, nausea, and stiff neck. Blisters are seen in the throat that are approximately 2 mm in size and surrounded by an intense erythema. These lesions may coalesce, and some may ulcerate. The course is usually 7 to 10 days.

The cause of herpangina is primarily coxsackievirus A, but echovirus types have also been isolated from sporadic cases.

DIFFERENTIAL DIAGNOSIS

Aphthous stomatitis, drug eruption, primary herpes gingivostomatitis, and hand-foot-and-mouth disease, which is another related viral condition, must be differentiated.

TREATMENT

Soothing mouthwashes and antipyretics are used.

ECHOVIRUS INFECTIONS

ECHO is an acronym for *enteric cytopathic human orphan*, the label given to the virus before it was known to be causative of any disease.

Echovirus Exanthem

The complaints include fever, nausea, vomiting, diarrhea, sore throat, cough, and stiff neck. A measles-like eruption occurs in one third of cases. Small erosions may develop on the mucous membranes of the cheek. Echoviruses 9 and 4 have been isolated from most cases with skin lesions.

TREATMENT

Treatment is symptomatic. The infection usually lasts 1 to 2 weeks.

BIBLIOGRAPHY

Bialecki C, Feder HM, Grant-Kels JM. The six classic exanthems: a review and update. J Am Acad Dermatol 1989; 21:891.

Cohen BA, Honig P, Androphy E. Anogenital warts in children. Arch Dermatol 1990;126:1575.

Drake LA, Ceilley RI, et al. Guidelines of care for warts: Human papillomavirus. J Am Acad Dermatol 1995;32:1.

Drugs for non-HIV viral infections. Med Lett Drugs Ther 1994;36:27.

Edwards L, Ferenczy A, Eron L, et al. Self-administered topical 5% imiquimod cream for external anogenital warts. Arch Dermatol 1998;134:25.

Genital Herpes Simplex Virus (HSV) Infection. Arch Dermatol 1998;134.

Goh CL, Khoo L. A retrospective study of the clinical presentation and outcome of herpes zoster in a tertiary dermatology outpatient referral clinic. Int J Dermatol 1997;36:667.

Gross G, Von Krogh G. Human papillomavirus infections in dermatovenereology. Boca Raton, FL, CRC Press, 1997.

Kost RG, Straus SE. Postherpetic neuralgia: Pathogenesis, treatment, and prevention. N Engl J Med 1996;335:1.

Ling MR. Therapy of genital papillomavirus infections: II. Methods of treatment. Int J Dermatol 1992;31:769.

Majewski S, Joblonska S. Human papillomavirus-associated tumors of the skin and mucosa. J Am Acad Dermatol 1997;36:5.

Myskowski, PL. Molluscum contagiosum: New insights, new directions. Arch Dermatol 1997;133:1039.

Pereira FA. Herpes simplex: Evolving concepts. J Am Acad Dermatol 1996;35:4.

Solomon AR, et al. The Tzanck smear in the diagnosis of cutaneous herpes simplex. JAMA 1984;251:633.

Cutaneous Diseases Associated with Human Immunodeficiency Virus

M. Joyce Rico, M.D.,* and Neil S. Prose, M.D.†

Despite rapid advances in the treatment of human immunodeficiency virus (HIV) and improved survival of patients with acquired immunodeficiency syndrome (AIDS), patients infected with HIV develop numerous skin conditions that may present to the primary care physician or dermatologist. The dermatologic conditions in these patients represent both common diseases that may have atypical clinical presentations and unusual cutaneous disorders. Changes in behavior and in treatment have altered the incidence of some conditions seen in these patients; nevertheless, patients with HIV continue to develop skin diseases throughout their disease course. In this chapter, we review the mucocutaneous diseases that are seen in patients infected with HIV.

EPIDEMIOLOGY

AIDS is the end result of infection with HIV, a retrovirus that is transmitted either by sexual contact, sharing contaminated needles, or trans-fusion of infected blood or blood products. After inoculation, HIV enters cells of the immune systemic through the CD4 receptor on T-helper lymphocytes. Once inside the cells, the virus may remain latent or proliferate and divide. Patients begin to manifest signs and symptoms of HIV infection months to years after exposure, although infected individuals typically have serologic evidence of infection shortly after exposure. The Centers for Disease Control (CDC) has established criteria for the diagnosis of AIDS. These include several conditions with dermatologic manifestations, such as Kaposi's sarcoma and chronic mucocutaneous herpes simplex.

Since its inception, AIDS has primarily affected homosexual or bisexual males, intravenous drug users, patients who received HIV-contaminated blood or blood products, and the heterosexual partners of those with AIDS or at risk for AIDS. Casual household transmission of the virus does not occur.

In the United States, the rate of HIV infection in women and children is increasing rapidly, particularly among minorities. The majority of children with HIV infection are the infants of mothers with the disease; a small percentage of children with AIDS are the recipients of contaminated blood or blood products. Recent studies suggest that the incidence of perinatal transmission ranges from 15 to 35% and can be decreased by appropriate diagnosis and treatment of HIV-infected women during pregnancy.

*Associate Professor, Department of Dermatology, New York University; Chief, Dermatology Service, New York VA Medical Center, New York, New York

†Associate Professor, Departments of Medicine (Dermatology) and Pediatrics, Duke University Medical Center, Durham, North Carolina

HIV infection is a worldwide epidemic. The greatest number of deaths from AIDS have occurred in sub-Saharan Africa, and the prevalence of HIV infection is increasing most rapidly in southeast Asia. Worldwide, it is estimated that 30 to 40 million people will be infected with HIV by the end of the decade. Although the incidence of AIDS and deaths from AIDS has declined in the United States, the number of patients infected with HIV continues to increase. In the United States, public health efforts have focused on earlier diagnosis and treatment, which have led to improvements in survival.

RELEVANCE TO DERMATOLOGY

The role of the dermatologist in caring for patients with AIDS should not be underestimated. Mucocutaneous eruptions occur frequently in patients with HIV infection and are a major source of morbidity. Several prospective studies have shown the prevalence of skin diseases in patients with HIV infection to range between 85 and 100%. The vast majority of patients with AIDS present with dermatologic complaints that are not specific for HIV infection. In the early days of the epidemic the most frequent diagnoses were oral candidiasis, seborrheic dermatitis, xerosis, fungal infections, and Kaposi's sarcoma. Although Kaposi's sarcoma has decreased in incidence, inflammatory and infectious cutaneous diseases, particularly viral and fungal infections, remain prevalent.

MUCOCUTANEOUS DISEASES ASSOCIATED WITH HIV INFECTION
(Fig. 18-1)

Infections and Infestations

VIRAL INFECTIONS

Herpes simplex virus (HSV) infections, and in particular chronic perianal herpes, was one of the first noted complications of HIV infection and remains a cause of significant morbidity. These patients may have persistent or recurrent painful ulcers, sometimes in the absence of vesicles, involving the genitalia, groin, perianal area, or other mucocutaneous surfaces. Acyclovir-resistant HSV has been described in HIV-infected patients with chronic, persistent disease. Foscarnet may be helpful in these resistant cases. In children, chronic or recurrent herpetic gingivostomatitis can significantly impede adequate oral in-

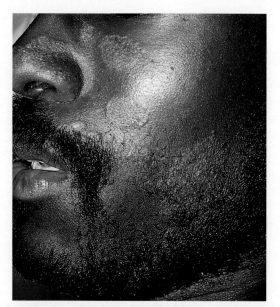

Figure 18-1. Seborrheic dermatitis. Annular scaling plaques on the nasolabial fold and cheeks. (*Drs. J. Rico and N. Prose*)

take. Herpes simplex virus ulcers can become a portal of entry or transmission site for HIV.

Infection with varicella-zoster virus may result in several different clinical manifestations. The occurrence of chickenpox in children or adults with HIV infection may result in disseminated cutaneous disease with systemic manifestations. These patients require treatment with systemic antiviral agents such as acyclovir, famciclovir, and valacyclovir. Herpes zoster ("shingles") is not uncommon in adults and children with HIV infection and may be the initial manifestation of HIV infection (Fig. 18-2). The occurrence of zoster in a patient at risk for HIV infection should prompt the provider to suggest appropriate counseling and testing for HIV. Chronic ecthymatous varicella-zoster virus infection develops either in patients with AIDS and a previous history of varicella-zoster exposure or in children with HIV infection and varicella (Fig. 18-3). Patients may present either with dermatomal vesicles that subsequently ulcerate and disseminate or with frank ulcers. These lesions are often recalcitrant to therapy and may heal with scarring. Dissemination of both herpes simplex and herpes zoster to extracutaneous sites has been reported.

Molluscum contagiosum in patients with HIV infection often occurs in the beard area and may present as disfiguring papules, plaques, or tumors; disseminated cutaneous disease may also

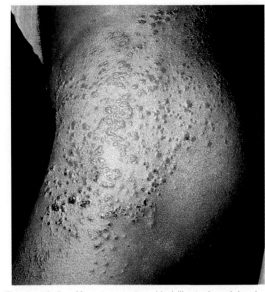

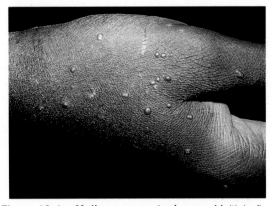

Figure 18-4. **Molluscum contagiosum.** Multiple firm white papules scattered over the dorsal hand and forearm in a Haitian man with AIDS. (*Drs. J. Rico and N. Prose*) (*Owen/Galderma*)

Figure 18-2. **Herpes zoster.** Umbilicated vesicles in a dermatomal distribution in a man with AIDS. (*Drs. J. Rico and N. Prose*) (*Owen/Galderma*)

FUNGAL INFECTIONS

The most common mucocutaneous eruption in patients infected with HIV is oral candidiasis (Fig. 18-7) or thrush. A number of these patients may develop esophageal involvement with characteristic ulcerations visible on endoscopy or barium swallow. Moniliasis involving the diaper area is a significant problem in children with AIDS. Candida paronychia has also been reported.

be seen (Fig. 18-4). Human papillomavirus infection, particularly condyloma acuminata (Fig. 18-5), may present as large, fungating lesions. Widespread flat warts have been observed. Oral hairy leukoplakia (Fig. 18-6), a mixed infection of Epstein–Barr virus and human papillomavirus, is usually asymptomatic and presents as filiform white papules or corrugated plaques on the lateral sides of the tongue. Complex viral and fungal lesions involving the skin may be hyperkeratotic, vegetating, or ulcerative in appearance. Herpesvirus, papillomavirus, and fungal elements have been cultured or observed on biopsy.

Cutaneous fungal infections may occur as extensive scaling papules and plaques or involve atypical sites. In the adult population, fungal infection of the nails is common; proximal white subungual onychomycosis is seen with particular frequency in patients with HIV infection. Disseminated deep fungal infections, including cryptococcosis, histoplasmosis, coccidiomycosis,

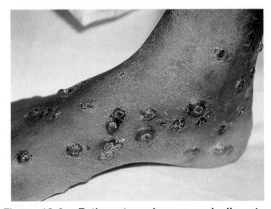

Figure 18-3. **Ecthymatous herpes varicell-zoster.** Crusted erosions and blisters on the foot of a patient with AIDS. (*Drs. J. Rico and N. Prose*) (*Owen/Galderma*)

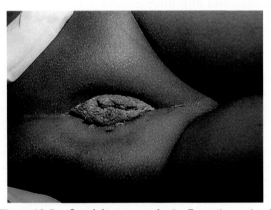

Figure 18-5. **Condyloma acuminata.** Fungating perianal warts in a child infected with HIV. (*Drs. J. Rico and N. Prose*)

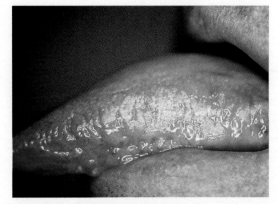

Figure 18-6.   Oral hairy leukoplakia. Filamentous white papules on the sides of the tongue. (*Drs. J. Rico and N. Prose*) (*Owen/Galderma*)

and blastomycosis, may present with skin involvement in patients with AIDS. These patients may present with ulcers, plaques, or nodules; biopsy for routine histology and culture, as well as touch preparations are necessary to establish the diagnosis.

OTHER INFECTIONS AND INFESTATIONS

Infants and children with AIDS are particularly at risk for bacterial infections; cutaneous bacterial diseases including cellulitis and impetigo are frequent. In adults, acneiform eruptions and extensive folliculitis have been reported. Mycobacteria may involve the skin in patients with AIDS either as a primary cellulitis with *Mycobacterium avium-intracellulare* or other mycobac-

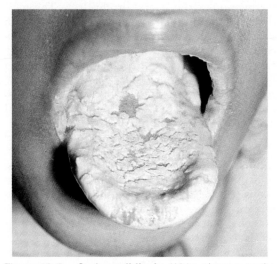

Figure 18-7.   Oral candidiasis. White plaques on the tongue of a child with AIDS. (*Drs. J. Rico and N. Prose*)

terium, or with secondary spread of *M. tuberculosis* as in scrofula.

Syphilis, like HIV infection, is a sexually transmitted disease that predominately affects young adults. Patients with AIDS who are homosexual or bisexual or are intravenous drug users are at increased risk for syphilis. Rarely, patients coinfected with syphilis and HIV may be serologically negative for syphilis (RPR, FTA) despite active infection. Several patients with early HIV and syphilis have failed to respond to standard antibiotic regimens, and appropriate serologic follow-up is advised for all patients with syphilis. Those caring for patients with HIV infection or syphilis are urged to review the CDC recommendations for diagnosis and treatment.

Bacillary angiomatosis is a unique illness characterized by the development of fever, chills, weight loss, and numerous angiomatous nodules. The etiologic agent is *Bartonella*, the same organism that causes cat-scratch disease. Treatment with oral erythromycin, or other antibiotics including doxycycline or ciprofloxacin, leads to the rapid resolution of both skin lesions and systemic symptoms.

Atypical forms of scabies have been reported in both adults and children with AIDS. The rash tends to be highly pruritic, and patients may present with widespread, keratotic papules, similar clinically to Norwegian scabies.

Inflammatory Disorders

A flu-like illness may occur at the time of acute seroconversion. An evanescent morbilliform rash has been associated with this syndrome. Seborrheic dermatitis is seen in up to 50% of patients with HIV infection. Clinically, seborrheic dermatitis in these patients tends to be more florid and less responsive to therapy than in the nonimmunocompromised host. Psoriasis and Reiter's disease have been reported in 1 to 5% of patients infected with HIV. Psoriasis may flare in those with previously stable plaque type disease, or develop de novo. Reiter's disease (Fig. 18-8), manifested by psoriasiform dermatitis, keratoderma blennorrhagica, seronegative spondyloarthropathy, urethritis, balanitis, uveitis, or conjunctivitis, is more common in patients with AIDS and is associated with the histocompatibility locus antigen B-27. Drug eruptions, particularly due to trimethoprim/sulfamethoxazole (Fig. 18-9) and other antibiotics, are common in patients with AIDS. Generalized granuloma an-

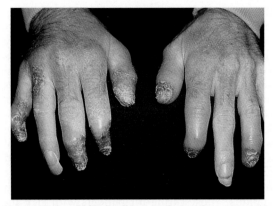

Figure 18-8. Reiter's disease. Psoriasiform dermatitis involving the distal fingers. Note the joint changes due to active arthritis. (*Drs. J. Rico and N. Prose*)

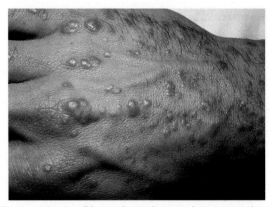

Figure 18-10. Disseminated granuloma annulare. Discrete annular pink papules on the dorsal hand. (*Drs. J. Rico and N. Prose*)

nulare (Fig. 18-10) may be seen with widespread annular dermal papules. Additional inflammatory skin disorders that may be associated with HIV infection include acute and chronic photoeruptions, porphyria cutanea tarda, vasculitis, pyoderma gangrenosum, calciphylaxis, and erythema elevatum diutinum. Papular eruption of HIV infection was described by James et al. as multiple, 2- to 5-mm, flesh-colored papules on the face, neck, and upper thorax, which are often pruritic. Pruritus may be one of the initial symptoms of HIV infection and is often incapacitating. Patients may present with excoriations, lesions of lichen simplex chronicus, prurigo nodularis, or minimal skin changes. Xerosis, which is not specific for HIV infection and can be seen in a variety of chronic illnesses, has been reported in up to 30% of patients with HIV infection.

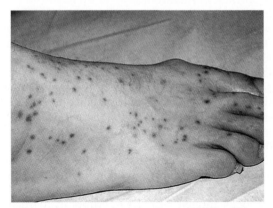

Figure 18-9. Leukocytoclastic vasculitis. Palpable purpura on the foot. This patient developed vasculitis after receiving trimethoprim-sulfamethoxazole. (*Drs. J. Rico and N. Prose*)

Patients with AIDS and chronic diarrhea or AIDS-wasting syndrome, particularly children, are at risk for cutaneous manifestations of nutritional deficiencies. Scurvy, acrodermatitis enteropathica, and cutaneous manifestations of B vitamin deficiency have been reported.

Neoplasms

Disseminated Kaposi's sarcoma was one of the initial manifestations of HIV infection; the first cases were reported in 1980 in previously healthy homosexual and bisexual men. Since then, Kaposi's sarcoma has remained a disease predominately seen in that subgroup of patients and has been infrequently reported in those who acquire the disease through heterosexual contact, intravenous drug users, or children. The incidence of Kaposi's sarcoma among patients with HIV infection has decreased steadily, and currently fewer than 15% of patients with HIV infection develop Kaposi's sarcoma. Kaposi's sarcoma is associated with herpesvirus 8 (HHV-8). In one recent study, approximately 50% of homosexual men coinfected with HIV and HHV-8 developed Kaposi's sarcoma within 10 years.

Disseminated Kaposi's sarcoma associated with AIDS differs from classical Kaposi's sarcaoma in that the majority of patients present with multiple, often widespread, red or violaceous papules, plaques, or tumors involving the integument and mucosa (Fig. 18-11). Visceral involvement occurs in 25%, and may result in systemic hemorrhage. The lesions generally are asymptomatic; however, patients may complain of pruritus or pain, and large lesions may ulcerate. The treatment of isolated lesions by excision,

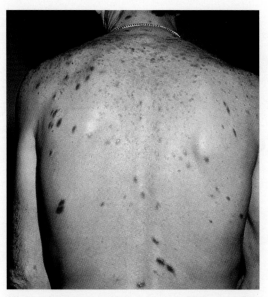

(A) Disseminated Kaposi's sarcoma: Multiple red to brown papules and plaques distributed along the skin tension lines in a homosexual man with AIDS.

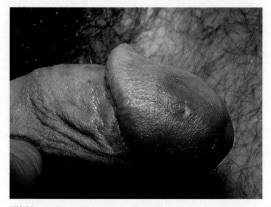

(B) Kaposi's sarcoma: an ill-defined purple plaque on the glans penis of a homosexual man with AIDS.

Figure 18-11. **Cutaneous diseases associated with HIV infection.** (Drs. J. Rico and N. Prose)

cryotherapy, or local radiation may offer palliation or cosmetic improvement. Doxcil (liposomal adinomycin) is a beneficial systemic agent given intravenously for advanced disease.

B-cell lymphoma, which commonly involves the central nervous system in patients with AIDS, has been rarely reported to involve skin. Patients may present with small, ulcerated papules or nodules. Despite anecdotal reports, there is no clear evidence for an increase in other cutaneous malignancies, such as basal cell carcinoma, squamous cell carcinoma or melanoma, among patients with HIV infection.

SUMMARY

HIV infection is characterized by a wide variety of mucocutaneous manifestations. Several of these skin diseases, such as Kaposi's sarcoma and oral hairy leukoplakia, are very frequently associated with HIV infection. The majority of the patients, however, develop common dermatoses that are distinguished by their persistence, frequent recurrence, or poor response to therapy. As treatment modalities to prevent the development of opportunistic infections and for HIV infection become available, the early diagnosis of this disease becomes increasingly important. For this reason, the clinical dermatologist must become familiar with the cutaneous disease that may signal the presence of HIV-related illness.

BIBLIOGRAPHY

Cockerell CJ. Bacillary angiomatosis and related diseases caused by Rochalimaea. J Am Acad Dermatol 1995;32:783.

Coopman SA, Johnson RA, Stern RS. Cutaneous diseases and drug reactions in HIV infection. N Engl J Med 1993;328:1670.

Grossman ME. Cutaneous manifestations of infection in the immunocompromised host. Baltimore, Williams & Wilkins, 1996.

Kerschmann R, Berger T, et al. Cutaneous presentations of lymphoma in human immunodeficiency virus disease. Arch Dermatol 1995;131.

Martin JH, Ganem DE, Osmond DH, et al. Sexual transmission and the natural history of human herpesvirus 8 infection. N Engl J Med 1998;338:948.

Murakawa GJ, Kerschmann R, Berger T. Cutaneous cryptococcus infection and AIDS. Arch Deramtol 1996;132:545.

MMWR. Diagnosis and reporting of HIV and AIDS in states with integrated HIV and AIDS surveillance: United States, January 1994–June 1997. MMWR 1998;47:309.

MMWR. Recommendations for diagnosing and treating syphilis in HIV-infected patients. Arch Dermatol 1989;125:15.

Myers SA, Prose NS, Bartlett JA. Progress in the understanding of HIV infection: An overview. J Am Acad Dermatol 1993;29:1.

Prose NS. Cutaneous manifestations of HIV infection in children. Dermatol Clin 1991;9:543.

Rico MJ, Myers SA, Sanchez M. Guidelines of care: Dermatologic conditions in patients infected with human immunodeficiency syndrome. J Am Acad Dermatol 1997;37:450.

Rosatelli JB, Machado AA, Roselino AM. Dermatoses among Brazilian HIV-positive patients: Correlation with the evolutionary phases of AIDS. Int J Deramtol 1997;36:729.

Zalla M. Kaposi's sarcoma. Dermatol Surg 1996;22:274.

19

Dermatologic Mycology

Fungi can be present as part of the normal flora of the skin or as abnormal inhabitants. Dermatologists are concerned with the abnormal inhabitants, or pathogenic fungi. However, so-called nonpathogenic fungi can proliferate and invade immunosuppressed persons.

Pathogenic fungi have a predilection for certain body areas; most commonly they infect the skin, but the lungs, the brain, and other organs can also be infected. Pathogenic fungi can invade the skin *superficially* and *deeply* and are thus divided into these two groups.

SUPERFICIAL FUNGAL INFECTIONS

The superficial fungi live on the dead horny layer of the skin and elaborate an enzyme that enables them to digest keratin, causing the superficial skin to scale and disintegrate, the nails to crumble, and the hairs to break off. The deeper reactions of vesicles, erythema, and infiltration are presumably due to the fungi liberating an exotoxin. Fungi are also capable of eliciting an allergic or id reaction.

When a skin scraping, a hair, or a culture growth is examined with the microscope in a wet preparation (see Chap. 2 and Fig. 2-1), the two structural elements of the fungi are seen: the spores and the hyphae.

Spores are the reproducing bodies of the fungi. Sexual and asexual forms occur. Spores are rarely seen in skin scrapings.

Hyphae are threadlike, branching filaments that grow out from the fungus spore. The hyphae are the identifying filaments seen in skin scrapings in potassium hydroxide (KOH) solution.

Mycelia are matted clumps of hyphae that grow on culture plates.

Culture media vary greatly in content, but modifications of Sabouraud's dextrose agar are used to grow the superficial fungi (see Fig. 2-2). Sabouraud's agar and corn meal agar are both used to identify the deep fungi. Hyphae and spores grow on the media, and identification of the species of fungi is established by the gross appearance of the mycelia, the color of the substrate, and the microscopic appearance of the spores and the hyphae when a sample of the growth is placed on a slide. Some media show a color change when pathogenic fungi are isolated.

Classification

The latest classification divides the superficial fungi into three genera: *Microsporum, Epidermophyton,* and *Trichophyton.* Species of only two of these invade the hair: *Microsporum* and *Tricho-*

TABLE 19-1
RELATIONSHIP OF FUNGI TO BODY AREAS

Fungus	Feet and Hands	Nails	Groin	Smooth Skin	Scalp	Beard
Microsporum species						
M. audouini	0	0	0	Uncommon	Uncommon	0
M. canis	0	0	0	Common	Uncommon	Rare
M. gypseum	0	0	0	Rare	Rare	0
Epidermophyton species						
E. floccosum	Moderately common	Rare	Common	Moderately common	0	0
Trichophyton species						
Endothrix species						
T. schoenleini	0	Rare	0	Rare	(Favus) rare, especially tropics	0
T. violaceum	0	Rare	0	0	Rare	Rare
T. tonsurans	0	Rare	0	Rare	Moderately common	0
Ectothrix species						
T. mentagrophytes	Common	Moderately common	Common	Rare	Rare	Moderately common
T. rubrum	Common	Common	Moderately common	Rare	0	Rare
T. verrucosum	0	0	0	Rare	Rare	Rare

phyton. As seen in a KOH preparation, *Microsporum* species cause an ectothrix infection of the hair shaft, whereas *Trichophyton* species cause either an ectothrix or an endothrix infection. The ectothrix fungi cause the formation of an external spore sheath around the hair, whereas the endothrix fungi do not. The filaments of mycelia penetrate the hair in both types of infection.

The species of fungi is correlated with the clinical diseases in Table 19-1. The organism causing tinea versicolor is not included in this table because it does not liberate a keratolytic enzyme.

SAUER NOTES

Since the discovery of specific systemic antifungal agents many physicians have believed that (1) these agents are indicated for every fungus infection and (2) most skin diseases are due to a fungus, so they should treat the patient with the antifungal agent and make a diagnosis later. Both of these assumptions are erroneous.

1. Correct diagnosis of a fungal infection is necessary. An oral antifungal drug should not be prescribed for a patient if the diagnosis has not been confirmed. Systemic antifungal agents are of no value in treating atopic eczema, contact dermatitis, psoriasis, pityriasis rosea, and so on.

2. Except for tinea of the scalp and nails, true fungal infections are noticeably improved after only 1 to 2 weeks of oral antifungal therapy. If there is no improvement, the diagnosis of the dermatosis as a fungus disease is erroneous and the therapy should be stopped.

(display continues on page 200)

3. An adequate dosage is necessary, including (1) the correct daily dose for the particular type of fungal infection and (2) the correct duration of such dosage.

4. In general, systemic antifungal therapy should not be used to treat tinea of the feet. The recurrence rate after completion of therapy is very high.

5. Candidal infections should not be treated with oral griseofulvin. Very commonly, candidal intertrigo of the groin or candidal paronychias are erroneously treated with griseofulvin. Griseofulvin is of no value in these conditions. Because it is a penicillin-related drug, it usually aggravates the candidiasis.

6. Tinea versicolor does not respond to oral griseofulvin therapy.

7. So-called fungal infection of the ear does not respond to oral antifungal therapy. Most external ear diseases are not caused by a fungus (see External Otitis, Chap. 11).

Clinical Classifications

Superficial fungal infections of the skin affect various sites of the body. The clinical lesions, the species of fungi, and the therapy vary for these different sites. Therefore, fungal diseases of the skin are classified, for clinical purposes, according to the location of the infection. These clinical types are as follows:

- Tinea of the feet (tinea pedis)
- Tinea of the hands (tinea manus)
- Tinea of the nails (onychomycosis)
- Tinea of the groin (tinea cruris)
- Tinea of the smooth skin (tinea corporis)
- Tinea of the scalp (tinea capitis)
- Tinea of the beard (tinea barbae)
- Dermatophytid
- Tinea versicolor (see Chap. 14)
- Tinea of the external ear (see External Otitis, Chap. 11).

There is a predilection for certain sites of tinea in which the frequency varies with the age of the patient. This is outlined in Table 19-2.

Tinea of the Feet
(Figs. 19-1–19-3)

Tinea of the feet (athlete's foot, fungal infection of the feet, ringworm of the feet) is a very common skin infection. Many persons have the disease and are not even aware of it. The clinical appearance varies.

PRIMARY LESIONS. *Acute form*: Blisters occur on the soles and the sides of feet or between the toes. *Chronic form*: Lesions are dry and scaly.

SECONDARY LESIONS. Bacterial infection of the blisters is very common; maceration and fissures are also seen.

COURSE. Recurrent acute infections can lead to a chronic infection. If the toenails become infected, a cure is highly improbable, because this focus is very difficult to eradicate.

The species of fungus influences the response to therapy. Most vesicular, acute fungal infections are due to *T. mentagrophytes* and respond readily to correct treatment. The chronic scaly type of infection is usually due to *T. rubrum* and is exceedingly difficult, if not impossible, to cure.

CONTAGIOUSNESS. Experiments have shown that there is a susceptibility factor necessary for infection. Males are much more susceptible than females, even when the latter are exposed.

LABORATORY FINDINGS. KOH-ink preparations of scrapings and cultures on Sabouraud's media serve to demonstrate the presence of fungi

TABLE 19-2
SITES OF TINEA IN RELATIONSHIP TO AGE-GROUPS

Tinea Site	Children (0–16 yr)	Adults
Tinea capitis (scalp)	Common	Very rare
Tinea corporis (body)	Common	Fairly common
Tinea cruris (groin)	Rare	Common (esp. males)
Tinea pedis (feet)	Rare (mimics eczema)	Very common
Onychomycosis (nails)	Very rare	Very common

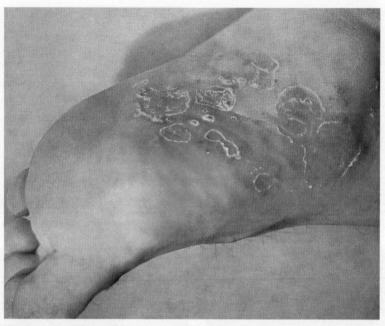

Figure 19-1. **Tinea of the foot.** This dry, scaly form of fungus infection is usually due to *T. rubrum.* (Smith Kline & French Laboratories)

and the specific type. A KOH preparation is a very simple office procedure and should be resorted to when the diagnosis is uncertain or the response to therapy is slow (see Chap. 2).

DIFFERENTIAL DIAGNOSIS

Contact dermatitis: Due to shoes, socks, gloves, foot powder usually on dorsum of feet or hands; history of new shoes or new foot powder; fungi not found (see Chap. 9).

Atopic eczema: Especially on dorsum of toes in children; quite chronic; usually in winter; very pruritic; atopic family history; on dorsum of toes; fungi not found (see Chap. 9 and Fig. 33-24).

Psoriasis: Affects soles and palms; rarely pustular, thickened, well-circumscribed lesions; psoriasis elsewhere on body; fungi not found (see Chap. 14).

Pustular bacterid: Pustular lesions only; chronic; resistant to local therapy; fungi not found.

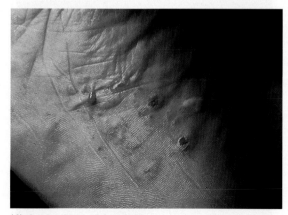

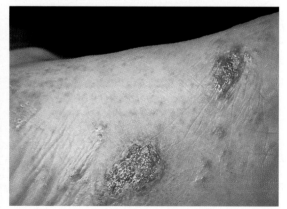

(*A*) Acute tinea of foot with secondary bacterial infection.

(*B*) Acute tinea of sole of foot of *T. mentagrophytes* type.

Figure 19-2. **Tinea of the foot.** *(Schering Corp.)*

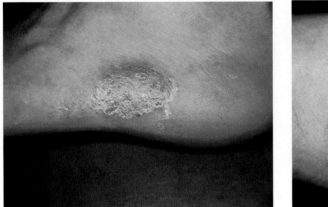

(*A*) Chronic tinea of side of foot.

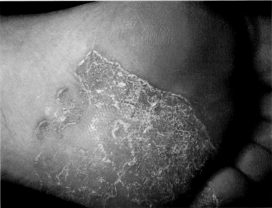

(*B*) Chronic tinea of sole due to *T. rubrum*.

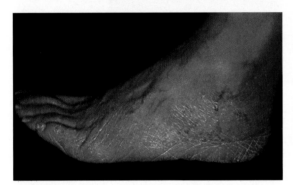

(*C*) Chronic extensive tinea on patient on corticosteroids.

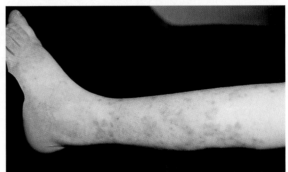

(*D*) Chronic tinea extending up leg.

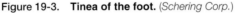

Figure 19-3. **Tinea of the foot.** (*Schering Corp.*)

This condition may be associated with a focus of infection, as in tonsil, teeth, or gallbladder.

Hyperhidrosis of feet: Can be severe and cause white, eroded maceration of the soles, accompanied by a foul odor. Zeasorb AF powder is helpful, as is Drysol solution.

Symmetric lividity of the soles (Fig. 19-4): Rather common condition of the soles of the feet characterized by the presence of patches of macerated, whitish, sharply defined, odoriferous skin associated with hyperhidrosis.

Pitted keratolysis (keratolysis plantare sulcatum): Produces circular areas of erosions with a punched-out appearance on the soles of the feet; associated with hyperhidrosis; filamentous, gram-positive, branching microorganisms are found on skin scrapings caused by corynebacterium. Topical or systemic erythromycin is usually beneficial.

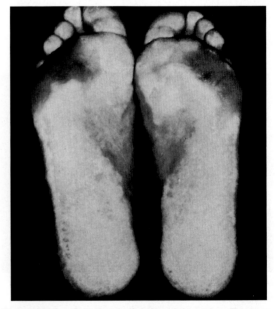

Figure 19-4. **Symmetric lividity of the soles.** This is associated with hyperhidrosis.

TREATMENT

ACUTE INFECTION. An acute vesicular, pustular fungal infection of 2 weeks' duration is present on the soles of the feet and between the toes in a 16-year-old boy. This clinical picture is usually due to the organism *T. mentagrophytes*.

FIRST VISIT

1. The fear of the infectiousness of athlete's foot should be minimized but normal cleanliness emphasized, including the wearing of slippers over bare feet, wiping the feet last after a bath (not the groin last), and changing socks daily (white socks are not necessary).
2. Débridement. The physician or the patient should snip off the tops of the blister with small scissors. This enables the pus to drain out and allows the medication to reach the organisms. The edges of any blister should be kept trimmed, since the fungi spread under these edges. This débridement is followed by a foot soak.
3. Burow's solution soak
   Sig: 1 packet of Domeboro powder to 1 quart of warm water. Soak feet for 10 minutes b.i.d. Dry skin carefully afterward.
4. Antifungal cream   15.0
   Miconazole (Monistat-Derm, Micatin), clotrimazole (Lotrimin, Mycelex), econazole (Spectazole), ketoconazole (Nizoral), ciclopirox (Loprox), oxiconazole (Oxistat), naftifine (Naftin), terbenifine (Lamisil), sulconazole (Exelderm), butenafine (Mentax), and tolnaftate (Tinactin) (see Table 19-3 for detailed list of antifungal agents).
   Sig: Apply b.i.d. locally to feet after soaking.
   Sig: Apply b.i.d. locally for long term.
5. Rest at home for 2 to 4 days may be advisable, if severe.
6. Place small pieces of cotton sheeting or cotton between the toes when wearing shoes.

SAUER NOTES

A favorite medication of mine for tinea of the feet and body is

Sulfur, ppt.	5%
Hydrocortisone	1%
Antifungal cream q.s.	30.0

Five days later, the secondary infection and blisters should have decreased.

SUBSEQUENT VISITS

1. The soaks may be continued for another 3 days or stopped if no marked redness or infection is present.
2. The previously described salve is continued or the following salves are substituted: A combination of an antifungal cream and a corticosteroid, as in Lotrisone cream, is beneficial. Antifungal solutions, such as Lotrimin or Mycelex or Loprox are quite effective. Apply a few drops on affected skin and rub in.
3. Antifungal powder q.s.   45.0
   Zeasorb AF, Micatin, Tinactin, Desenex, Enzactin, and Sopronal
   Sig: Supply in powder can. Apply small amount to feet over the salve and to the shoes in the morning.
4. Systemic antifungal therapy. These forms of oral treatment are not recommended for acute tinea of the feet because (1) response to oral agents is slow for these acute and rather disabling cases; (2) the recurrence rate is very high; and (3) the cost of oral therapy is much greater than that of the more rapidly effective local therapy.

CHRONIC INFECTION. A patient presents with chronic, scaly, thickened fungal infection of 4 years' duration. In the past week a few small tense blisters on the sole of the feet had developed. This type of clinical picture probably is due to the organism *T. rubrum*.

FIRST VISIT

1. The patient is told that the acute flare-up (the blisters) can be cleared but that it will be difficult and time-consuming to cure the chronic infection. If the toenails are found to be infected, the prognosis for cure is even poorer. (See Tinea of the Nails later in this chapter.)
2. The blisters are débrided and trimmed with manicure scissors.
3. Any of the antifungal creams,
   Sig: Apply locally to soles b.i.d., *or*
   Antifungal solution   10.0
   Sig: Rub in a few drops b.i.d.

204 CHAPTER 19 DERMATOLOGIC MYCOLOGY

TABLE 19-3
MEDICATIONS USED AGAINST FUNGI AND CANDIDA

Antifungal Agent	Route of Administration	Organism Responsive	Side Effects
Allylamines			
Naftifine (Naftin)	Cream, gel	Dermatophytes (fungicidal)	Rare
Terbinafine (Lamisil)	Cream, oral (not *m. canis*), spray	Dermatophytes (fungicidal), tinea versicolor	Rare
Benzylamines			
Butenafine HCl (Mentax)	Cream	Dermatophytes (fungicidal)	Rare
Azoles			
Clotrimazole (Mycelex, Lotrimin)	Cream, solution, troches, suppositories	Dermatophytes, *Candida*, tinea versicolor	Rare
Econazole (Spectazole)	Cream	Dermatophytes, *Candida*, tinea versicolor, gram-positive bacteria	Rare
Fluconazole (Diflucan)	Oral	*Candida*, cryptococcosis, Dermatophytes	Rare
Itraconazole (Sporanox)	Oral (with food)	Dermatophytes, sporotrichosis, *Candida*, tinea versicolor, some deep fungi	Rare liver toxicity
Ketocanazole (Nizoral)	Cream, shampoo, oral (empty stomach, acidic ph)	Some deep fungi, dermatophytes, *Candida*, tinea versicolor	>1 in 10,000 liver toxicity, antitetosterone
Miconazole (Micatin, Monistat)	Cream, aerosol, suppositories, Zeasorb AF powder	Dermatophytes, *Candida*, tinea versicolor	Rare
Oxiconazole (Oxistate)	Cream	Dermatophytes, *Candida*, tinea versicolor	Rare
Sulconazole (Exelderm)	Cream, solution	Dermatophytes, *Candida*, tinea versicolor	Rare
Polyenes			
Amphotericin B (Fungizone, Abelcet)	Intravenous	Deep fungi, *Candida* in life-threatening situations	Renal toxicity common, thrombophlebitis, hypokalemia
Nystatin (Mycostatin)	Cream, ointment, powder, oral (not absorbed), pastilles, with triam-cinolone (mycolog II cream, ointment)	*Candida*	Rare
Miscellaneous			
Flucytosine (Ancobon)	Oral, usually given with amphotericin B	Deep fungi, *Candida*	Liver, bone marrow, gastrointestinal and renal toxicity
Griseofulvin (Gris-Peg, Fulvicin, Grifulvin)	Oral (evening with fatty meal) tablets, suspension	Dermatophytes	Rare, headaches, Antabuse effect
Selenium sulfide (Selsun, Head and Shoulders Intensive Treatment)	Shampoo (sometimes used as lotion)	Tinea versicolor	Irritation
SSKI (saturated solution of potassium iodide)	Oral	Sporotrichosis	Gastrointestinal toxicity, bitter taste, goiter if long-term
Tolnaftate (Tinactin)	Cream	Dermatophytes	Rare
Undecylenic acid (Desenex)	Cream	Dermatophytes	Rare

1. Systemic antifungal therapy: This type of oral therapy is not recommended for chronic tinea of the feet. But the patient may have heard or read about the "pill for athlete's feet," so it would be wise for you to discuss this with the patient. If you mention that you cannot guarantee a cure, even after months of taking a large quantity of rather expensive pills, most patients will be content with keeping the chronic infection in an innocuous state with sporadic local therapy.
2. However, if after you have explained about the poor results and the expense of therapy, the patient still wants to try oral therapy, then consider the systemic antifungal agents listed in the following section on Tinea of the Hands and in Table 19-3. Long-term therapy is indicated, with appropriate monitoring of the patient.

Tinea of the Hands
(Fig. 19-5)

A primary fungal infection of the hand or hands is quite rare. In spite of this fact, the diagnosis of "fungal infection of the hand" is commonly applied to cases that in reality are contact dermatitis, atopic eczema, pustular bacterid, or psoriasis. The best differential point is that tinea of the hand usually is seen only on one hand, not bilaterally.

SAUER NOTE

Because tinea of one hand is usually found with tinea of both feet, this is commonly called "one-hand, two-foot disease."

PRIMARY LESIONS. *Acute form*: Blisters on the palms and the fingers are seen at the edge of red areas. *Chronic form*: Lesions are dry and scaly; usually there is a single patch, not separate patches.

SECONDARY LESIONS. Bacterial infection is rather unusual.

COURSE. This gradually progressive disease spreads to fingernails. It usually is nonsymptomatic.

LABORATORY FINDINGS. KOH-ink preparations reveal mycelia, or cultures on Sabouraud's media grow the fungus (see Chap. 2).

DIFFERENTIAL DIAGNOSIS

Contact dermatitis of hands: Due to soap, detergents, and other irritants; usually bilateral, periodic, more vesicular, and less frequently chronic; fungi not found (see Chap. 9).
Atopic eczema: History of atopy in patient or family; bilateral; periodic; fungi not found (see Chap. 9).
Psoriasis: See thick patch or patches in palms of menopausal women, usually bilateral; occasionally see psoriasis elsewhere; fungi not found (see Chap. 14).
Pustular bacterid: Pustular lesions only; periodic and chronic; resistant to local therapy; fungi not found.
Dyshidrosis of palms: Recurrent; seasonal incidence; mainly vesicular on the sides of the fingers: not scaly; bilateral; related to atopic eczema; fungi not found.

TREATMENT

A man presents with scaly thickening of one palm of 8 years' duration. His fingernails are not involved. Itching is noted slightly at times.

1. Antifungal creams, especially naftifine (Naftin), terbinafine (Lamisil) cream, or butenafine (Mentax) may control or occasionally cure the tinea of the hand.
2. Systemic therapy (see Table 19-3). The following medicines are all expensive, especially because therapy must be continued, as for hand tinea, for several months. Appropriate monitoring of the patient during therapy is necessary. There are also drug interactions that can occur.
   a. Griseofulvin (Gris-Peg, 250 mg; Fulvicin P/G, 330 mg; Grisactin, 330 mg; Grifulvin, 330 mg)
   Sig: 1 tablet t.i.d after meals for at least 8 weeks, and probably for 4 to 6 months.
   Comment: Griseofulvin commonly causes headaches in the first few days of therapy. It is a penicillin derivative.
   b. Ketoconazole (Nizoral), 200 mg (rarely 400 mg)
   Sig: 1 tablet once a day for 3 to 4 months.
   Comment: Hepatotoxicity has been rarely reported with ketoconazole therapy, also impotence.

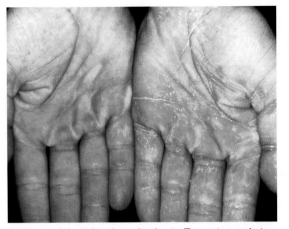

(*A*) Tinea of the left palm only, due to *T. mentagrophytes*.

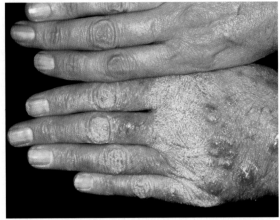

(*B*) Deep tinea of left hand, due to *T. mentagrophytes*.

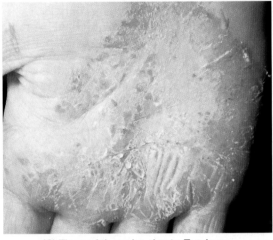

(*C*) Tinea of the palm, due to *T. rubrum*.

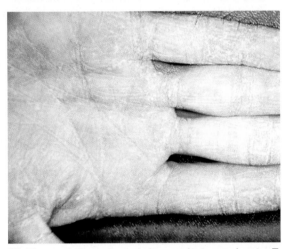

(*D*) Tinea of the palm, of dry, scaly type, due to *T. rubrum*.

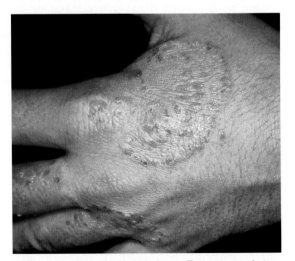

(*E*) Tinea on dorsum of hand, due to *T. mentagrophytes*, in a diabetic, age 15 years.

Figure 19-5.   **Tinea of the hand.** Tinea of the hand usually affects only one hand, but both feet. Thus, it is called "one-hand, two-foot syndrome." (*Duke Laboratories, Inc.*)

c. Itraconazole (Sporanox) capsule, 100 mg. 200 mg b.i.d. for 7 days, repeated once a month for 3 to 4 months. Monitoring for rare liver toxicity must be done. Drug interactions are numerous.

d. Fluconazole (Diflucan) has not been approved for superficial dermatophyte therapy. It may be effective in doses of 200 mg per week for 1 to 3 months. Drug interactions are numerous. It is expensive.

e. Terbinafine (Lamisil) 250 mg.
Sig: 1 tablet each day for 1 to 3 months. It is expensive.

SAUER NOTE

Most superficial fungus infections have an initial rapid response to systemic therapy. In a few days, there is evidence of healing and less itching. If this does not occur, then it is possible that the diagnosis of tinea is incorrect and other therapy should be instituted.

Tinea of the Nails
(Fig. 19-6; see Fig. 28-9)

Tinea of the toenails is very common, but tinea of the fingernails is uncommon. Tinea of the toenails is almost inevitable in patients who have recurrent attacks of tinea of the feet. Once developed, the infected nail serves as a resistant focus for future skin infection.

PRIMARY LESIONS. Distal and lateral detachment of the nail occurs with subsequent thickening and deformity.

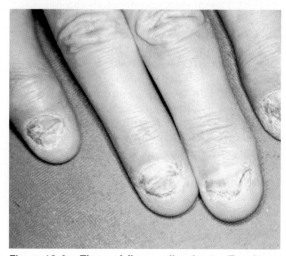

Figure 19-6. Tinea of fingernails, due to *T. rubrum*. *(Duke Laboratories, Inc.)*

SECONDARY LESIONS. Bacterial infection can result from the pressure of shoes on the deformed nail and surrounding skin. Ingrown toenails are another undesirable consequence.

DISTRIBUTION. The infection usually begins in the fifth toenail and may remain there or spread to involve the other nails.

COURSE. *Tinea of the toenails can rarely be cured.* Aside from the deformity, ingrown toenail (especially in diabetes mellitus and marked vascular or neurologic compromise to the feet) and an occasional mild flare-up of acute tinea, treatment is not necessary. Progression is slow, and spontaneous cures are rare.

Tinea of the fingernails can be treated, but the treatment usually takes months.

ETIOLOGY. This type of tinea is usually due to *T. rubrum* and, less importantly, to *T. mentagrophytes*.

LABORATORY FINDINGS. These organisms can be found in a KOH preparation of a scraping and occasionally can be grown on culture media. The material should be gathered from the most proximal debris under the nail plate. It is often difficult to obtain a positive test.

DIFFERENTIAL DIAGNOSIS

See also Chap. 28, Diseases Affecting the Nails.

Nail injury: A history of the injury must be obtained(Jogger's nails or pseudoonychomycosis), although tinea infection often starts in an injured nail; fungi are absent.

Psoriasis of fingernails: Pitting, red areas occur under nail with resulting detachment; psoriasis is elsewhere, usually; no fungi are found (see Chap. 14).

Psoriasis of toenails: This may be impossible to differentiate from tinea, because many psoriatic nails have some secondary fungal invasion.

Candidiasis of fingernails: Common in people who frequently wash their hands; paronychial involvement common; *Candida* found (see later in this chapter).

Green nails: This fingernail infection yields *Candida albicans* and *Pseudomonas aeruginosa* most commonly. Clinically, there is a distal detachment of the nail plate, with underlying greenish black debris. For cure, complete débridement of the detached part of the nail is necessary, plus local antifungal therapy.

TREATMENT

TINEA OF THE FINGERNAILS. A young salesman presents with a fungal infection in three fingernails of his left hand of 9 months' duration. The surrounding skin shows mild redness and scaling.

1. Griseofulvin therapy (see earlier and Table 19-3). Griseofulvin ultrafine type, 250 to 330 mg or equivalent
   Sig: 1 tablet b.i.d. or t.i.d. for 9 months.
   Comment: Therapy is stopped when there is no clinical evidence of infection (crumbling, thickening of nail plate, or subungual debris) and no cultural or KOH-ink mount evidence of fungi.
2. Ketoconazole (Nizoral) therapy. If the patient and the physician are aware of the possibility of liver and other toxicity, then a 200-mg tablet once a day for 9 months might be curative. Close patient monitoring is necessary. Many drug interactions, very expensive.
3. Itraconazole (Sporanox) therapy has been reported to be curative, 200 mg b.i.d. for 7 days, repeated monthly for 4 to 6 months. Available as a Pulse Pak. Many drug interactions.
4. Terbinafine (Lamisil) 250 mg a day for 3 months. Very expensive.

TINEA OF THE TOENAILS. A 45-year-old woman presents with three infected toenails on the right foot and two on the left foot. These are causing mild pain when she wears certain tight-fitting shoes. Scaliness of soles of feet is also evident.

1. Griseofulvin or ketoconazole therapy. This oral therapy is not effective or indicated for tinea of the toenails. Apparently some dermatologists have cured cases after oral therapy was continued for several years or when oral therapy was combined with evulsion of the toenails. The only time such therapy for toenails is prescribed, in our practice, is when the patient understands the problem but still wants to attempt a cure or a cosmetic improvement. At least 12 months of griseofulvin therapy is necessary. Women respond to this therapy better than men.
2. Itraconazole (Sporanox) may be used. A dosage of 200 mg b.i.d. for 7 days, repeated monthly for 4 to 8 months, has been suggested. A Pulse Pak is available. Drug interactions must be watched for. Monitoring of the patient is necessary for rare liver toxicity. Very expensive
3. Terbinafine (Lamisil) 250 mg a day for 3 or 4 months. Very expensive.

4. Antifungal solution, 15 mL. For the patient who wants to "do something," applications two to four times a day for months might help some mild cases. One can combine this therapy with débridement of the nails. These solutions include Fungi-Nail, Fungoid, and Loprox.
5. Débriding of thick nails by patient, dermatologist, or podiatrist offers obvious relief from discomfort. This can be accomplished by the use of nail clippers or filing or picking away with a scalpel blade or a motor-driven drill.
6. Surgical evulsion of the toenail is rarely curative. As stated previously, this surgical approach can be combined with oral systemic therapy with probable enhancement of the end result.

Tinea of the Groin
(Fig. 19-7)

Tinea of the groin is a common, itching, annoying fungal infection appearing usually in men and often concurrently with tinea of the feet. Home remedies often result in a contact dermatitis that adds "fuel to the fire."

PRIMARY LESIONS. Bilateral, fan-shaped, red, scaly patches with a sharp, slightly raised border occur. Small vesicles may be seen in the active border.

SECONDARY LESIONS. Oozing, crusting, edema, and secondary bacterial infection are evident. In chronic cases lichenification may be marked. Lichen simplex chronicus can develop.

DISTRIBUTION. The infection affects the crural fold, extending to involve the scrotum, penis, thighs, perianal area, and buttocks.

COURSE. The type of fungus influences the course, but most acute cases respond rapidly to treatment. Other factors that affect the course and recurrences are obesity, hot weather, sweating, and chafing garments.

ETIOLOGY. Tinea of the groin is commonly due to the fungi of tinea of the feet, *T. rubrum*, and *T. mentagrophytes*, and also to the fungus *E. floccosum*.

CONTAGIOUSNESS. This is minimal, even between husband and wife.

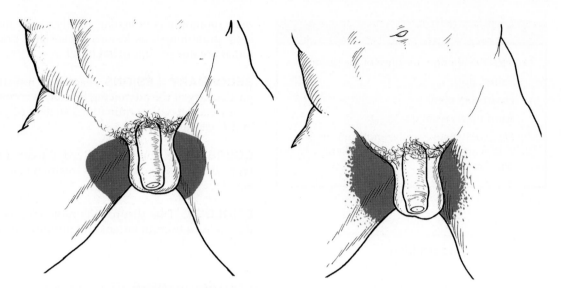

Figure 19-7. Dermagrams for comparison of tinea of crural area and candidiasis of crural area.
(*Left*) Tinea of crural area. Note sharp border of lesions. (See also Fig. 19-18). (*Right*) Candidiasis of crural area. Note indefinite border with satellite pustule-like lesions as edge. Candiadiasis can also involve the scrotum. (See also Fig. 19-14.)

LABORATORY FINDINGS. The organism is found in KOH preparations of scrapings and can be grown on culture. Material is taken from the active border (see Chap. 2).

DIFFERENTIAL DIAGNOSIS

Candidiasis: No sharp border; fine scales, oozing, redness, satellite pustule-like lesions at edges; more common in obese females; *Candida* found (see later in this chapter and Figs. 19-12–19-15).

Contact dermatitis: Often coexistent but can be separate entity; new contactant history; no fungi found; no active border (see Chap. 9).

Prickly heat: Pustular, papular; no active border, no fungi; may also be present with tinea.

Lichen simplex chronicus: Unilateral, usually; may have resulted from old chronic tinea; no fungi (see Chap. 11).

Psoriasis: Usually unilateral; may or may not have raised border; psoriasis elsewhere; no fungi (see Chap. 14).

Erythrasma: Faint redness, fine scaling with no elevated border, also seen in axilla and webs of toes; coral reddish fluorescence under Wood's light; due to a diphtheroid organism called *Corynebacterium minutissimum* (see Chap. 15).

Bowen's Disease or Extramammory Paget's Disease: Consider these diagnoses if unilateral and recalcitrant to therapy; biopsy necessary to make these diagnoses.

TREATMENT

Oozing, red dermatitis with sharp border occurring in crural area of young man.

1. Because the infection usually comes from chronic tinea of the feet, to prevent recurrences, advise the patient to dry the feet last and not the groin area last when taking a bath.
2. Vinegar wet packs
   Sig: ½ cup of white vinegar to 1 quart of warm water. Wet the sheeting or thin toweling and apply to area for 15 minutes twice a day.
3. Antifungal cream 15.0
   Sig: Apply b.i.d. locally (see Table 19-3).
4. Griseofulvin oral therapy
   Griseofulvin ultrafine types, 250 to 330 mg
   Sig: 1 tablet b.i.d. for 6 to 8 weeks for extensive case.
5. Ketoconazole, itraconazole or terbinafine therapy may also be used.

SAUER NOTE

An effective therapy for tinea of the groin is:

Sulfur, ppt.	5%
Hydrocortisone	1%
Antifungal cream q.s.	15.0

Sig: Apply b.i.d. locally, and continue for 7 days after apparently clear ("therapy-plus" routine).

Tinea of the Smooth Skin
(Figs. 19-8 and 19-9; see Fig. 33-30C)

The familiar ringworm of the skin is most common in children partially because of their intimacy with animals and other children. The lay public believes that *most* skin conditions are "ringworm," and many physicians erroneously agree with them.

PRIMARY LESIONS. Round, oval, or semicircular scaly patches have a slightly raised border that commonly is vesicular. Rarely, deep, ulcerated, granulomatous lesions (Majocchi's granuloma) are due to superficial fungi.

SECONDARY LESIONS. Bacterial infection, particularly at the advancing border, is common in association with certain fungi, such as *M. canis* and *T. mentagrophytes*.

COURSE. Infection is short lived, if treated correctly. It seldom recurs unless treatment is inadequate.

ETIOLOGY. This disorder is most commonly due to *M. canis* from kittens and puppies and less commonly due to *E. floccosum* and *T. mentagrophytes* from groin and foot infections.

CONTAGIOUSNESS. The incidence is high.

LABORATORY FINDINGS. This is the same as for previously discussed fungal diseases.

DIFFERENTIAL DIAGNOSIS

Pityriasis rosea: History of herald patch; sudden shower of oval lesions; fungi not found (see Chap. 14).

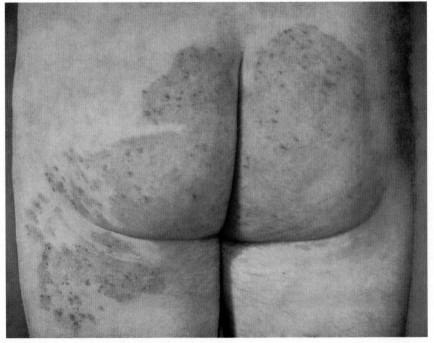

Figure 19-8. Tinea of the smooth skin. This infection on the buttocks had spread from the crural region. (*Smith Kline & French Laboratories*)

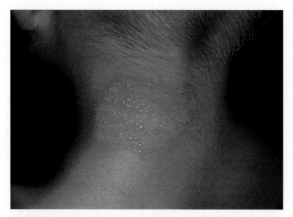

(*A*) Tinea of posterior neck area probably due to *T. ver-rucosum*.

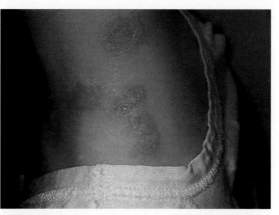

(*B*) Tinea of side of neck due to *T. mentagrophytes*.

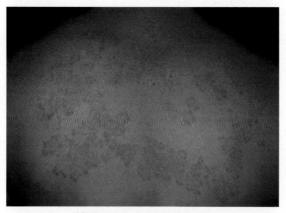

(*C*) Extensive tinea of back.

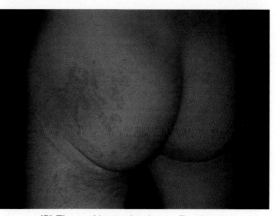

(*D*) Tinea of buttocks due to *T. rubrum*.

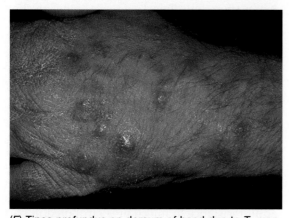

(*E*) Tinea profundus on dorsum of hand due to *T. men-tagrophytes*.

Figure 19-9. **Tinea of smooth skin.** (*Ortho Pharmaceutical Corp.*)

Impetigo: Vesicular, honey-colored, crusted; most commonly on face; no fungi found (see Chap. 15).

Contact dermatitis: No sharp border or central healing; may be coexistent with ringworm worsened by overtreatment (see Chap. 9).

TREATMENT

A child has several 2- to 4-cm scaly lesions on his arms of 1 week's duration. He has a new kitten that he holds and plays with.

1. Examine the scalp, preferably with a Wood's light, to rule out scalp infection.
2. Advise the mother regarding moderate isolation procedures in relation to the family and others.
3. Antifungal salve q.s.   15.0
   Sig: Apply b.i.d. locally (see Table 19-3).

SUBSEQUENT VISIT OF RESISTANT CASE OR A NEW WIDESPREAD CASE: GRISEOFULVIN ORAL THERAPY

Griseofulvin (ultrafine types) can be given in tablet or oral suspension form. The usual dose for children is 165 mg b.i.d., but the pharmaceutical company's product information sheet should be consulted. Therapy should be maintained for 3 to 6 weeks or until lesions are gone. Occasionally, a higher dose is needed in deeper forms of infection.

Tinea of the Scalp
(Fig. 19-10; see also Fig. 33-30 A,B)

Tinea of the scalp is the most common cause of patchy hair loss in children (Fig. 19-10). Endemic cases are with us always, but epidemics, usually due to the human type, were, until the discovery of griseofulvin, the real therapeutic problem. Griseofulvin orally finds its greatest therapeutic usefulness and triumph in the management of tinea of the scalp. Before griseofulvin, children with the human type of scalp tinea had to be subjected to traumatic shampoos and salves for weeks or months, or they had to be epilated by x-ray. Often they were kept out of school for this entire period of therapy.

Ketoconazole, terbinafine, or itraconazole systemic therapy is available for griseofulvin-resistant cases, if these truly occur in tinea of the scalp.

Tinea capitis infections can be divided into two clinical types: (1) *noninflammatory* and (2) *inflammatory*. The treatment, the cause, and the course vary for these two types.

Noninflammatory Type

PRIMARY LESIONS. Grayish, scaly, round patches with broken-off hairs are seen, causing balding areas. The size of the areas varies.

SECONDARY LESIONS. Bacterial infection and id reactions are rare. A noninflammatory patch can become inflamed spontaneously or as the result of strong local treatment. Scarring almost never occurs. "Black dot" hairs (short broken-off hairs) are seen with *T. tonsurans* infection.

DISTRIBUTION. The infection is most common in the posterior scalp region. Body ringworm from the scalp lesions is common, particularly on the neck and the shoulders.

SAUER NOTES

1. Examine the scalp in any child who has body ringworm.
2. Perform hair KOH mounts, cultures, or Wood's light examination of suspicious scalp areas.
3. Inquire about siblings having similar scalp lesions.

COURSE. The incubation period in and on the hair is short, but clinical evidence of the infection cannot be expected less than 3 weeks after inoculation. Parents often do not notice the infection for another 3 weeks to several months, particularly in girls. Spontaneous cures are rare in 2 to 6 months but after that time occur with greater frequency. Some cases last for years, if untreated. Recurrence of the infection after the cure of a previous episode is possible, because adequate immunity does not develop.

AGE GROUP. Infection of the noninflammatory type is most common between the ages of 3 and 8 years and is rare after the age of puberty. This adult resistance to infection is attributed in part to the higher content of fungistatic fatty acids in the sebum after puberty. This research laboratory finding had great therapeutic significance, and the direct outgrowth was the development of Desenex, and other fatty-acid ointments and powders.

T. tonsurans infection is seen mainly in African-American urban preadolescent children

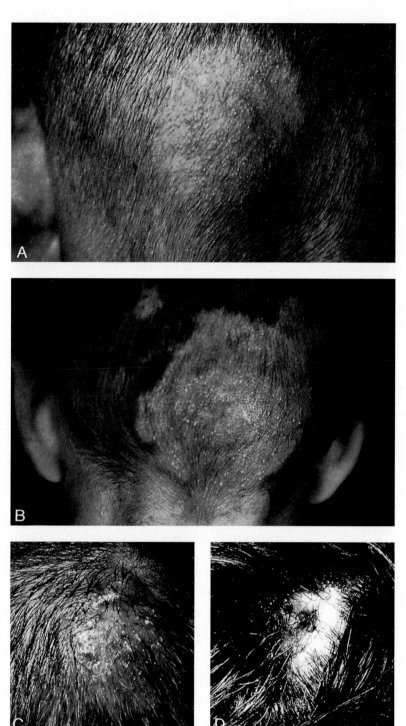

(*A*) Due to *M. audouini*. Note absence of visible inflammation.

(*B*) Due to *T. tonsurans*. Wood light examination revealed no fluorescence.

(*C*) Due to *T. mentagrophytes*. Note inflammation.

(*D*) Favus, due to *T. shoenleini*, of 11 years' duration.

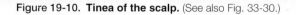

Figure 19-10. **Tinea of the scalp.** (See also Fig. 33-30.)

(often females who braid their hair). Spontaneous cures at puberty, particularly for girls, do not always occur.

ETIOLOGY. The noninflammatory type of scalp ringworm is caused most frequently by *T. tonsurans* and occasionally by *M. canis* and *M. audouini*. *M. audouini* and *T. tonsurans* are anthropophilic fungi (human-to-human passage only), whereas *M. canis* is a zoophilic fungus (animals are the original source, mainly kittens and puppies).

CONTAGIOUSNESS. The case can be a part of a large urban epidemic.

LABORATORY FINDINGS. *Wood's light examination of the scalp hairs* is an important diagnostic test, but hairs infected with *T. tonsurans* do not fluoresce. The Wood's light is a specially filtered long-wavelength ultraviolet light. The hairs infected with *M. audouini* and *M. canis* fluoresce with a bright yellowish green color (see Fig. 33-30). The bright fluorescence of fungus-infected hairs is not to be confused with the white or dull yellow color emitted by lint particles or sulfur-laden scales.

Microscopic examination of the infected hairs in 20% KOH solution shows an ectothrix arrangement of the spores when due to the *Microsporum* species and endothrix spores when due to *T. tonsurans*. Culture is necessary for species identification (see Fig. 2-2). The cultural characteristics of the various fungi can be found in many larger dermatologic or mycologic texts and are not presented here.

TREATMENT

<u>PROPHYLACTIC</u>

1. Infected children can attend school, provided that they wear cotton stockinette caps at all times (no swapping allowed) and present a note from the physician every 3 weeks stating that they are under a physician's care. Infected children should be restricted from theaters, churches, and other public places. Community health departments should be consulted for specific rulings.
2. All susceptible schoolchildren are inspected with a Wood's light by a school nurse every 4 weeks during an epidemic.
3. Hair is washed after every haircut by a barber or beautician.

4. Parents and teachers are educated on methods of spread of disease, particularly during an epidemic.
5. Suggestions should be given for provision for individual storage of clothing, particularly caps, in school and home.

<u>ACTIVE</u>

1. Griseofulvin oral therapy. The ultrafine types of griseofulvin (Fulvicin U/F, Fulvicin P/G, Gris-Peg, Grifulvin V, and Grisactin) can be administered in tablet form or liquid suspension (not all brands available in liquid form). The usual dose for a child aged 4 to 8 is 250 mg b.i.d., but some require a larger dose. The duration of therapy is usually 6 to 8 weeks. Both dose and duration have to be individualized and based on clinical, Wood's light, or culture response.
2. Ketoconazole, terfinafine, itriconazole or fluconazole oral therapy. This type of therapy is usually not indicated or necessary, but regimens are effective and preferred by some.
3. Selenium sulfide (Selsun) Shampoo is sporicidal and may help decrease the spread of infection.
4. Manual epilation of hairs. Near the end of therapy, the remaining infected and fluorescent hairs can be plucked out, or the involved area can be shaved closely. This will eliminate the infected distal end of the growing hair.

Inflammatory Type

PRIMARY LESIONS. Pustular, scaly, round patches with broken-off hairs are found, resulting in bald areas.

SECONDARY LESIONS. Bacterial-like infection is common. When the secondary reaction is marked, the area becomes swollen and tender. This inflammation is called a *kerion*. Minimal scarring sometimes remains.

DISTRIBUTION. Any scalp area is involved. Concurrent body ringworm infection is common.

COURSE. Duration is much shorter than the noninflammatory type of infection. Spontaneous cures will result after 2 to 4 months in many cases, even if untreated, except for the *T. tonsurans* type.

ETIOLOGY. The inflammatory type of scalp ringworm is most commonly caused by *T. ton-*

surans and *M. canis* and rarely by *M. audouini*, *M. gypseum*, *T. mentagrophytes*, and *T. verrucosum*. *T. tonsurans*, *M. audouini*, and *T. mentagrophytes* are anthropophilic (coming from humans); *M. canis* and *T. verrucosum* are zoophilic (passed from infected animals); and *M. gypseum* is geophilic (coming from the soil).

CONTAGIOUSNESS. The incidence is high in children and farmers. It is mainly endemic, except for cases due to *M. audouini*.

LABORATORY FINDINGS. Microscopic examination of the infected hairs in 20% KOH solution shows an ectothrix arrangement of the spores, but *T. tonsurans* shows endothrix spores. The hairs infected with *M. canis* and *M. audouini* fluoresce with a bright yellowish green color under the Wood's light.

DIFFERENTIAL DIAGNOSIS
(Table 19-4)

TREATMENT

PROPHYLACTIC

This is the same as for noninflammatory cases.

ACTIVE

1. Griseofulvin oral therapy (as under noninflammatory type).
2. Local therapy. For some mild cases of the inflammatory type, or where drug expense is a factor, local therapy can be used with good results.

Bactroban ointment   15.0
Sig: Apply locally b.i.d. The scalp and the hair should be shampooed nightly.
3. If kerion is severe, with or without griseofulvin therapy:
   a. Burow's solution wet packs.
      Sig: 1 Domeboro packet to 1 pint of warm water. Apply soaked cloths for 15 minutes twice a day.
   b. Antibiotic therapy orally helps to eliminate secondary bacterial infection.

Tinea of the Beard
(Fig. 19-11)

Fungal infection is a rare cause of dermatitis in the beard area. Farmers occasionally contract it from infected cattle. Any presumed bacterial infection of the beard that does not respond readily to proper treatment should be examined for fungi.

PRIMARY LESIONS. Follicular, pustular, or sharp-bordered ringworm-type lesions or deep, boggy, inflammatory masses are seen.

SECONDARY LESIONS. Bacterial infection is common. Scarring is unusual.

ETIOLOGY. See Table 19-1.

DIFFERENTIAL DIAGNOSIS

Bacterial folliculitis: Acute onset, rapid spread; no definite border; responds rather rapidly to antibiotic therapy; no fungi found on examination of hairs or culture (see Chap. 15).

TABLE 19-4
DIFFERENTIAL DIAGNOSIS OF SCALP DERMATOSES

Dermatosis	Wood's Light	Scales	Redness	Hair Loss	Remarks
Tinea capitis	±	Dry or crusted	Uncommon	Yes	Back of scalp, child
Alopecia areata (see Chap. 27)	—	None	No	Yes	Exclamation point hairs at edges
Seborrheic dermatitis (see Chap. 13)	—	Greasy	Yes	No	Diffuse scaling
Psoriasis (see Chap. 14)	—	Thick and dry	Yes	No	Look at elbows knees, and nails
Trichotillomania (see Chap. 27)	—	None	No	Yes	Psychoneurotic child
Pyoderma (see Chap. 15) (with or without lice)	—	Crusted	yes	Occasional	Poor hygiene

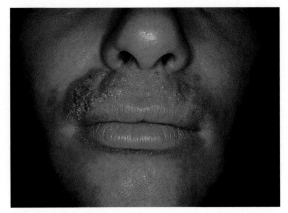

Figure 19-11. Tinea of the beard. Due to *T. mentagrophytes*.

TREATMENT

A farmer presents with a quarter-sized, boggy, inflammatory, pustular mass on his chin of 3 weeks' duration.

1. Have veterinarian inspect cattle if farmer is not aware of source of infection.
2. Burow's solution wet packs
   Sig: 1 Domeboro packet to 1 pint of hot water. Apply wet cloths to area for 15 minutes t.i.d.
3. Antifungal cream q.s.   15.0
   Sig: Apply locally b.i.d.
4. Griseofulvin oral therapy. The usual dose of griseofulvin, ultrafine type, for an adult is 250 to 330 mg b.i.d. for 6 to 8 weeks or longer, depending on clinical response or negative Sabouraud's culture.
5. Other oral antifungals can be used.

Dermatophytid

During an acute episode of any fungal infection, an id eruption can develop over the body. This is a manifestation of an allergic reaction to the fungal infection. The most common id reaction occurs on the hands during an acute tinea infection on the feet. To assume a diagnosis of an id reaction, the following criteria should be followed: (1) The primary focus should be acutely inflamed or infected with fungi, not chronically infected; (2) the id lesions must not contain fungi; and (3) the id eruption should disappear or wane after adequate treatment of the acute focus.

PRIMARY LESIONS. Vesicular eruption of the hands (primary lesion on the feet) and papulofollicular eruption on body (primary lesion commonly is scalp kerion) are found; pityriasis rosea-like id eruptions and others are seen less commonly.

SECONDARY LESIONS. Excoriation and infection occur, when itching is severe, which is unusual.

TREATMENT

1. Treat the primary focus of infection.
2. For a vesicular id reaction on the *hands*:
   Burow's solution soaks
   Sig: 1 Domeboro packet to 1 quart of cool water. Soak hands for 15 minutes b.i.d.
3. For an id reaction on the *body* that is moderately pruritic:
   Aveeno oatmeal bath
   Sig: 1 packet of Aveeno to 6 to 8 inches of cool water in a tub, once daily.
   Hydrocortisone 1% lotion   120.0
   Sig: Apply locally b.i.d.
   Comment: Menthol 0.25%, phenol 0.5%, or camphor 2% could be added to this lotion.
4. For a severely itching, *generalized* id eruption:
   Prednisone, 10 mg, or related corticosteroid tablets   #30
   Sig: 1 tablet q.i.d. for 2 days, then 2 tablets every morning for 7 days (or longer if necessary).

DEEP FUNGAL INFECTIONS

Those fungi that invade the skin deeply and go into living tissue are also capable of involving other organs. Only the skin manifestations of these deeply invading fungi are discussed here.

The following diseases are included in this group of deep fungal infections (other, rarer, deep mycotic diseases are found in the Dictionary–Index and in Chap. 35):

- Candidiasis
- Sporotrichosis (see Fig. 35-19)
- North American blastomycosis (see Fig. 19-17)

Systemic fungus infections that were extremely rare are now being seen more frequently in those patients who are immunocompromised, such as patients on chemotherapy, organ transplant cases, and those with the acquired immunodeficiency syndrome.

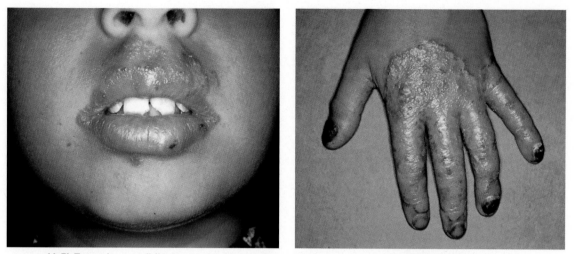

(*A,B*) Extensive candidiasis around the mouth and on dorsum of hand in child with Addison's disease.

Figure 19-12. **Candidal infections.** (*Herbert Laboratories*)

Candidiasis

(Figs. 19-12–19-14; see Figs. 18-7, 33-4A–B, and 33-17)

Candidiasis (moniliasis) is a fungal infection caused by *Candida albicans* that produces lesions in the mouth, the vagina, the skin, the nails, the lungs, or the gastrointestinal tract or occasionally a septicemia. The latter condition is seen in patients who are on long-term, high-dose antibiotic therapy and in those who are immunosuppressed. Because *C. albicans* exists commonly as a harmless skin inhabitant, the laboratory findings of this organism are not adequate proof of its pathogenicity and etiologic role. *Candida* organisms commonly seed preexisting disease conditions. Concern here is with the *cutaneous* and the *mucocutaneous* candidal diseases. The following classification is helpful.

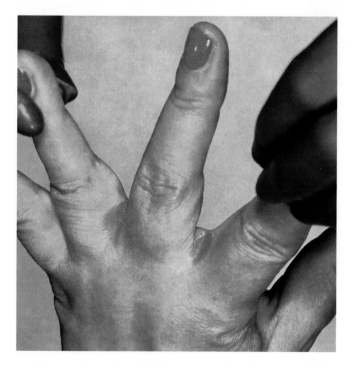

Figure 19-13. **Candidal intertrigo of the webs of the fingers.** (*Smith Kline & French Laboratories*)

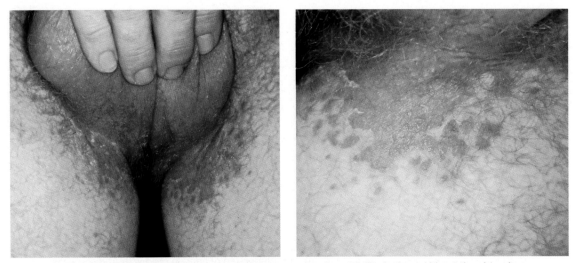

(*A,B*) Candidal intertrigo of crural area and close-up showing satellite lesions without the sharp border as seen in tinea cruris.

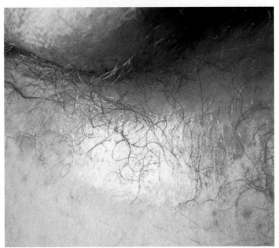

(*C*) Moist candidal intertrigo of crural area.

Figure 19-14. **Candidal infections.** (*Herbert Laboratories*)

CUTANEOUS CANDIDIASIS

1. Localized diseases
   a. Candidal paronychia (see Fig. 28-3B). This common candidal infection is characterized by the development of painful, red swellings of the skin around the nail plate. In chronic infections the nail becomes secondarily thickened and hardened. Candidal paronychia is commonly seen in housewives and those persons whose occupations predispose to frequent immersion of the hands in water.

   This nail involvement is to be differentiated from *superficial tinea of the nails* (the candidal infection usually does not cause the nail to lose its luster or to become crumbly, and debris does not accumulate beneath the nail, except in chronic mucocutaneous candidiasis) and from *bacterial paronychia* (this is more acute in onset and throbs with pain and may drain pus).
   b. Candidal intertrigo (Fig. 19-15; see Figs. 19-7 and 19-14). This moderately common condition is characterized by red, eroded patches, with scaly, pustular or pustulovesicular lesions, with an indefinite border of satellite pustules. The most common sites are axillae, inframammary areas, umbilicus, genital area, anal area, and webs

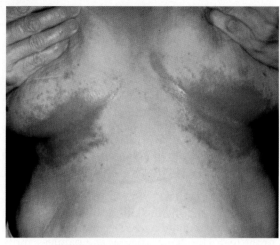

(*A*) Candidal intertrigo under breasts.

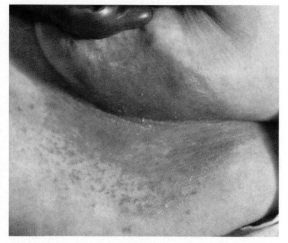

(*B*) Note the lack of a definite border to the eruption, which distinguishes it from a tinea infection.

Figure 19-15. **Candidal intertrigo under the breast.** (*Smith Kline & French Laboratories*)

of toes and fingers. Obesity, diabetes, and systemic antibiotics predispose to the development of this intertriginous type.

Candidal intertrigo is to be differentiated from *superficial tinea infections*, which are not as red and eroded, and from *seborrheic dermatitis* or *psoriasis*.

2. Generalized cutaneous candidiasis (see Figs. 33-4 and 33-17). This rare infection involves the smooth skin, mucocutaneous orifices, and intertriginous areas. It follows in the wake of general debility, as seen in immunosuppressed patients, and was very resistant to treatment before the discovery of ketoconazole and, more recently, fluconazole and itriconazole.

MUCOUS MEMBRANE CANDIDIASIS
(see Fig. 19-12A)

1. *Oral candidiasis (thrush and perlèche).* Thrush is characterized by creamy white flakes on a red, inflamed mucous membrane. The tongue may be smooth and atrophic, or the papillae may be hypertrophic, as in the condition labeled "hairy tongue." Therapy with Mycostatin pastilles (lozenges) or Mycelex troches is effective. Perlèche is seen as cracks or fissures at the corners of the mouth and is usually associated with candidal disease elsewhere and rarely a dietary deficiency (usually B12 deficiency). Thrush is seen commonly in immunosuppressed patients.

A noncandidal, clinically similar condition is commonly seen in *elderly persons with ill-fitting dentures* in whom the corners of the mouth override. Oral candidiasis is also to be differentiated from allergic conditions, such as those due to toothpaste or mouthwash.

2. *Candidal vulvovaginitis.* The clinical picture is an oozing, red, sharply bordered skin infection surrounding an inflamed vagina that contains a buttermilk-like discharge. This type of candidal infection is frequently seen in pregnant women, diabetics, and those who have been on antibiotics systemically.

It is to be differentiated from an *allergic condition* or from *trichomonal* or *chlamydial vaginitis*.

LABORATORY FINDINGS. Skin or mucous-membrane scrapings placed in 20% KOH solution and examined with the high-power microscope lens reveal small, oval, budding, thin-walled, yeast-like cells with occasional mycelia. Culture on Sabouraud's media produces creamy dull-white colonies in 4 to 5 days. Further cultural studies on corn meal agar are necessary to identify the species as *C. albicans*.

TREATMENT

CASE 1

Candidal paronychia of two fingers is seen in a 37-year-old male bartender.

1. Advise the patient to avoid exposure of his hands to soap and water by wearing cotton

gloves under rubber gloves, hiring a dish-washer, and so on.

2. Antifungal imidazole-type solution (Lotrimin or Mycelex solution 1%)   15.0
   or Fungi-Nail   15.0
   Sig: Apply to base of nail q.i.d. Continue treatment for several weeks.
3. At night, apply:
   Lotrisone cream   15.0
   Sig: Apply locally h.s.

CASE 2

Candidal intertrigo of inframammary and crural region is seen in an elderly obese woman.

1. Advise the patient to wear pieces of cotton sheeting under breasts to keep the apposing tissues drier. Frequent bathing with thorough drying is helpful. Use of antibacterial soap should be avoided.
2. Sulfur, ppt.   5%
   Hydrocortisone   1%
   Mycostatin cream q.s.   30.0
   Sig: Apply locally t.i.d.
3. Powder can be used over cream:
   Mycostatin dusting powder q.s.   15.0
   Sig: Apply locally t.i.d.

CASE 3

Candidal vulvovaginitis is found in a woman who is 6 months pregnant.

1. Mycostatin vaginal tablets, 100,000 units #20
   Sig: Insert 1 tablet b.i.d. in vagina.
2. Monistat-Derm lotion, or
   Sulfur, ppt.   5%
   Hydrocortisone   1%
   Mycostatin cream q.s.   30.0
   Sig: Apply locally b.i.d. to vulvar skin.
3. Diflucan (fluconazole)
   150 mg tablet. Single dose p.o. Can repeat for resistant cases.

SAUER NOTE

Do not treat a candidal infection with oral griseofulvin. This intensifies the candidal infection.

KETOCONAZOLE (NIZORAL), ITRICONAZOLE (SPORANOX) OR FLUCONAZOLE (DIFLUCAN) THERAPY. This systemic therapy is rarely indicated for routine candidal infections. For *chronic* mucocutaneous candidiasis, ketoconazole and fluconazole can heal dramatically.

Dosage information is provided in the package insert. The patient must be monitored carefully.

Sporotrichosis *(see Chap. 35)*
(Fig. 19-16; see fig. 35-19)

Sporotrichosis is a granulomatous fungal infection of the skin and the subcutaneous tissues. Characteristically, a primary chancre precedes more extensive skin involvement. Invasion of the internal viscera is rare (see Chap. 35).

PRIMARY LESION. A sporotrichotic chancre develops at the site of skin inoculation, which is commonly the hand and less commonly the face or the feet. The chancre begins as a painless, movable, subcutaneous nodule that eventually softens and breaks down to form an ulcer.

SECONDARY LESIONS. Within a few weeks subcutaneous nodules arise along the course of the draining lymphatics and form a chain of tumors that develop into ulcers. This is the classic clinical picture, of which there are variations.

COURSE. The development of the skin lesions is slow and rarely affects the general health.

ETIOLOGY. The causative agent is *Sporothrix schenckii*, a fungus that grows on wood and in the soil. It invades open wounds and is an occupational hazard of farmers (especially sphagnum moss), gardeners (especially roses), laborers, and miners.

LABORATORY FINDINGS. Cultures of the purulent material from unopened lesions readily grow on Sabouraud's media. The organism is difficult to see, even with special stains or tissue examination from a biopsy.

DIFFERENTIAL DIAGNOSIS

Any of the skin granulomas should be considered, such as *pyodermas, syphilis, tuberculosis, sarcoidosis*, and *leprosy*. An *ioderma* or *bromoderma* can cause a similar clinical picture.

TREATMENT

1. Saturated solution of potassium iodide, 60.0 mL
   Sig: On the first day, 10 drops t.i.d., p.c. added to milk or water; second day, 15 drops t.i.d.; third day, 20 drops t.i.d. and increase until 30 to 40 drops t.i.d. is given.

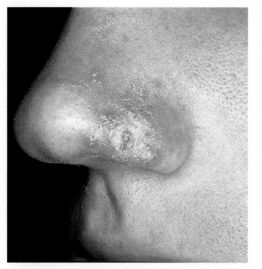 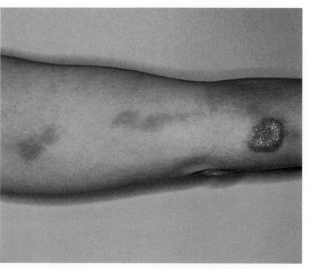

(*A*) Sporotrichotic primary lesion on the nose. (*B*) Sporotrichotic chancre on arm with subcutaneous nodules.

Figure 19-16. **Deep fungus infections.** (*Stiefel Laboratories [in part]*)

Comment: The initial doses may be smaller and the increase more gradual if one is concerned about tolerance. Gastric irritation and ioderma should be watched for. There is a very bitter taste. This very specific treatment must be continued for 1 month after apparent cure.

2. Ketoconazole (Nizoral), 200 mg
   Sig: 2 tablets a day for 8 weeks.
   Comment: Some cases are not helped. The patient must be monitored closely.
3. Itraconazole (Sporanox), 100 mg
   Sig: 1 tablet daily for 4 to 6 weeks.
   Comment: Patient should be monitored for rare liver toxicity.

North American Blastomycosis
(*Fig. 19-17*)

Two cutaneous forms of this disease are seen: (1) primary cutaneous blastomycosis and (2) secondary localized cutaneous blastomycosis.

Primary cutaneous blastomycosis occurs in laboratory workers and physicians after accidental inoculation. A primary chancre develops at the site of the inoculation, and the regional nodes enlarge. In a short time the primary lesion and nodes heal spontaneously and the cure is complete.

The following discussion is confined to the *secondary cutaneous form*. Systemic blastomycosis is rarer than the cutaneous forms but is seen occasionally in immunosuppressed patients.

PRIMARY LESION (SECONDARY, LOCALIZED, CUTANEOUS FORM). The lesion begins as a papule that ulcerates and slowly spreads peripherally, with a warty, pustular, raised border. The face, the hands, and the feet are involved most commonly.

SECONDARY LESION. Central healing of the ulcer occurs gradually, with resultant thick scar.

COURSE. A large lesion develops over several months. Therapy is moderately effective on a long-term basis. Relapses are common.

ETIOLOGY. The fungus *Blastomyces dermatitidis* is believed to invade the lungs primarily and the skin secondarily as a metastatic lesion. High native immunity prevents the development of more than one skin lesion. This immunity is low in the rare systemic form of blastomycosis in which multiple lesions occur in the skin, the bones, and other organs. This fungal disease affects adult males most frequently.

LABORATORY FINDINGS. The material for a 20% KOH solution mount is collected from the pustules at the border of the lesion. Round, budding organisms can be found in this manner or in a culture mount. A chest roentgenogram is indicated in every case.

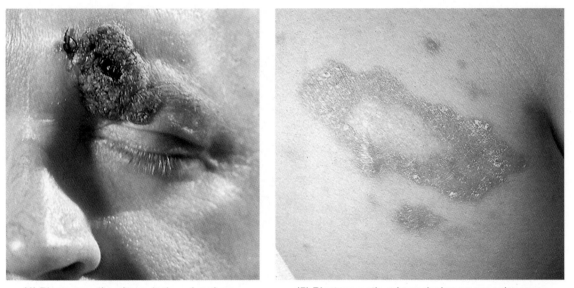

(*A*) Blastomycotic primary lesion of eyebrow.   (*B*) Blastomycotic primary lesion on scapular area.

Figure 19-17.   **Deep fungus infections.** (*Stiefel Laboratories [in part]*)

DIFFERENTIAL DIAGNOSIS

Consider any of the granuloma-producing diseases, such as *tuberculosis, syphilis, iodide* or *bromide drug eruption, pyoderma,* and *neoplasm.*

TREATMENT

1. Surgical excision and plastic repair of early lesions is effective.
2. Amphotericin B suppresses the chronic lesion more effectively than any other drug. It is administered by intravenous infusion, daily, in varying schedules, which are described in larger texts or reviews. Abelcet is a safer more effective form of this drug.
3. Ketoconazole or itraconazole therapy on a long-term basis is also beneficial. Higher than normal dosages for a longer period of time are necessary for immunosuppressed patients.

BIBLIOGRAPHY

Barranco V. Proceedings and transactions, Second Internations Symposium on Onychomycosis. Int J Dermatol 1997; 36.

Drake LA, Dinehart SM, et al. Guidelines of care for superficial mycotic infections of the skin: Mucocutaneous candidiasis. J Am Acad Dermatol 1996; 34:287.

Drake LA, Dinehart SM, et al. Guidelines of care for superficial mycotic infections of the skin: Tinea corporis, tinea cruris, tinea faciei, tinea manuum, and tinea pedis. J Am Acad Dermatol 1996; 34:2.

Elewski BE. Cutaneous fungal infections, ed 2. Boston, Blackwell Science 1998.

Herbert AA. Tinea capitis. Arch Dermatol 1988; 124:1554.

Gupta AK, Shear NH. Terbinafine: An update. J Am Acad Dermatol 1997; 37:979.

Hochman LG, Scher RK, Meyerson MS, et al. The safety and efficacy of oral fluconazole in the treatment of onychomycosis. J Geriatr Dermatol 1993; 1:169.

Jacobs PH, Nall L. Systemic antifungals. Cutis 1993; 52:165.

Mooney MA, Thomas I, Sirois D. Oral candidosis. Int J Dermatol 1995; 34:759.

Odom R. Pathophysiology of dermatophyte infections. J Am Acad Dermatol 1993; 28:S2.

Proceedings of the International Summit on Cutaneous Antifungal Therapy and Mycology Workshop, San Francisco, CA. J Am Acad Dermatol Suppl 1994; 31.

Proceedings of a symposium, Onychomycosis: Issues and Observations, Chicago, IL. J Am Acad Dermatol Suppl 1995; 35:3.

Radentz WH. Opportunistic fungal infections in immunocompromised hosts. J Am Acad Dermatol 1989; 20:989.

Schwartz RA, Janniger CK. Tinea capitis. Cutis 1995; 55:29.

Smith EB. Topical antifungal drugs in the treatment of tinea pedis, tinea cruris, and tinea corporis. J Am Acad Dermatol 1993; 28:S24.

Sugar AM, Lyman CA. A Practical guide to medically important fungi and the diseases they cause. Philadelphia, Lippincott–Raven Publishers, 1997.

Systemic antifungal drugs. Med Lett 1997; 39:1009.

20

Granulomatous Dermatoses

When considered singularly, granulomatous diseases are uncommon, but when all of them are considered together, they form a group that is interesting, varied, and ubiquitous.

A granuloma is a focal chronic inflammatory response to tissue injury manifested by a histologic picture of an accumulation and proliferation of leukocytes, principally of the mononuclear type and its family of derivatives, the mononuclear phagocyte system. The immunologic components in granulomatous inflammation originate from cell-mediated or delayed hypersensitivity mechanisms controlled by thymus-dependent lymphocytes (T lymphocytes). Five groups of granulomatous inflammations have been promulgated (Hirsh and Johnson, 1984):

Group 1 is the *epithelioid granulomas*, which include sarcoidosis, tuberculosis in certain forms, tuberculoid leprosy, tertiary syphilis, zirconium granuloma, beryllium granuloma, mercurial granuloma, and lichen nitidus.

Group 2, *histiocytic granulomas*, include lepromatous leprosy, histoplasmosis, and leishmaniasis.

Group 3 is the group *of foreign-body granulomas*, including endogenous products (*e.g.,* hair, fat, keratin), minerals (*e.g.,* tattoos, silica, talc), plant and animal products (*e.g.,* cactus, suture, oil, insect parts), and synthetic agents such as synthetic hair.

Group 4 is the *necrobiotic/palisading granulomas*, such as granuloma annulare, necrobiosis lipoidica, rheumatoid nodule, rheumatic fever nodule, cat-scratch disease, and lymphogranuloma venereum.

Group 5 is the *mixed inflammatory granulomas*, including many deep fungus infections such as blastomycosis and sporotrichosis, mycobacterial infections, granuloma inguinale, and chronic granulomatous disease.

Most of these diseases are discussed with their appropriate etiologic classifications in the Dictionary–Index. Two of these granulomatous inflammations are discussed in this chapter: *sarcoidosis*, which is an epithelioid granuloma in group 1, and *granuloma annulare*, which is in group 4 of necrobiotic/palisading granulomas.

SARCOIDOSIS
(Fig. 20-1; see Fig. 26-16)

Sarcoidosis is an uncommon systemic granulomatous disease of unknown cause that affects skin, lungs, lymph nodes, liver, spleen, parotid glands, and eyes. Less commonly involved organs indicative of more severe disease are the central nervous system, heart, bones, and upper respiratory tract. Any one of these organs or all of them may be involved with sarcoid granulomas. Lymphadenopathy is the single most common

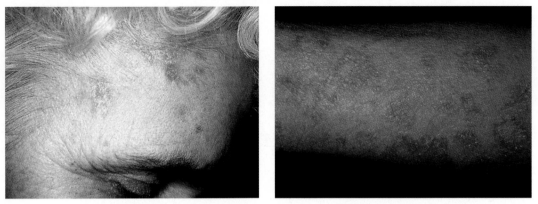

(A) Sarcoid of the forehead.   (B) Sarcoid on the forearm.

Figure 20-1.   **Sarcoidosis.** (*Hoechst-Roussel Pharmaceuticals Inc.*)

finding. African-Americans are affected more often than Caucasians. Only the skin manifestations of sarcoidosis are discussed here.

PRIMARY LESIONS. The superficial lesions consist of reddish papules, nodules, and plaques, which may be multiple or solitary and of varying size and configuration. Annular forms of skin sarcoidosis are common. These superficial lesions usually involve the face, the shoulders, and the arms. Infiltration of sarcoidal lesions frequently occurs at scar sites. Subcutaneous nodular forms and telangiectatic, ulcerative, erythrodermic, and ichthyosiform types are rare. Lupus pernio is most often seen in African-American females. It is often associated with chronic systemic disease.

SECONDARY LESIONS. Central healing can result in atrophy and scarring.

COURSE. Most cases of sarcoidosis run a chronic but benign course with remissions and exacerbations. Spontaneous "cure" is not unusual.

Erythema nodosum is characteristic of acute benign sarcoidosis (see Chap.12). Lupus pernio (indurated violaceous lesions on ears, nose, lips, cheeks, and forehead) and plaques are characteristic of chronic, severe, systemic disease.

ETIOLOGY. The exact cause is unknown, but the clinicopathologic picture undoubtedly can be caused by several agents, including bacteria, fungi, and certain inorganic agents.

LABORATORY FINDINGS. The histopathology is quite characteristic and consists of epithelioid cells surrounded by Langhans' giant cells, CD4 lymphocytes, some CD8 lymphocytes, and mature macrophages. No acid-fast bacilli are found, and caseation necrosis is absent. The Kveim test, using sarcoidal lymph node tissue, is positive after several weeks. Tuberculin-type skin tests are negative (anergic). The total blood serum protein is high and ranges from 7.5 to 10.0 grams/dL, mainly because of an increase in the globulin fraction.

Angiotensin-converting enzyme (ACE) deficiency may be noted.

Differential Diagnosis

Other granulomatous diseases: These can be ruled out by biopsy and other appropriate studies.
Silica granulomas: Histologically similar; a history of such injury can usually be obtained.

Treatment

Time appears to cure or cause remission of most cases of sarcoidosis, but corticosteroids and immunosuppressant drugs may be indicated for extensive cases. Hydroxychloroquine and methotrexate may be beneficial.

GRANULOMA ANNULARE
(*Fig. 20-2; see Fig. 18-10*)

Granuloma annulare is a moderately common skin problem. The usually encountered ring-shaped, red-bordered lesion is often mistaken for

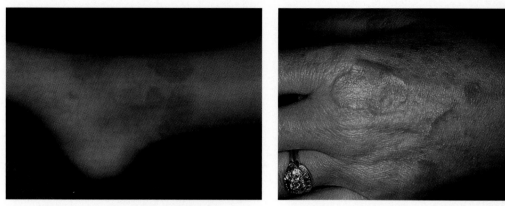

(*A*) Granuloma annulare on ankle area.   (*B*) Granuloma annulare on dorsum of hand.

Figure 20-2.   Granulomas. (*Hoechst-Roussel Pharmaceuticals Inc.*)

ringworm by the inexperienced. Several clinical variations exist. The two most common are the *localized form* and *the generalized form.*

Females with granuloma annulare predominate over males in a ratio of 2.5 to 1. No ages are exempt, but the localized form is usually seen in patients in the first three decades of life and the generalized form in patients in the fourth through seventh decades. A granuloma annulare-like eruption has been reported in HIV-positive and chronic Epstein-Barr–positive patients.

PRIMARY LESIONS. In both the *localized form* and the *generalized form* the lesion is a red asymptomatic papule with no scaling. The papule may be solitary. Most frequently the lesion assumes a ring-shaped or arcuate configuration of papules that tends to enlarge centrifugally. Rarely are the rings over 5 cm in diameter. In the *localized form* of granuloma annulare the lesions appear mainly over the joints on hands, arms, feet, and on legs. In the *generalized form* there may be hundreds of the red or tan papular circinate lesions on the extremities and on the trunk.

SECONDARY LESIONS. On healing, the red color turns to brown before the lesions disappear.

COURSE. Both forms of granuloma annulare can resolve spontaneously after one to several years, but the generalized form is more long-lasting.

ETIOLOGY. The cause is unknown. An immune-complex vasculitis or a cell-mediated immunity has been proposed to be a factor in the disease, as has trauma.

LABORATORY FINDINGS. The histopathology is quite characteristic. The middle and upper dermis have focal areas of altered collagenous connective tissue surrounded by an infiltrate of histiocytic cells and lymphocytes. In some cases these cells infiltrate between the collagen bundles, giving a palisading effect. The term *necrobiosis* has been used to describe these changes. Some believe that the generalized form of granuloma annulare is associated with a higher incidence of diabetes mellitus.

Differential Diagnosis

Tinea corporis: Usually itches and has a scaly red border; the fungus can be demonstrated with a potassium hydroxide scraping or Sabouraud culture (see Chap. 19).
Lichen planus, annular form: Characterized by violaceous flat-topped papules with Wickham's striae; mucous membrane lesions are often seen (see Chap. 14).
Secondary syphilis: Can be clinically similar but has a positive serology (see Chap. 16).
Other granulomatous diseases: Can usually be distinguished by biopsy.

There is a *subcutaneous form of granuloma annulare* that is difficult to separate histologically from the *rheumatoid nodule* or a soft tissue tumor.

Treatment

LOCALIZED FORM. Many cases respond to the application of a corticosteroid cream covered for 8 hours a day with an occlusive dressing such as Saran Wrap. Intralesional corticosteroids are effective for a case with only a few lesions. Light liquid nitrogen therapy is sometimes beneficial.

GENERALIZED FORM. Numerous remedies have been tried with anecdotal benefit. Dapsone and hydroxychloroquine have been used.

BIBLIOGRAPHY

Hirsh BC, Johnson WC. Concepts of granulomatous inflammation. Int J Dermatol 1984;23:90.

Kerdel FA, Moschella SL. Sarcoidosis. J Am Acad Dermatol 1984;11:1.

Mana J, Marcoval J, et al. Cutaneous involvement in sarcoidosis. Arch Dermatol 1997;133:882.

Newman LS, Rose CS, Maier LA. Sarcoidosis. N Engl J Med 1997;336:17.

Smith MD, Downie JB, DiCostanzo D. Granuloma annulare. Int J Dermatol 1997;36:326.

21

Dermatologic Parasitology

Dermatologic parasitology is a very extensive subject and includes the dermatoses due to three main groups of organisms: protozoa, helminths, and arthropods.

The *protozoal dermatoses* are exemplified by the various forms of trypanosomiasis and leishmaniasis (see Chap. 35).

Helminthic dermatoses include those due to roundworms (ground itch, creeping eruption, filariasis, and other rare tropical diseases) and those due to flatworms (schistosomiasis, swimmer's itch, and others) (see Chap. 35).

Arthropod dermatoses are divided into those caused by two classes of organisms: the arachnids (spiders, scorpions, ticks, and mites) and the insects (lice, bugs, flies, moths, beetles, bees, and fleas). Lyme disease is caused by a spirochete that is transmitted by a tick and is discussed in Chap. 16.

In this chapter *scabies*, caused by a mite, and *pediculosis*, caused by lice, are discussed.

Flea bites, chigger bites, creeping eruption, swimmer's itch, and *tropical dermatoses* are discussed in Chap. 35, "Tropical Diseases of the Skin."

SCABIES

(Figs. 21-1 and 21-2; see Fig. 35-9)

Scabies is usually more prevalent in a populace ravaged by war, famine, or disease, when personal hygiene becomes relatively unimportant.

However, there are unexplained cyclic epidemics of this parasitic infestation. In the 1970s and 1980s such a cycle plagued Americans. In normal times scabies is rarely seen except in schoolchildren, among the elderly in nursing care centers, or in poorer populations under crowded conditions. It can be a sexually transmitted disease.

SAUER NOTES

1. Scabies should be ruled out in any generalized excoriated eruption.
2. The patient should always be asked if other members of the household itch.

PRIMARY LESIONS. A burrow caused by the female of the mite *Sarcoptes scabiei* (Fig. 21-2) measures approximately 2 mm in length and can be hidden by the secondary eruption. Small vesicles may overlie the burrows. *Scabies incognito* is a form of the disease in which the burrows are not easily identified. *Norwegian*, or *keratotic*, *scabies* occurs in immunosuppressed patients. Hundreds of organisms create a psoriasiform dermatitis.

SECONDARY LESIONS. Excoriations of the burrows may be the only visible pathologic process. In severe, chronic cases, bacterial infection may

227

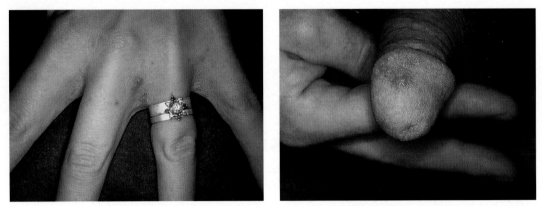

(A) Scabies on the hand.

(B) Scabies on the penis.

Figure 21-1. **Scabies.** (*Hoechst-Roussel Pharmaceuticals*)

be extensive and may take the form of impetigo, cellulitis, or furunculosis.

Residual nodular lesions may persist as an allergic reaction for many weeks or months after the organism is eliminated. They are often recalcitrant to therapy and topical, intralesional, and even systemic corticosteroids may be necessary. Nodular scabies is not contagious.

DISTRIBUTION. Most commonly the excoriations are seen on the lower abdomen and the back, with extension to the pubic and the axillary areas, the legs (ankles especially), the arms (flexor wrists especially), and the webs of the fingers.

SUBJECTIVE COMPLAINTS. Itching is intense, particularly at night, when the patient is warm and in bed and the mite is more active. However, many skin diseases itch worse at night, presumably due to a lower itch threshold when relaxation occurs.

COURSE. The mite can persist for months and years ("7-year itch") in untreated persons.

CONTAGIOUSNESS. Other members of the household or intimate contacts may or may not have the disease, depending on exposure and the severity of the infestation.

LABORATORY FINDINGS. The female scabies mite, ova, and fecal pellets may be seen in curetted burrows examined under the low-power magnification of the microscope (see Fig. 21-2). Potassium hydroxide (20% solution) can be used to clear the tissue, as with fungus smears. Another method of collection is to scrape the burrow through immersion oil and then transfer the scrapings to the microscopic slides. Skill is necessary to uncover the mite by curetting or scraping.

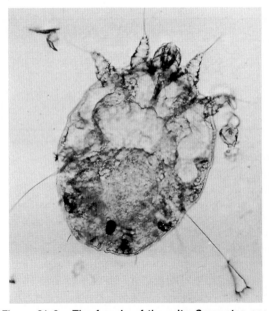

Figure 21-2. **The female of the mite *Sarcoptes scabiei.*** The small, oval, black body near the anal opening is a fecal pellet. Proximal to it is a vague, much larger, oval, pale-edged mass—an egg. (*Dr. H. Parlette*)

Differential Diagnosis

Pyoderma: Rule out concurrent parasitic infestation; positive history of diabetes mellitus; only mild itching (see Chap. 15).
Pediculosis pubis: Lice and eggs on and around hairs; distribution different (see following section).

Winter itch: No burrows; seasonal incidence; elderly patient, usually; worse on legs and back (see Chap. 11).

Dermatitis herpetiformis: Vesicles, urticaria; excoriated papules; eosinophilia; no burrows (see Chap. 22).

Neurotic excoriations: Nervous person; patient admits picking at lesions; present in areas where patient can easily reach; no burrows; characteristic white scars indicate a prolonged illness.

Parasitophobia: Usually the patient brings to the office pieces of skin and debris; showing the patient the debris under a microscope helps to convince him or her of the absence of parasites. This is a difficult problem to manage. Pimozide (Orap) can be used by a physician experienced in its use.

Treatment

ADULTS AND OLDER CHILDREN

1. Inspect or question concerning itching in other members of the family or intimate contacts to rule out infestation in them. Any infested household members must be treated at the same time as the patient to prevent "ping-pong" infestation.
2. Instruct patient to bathe thoroughly, scrubbing the involved areas with a brush.
3. Permethrin (Elimite, Acticin) 5% cream   60.0
or Lindane lotion (Kwell)   120.0
Sig: Apply to the entire body from the neck down. Repeat therapy in 1 week.
4. After 24 hours bathe carefully and change to clean clothes and bedding.

SAUER NOTES

1. I have the patient *repeat* the medication application in 1 week, leaving it on again for 24 hours.
2. Tell the patient that the itching can persist for weeks.
3. Treat all household and sexual contacts (itching or not).

5. Washing, dry cleaning, or ironing of clothes or bedding is sufficient to destroy the mite. Sterilization is unnecessary.
6. Itching may persist for a few days, even for 2 to 3 weeks or longer, in spite of the destruction of the mite. For this apply b.i.d.:

a. Crotamiton (Eurax) cream q.s.   60.0
Comment: This cream has scabicidal power and antipruritic action combined.
b. Corticosteroid systemic therapy may be indicated for 10 to 14 days.
7. If itching persists after 4 weeks, reexamine the patient carefully, and repeat the KOH preparation to be sure reinfestation or inadequate treatment has not occurred. It takes a lot of reassurance to convince these itchy patients that they are not still infested with scabies.
8. Oral ivermectin is a therapy advocated by some authors.

NEWBORNS AND INFANTS

1. General instructions are as above.
2. Lindane lotion used in newborns and infants has caused convulsions.
3. Elimite or Eurax cream   60.0
Sig: Apply b.i.d. locally to affected areas only, *or*
4. Sulfur, ppt.   5%
Water-washable cream base q.s.   60.0
Sig: Apply b.i.d. to affected areas.
5. Younger than 1 year of age the mite may occur above the neck.

PEDICULOSIS

Lice infestation affects persons of all ages, but usually those in the lower income strata are affected most often because of lack of cleanliness and infrequent changes of clothing. It is also seen as a sexually transmitted disease.

Three clinical entities are produced: (1) infestation of the hair by the head louse *Pediculus humanus capitis*, (2) infestation of the body by *P. humanus corporis*, and (3) infestation of the pubic area by the pubic louse *Pthirus pubis* (Fig. 21-3). Because lice bite the skin and live on the blood, it is impossible for them to live without human contact. The readily visible oval eggs or nits are attached to hairs or to clothing fibers by the female louse. After the eggs hatch, the newly born lice mature within 30 days. Then the female louse can live for another 30 days and deposit a few eggs daily.

PRIMARY LESIONS. The bite is not unusual but is seldom seen because of the secondary changes produced by the resulting intense itching. In the *scalp* and *pubic forms* the nits are found on the hairs, but the lice are found only occasionally. In

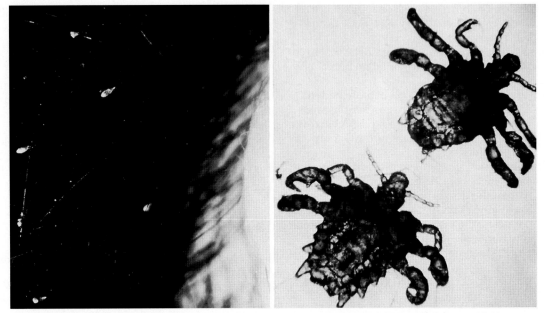

Figure 21-3. Pediculosis. (*Left*) Nits on scalp hair behind ear. (*Dr. L. Hyde*) (*Right*) Pubic louse or *Pthirus pubis* as seen with the 7.5× lens of a microscope. (*Dr. J. Boley*)

the *body form* the nits and the lice can be found after careful searching in the seams of the clothing.

SECONDARY LESIONS. In the *scalp form* the skin is red and excoriated, with such severe secondary bacterial infection, in some cases, that the hairs become matted together in a crusty, foul-smelling "cap." Regional lymphadenopathy is common. A morbilliform rash on the body, an id reaction, is seen in longstanding cases.

In the *body form* linear excoriations and secondary infection, seen mainly on the shoulders, the belt line, and the buttocks, mask the primary bites.

In the *pubic form* the secondary excoriations are again dominant and produce some matting of the hairs. This louse can also infest body, axillary, and eyelash hairs. An unusual eruption on the abdomen, the thighs, and the arms, called *maculae cerulea*, because of the bluish gray, pea-sized macules, can occur in chronic cases of pubic pediculosis.

Differential Diagnosis

PEDICULOSIS CAPITIS

Bacterial infection of the scalp: Responds rapidly to correct antibacterial therapy (see Chap. 15).

> **SAUER NOTE**
>
> All cases of scalp pyoderma must be examined closely for a primary lice infestation.

Seborrheic dermatitis or dandruff: The scales of dandruff are readily detached from the hair, but oval nits are not so easily removed (see Chap. 13).
Hair casts (pseudonits): Resemble nits but can be pulled off more easily; no eggs are seen on microscopic examination.

PEDICULOSIS CORPORIS

Scabies: May be small burrows; distribution of lesions different; no lice in clothes (see beginning of this chapter).
Senile or winter itch: History helpful; dry skin, aggravated by bathing; will not find lice in clothes (see Chap. 11).

PEDICULOSIS PUBIS

Scabies: No nits; burrows in pubic area and elsewhere (see beginning of this chapter).
Pyoderma secondary to contact dermatitis from condoms, contraceptive jellies, new underwear,

douches: History important; acute onset, no nits (see Chap. 15).

Seborrheic dermatitis, when in eyebrows and eyelashes: No nits found (see Chap. 13).

Treatment

<u>P</u>EDICULOSIS <u>C</u>APITIS

1. Shampoos or rinses
   a. Permethrin (Nix) creme rinse   60.0
   Sig: Use as a rinse for 10 minutes after shampooing. Only one application is necessary.
   b. Lindane (Kwell) shampoo   60.0
   Sig: Shampoo and comb hair thoroughly. Leave on the hair for 4 minutes. Shampoo again in 3 days.
   c. Pyrethrins (RID)   60.0
   Sig: Apply to scalp for 10 minutes and rinse off. Apply again in 7 days (nonprescription).
   d. Step Two (formic acid) solution (obtainable without a prescription) can be used to help remove nits from the hair.
   e. Permethrin 5% (Elimite) Cream   60.0
   Leave on overnight under shower cap. May be the most effective topical treatment of all for recalcitrant cases.
   f. A single oral dose of ivermectin (Stromectol), 200 micrograms/kg, repeated in 10 days may be the most effective oral agent in persistent cases. Some authors are concerned about the safety of this therapy.
2. For secondary scalp infection:
   a. Trim hair as much as possible and agreeable with the patient.
   b. Shampoo hair once a day with an antiseborrhea-type shampoo.
   c. Bactroban or Polysporin ointment   15.0
   Sig: Apply to scalp b.i.d.
3. Change and clean bedding and headwear after 24 hours of treatment. Storage of headwear for 30 days will destroy the lice and the nits.

<u>P</u>EDICULOSIS <u>C</u>ORPORIS

1. Calamine lotion q.s.   120.0
   Sig: Apply locally b.i.d. for itching. (The lice and the nits are in the clothing.)
2. Have the clothing laundered or dry cleaned. If this is impossible, dusting with 10% lindane powder kills the parasites. Care should be taken to prevent reinfestation. Storage of clothing in a plastic bag for 30 days kills both nits and lice.

<u>P</u>EDICULOSIS <u>P</u>UBIS

Treatment is the same as for the scalp form.

BIBLIOGRAPHY

Buntin DM, Rosen T, Lesher JL, et al. Sexually transmitted diseases: viruses and ectoparasites. J Am Acad Dermatol 1991;25:527.

Centers for Disease Control. Scabies in health-care facilities: Iowa. Arch Dermatol 1988;124:837.

Goddard J. Physician's guide to arthropods of medical importance, ed. 2. 1996.

Mumcuoglu KY, Klaus S, Kafka D, et al. Clinical observations related to head lice infestation. J Am Acad Dermatol 1991;25:248.

Taplin D, Meinlsing TL. Pyrethrins and pyrethroids in dermatology. Arch Dermatol 1990;126:213.

22

Bullous Dermatoses

To medical students and practitioners alike, the bullous skin diseases appear most dramatic. One of these diseases, pemphigus, is undoubtedly greatly responsible for the aura that surrounds the exhibition and the discussion of an unfortunate patient with a bullous disease. Happy would be the instructor who could behold such student interest when a case of acne or hand dermatitis is being presented.

In almost all cases of bullous diseases, it is necessary to examine a fresh tissue biopsy specimen for deposits of immune reactants, immunoglobulins, and complement components, at or near the basement membrane zone. Routine histologic examination of a formalin-fixed biopsy specimen is, of course, also usually indicated (see Chap. 10).

Three bullous diseases are discussed in this chapter: *pemphigus vulgaris, dermatitis herpetiformis,* and *erythema multiforme bullosum.* However, other bullous skin diseases do occur, and in this introduction they are differentiated from these three.

BULLOUS IMPETIGO. The name *pemphigus neonatorum* has been attached to this pyodermic skin infection because of the resemblance of the large bullae in this disease to pemphigus. This term should be abandoned. Bullous impetigo is to be differentiated from the other bullous diseases by its occurrence in infants and children, rapid development of the individual bullae, pres-

ence of impetigo lesions in siblings, bacterial culture positive for staphylococcus aureus, and rapid response to antibiotic therapy (see Chaps. 15 and 33).

CONTACT DERMATITIS DUE TO POISON IVY OR SIMILAR PLANTS. Bullae and vesicles are seen in linear configuration. A history of pulling weeds or burning brush is usually obtained, and a past history of poison ivy or related dermatitis is common. The duration of disease is 10 to 14 days (see Chap. 9).

DRUG ERUPTION. Elicit drug history (particularly of sulfonamides and iodides). The eruption usually clears on discontinuing drugs. Bullae appear rapidly (see Chap. 9).

EPIDERMOLYSIS BULLOSA. *(See Fig. 31-3).* This rare, chronic, hereditary skin disease is manifested by the formation of bullae, usually on the hands and the feet, following trauma. The full clinical and immunologic spectra of these diseases have not been completely defined.

The *simple form* (epidermolysis bullosa simplex) of dominant inheritance can begin in infancy or adulthood with the formation of tense, slightly itching bullae at the sites of pressure, which heal quickly without scarring. Forced marches or jogging can initiate this disease in patients who have the heredity factor. Such cases are usually treated erroneously as athlete's foot.

The disease is worse in the summer or may be present only at this time.

The *dystrophic form* of recessive inheritance begins in infancy and as time elapses the bullae become hemorrhagic, heal slowly, and leave scars that can amputate digits; death can result from secondary infection and metastatic squamous cell carcinomas. Mucous membrane lesions are more common in the dystrophic form than in the simple form. Treatment is supportive. Gene therapy may be a future modality. Surgical dressings and skin substitutes (Apligraft) are an important part of care.

A lethal, nonscarring form is of recessive inheritance also but is usually fatal within a few months (see Chap. 31).

FAMILIAL BENIGN CHRONIC PEMPHIGUS (HAILEY-HAILEY DISEASE). This is a rare, hereditary bullous eruption that is most common on the neck and in the axillae. It can be distinguished from pemphigus by its chronicity and benign nature and by its histologic picture (see Chap. 31). Some consider this disease to be a bullous variety of *keratosis follicularis (Darier's disease).*

PORPHYRIA. The congenital erythropoietic type and the chronic hepatic type (porphyria cutanea tarda) commonly have bullae on the sun-exposed areas of the body. See Dictionary–Index under *Porphyria* and also Chap. 30.

BULLOUS PEMPHIGOID. *(See Figs. 34-10 and 34-13A).* This chronic bullous eruption most commonly occurring in elderly adults is usually not fatal. It is differentiated from *Pemphigus vulgaris* by the histologic presence of subepidermal bullae without acantholysis and quite specific immunofluorescent autoantibodies in the basement membrane zone; from *erythema multiforme* by its chronicity, absence of iris lesions, and histology; and from *dermatitis herpetiformis* by the absence of response to sulfapyridine or dapsone therapy (some bullous pemphigoid cases do respond to this therapy) and by histology.

CICATRICIAL PEMPHIGOID. *(See Fig. 34-13).* This disabling but nonfatal bullous eruption of the mucous membranes most commonly involves the eyes. As the result of scarring, which is characteristic of this disease and separates it from true pemphigus, the eyesight is eventually lost. Over 50% of the cases have skin lesions. Histologically, the bullae are subepidermal and do not show acantholysis. There is quite a bit of immunologic similarity between this disease and bullous pemphigoid.

LINEAR IgA BULLOUS DISEASE. Most of the children and adults with this disease differ from classic dermatitis herpetiformis in the morphology and distribution of their lesions, have a poorer response to dapsone, and have linear IgA antibasement membrane zone antibodies.

INCONTINENTIA PIGMENTI. The first stage of this rare disease of infants manifests itself with bullous lesions, primarily on the hands and feet. See Chap. 33.

TOXIC EPIDERMAL NECROLYSIS. This rare disease is characterized by large bullae and a quite generalized Nikolsky's sign, in which large sheets of epidermis become detached from the underlying skin. The mucous membranes are frequently involved. The patient is toxic. Adults are most commonly affected. In many instances it is difficult to separate this disease clinically from severe erythema multiforme-like disease (*Stevens-Johnson syndrome*). Drugs are usually the causative factor. Most commonly implicated are sulfonamides, anticonvulsants, and non-steroidal anti-inflammatory drugs. There may be a genetic predisposition to this bullous drug reaction. Therapy is supportive, and an appreciable number of cases are fatal.

STAPHYLOCOCCAL SCALDED SKIN SYNDROME. Clinically, this disorder is similar to toxic epidermal necrolysis but has been separated from this disease because of the finding that phage group 2 *Staphylococcus aureus* is the usual cause. In newborns, this formerly was known as *Ritter von Ritterschein's disease.* It also occurs in children and rarely adults. The prognosis is very favorable.

IMPETIGO HERPETIFORMIS. One of the rarest of skin diseases, this disease is characterized by groups of pustules mainly seen in the axillae and the groin, high fever, prostration, severe malaise, and, generally, a fatal outcome. It occurs most commonly in pregnant or postpartum women. It can be distinguished from *pemphigus vegetans* or *dermatitis herpetiformis* by the fact that these diseases do not produce such general, acute, toxic manifestations.

In spite of high medical student and general practitioner interest in the bullous skin conditions, the diagnosis and the management of the three main diseases, particularly pemphigus vulgaris and dermatitis herpetiformis, should be in the realm of the dermatologist. In this chapter the salient features of these diseases are presented, with therapy skimmed over lightly.

PEMPHIGUS VULGARIS
(Fig. 22-1; see also Figs. 3-1F, 34-13C–D, and Chap. 10)

Pemphigus vulgaris is rare. These patients are miserable, odoriferous, and debilitated. Before the advent of corticosteroid therapy, the disease was fatal.

PRIMARY LESIONS. The early lesions of pemphigus are small vesicles or bullae on apparently normal skin. Redness of the base of the bullae is unusual. Without treatment, the bullae enlarge and spread, and new ones balloon up on different areas of the skin or the mucous membranes. Rarely, mucous membrane lesions may be the main or only manifestation of the disease. Rupturing of the bullae leaves large eroded areas. Nikolsky's sign is positive; that is, a top layer of the skin adjacent to a bulla readily separates from the underlying skin after firm but gentle pressure.

SECONDARY LESIONS. Bacterial infection with crusting is marked and accounts, in part, for the characteristic mousy odor. Lesions that heal spontaneously or under therapy do not leave scars.

COURSE. When untreated, pemphigus vulgaris can be rapidly fatal or assume a slow lingering course, with debility, painful mouth and body erosions, systemic bacterial infection, and toxemia. Spontaneous temporary remissions do occur without therapy. The following clinical variations of pemphigus also exist:

Pemphigus vegetans is characterized by the development of large granulomatous masses in the intertriginous areas of the axillae and the groin. Secondary bacterial infection, although often present in all cases of pemphigus, is most marked in this form. Pemphigus vegetans is to be differentiated from a granulomatous *ioderma* or *bromoderma* (see Chap. 9) and from *impetigo herpetiformis* (see beginning of this chapter).

Pemphigus foliaceus appears as a scaly, moist, generalized exfoliative dermatitis. The characteristic mousy odor of pemphigus is dominant in this variant, which is also remarkable for its chronicity. The response to corticosteroid therapy is less favorable in the foliaceus form than in the other types. (See also Chap. 35 for a Brazilian form.)

Pemphigus erythematosus clinically resembles a mixture of pemphigus vulgaris, seborrheic dermatitis, and lupus erythematosus. The distribution of the red, greasy, crusted, and eroded lesions is on the butterfly area of the face, the sternal area, the scalp, and occasionally in the mouth. The course is more chronic than for pemphigus vulgaris, and remissions are common.

Some dermatologists believe that pemphigus foliaceus and pemphigus erythematosus may be distinct diseases from pemphigus vulgaris and vegetans.

ETIOLOGY. The cause of pemphigus vulgaris is unknown, but autoimmunity is a factor. Some cases are associated with underlying malignancy

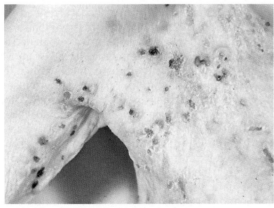

(*A*) Pemphigus vulgaris on anterior chest and right arm areas.

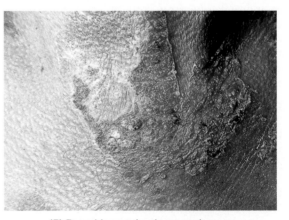

(*B*) Pemphigus vulgaris on neck area.

Figure 22-1. **Bullous dermatoses.** (*Roche Laboratories*)

(*paraneoplastic pemphigus*). Paraneoplastic pemphigus has unique immunofluorescent findings and is usually rapidly fatal. Human herpesvirus 8 has been isolated from the skin lesions of some patients.

LABORATORY FINDINGS. The histopathology of early cases is characteristic and serves to differentiate most cases of pemphigus vulgaris from dermatitis herpetiformis and the other bullous diseases. Acantholysis, or separation of intercellular contact between the keratinocytes, is characteristic. The bulla is intraepidermal. Cytologic smears (Tzanck test) for diagnosis of pemphigus vulgaris reveal numerous rounded acantholytic epidermal cells with large nuclei in condensed cytoplasm. Antiepithelial auto-antibodies against the intercellular substance are found by direct and indirect immunofluorescent tests. Fresh tissue biopsy specimens taken from noninvolved skin best show immunoglobulins. Indirect tests are performed on serum.

Differential Diagnosis

See introduction to this chapter and also *dermatitis herpetiformis* and *erythema multiforme bullosum*.

Treatment

1. If possible, a dermatologist or an internist should be called in to share the responsibility of the care.
2. Hospitalization is necessary for the patient with large areas of bullae and erosions. Mild cases of pemphigus can be managed in the office.
3. Prednisone, 10 mg   #100
   Sig: One or 2 tablets q.i.d. until healing occurs; then reduce the dose slowly as warranted.
   Comment: Very high doses of prednisone may be needed to produce a remission in severe cases.
4. Local therapy is prescribed to make the patient more comfortable and to decrease the odor by reducing secondary infection. This can be accomplished by the following, which must be varied for individual cases:
   a. Potassium permanganate crystals   60.0
   Sig: Place 2 teaspoonfuls of the crystals in the bathtub with approximately 10 inches of lukewarm water.

Comment: To prevent crystals from burning the skin they should be dissolved completely in a glass of water before adding to the tub. The solution should be made fresh daily. The tub stains can be removed by applying acetic acid or "hypo" solution.
   b. Talc   120.0
   Sig: Dispense in powder can. Apply to bed sheeting and to erosions twice a day (called a "powder bed").
   c. Polysporin, Bactroban, or other antibiotic ointment q.s.   60.0
   Sig: Apply to small infected areas b.i.d.
5. Supportive therapy should be used when necessary. This includes vitamins, iron, blood transfusions, and oral antibiotics. Dapsone therapy can be used with benefit in some cases as a corticosteroid-sparing agent. Methotrexate and other immunosuppressive therapy are also being used.
6. Nursing care of the highest caliber is a prerequisite for the severe case of pemphigus with generalized erosions and bullae. The nursing personnel should be told that this disease is not contagious or infectious. A "burn unit" when available in a hospital may be the best place for local care.

DERMATITIS HERPETIFORMIS
(Fig. 22-2)

Dermatitis herpetiformis is a rare, chronic, markedly pruritic, papular, vesicular, and bullous skin disease of unknown etiology. It is probably an autoimmune disease and activated via the alternate complement pathway. The patient describes the itching of a new blister as a burning itch that disappears when the blister top is scratched off. The severe scratching results in the formation of excoriations and papular hives, which may be the only visible pathology of the disease. Individual lesions heal, leaving an area of hyperpigmentation that is very characteristic. The typical distribution of the blisters or excoriations is on the scalp, sacral area, scapular area, forearms, elbows, and thighs. In severe cases, the resulting bullae may be indistinguishable from pemphigus or bullous pemphigoid.

The duration of dermatitis herpetiformis varies from months to as long as 40 years, with periods of remission scattered in between. The illness is associated with *nontropical sprue*.

Laboratory tests should include fixed tissue and fresh tissue biopsy. The latter shows in most

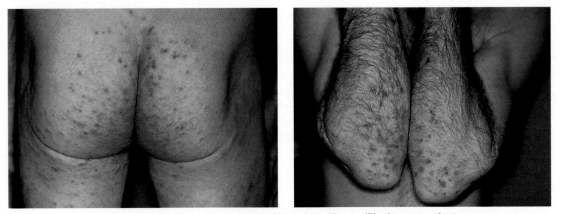

Dermatitis herpetiform on buttocks (*A*) and on elbows (*B*) of same patient.
Figure 22-2. Bullous dermatoses. (*Roche Laboratories*)

cases granular IgA in the dermal papillae, along with the third component of complement (C3). The finding of endomysial antibodies in the blood is highly specific for the disease. A blood cell count usually shows an eosinophilia.

Herpes gestationis (see Fig. 26-11D–E) is a vesicular and bullous disease that occurs in relation to pregnancy. It usually develops during the second or the third trimester and commonly disappears after birth, only to return with subsequent pregnancies. The histologic features are believed significantly distinctive so that this disease can be separated from dermatitis herpetiformis. Immunologic findings of C3 bound to the basement membrane of the epidermis and occasional IgG deposition may be significant. Therapy with systemic corticosteroids is usually indicated.

Differential Diagnosis

Pemphigus vulgaris: Large, flaccid bullae; mouth involvement more common; debilitating course; biopsy specimen quite characteristic; eosinophilia is uncommon (see Pemphigus, at beginning of chapter).

Erythema multiforme bullosum: Bullae usually arise on a red, iris-like base; burning itch is absent; residual pigmentation is minor; course is shorter (see following section for a discussion of this disease).

Neurotic excoriations: If this diagnosis is being considered, it is very important to rule out dermatitis herpetiformis. In a case of neurotic excoriations one usually does not find scalp lesions, blisters, or eosinophilia. The skin biopsy is helpful.

Scabies: No vesicles (rarely can occur) or bullae; burrows and lesions are found in other members of the household (see Chap. 21). KOH scraping is diagnostic.

Subcorneal pustular dermatosis: Rare, chronic dermatosis characterized by an annular and serpiginous arrangement of pustules and vesiculopustules on the abdomen and the groin and in the axillae. Histopathologically, the pustule is found directly beneath the stratum corneum. Dapsone (avlosulfone) or sulfapyridine therapy is effective.

Treatment

A dermatologist should be consulted to establish the diagnosis and to outline therapy. This would consist of local and oral measures to control itching and a course of one of the following quite effective drugs: sulfapyridine (0.5 gram q.i.d.) or dapsone (25 mg t.i.d.). Rapid response to these medicines should make the diagnosis suspect. These initial doses should be decreased or increased dpending on the patient's response. These drugs can be toxic, and the patient must be under the close surveillance of the physician. A diet that is gluten-free and low in iodine and bromine is beneficial for an appreciable number of patients. This is a difficult diet to follow.

ERYTHEMA MULTIFORME BULLOSUM
(*Fig. 22-3*)

Erythema multiforme bullosum has a clinical picture and course distinct from that of erythema

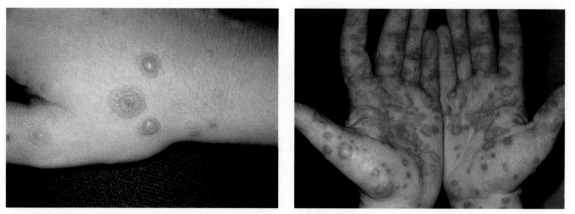

Erythema multiforme bullosum on dorsum of hand (*A*) and on palms (*B*) 5 days later on same patient.

Figure 22-3. **Bullous dermatoses.** (*Roche Laboratories*)

multiforme (see Chap. 12). Many drugs can cause an erythema multiforme bullosum-like picture, but then this manifestation should be labeled a "drug eruption."

True erythema multiforme bullosum has no known cause. Clinically, one sees large vesicles and bullae usually overlying red, iris-like macules. The lesions most commonly appear on the arms, the legs, and the face but can occur elsewhere, including, on occasion, the mouth. Erythema multiforme bullosum can last from days to months.

Slight malaise and fever may precede a new shower of bullae, but for the most part the patient's general health is unaffected. Itching may be mild or severe enough to interfere with sleep.

When the characteristic iris lesions are absent, it is difficult to differentiate this bullous eruption from early *pemphigus vulgaris, dermatitis herpetiformis,* and *bullous hives.* However, the histopathology is often helpful.

Treatment

These patients should be referred to a dermatologist or an internist to substantiate the diagnosis and initiate therapy. Corticosteroids orally and by injection are the single most effective drugs in use today. For widespread cases requiring hospitalization, the local care is similar to that for pemphigus.

BIBLIOGRAPHY

Ahmed AR, Kurgis BS, Rogers RS III. Cicatricial pemphigoid. J Am Acad Dermatol 1991;24:987.

Avakian R, Flowers FF, Araujo OE, et al. Toxic epidermal necrolysis. J Am Acad Dermatol 1991;25:69.

Bastuji-Gavin S, Rzany B, Stern RS, et al. Clinical classification of cases of toxic epidermal necrolysis, Stevens-Johnson syndrome, and erythema multiforme. Arch Dermatol 1993;129:92.

Bystrun JC, Steinman NM. The adjuvant therapy of pemphigus. Arch Deramtol 1996;132:203.

Diaz LA, Sampaio SA, Rivitti EA, et al. Endemic pemphigus foliaceus (fogo selvagem). J Am Acad Dermatol 1989;20:657.

Fine JD. Management of acquired bullous skin disease. N Engl J Med 1995;333:22.

Hall RP III. Dermatitis herpetiformis. Prog Dermatol 1992;2:1.

Helm KF, Peters MS. Immunodermatology update: The immunologically mediated vesiculobullous diseases. Mayo Clin Proc 1991;66:187.

Korman NJ. Bullous pemphigoid. The latest in diagnosis, prognosis, and therapy. Arch Dermatol 1998;134:1137.

Rogers RS III. Bullous pemphigoid: Therapy and management. J Geriatr Dermatol 1995;3:91.

Schwartz RA. Toxic epidermal necrolysis. Cutis 1997;59.

Wojnarowska F, Briggaman RA. Management of blistering diseases. New York, Raven Press, 1990.

Zemstov A, Neldner KH. Successful treatment of dermatitis herpetiformis with tetracycline and nicotinamide in a patient unable to tolerate dapsone. J Am Acad Dermatol 1993;28:505.

23

Exfoliative Dermatitis

As the term implies, exfoliative dermatitis is a generalized scaling eruption of the skin. The causes are many. This diagnosis should never be made without additional qualifying etiologic terms.

This is a rare skin condition, but many general physicians, residents, and interns see these cases because the patients are occasionally hospitalized. Hospitalization serves two purposes: (1) to perform a diagnostic workup, because the cause, in many cases, is difficult to ascertain; and (2) to administer intensive therapy under close supervision.

Classification of the cases of exfoliative dermatitis is facilitated by dividing them into primary and secondary forms.

PRIMARY EXFOLIATIVE DERMATITIS

These cases develop in apparently healthy persons from no ascertainable cause.

SKIN LESIONS. Clinically, it is impossible to differentiate this primary form from the one in which the etiology is known or suspected. Various degrees of scaling and redness are seen, ranging from fine, generalized, granular scales with mild erythema to scaling in large plaques, with marked erythema (generalized erythroderma) and lichenification. Widespread lymphadenopathy is usually present. The nails become thick and lusterless, and the hair falls out in varying degrees.

SUBJECTIVE COMPLAINT. Itching, in most cases, is intense.

COURSE. The prognosis for early cure of the disease is poor. The mortality rate is high in older patients due to generalized debility and secondary infection.

ETIOLOGY. Various authors have studied the relationship of lymphomas to cases of exfoliative dermatitis. Some believe the incidence to be low, but others state that from 35% to 50% of these exfoliative cases, particularly those in patients older than the age of 40 years, are the result of *lymphomas*. However, years may pass before the lymphoma becomes obvious.

LABORATORY FINDINGS. There are no diagnostic changes, but the patient with a usual case has an elevated white blood cell count with eosinophilia. Biopsy of the skin is not diagnostic in the primary type. Biopsy of an enlarged lymph node, in either the primary or the secondary form, reveals *lipomelanotic reticulosis (dermatopathic lymphadenopathy)*.

Treatment

A 50-year-old man presents with a generalized, pruritic, scaly, erythematous eruption that he has had for 3 months.

238

<u>FIRST VISIT</u>

1. A general medical work-up is indicated.
2. A high-protein diet should be prescribed because these patients have an increased basal metabolic rate and catabolize protein.
3. Bathing instructions are variable. Some patients prefer a daily cool bath in a colloid solution for relief of itching (one box of soluble starch or 1 cup of Aveeno to 10 inches of water). For most cases, however, generalized bathing dries the skin and intensifies the itching.
4. Provide extra blankets for the bed. These patients lose a lot of heat through their red skin and consequently feel chilly.
5. Locally, an ointment is most desired, but some patients prefer an oily liquid. Formulas for both follow:
   a. White petrolatum   240.0
   or a generic corticosteroid ointment, such as triamcinolone 0.025% ointment   240.0
   Sig: Apply locally b.i.d.
   b. Zinc oxide   40%
   Olive oil q.s.   240.0
   Sig: Apply locally with hands or a paintbrush b.i.d.
   Comment: Antipruritic chemicals can also be added to this.

6. Oral antihistamine, for example:
   Chlorpheniramine, 8 or 12 mg   #100
   Sig: 1 tablet b.i.d. for itching. Warn patient of possible drowsiness.

<u>SUBSEQUENT VISITS</u>

1. Systemic corticosteroids. For resistant cases the corticosteroids have consistently provided more relief than any other single form of therapy. Any of the preparations can be used; for example:
   Prednisone, 10 mg   #100
   Sig: 4 tablets every morning for 1 week, then 2 tablets every morning.
   Comment: Regulate dosage as indicated.
2. Systemic antibiotics may or may not be indicated.

SECONDARY EXFOLIATIVE DERMATITIS
(Fig. 23-1)

Most patients with secondary exfoliative dermatitis have had a previous skin disease that became generalized because of overtreatment or for unknown reasons. There always remain a few

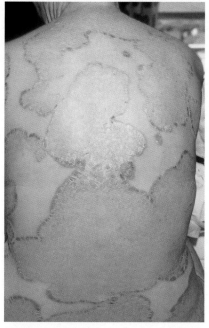

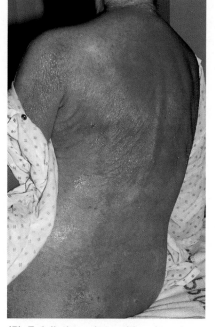

(*A*) Only at the edge of the large plaques is there a suggestion of psoriasis as the underlying diagnosis.

(*B*) Exfoliative dermatitis due to a Dilantin drug eruption.

Figure 23-1. **Exfoliative dermatitis.**

cases of exfoliative dermatitis in which the cause is unknown but suspected.

SKIN LESIONS. The clinical picture of this secondary form is indistinguishable from the primary form unless some of the original dermatitis is present.

SAUER NOTES

1. From the history, ascertain where the exfoliative eruption *began* on the body. This information can aid in establishing the cause.

2. Look at the edge of an advancing exfoliative dermatitis for the characteristic lesions of the *primary* disease, if present.

3. As the exfoliative dermatitis becomes more widespread the characteristics of the original skin disease become less obvious or completely disappear. History, therefore, may be critical in making the correct diagnosis.

COURSE. The prognosis in the secondary form is better than for the primary form, particularly if the original cause is definitely known and more specific therapy can be administered.

ETIOLOGY AND TREATMENT. A list follows of the more common causes of secondary ex-foliative dermatitis.

The treatment of these cases consists of a combination of that listed for the primary form of exfoliative dermatitis plus the cautious institution of stronger therapy directed toward the original causative skin condition. This therapy should be reviewed in the section devoted to the specific disease.

- Contact dermatitis (see Chap. 9)
- Drug eruption (see Chap. 9)
- Psoriasis (see Chap. 14)
- Atopic eczema (see Chap. 9)
- Pyoderma with id reaction (see Chap. 15)
- Fungal disease with id reaction (see Chap. 19)
- Seborrheic dermatitis (see Chap. 13)
- T-cell lymphoma (see Chap. 32). A useful rule is that 50% of all patients older than age 50 years who have an exfoliative dermatitis have a lymphoma. The *Sézary syndrome* form of lymphoma is a rare cause of exfoliative dermatitis.
- Internal cancer, leukemia, and other lymphomas can be causative.

BIBLIOGRAPHY

Botella-Estrada R, Sanmartin O, Oliver V, et al. Erythroderma. Arch Dermatol 1994;130:1503.

Pal S, Haroon TS. Erythroderma: A clinico-etiologic study of 90 cases. Int J Dermatol 1998;37:104.

Wilson DC, Jester JD, King LE Jr. Erythroderma and exfoliative dermatitis [review]. Clin Dermatol 1993;11:67.

24

Pigmentary Dermatoses

There are two variants of pigmentation of the skin: hyperpigmentation and hypopigmentation. The predominant skin pigment discussed in this chapter is melanin, but other pigments can be present in the skin. A complete classification of pigmentary disorders appears at the end of this chapter.

The melanin-forming cells and their relationship to the tyrosine-tyrosinase enzyme system are discussed in Chap. 1.

The common clinical example of abnormal hyperpigmentation is *chloasma*, but secondary melanoderma can result from many causes.

The most common form of hypopigmentation is *vitiligo*, but secondary leukoderma does occur.

CHLOASMA (MELASMA)
(Fig. 24-1)

CLINICAL LESIONS. An irregular hyperpigmentation of the skin that varies in shades of brown is seen.

DISTRIBUTION. The lesions usually occur on the sides of the face, the forehead, and the sides of the neck.

COURSE. The disorder is slowly progressive, but remissions do occur. It is more obvious in the summer.

ETIOLOGY. The cause is unknown, but some cases appear during pregnancy (called "mask of pregnancy") or with chronic illness. There is an increased incidence of chloasma in women taking contraceptive, postmenopausal, or fertility hormones. To be nosologically correct, such cases should be labeled *drug eruption, hyperpigmentation, due to hormones*. A lay term for chloasma is "liver spots," but there is no association with liver pathology. The melanocyte-stimulating hormone of the pituitary may be excessive and affect the tyrosine–tyrosinase enzyme system.

Differential Diagnosis

The causes of *secondary melanoderma* should be ruled out (see end of this chapter).

Treatment

1. The patient should not be promised great therapeutic results. Most cases associated with pregnancy slowly fade or disappear completely after delivery. The pigmentation may be prolonged if the patient elects to breastfeed.
2. For a mild case in an unconcerned patient, cosmetic coverage can be adequate. Dermablend or Lydia O'Leary Covermark are two useful products.

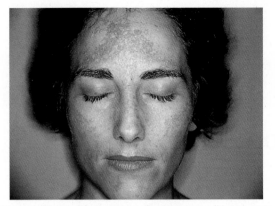

Figure 24-1. Pigmentary dermatoses. (*Neutrogena Skin Care Institute*) Cloasma of face.

3. Sunlight intensifies the pigmentation, so a sunscreen should be added to the routine.
4. Hydroquinone preparations (any of the following):

Melanex solution 3%	30.0
Lustra Cream 4%	
Eldopaque Forte cream (tinted)	30.0
Solaquin Forte cream (nontinted)	30.0

Sig: Apply locally b.i.d. Stop if irritation develops.
Comment: The treatment with any of these hydroquinone preparations should be continued for at least 3 months. Response to therapy is slow. The two latter preparations also contain a sunscreen.
5. Retinoic acid (Retin-A cream or gel) can slowly decrease the pigmentation, if tolerated.
6. NeoStrata gel (with glycolic acid and hydroquinone) is beneficial.

VITILIGO
(*Fig. 24-2*)

CLINICAL LESIONS. Irregular areas of depigmented skin are occasionally seen with a hyperpigmented border. There is a segmental variety that has pigment loss in a dermatomal (especially trigeminal) distribution.

DISTRIBUTION. Most commonly the lesions occur on the face and the dorsum of hands and feet, but they can occur on all body areas.

COURSE. The disease is slowly progressive, but remissions and changes are frequent. It is more obvious during the summer because of the tanning of adjacent normal skin.

ETIOLOGY. The cause is unknown but believed by some to be an autoimmune disease. Heredity is a factor in some cases. Autoimmune diseases, especially thyroiditis, can be associated with vitiligo.

Differential Diagnosis

Causes of *secondary hypopigmentation* need to be ruled out (see end of this chapter and Fig. 24-3).

Treatment

A young woman with large depigmented patches on her face and dorsum of hands asks if something can be done for her "white spots." Her sister has a few lesions.

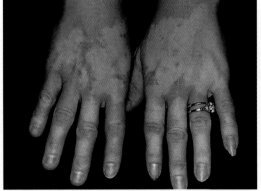

(*A*) Vitiligo of hands in a Caucasian patient.

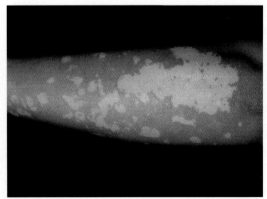

(*B*) Vitiligo of forearm in an African-American patient.

Figure 24-2. Pigmentary dermatoses. (*Neutrogena Skin Care Institute*)

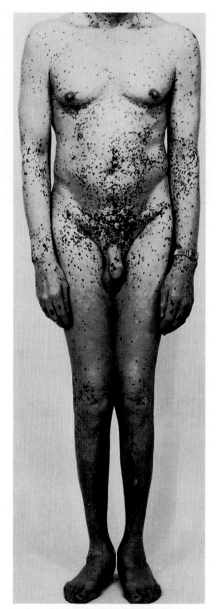

Figure 24-3. Secondary hypopigmentation. A marked example of loss of pigment that occurred in an African-American man following healing of an exfoliative dermatitis. Corticosteroids were used in the therapy.

Cosmetics: The use of the following covering or staining preparations is recommended: pancake-type cosmetics, such as Covermark, by Lydia O'Leary; Vitadye (Elder); dihydroxyacetone containing self-tanning creams, gels, and foams; walnut-juice stain; or potassium permanganate solution in appropriate dilution. Many patients with vitiligo

become quite proficient in the application of these agents.

Corticosteroid cream therapy: This is effective for early mild cases of vitiligo, especially when one is mainly concerned with face and hand lesions. Betamethasone valerate cream 0.1% (Valisone cream) can be prescribed for use on the hands for 4 months or so and for use on the face for only 3 months. It should not be used on the eyelids or as full-body therapy.

Sun avoidance: Suntanning should be avoided because this accentuates the normal pigmentation and makes the nonpigmented vitiligo more noticeable. The white areas of vitiligo are more susceptible to sunburn.

If the patient desires a more specific treatment, the following can be suggested, with certain reservations:

Psoralen derivatives: For many years, Egyptians along the Nile River chewed certain plants to cause the disappearance of the white spots of vitiligo. Extraction of the chemicals from these plants revealed the psoralen derivatives to be the active agents, and one of these, 8-methoxypsoralen (8-MOP), was found to be the most effective. This chemical is available as Oxsoralen in 10-mg capsules and also as a topical liquid form. The oral form is to be ingested 2 hours before exposure to measured sun radiation. The package insert should be consulted. Our results with this long-term therapy have been very disappointing.

Trisoralen is a synthetic psoralen in 5-mg tablets. The recommended dosage is 2 tablets taken 2 hours before measured sun exposure for a long-term course. Detailed instructions accompany the package. Some dermatologists believe this therapy to be more effective than Oxsoralen.

A short 2-week course of Oxsoralen capsules (20 mg/day) has been advocated for the purpose of acquiring a better and quicker *suntan*. The value of such a course has been questioned. The sun exposure must be gradual. *Oral psoralens plus self-administered UVA or UVB in "tanning booths" can produce severe burns, which may be fatal.*

PUVA therapy: The combination of topical or oral psoralen therapy with UVA radiation has been somewhat successful in repigmenting vitiligo. The psoralen can be given orally, topically, or as a bath. Precautions concerning photoaging and skin cancer apply.

Depigmentation therapy: In the hands of experts, monobenzyl ether of hydroquinone (Benoquin) can be used to remove skin pigment to even out the patient's skin color.

Skin grafting: Autologous minigrafting and other similar surgical procedures have been used with success by some.

Surgical therapy: Various grafting procedures are valuable in recalcitrant disease. Epidermal or full thickness autographs have been advocated by some authors.

Classification of Pigmentary Disorders

MELANIN HYPERPIGMENTATION OR MELANODERMA

1. Chloasma (melasma) (see Fig. 24-1)
2. Incontinentia pigmenti
3. Secondary to skin diseases
   a. Chronic discoid lupus erythematosus
   b. Tinea versicolor
   c. Stasis dermatitis
   d. Lichen planus
   e. Fixed drug eruption
   f. Many cases of dermatitis in African-Americans and other dark-skinned individuals (see Fig. 24-3)
   g. Scleroderma
   h. Porphyria cutanea tarda (Fig. 24-4)
   i. Dermatitis herpetiformis
4. Secondary to external agents
   a. X-radiation
   b. Ultraviolet light
   c. Sunlight

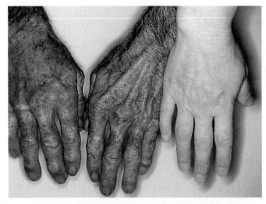

Figure 24-4. Pigmentary dermatoses. (*Neutrogena Skin Care Institute*) Porphyria cutanea tarda hyperpigmentation.

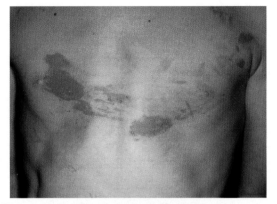

Figure 24-5. Pigmentary dermatoses. (*Neutrogena Skin Care Institute*) Berlock dermatitis: photosensitivity reaction from mother's perfume, age 7 years.

   d. Tars
   e. Photosensitizing chemicals, as in cosmetics, causing development of clinical entities labeled as Riehl's melanosis, poikiloderma of Civatte on the sides of the neck due to chronic sun exposure, berlock dermatitis (Fig. 24-5), and others
5. Secondary to internal disorders
   a. Addison's disease (see Fig. 26-1)
   b. Chronic liver disease
   c. Pregnancy
   d. Hyperthyroidism
   e. Internal carcinoma causing malignant form of acanthosis nigricans
   f. Hormonal influence on benign acanthosis nigricans
   g. Intestinal polyposis causing mucous membrane pigmentation (Peutz-Jeghers syndrome)
   h. Albright's syndrome
   i. Schilder's disease
   j. Fanconi's syndrome, ie., HIV-positive patients
6. Secondary to drugs such as adrenocorticotropic hormone, estrogens, progesterone, melanocyte-stimulating hormone

NONMELANIN PIGMENTATIONS

1. Argyria due to silver salt deposits
2. Arsenical pigmentation due to ingestion of inorganic arsenic, as in Fowler's solution and Asiatic pills
3. Pigmentation from heavy metals such as bismuth, gold, and mercury
4. Tattoos

5. Black dermographism, the common bluish black or green stain seen under watches and rings in certain persons from the deposit of the metallic particles reacting with chemicals already on the skin
6. Hemosiderin granules in hemochromatosis or pigmented purpuric eruptions (see Chap. 12).
7. Bile pigments from jaundice
8. Yellow pigments following atabrine and chlorpromazine ingestion
9. Carotene coloring in carotenemia
10. Homogentisic acid polymer deposit in ochronosis
11. Minocycline hyperpigmentation (characteristic histopathology) diffuse and also localized at scar sites (and rarely teeth).

HYPOPIGMENTATION

1. Albinism
2. Vitiligo
3. Leukoderma or acquired hypopigmentation (Fig. 24-6)
   a. Secondary to skin diseases such as tinea versicolor, chronic discoid lupus erythematosus, localized scleroderma, psoriasis, secondary syphilis, pinta, etc. (see Fig. 24-3)
   b. Secondary to chemicals such as mercury compounds, monobenzyl ether of hydroquinone, and cortisone-type drugs given intralesionally, especially in African-Americans (see Fig. 24-6)
   c. Secondary to internal diseases, such as hormonal diseases, and in Vogt-Koyanagi syndrome

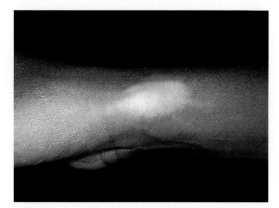

Figure 24-6. **Pigmentary dermatoses.** (*Neutrogena Skin Care Institute*) Leukoderma on wrist from corticosteroid intralesionally in a black patient.

   d. Associated with pigmented nevi (halo nevus or leukoderma acquisitum centrifugum)

BIBLIOGRAPHY

Boersma BR, Westerhof W, Bos JD. J Am Acad Dermatol 1995;33:6.

Drake LA, Dinehart SM, Farmer ER, et al. Guidelines of care for vitiligo. J Am Acad Dermatol 1996;35:620.

Fulk CS. Primary disorders of hyperpigmentation. J Am Acad Dermatol 1984;10:1.

Kovacs SO. Vitiligo. J Am Acad Dermatol 1998;38:5.

Levine N. Pigmentation and pigmentary disorders. Boca Raton, FL, CRC Press, 1994.

Nordlund JJ, Boissy R, et al. The pigmentary system: Physiology and pathophysiology. 1998.

25

Collagen Diseases

The diseases commonly included in this group are *lupus erythematosus, scleroderma*, and *dermatomyositis*. The skin manifestations are usually a dominant feature of these diseases, but in some cases, particularly systemic lupus erythematosus, skin lesions may be absent. Rheumatoid arthritis and periarteritis nodosa are often included in the collagen disease group but are only occasionally accompanied by skin lesions, usually of the erythema multiforme-like group (see Chap. 12).

The onset of the collagen diseases is insidious, and the prognosis as to life is serious. It is not unusual to attach the label of "collagen disease" to a patient who has only minimal subjective and objective findings (malaise, weakness, vague joint and muscle pains, antibody and immunologic abnormalities, biologic false-positive serology, and high sedimentation rate), with the realization by the physician that months and years have to elapse before a more exacting diagnosis of one of the previously mentioned diseases can be made.

Considerable advances have been made in the laboratory testing directed toward differentiation of the several collagen diseases. The LE cell test was the first test developed, but it has been superseded by the antinuclear antibody (ANA) test, fluorescent ANA test, anti-DNA, and many more complicated serologic and tissue tests (see Chap. 10).

If the ANA test is positive in a patient, then the fluorescent ANA test is usually indicated. The pattern of nuclear fluorescence, as well as the dilution of a serum at which fluorescence is lost, may provide important diagnostic and prognostic information.

For completeness and for a better understanding of these patterns, consult Chapter 10.

LUPUS ERYTHEMATOSUS
(Figs. 25-1–25-3)

Discoid lupus erythematosus, subacute lupus erythematosus, and systemic lupus erythematosus are clinically distinct but basically related diseases. The three diseases differ in regard to characteristic skin lesions, subjective complaints, other organ involvement, blood and tissue test findings, response to treatment, and eventual prognosis. However, rare cases of clinically classic discoid lupus erythematosus show laboratory evidence of the pathology seen with the systemic form of lupus erythematosus and can terminate as the disseminated disease. Certain early borderline cases are difficult to categorize, and some *subacute* forms may develop into the systemic disease. The variations of the three forms of lupus erythematosus are shown in Table 25-1.

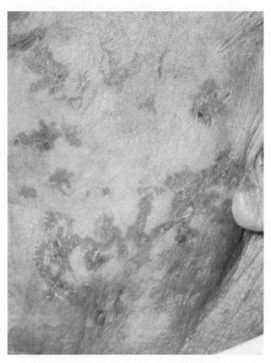

A

Figure 25-1. **Lupus erythematosus.** (*A*) Chronic discoid lupus erythematosus on the cheek of an elderly man. (*K.C.G.H., Truman Medical Center; Smith Kline & French Laboratories*) (*B*) Chronic discoid lupus erythematosus. (*Burroughs Wellcome Co.*)

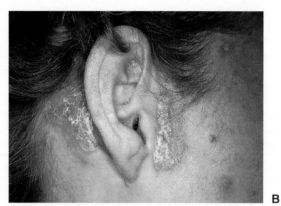
B

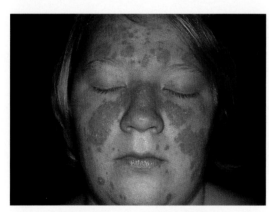

(*A*) Subacute lupus erythematosus.

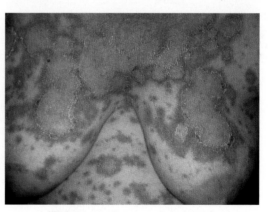

(*B*) Subacute lupus erythematosus.

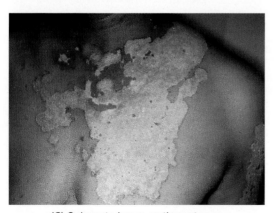

(*C*) Subacute lupus erythematosus.

Figure 25-2. **Lupus erythematosus.** (*Burroughs Wellcome Co.*)

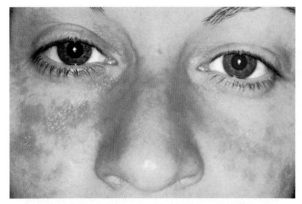 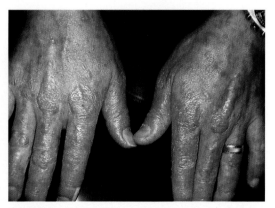

(A) Systemic lupus erythematosus showing classic "butter-fly" eruption. *(Drs. S. Wilson and W. Larson; Smith Kline & French Laboratories)*

(B) Systemic lupus erythematosus of hands. *(Burroughs Wellcome Co.)*

Figure 25-3. **Lupus erythematosus.**

TABLE 25-1
COMPARISON OF THE THREE FORMS OF LUPUS ERYTHEMATOSUS

Parameter	Discoid	Subacute	Systemic
Primary lesions	Red, scaly, thickened, well-circumscribed patches with enlarged follicles and elevated border	Papulosquamous psoriasiform lesions or annular lesions often with central depigmentation	Red, mildly scaly, diffuse, puffy lesions; purpura is also seen; bullae occur rarely
Secondary lesions	Atrophy, scarring, and pigmentary changes	Usually nonscarring but can heal with vitiliginous white areas	No scarring; mild hyperpigmentation
Distribution	Face, mainly in "butterfly" area but also on scalp, ears, arms, and chest; may not be symmetric	Areas of sun exposure (face, trunk, extremities); symmetric	Face in "butterfly" area, arms, fingers, and legs; usually symmetric
Course	Very chronic, with gradual progression; slow healing under therapy; no effect on life	Marked photosensitivity in most patients; many develop signs of systemic lupus erythematosus (50%); usually does not affect life span; chronic but often responds well to treatment	Acute onset with fever, rash, malaise, and joint pains; most cases respond rather rapidly to corticosteroid and supportive therapy, but the prognosis for life is poor
Season	Aggravated by intense sun exposure or radiation therapy	Same	Same
Sex incidence	Almost twice as common in females	Same	Same
Systemic pathology	None obvious	Arthritis common (75%), but central nervous system and renal disease (10%) are uncommon	Nephritis, arthritis, epilepsy, pancarditis, hepatitis and so on
Laboratory findings	Biopsy characteristic in classic case; antinuclear antibody and related tests are negative, as are other laboratory tests; direct band test on fresh tissue of involved skin is positive	RO (SS-A) antigen often positive (70%)	Biopsy is useful, especially fresh tissue immunofluorescent studies, which may be positive in involved skin, sun-exposed skin or non-sun-exposed skin; leukopenia, anemia, albuminuria, increased sedimentation rate, positive antinuclear antibody test, and biologic false-positive serologic test for syphillis are found.

Discoid Lupus Erythematosus
(See Fig. 25-1)

DIFFERENTIAL DIAGNOSIS

Systemic lupus erythematosus: See Table 25-1.
Subacute lupus erythematosus: See Table 25-1.
Polymorphous light eruption: Many cases are grossly and histologically similar to systemic or discoid lupus erythematosus but get history of presence only in summer; response is faster to antimalarial drugs and locally applied sunscreening agents.
Seborrheic dermatitis: Lesions greasy, red, scaly, associated with scalp dandruff; occurs in eyebrows and scalp without hair loss; response is rapid to antiseborrheic local therapy, and sunlight tends to improve seborrhea (see Chap. 13).
Any cutaneous granulomas: Such as sarcoidosis (see Chap. 20), secondary and tertiary syphilis (see Chap. 16), and lupus vulgaris (see Chap. 15).

Cases with scarring alopecia (see Fig. 27-6) are to be differentiated from *alopecia cicatrisata* (see Chap. 27), *old tinea capitis of endothrix type* (see Chap. 19), *lichen planus* (see Chap. 14), and *folliculitis decalvans* (see Chap. 27).

TREATMENT

A young woman presents with two red, scaly, dime-sized lesions on her right cheek of 3 months' duration.

1. Laboratory work-up should include a complete blood cell count, urinalysis, serology, ANA and related tests, sedimentation rate and, usually, a biopsy. The blood tests should be normal, but the biopsy of fixed tissue and fresh tissue is rather characteristic of discoid lupus. The fresh tissue shows positive direct immunofluorescence at the dermal–epidermal junction (positive lupus band test). The serum test for ANA is usually negative.
2. Fluorinated corticosteroid cream   15.0
   Sig: Apply b.i.d. locally to lesions. Do not use fluorinated corticosteroids creams on the face for long periods of time because atrophy and telangiectasia can develop.
3. Sunscreen cream with a sun protective factor (SPF) of 15 or more.
   Sig: Apply to face as sunscreen for protection; reapply frequently and use year round.

Chloroquine and hydroxychloroquine are very effective drugs for this disease. However, because of an irreversible retinitis that has developed in rare patients on long-term therapy, periodic eye examinations usually at 6-month intervals by an ophthalmologist are recommended. Quinacrine can also be used but it does cause a yellow discoloration of skin.

Subacute (Cutaneous) Lupus Erythematosus
(see Fig. 25-2)

DIFFERENTIAL DIAGNOSIS

Systemic lupus erythematosus: Often involves kidneys and central nervous system; lesions less likely to be papulosquamous or annular; not as often associated with positive RO (SS-A) antigen.
Discoid lupus erythematosus: See Table 25-1.
Erythema annulare centrifigum: Often is singular lesion without follicular plugging or telangiectasia; lesions are circinate and may have fine adherent scale and clearing in center; may be related to underlying illness but not usually lupus erythematosus; ANA test is negative and patients are not photosensitive; skin biopsy may be diagnostic and direct immunofluorescence is negative (see Dictionary–Index).
Psoriasis: Silvery white, thick adherent scale usually improves with sun exposure; common on elbows, knees, scalp, and intertriginous locations; histology often nonspecific but negative lupus band; may be associated with arthritis (7%) but other organs spared and ANA test negative.
Vitiligo: Not associated with previous inflammatory stage and photosensitive only in areas of pigment loss; negative ANA blood test and not associated with arthritis.

TREATMENT

A young woman presents with photosensitivity, arthritis, and skin lesions thought to represent psoriasis. A blood test reveals SS-A antigen.

1. It is necessary to evaluate other organ systems (kidney, central nervous system, liver, lung) even though joint and skin diseases are probably the only involvement.
2. Photosensitivity drug eruption should be checked for and a potent sunscreen considered.
3. Topical corticosteroids and oral antimalarial agents are first-line therapies. Systemic corticosteroids and immunosuppressive drugs

(azathioprine, cyclophosphamide) should be used only in severe cases.

Systemic Lupus Erythematosus
(see Fig. 25-3)

DIFFERENTIAL DIAGNOSIS

Discoid lupus erythematosus: See Table 25-1.
Subacute cutaneous lupus erythematosus: See Table 25-1.
Polymorphous light eruption: Skin lesions similar in appearance; usually only in summer; no altered laboratory studies; more rapid response to antimalarial drugs.
Seborrheic dermatitis: Associated with scalp dandruff; responds to local antiseborrhea therapy (see Chap. 13).
Rosacea: Presence of acne-like lesions and telangiectasia on nose and butterfly area of cheeks, without systemic symptoms but may have associated eye abnormalities, may worsen with sun exposure (see Chap. 13).
Contact dermatitis: Due to cosmetics, paint sprays, vegetation, hand creams; acute onset with no systemic symptoms; history helpful (see Chap. 9).
Dermatomyositis: Muscle soreness and weakness (see at end of this chapter).
Drug eruption due to apresoline, hydralazine, procainamide, and others (see Chap 9): Can simulate systemic lupus; take history.
Mixed connective tissue disease: This is a distinct clinical syndrome sharing features of systemic lupus erythematosus, progressive systemic sclerosis, and polymyositis. A high titer of particulate fluorescent antinuclear antibody is significant.
Parvovirus B19 Infection: No discoid lesions or alopecia. No renal or cardiac involvement. Positive parvovirus B19 antibodies. If anemic have a low reticulocyte count.

TREATMENT

A young woman presents with diffuse red, puffy eruption on cheeks, nose, and forehead and at base of fingernails of 1 week's duration. She complains of malaise, fever, joint pains, headache, and ankle edema that has become progressively worse in the past 3 weeks.

The patient should have a complete diagnostic work-up and should be treated with corticosteroids, immunosuppressive agents, and any other supportive therapy, as indicated for the organs involved.

Photosensitizing drugs, such as some diuretics and sulfonamide therapy, may complicate the clinical picture. Preferably, patients with systemic lupus should be primarily under the care of an internist, with assistance from other specialists as needed.

Neonatal Lupus Erythematosus (see Fig. 33-18)

Polycyclic or psoriasiform lesions are present, mainly on the face, but disappear around 6 months of age. It is associated with cardiac conduction defects in 50% of cases and is the most common cause of neonatal heart block.

Anti-Ro(SS-A) antibodies are found. Most mothers have or will have signs of lupus erythematosus or Sjögren's syndrome.

SCLERODERMA
(Figs. 25-4–25-6)

As in lupus erythematosus, there are two forms of scleroderma that are clinically unrelated, except for some common histopathologic changes in the skin. *Localized scleroderma* (*morphea*) is a benign disease. *Diffuse scleroderma* (*systemic sclerosis*) is a serious disease.

Localized Scleroderma (Morphea)
(see Fig. 25-5)

Localized scleroderma is an uncommon skin disease of unknown etiology with extremely rare systemic involvement.

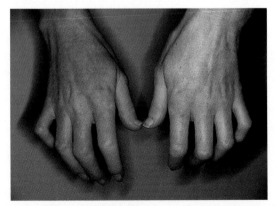

Figure 25-4. Scleroderma. Diffuse scleroderma of hands. (*Burroughs Wellcome Co.*)

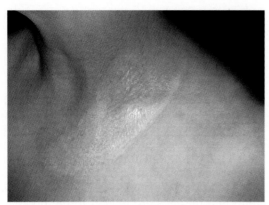

(A) Localized scleroderma of clavicular area.

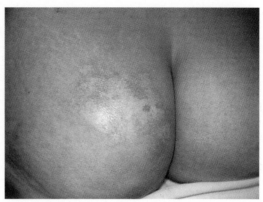

(B) Localized scleroderma of buttocks.

Figure 25-5. **Scleroderma.** (*Ortho Pharmaceutical Corp.*)

PRIMARY LESIONS. These are single or multiple, violaceous, firm, inelastic macules and plaques that enlarge slowly. The progressing border retains the violaceous hue, while the center becomes whitish and slightly depressed beneath the skin surface. Bizarre lesions occur, such as long linear bands on extremities, saber cut-type lesions in scalp, or lesions involving one side of the face or the body, causing *hemiatrophy* and rarely dental deformities and seizures when on the face (Fig. 25-6A).

SECONDARY LESIONS. Mild or severe scarring after healing is inevitable. Scalp lesions (*en coup de sabre* form) result in permanent hair loss (see Fig. 25-6A). Ulceration is rare.

DISTRIBUTION. Trunk, extremities, and head are most frequently involved.

ETIOLOGY. A possible etiology is *Borrelia burgdorferi*, but there are negative and positive findings regarding this agent as a cause and it seems to relate mainly to cases in Europe.

COURSE. Disability is confined to the area involved. Lesions may involute slowly and spontaneously. Relapses are rare.

DIFFERENTIAL DIAGNOSIS

Guttate macular form of localized scleroderma from *lichen sclerosus et atrophicus* (histopathology rather characteristic, but the two conditions may coexist).

Plaque type of localized scleroderma from *traumatic scars* (history important, no violaceous border).

Idiopathic atrophoderma of Pacini and Pierini (rare, no induration).

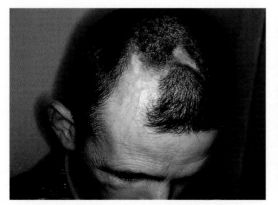

(A) Linear (en coup de sabre) scleroderma.

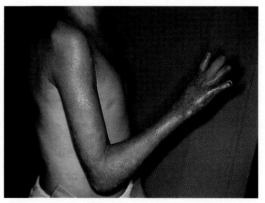

(B) Linear (hemiatrophy) scleroderma, age 8 years.

Figure 25-6. **Scleroderma.** (*Ortho Pharmaceutical Corp.*)

TREATMENT

No therapy is necessary for most mild cases. Reassurance with the correct diagnosis is very important. Time is the healer.

For extensive cases, a fluorinated corticosteroid cream applied twice daily locally for months, PUVA therapy, calcipotriene, all with appropriate precautions, is possibly beneficial.

Diffuse Scleroderma (Systemic Sclerosis)
(see Fig. 25-4)

Diffuse scleroderma is an uncommon systemic disease of unknown etiology that is characterized by a long course of progressive disability due primarily to lack of mobility of the areas and the organs that are affected. There are two clinical forms of this disease. In the *diffuse form* the skin becomes hidebound, the esophagus and the gastrointestinal tract semirigid, and the lungs and the heart fibrosed. In the *CREST form* (calcinosis, Raynaud's phenomenon, esophageal involvement, sclerodactyly, and telangiectasis), the course is relatively benign because of minimal internal organ involvement.

PRIMARY LESIONS. There is usually a long prodromal stage of swelling of the skin, with progressive limitation of movement. The early stage may or may not be associated with *Raynaud's phenomenon*, which is worse in the winter.

SECONDARY LESIONS. As months and years pass, the limitation of movement becomes marked, particularly of the hands, the feet, and the face. The skin becomes atrophic and hidebound and develops sensory, vasomotor, and pigmentary changes and, finally, ulcerations.

DISTRIBUTION. The skin of the hands, the feet, and the face is involved early, and in some rare cases the changes are confined only to the extremities ("acrosclerosis"). In most patients, however, the entire skin becomes involved, along with the internal organs.

COURSE. The prognosis is grave, and most patients die of the disease after years of disability. However, spontaneous or therapy-induced remissions can occur.

ETIOLOGY. Both forms have a high incidence of positive ANA. In 20% of patients with the diffuse form there is a positive Scl-70 antibody, while 20% of the patients with the CREST form have the centromere antibody.

SEX INCIDENCE. The disease is more common in females.

LABORATORY FINDINGS. Histologic examination of the skin shows generalized atrophy and hyalinization with entrapment of the eccrine glands in the scar tissue. The atrophic skeletal muscles lack the inflammatory component seen in dermatomyositis. The sedimentation rate is elevated early in the course of the disease. Other abnormal findings are related to the organs involved.

DIFFERENTIAL DIAGNOSIS

Dermatomyositis: Muscle tenderness, weakness, less scarring skin changes; muscle biopsy is characteristic (see Dermatomyositis, in the following section).
Early rheumatoid arthritis: Swelling of joints and overlying skin; radiographs are helpful in determining diagnosis, as is time itself; rheumatoid factor test is positive.

TREATMENT

No specific therapy is known. Protection of the skin from trauma, cold, and infection is important. Physiotherapy may prevent contractures. Sympathectomy produces temporary benefits in some patients. Chelating agents are reported helpful for patients with extensive calcification. Corticosteroids are not very beneficial.

DERMATOMYOSITIS
(Fig. 25-7)

The rarest of the three collagen diseases is dermatomyositis, which is characterized by an acute or insidious onset of muscle pain, weakness, fever, arthralgia, photosensitivity, and, in some cases, a puffy erythematous or heliotrope eruption, usually confined to the face and the eyelids. In older cases small 3×3-mm or so reddish papules develop on the knuckles of the fingers, known as Göttron's papules. Wire-loop shaped telangiectasias may occur on the proximal nail folds of the fingers.

Progression of the disease results in muscle atrophy and contractures, skin telangiectasia and atrophy, and generalized organ involvement, with death in 50% of cases. Dermatomyositis has a relationship to underlying adenocarcinoma.

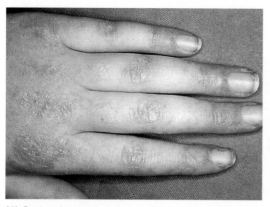

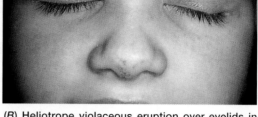

(*A*) Gottron's papules and erythema over knuckles in dermatomyositis.

(*B*) Heliotrope violaceous eruption over eyelids in dermatomyositis.

Figure 25-7. **Dermatomyositis.** (*Ortho Pharmaceutical Corp.*)

SEX INCIDENCE. It is more common in females.

LABORATORY FINDINGS. These include increased sedimentation rate, rather characteristic muscle changes on biopsy study, albuminuria, anemia, positive ANA test, and negative serologic test for syphilis. Degeneration of the muscles is accompanied by creatinuria and elevation of blood serum aldolase and creatine phosphokinase levels.

DIFFERENTIAL DIAGNOSIS

Systemic lupus erythematosus, diffuse scleroderma, photosensitivity reactions, erysipelas, polyneuritis, myasthenia gravis, and others must be differentiated.

TREATMENT

Removal of an associated adenocarcinoma (present in 20% of cases of dermatomyositis) may result in a remission. Rare vesicle formation may indicate an increased incidence of underlying cancer. Corticosteroid oral therapy, often in high doses as for systemic lupus erythematosus, and immunosuppressive agents, may cause a remission.

BIBLIOGRAPHY

Boyd AS, Neldner KH. Therapeutic options in dermatomyositis/polymyositis. Int J Dermatol 1994;33:240.

Callen JP, Tuffanelli DL, Provost TT. Collagen-vascular diseases: An update. J Am Acad Dermatol 1993;28:477.

Chlebus E, Wolska H, Blaszczyk M, Jablonska S. Subacute cutaneous lupus erythematosus versus systemic lupus erythematosus: Diagnostic criteria and therapeutic implications. J Am Acad Dermatol 1998;38:405.

Condemi JJ. The autoimmune diseases. JAMA 1992;268: 2882.

Dawkins MA, Jorizzo JL, et al. Dermatomyositis: A dermatology-based case series. J Am Acad Dermatol 1998;38: 397.

Farmer ER, Goltz RW, et al. Guidelines of care for scleroderma and sclerodermoid disorders. J Am Acad Dermatol 1996;35:4.

Perez MI, Kohn SR. Systemic sclerosis. J Am Acad Dermatol 1993;28:525.

Sontheimer RD. Cutaneous manifestations of rheumatic diseases. Baltimore, Williams & Wilkins, 1996.

Sontheimer RD. Lupus erythematosus: Clinicopathogenic correlations. Prog Dermatol 1990;24:1.

The Skin and Internal Disease

Warren R. Heymann, M.D.* and Robin M. Levin, M.D.†

A practicing dermatologist must be cognizant of how a particular skin disease relates to any potential systemic malady. On occasion, a cutaneous finding may alert the clinician to a previously undiagnosed systemic disease. It is the interplay between the skin and the internal organs that requires the physician to be aware of such relationships. We choose to demonstrate examples of cutaneous manifestations of systemic disease using an organ-system approach.

Cutaneous findings can be classified as specific or nonspecific. Specific changes (see Fig. 26-8A–C) demonstrate the same pathologic process as the internal disease and can, therefore, be diagnostic of the disease. Nonspecific changes (Figs. 26-1, 26-2, and see Fig. 26-8D), in contrast, are nondiagnostic because they do not contain the primary disease process. These changes, however, can be helpful in establishing the diagnosis only if all clinical data are considered. The following cases are a few examples of the myriad of systemic diseases with skin involvement.

*Head, Division of Dermatology, Associate Professor, Department of Clinical Medicine, Cooper Hospital/University Medical Center, UMDNJ-Robert Wood Johnson Medical School at Camden, Camden, New Jersey

†Chief Resident, Department of Dermatology, Cooper Hospital/University Medical Center, UMDNJ-Robert Wood Johnson Medical School at Camden, Camden, New Jersey

CARDIOLOGY

KAWASAKI'S SYNDROME. Kawasaki's syndrome, also known as mucocutaneous lymph node syndrome, is a self-limited systemic disorder of childhood. It has a propensity for coronary artery involvement with aneurysms, angina pectoris, or myocardial infarction in 15 to 20% of cases. The diagnosis of Kawasaki's syndrome is based on a constellation of clinical findings including fever, nonsuppurative cervical adenopathy, bilateral nonpurulent conjunctival injection, reddening and fissuring of the lips, "strawberry tongue," and several cutaneous findings. The skin changes begin with erythema of the palms and soles, which may spread to the trunk. Indurative edema and desquamation starting on the tips of the fingers and toes and around the nails is then noted. A polymorphous rash that can vary from maculopapular to morbilliform to scarlatiniform may also be present.

LEOPARD SYNDROME. Multiple lentigines syndrome is an autosomal dominant disorder with abnormalities of various clinical expression. Each letter in the name stands for a different abnormality that may be found in the syndrome:

Lentigines—multiple lentigines are present at birth and may cover the entire body, including the palms and soles, but sparing the lips and oral mucosa. The pigment can be seen in the iris and retina as well.

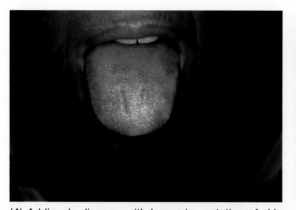

(*A*) Addison's disease, with hyperpigmentation of skin and tongue, in a Caucasian woman.

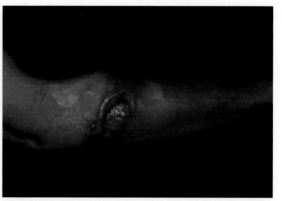

(*B*) Delusional excoriation on arm, "have to get the hairs out."

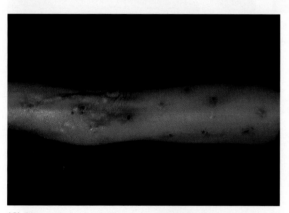

(*C*) Neurotic excoriations on the arm in a 47-year-old woman.

Figure 26-1.   Dermatoses due to internal disease.
(*Reed & Carnrick*)

Electrocardiogram conduction defects
Ocular telorism
Pulmonary stenosis
Abnormalities of the genitalia
Retardation of growth
Deafness (sensorineural)

SUBACUTE BACTERIAL ENDOCARDITIS.
Several cutaneous lesions can develop secondary to subacute bacterial endocarditis. These lesions vary in their frequency and have decreased in frequency with the advent of antibiotics. Petechiae and purpura can be found in the skin, conjunctiva (Roth spots), and oral mucosa. Splinter hemorrhages are found below the nail plate. Osler's nodes and Janeway's lesions can both present as hemorrhagic or erythematous macules, papules, or nodules but differ in their locations and symptoms. Osler's nodes are painful and found in the pulp of the distal digits or thenar eminences, whereas Janeway lesions

are nontender and located on the proximal aspects of the palms and soles.

ENDOCRINOLOGY

DIABETES MELLITUS. The cutaneous manifestations associated with diabetes mellitus can be correlated with metabolic derangements or chronic degenerative changes or have no relation to either of these problems (Fig. 26-3). Metabolic changes in patients with poorly controlled diabetes tend to cause a higher risk for the development of cutaneous bacterial, fungal, and yeast infections. Diabetic dermopathy—atrophic, circumscribed, brownish lesions on the anterior lower legs—or bullous diabeticorum—the spontaneous development of bullae on the extremities—as well as cutaneous neuropathies can be seen as a result of chronic degenerative changes. Necrobiosis lipoidica is seen in less than 1% of diabetics, but more than half of patients with necrobiosis

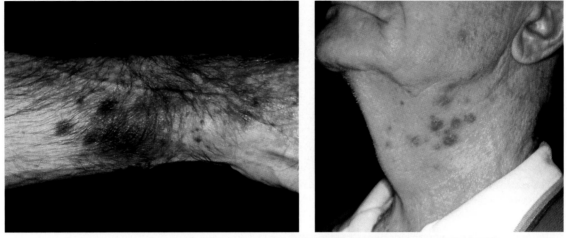

Purpura of arm (*A*) and folliculitis of neck (*B*) in same patient with myelogenous leukemia.

Figure 26-2. **Dermatoses associated with lymphomas.** (*Syntex Laboraties, Inc.*)

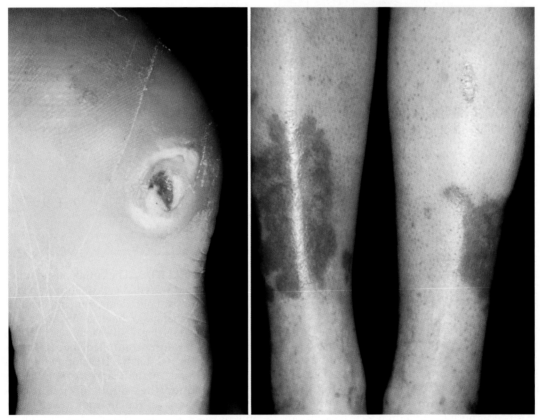

Figure 26-3. **Skin manifestations of diabetes mellitus.** (*Left*) Mal perforans of sole of foot of 3 years duration. (*Right*) Necrobiosis lipoidica diabeticorum on anterior tibial area of legs. (*Dermik Laboratories, Inc., and Smith Kline & French Laboratories*)

lipoidica have diabetes mellitus (Fig. 26-4). It is believed to occur without regard to metabolic derangements or chronic degenerative changes. Necrobiosis lipoidica begins as a sharply circumscribed dusky-red nodule. These lesions, typically seen on the anterior and lateral surfaces of the lower extremities, are chronic and indolent, and longstanding lesions may ulcerate.

THYROID DISEASE. Hypothyroidism and hyperthyroidism may create a variety of changes in the skin. In hyperthyroidism, the skin is warm, moist, and smooth due to vasodilatation of the cutaneous blood vessels. Persistent erythema of the face, elbows, and palms may be noted. Excessive sweating, especially of the palms and soles, a thin epidermis, altered texture of the hair, alopecia, onycholysis, and pretibial myxedema are also commonly observed. Pretibial myxedema consists of pink to skin-colored papules frequently on the anterior tibia and dorsal feet. A diffuse brawny edema may be noted with or without the nodules.

In hypothyroidism (Fig. 26-5), the skin is cold, dry, and pale from vasoconstriction of the cutaneous vessels. There is generalized thinning and hyperkeratosis of the epidermis with follicular plugging. Fine wrinkling and a yellowish discoloration are sometimes present. The hair is coarse, dry, brittle, and slow growing. Patchy or diffuse alopecia can be seen. Loss of the outer

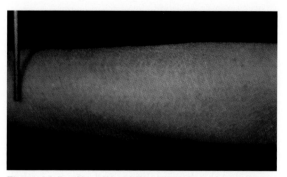

Figure 26-5.   **Hypothyroidism.** (*Reed and Carnick*) Year-round dry skin.

third of the eyebrow is a characteristic finding. Myxedema is also found but generally in a more diffuse distribution than seen in hyperthyroidism. The face lacks expression, with almost pathognomonic changes such as thickening of the lips, broadening of the nose, puffiness of the eyes, and drooping of the upper eyelids.

MULTIPLE MUCOSAL NEUROMA SYNDROME. Multiple mucosal neuroma syndrome is most likely a variant of multiple endocrine neoplasia, type IIB. In this syndrome, medullary thyroid carcinoma (MTC) and pheochromocytoma are associated with oral, nasal, upper gastrointestinal tract, and conjunctival neuromas. The skin lesions typically range from soft to firm intradermal nodules, which tend to precede the MTC. However, the MTC can occur in early childhood prior to the development of the neuromas. Additional skin findings include "blubbery" lips, lentigines, café-au-lait macules, and occasionally localized intense unilateral pruritus on the back (notalgia paresthetica).

GASTROENTEROLOGY

PSEUDOXANTHOMA ELASTICUM. Pseudoxanthoma elasticum is a genetic disorder of connective tissue characterized by progressive mineralization of elastic fibers. The disease manifests as angioid streaks on the retina, retinal hemorrhages, gastrointestinal bleeds, hypertension, and occlusive vascular disease secondary to the progressive calcification and fragmentation of the elastic fibers in the eye and blood vessels. Characteristic skin lesions also occur and tend to involve flexural sites. Yellowish papules that appear like a "plucked chicken" are seen on the neck, antecubital, popliteal, inguinal, axillary, and periumbilical areas. These lesions can also be seen in the oral, vaginal, and rectal mucosa.

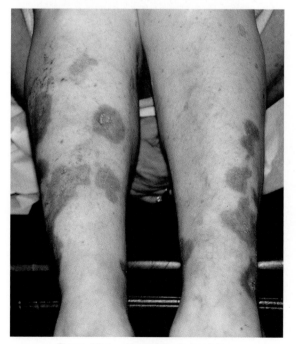

Figure 26-4.   **Necrobiosis lipoidica.**

ULCERATIVE COLITIS. Ulcerative colitis, an inflammatory disease of the intestines, is most commonly associated with pyoderma gangrenosum (Fig. 26-6), a destructive inflammatory skin disease. In pyoderma gangrenosum, a painful nodule or pustule breaks down to form an enlarging ulcer with a raised, undermined border and a boggy, necrotic base. Pyoderma gangrenosum has also been observed in association with Crohn's disease and many other systemic diseases, especially hematologic malignancies, monoclonal gammopathies, and various arthritides.

PEUTZ-JEGHERS SYNDROME. Peutz-Jeghers syndrome is an autosomal dominant disorder in which intestinal polyposis and extraintestinal hamartomatous and malignant neoplasms are seen in association with mucocutaneous pigmentation. Lentigines may be present at birth or develop in early childhood. They are almost always located on the oral mucosa but may appear on other sites including the lips, nose, eyelids, anus, nail bed, hands, and feet. The lesions appear as discrete brown, blue, or blue-brown macules. With increasing age, the cutaneous lesions may disappear, but the buccal mucosal lesions tend to persist into adulthood.

HEMATOLOGY—ONCOLOGY

INTERNAL MALIGNANCY. There are many different skin changes that can occur with internal malignancies. Some of these changes can be markers for many different malignancies, whereas other changes may be more specific markers for certain malignant neoplasms.

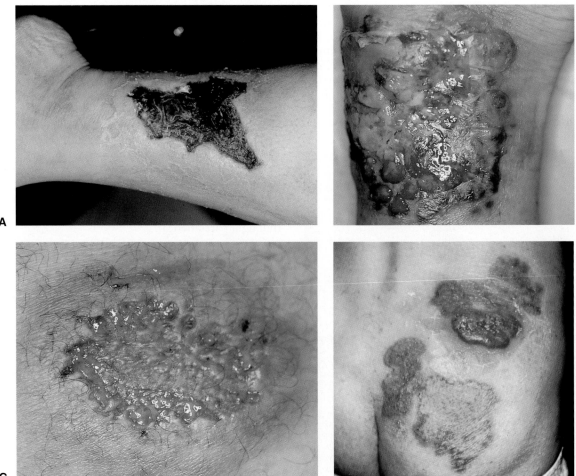

Figure 26-6. *(A–D)* **Pyoderman gangrenosum.** *(D: Schering Corp.)*

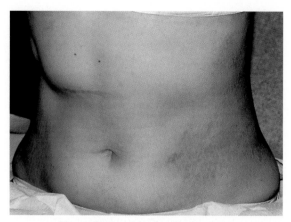

Figure 26-7. **Acquired icthoyosis.**

Acquired ichthyosis (Fig. 26-7), a hyperkeratosis or excessive scaling of the skin, is most often associated with lymphoma and has been reported in association with Hodgkin's lymphoma, mycosis fungoides, multiple myeloma, Kaposi's sarcoma, leiomyosarcoma, and breast, cervix, and lung cancer. It is most often a late manifestation of lymphoma but can precede the diagnosis by many years. Erythroderma is defined as a diffuse erythema or redness of the skin usually with induration and scaling. When associated with an internal malignancy, erythroderma is seen more commonly with hematologic malignancies, especially leukemia, lymphoma, and Sézary syndrome.

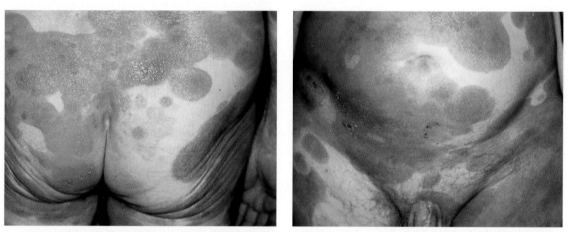

Mycosis fungoides in plaque stage of buttocks (*A*) and abdomen (*B*) of 79-year-old man.

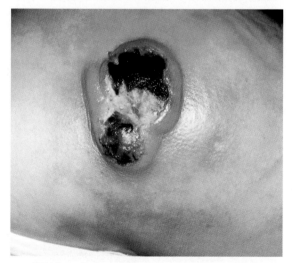

(*C*) Mycosis fungoides in tumor stage on thigh.

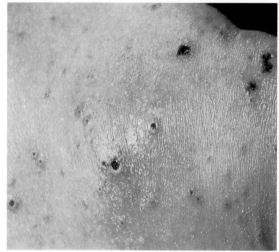

(*D*) Nonspecific pyoderma with lymphocytic leukemia.

Figure 26-8. **Dermatoses associated with lymphomas.** (*Syntex Laboraties, Inc.*)

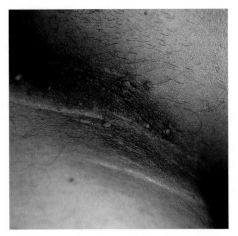

Figure 26-9. **Acanthosis nigricans.** The posterior neck.

ACUTE MONOCYTIC LEUKEMIA. Acute monocytic leukemia mostly affects adults. Cutaneous involvement includes gum hypertrophy and leukemia cutis. Leukemia cutis, a localized or disseminated infiltration of the skin by neoplastic leukocytes, usually presents as asymptomatic, small, raised, pinkish papules, nodules, or plaques on the trunk and extremities. Ulceronecrotic or hemorrhagic lesions may also be seen. Acute monocytic leukemia, myelomonocytic, and the T-cell leukemias have the highest incidence of leukemia cutis.

ACANTHOSIS NIGRICANS. (See Fig. 26-9.) Acanthosis nigricans can be benign or malignant. "Benign" forms may be seen in obese patients or associated with endocrinopathies such as insulin resistant diabetes mellitus. "Malignant" acanthosis nigricans is usually of sudden onset and is rapidly progressive but is otherwise clinically indistinguishable from benign acanthosis nigricans. Malignant acanthosis nigricans is most often associated with an adenocarcinoma, the large majority of which are of intraabdominal or gastric origin. Acanthosis nigricans appears as gray-brown, symmetric, velvety, papillomatous plaques. Increased skin markings, papillomas, and skin tags are also noted. It is commonly seen in the axilla, base of the neck, groin, antecubital fossa, dorsum of the hand, elbow, mucous membranes, vermilion border of the lips, eyelids, and periumbilical skin. Pruritus may be associated with acanthosis nigricans, especially in the malignant form.

INFECTIOUS DISEASE

LYME DISEASE. (See also Chap. 16.) Lyme borreliosis (Fig. 26-10), a vector-borne infection, can affect several organ systems. Cutaneous manifestations include erythema chronicum migrans (ECM), borrelial lymphocytoma (BL), and acrodermatitis chronica atrophicans (ACA). ECM is the principal cutaneous hallmark of Lyme disease. An initially homogenous erythema starts at the site of the tick bite and spreads in centrifugal fashion. The center may fade or clears leaving an annular erythema. BL, also known as lymphadenosis benigna cutis, often starts at or near the site of the tick bite. Some patients have a preceding or concomitant lesion of ECM. The classic lesion of BL is a solitary bluish-red nodule with regional lymphadenopathy. Sites of predilection include the earlobe, nipple and areola, scrotum, and nose. Lesions of ACA usually develop 6 months to 10 years after a tick bite. The connection between the two is rarely suspected by patients. ACA is a chronic dermatitis of the acral sites. The lesions often develop insidiously with a waxing and waning of edematous swelling and a bluish-red discoloration. As it progresses, the skin becomes atrophic, thin, and transparent. Nontender fibrotic bands and nodules later develop. This manifestation of Lyme disease seems more common in Europe.

HERPES ZOSTER. (See also Chap. 17.) Herpes zoster (Fig. 26-11A–C; see Figs. 17-4, 18-2, and 34-7C) is the result of reactivation of an endogenous infection with the varicella-zoster virus. Following an acute infection with varicella, the virus persists in a latent form in the sensory ganglia (dorsal root and trigeminal ganglia) for the lifetime of the individual. Upon reactivation, a vesicular eruption develops that is usually lim-

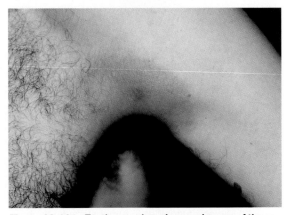

Figure 26-10. **Erythema chronicum migrans of the axilla.**

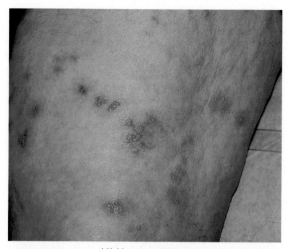

(*A*) Herpes zoster.

Figure 26-11.   Dermatoses due to internal disease.
(*Schering Corp.*)

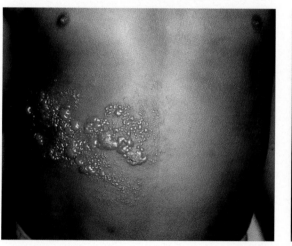 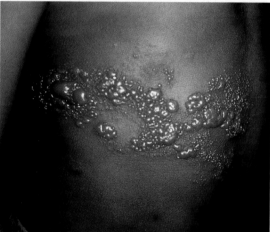

(*B,C*) Herpes zoster.

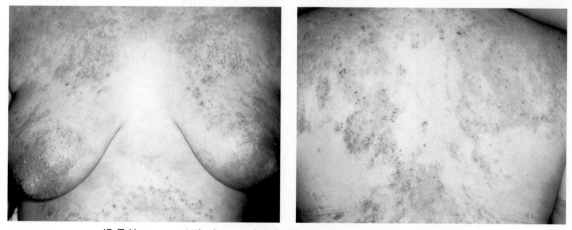

(*D,E*) Herpes gestationis associated with pregnancy (two different patients).

ited to a dermatome. The rash typically does not cross the midline and is limited to that part of the skin innervated by a single sensory ganglia. The disease is usually characterized by unilateral and dermatomal radicular pain and paresthesia that generally precedes the eruption by days and can range from itching, tingling, or burning to severe pain. Depending on the nerves involved, sensory and motor disorders may appear (*i.e.*, Ramsay Hunt syndrome with involvement of the geniculate ganglion).

SYPHILIS. (See also Chap. 16.) Syphilis is a communicable disease caused by the spirochete *Treponema pallidum*. An array of cutaneous manifestations are present in every stage of the disease, but other organ-system involvement varies with the stage as well as the mode of acquisition (*i.e.*, sexual transmission versus vertical transmis-

sion. Primary syphilis (see Figs. 16-1 and 16-2) presents as a syphilitic chancre—a firm, painless, eroded nodule at the site of entry of the treponeme. Eighty to ninety-five percent of cases of secondary syphilis (Fig. 26-12; see Figs. 16-3–16-5) develop generalized cutaneous eruptions termed *syphilids*, which can appear in a variety of ways including macular, maculopapular, papular, annular, and less frequently nodular and pustular eruptions. Mucous membrane lesions may also be seen. Condyloma lata (see Fig. 26-12C) are moist, macerated, cauliflower-like vegetations commonly seen in the genital and anal areas. Mucous patches are macerated, gray papules with denuded areas and can be seen anywhere in the mouth but especially on the tongue and lips. Tertiary syphilis (see Figs. 3-2, 16-6, 16-7), as in the other stages, shows a variety of skin lesions. Gummas are painless, pink to dusty-red nodules

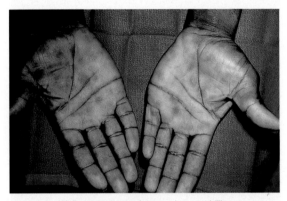

(A) Palm lesions of secondary syphillis.

Figure 26-12. **Syphilis.** Cutaneous markers of syphilis.

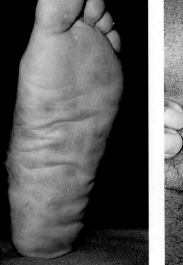

(B) Lesions of secondary syphillis on sole of foot.

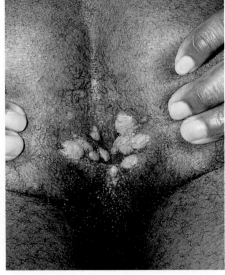

(C) Condyloma lata of secondary syphillis in the rectal area.

that can occur anywhere on the body and in almost any organ system. They tend to ulcerate, and larger ones can cause skin perforation, necrosis, and destruction of underlying structures.

NEPHROLOGY

FABRY'S DISEASE. Fabry's disease is an X-linked recessive inborn error of glycosphingolipid metabolism caused by a defect in the activity of the lysosomal enzyme, α-galactosidase A. The glycosphingolipid deposits primarily in the vascular endothelium, which leads to the major clinical manifestations, namely the cardiac, cerebral, and renal vascular manifestations. Cutaneous findings include acroparesthesias and hypohidrosis, but the characteristic skin lesion has led to the descriptive name for this disease: angiokeratoma corporis diffusum universale. Angiokeratomas can lead to the diagnosis of this disease during childhood as they may be one of the earliest manifestations. They begin as nonblanchable, punctate, red to blue-black angiectasias with slight hyperkeratosis in the larger lesions. With increasing age, these lesions increase in size and number. They tend to be most densely clustered between the umbilicus and the knees and are usually symmetrically distributed.

CHRONIC RENAL FAILURE/DIALYSIS. Several cutaneous changes are particularly prevalent in patients on dialysis. Generalized pruritus without a primary cutaneous eruption could be a sign of various underlying disorders including uremia or chronic renal failure. Dialysis seems to be an important trigger of pruritus. A bullous dermatosis that clinically looks like porphyria cutanea tarda has been described in patients on chronic hemodialysis. Several perforating disorders, which have come to be known as acquired perforating disease of dialysis/chronic renal failure, have also been associated with patients on dialysis. The perforating disorders consist of an alteration in a particular element of the connective tissue (*i.e.*, collagen or elastin), which is then extruded from the papillary dermis by transepithelial elimination. The lesions appear clinically as dome-shaped papules with keratotic centers on the trunk and extensor extremities.

HENOCH-SCHÖNLEIN PURPURA. (See also Chap. 12.) Henoch-Schönlein purpura is an IgA-mediated systemic vasculitis of the small blood vessels that affects the skin, joints, gastrointestinal tract, and kidneys (leukocytoclastic angiitis). Palpable purpura, predominantly of the legs and buttocks, occurs in almost every case and is the presenting sign in about half of the cases. Petechiae and ecchymoses may also be present. Urticarial and erythematous maculopapular lesions preceding the purpura have been described. A characteristic finding in children is painful edema of the face, scalp, ears, periorbital region, and extremities. Scrotal edema and bruising is seen in up to one third of male patients.

NEUROLOGY

NEUROFIBROMATOSIS. (See Chap. 31.) Neurofibromatosis (Fig. 26-13) is inherited in an autosomal dominant fashion. It comprises congenital and hamartomatous lesions of the central nervous system, bone, endocrine glands, eyes, and skin. Café-au-lait macules develop soon after birth and may be found anywhere on the body. These skin lesions can be seen in normal individuals, but individuals having six or more lesions 1.5 cm or greater have nearly always been found to have neurofibromatosis. Axillary freckling (Crowe's sign) is almost always diagnostic of neurofibromatosis. The principal dermatologic manifestation of this disease is cutaneous and subcutaneous tumors (neurofibromas). They vary in size and shape and range from a few to as many as 9,000.

TUBEROUS SCLEROSIS. (See Chap. 31.) Tuberous sclerosis is a congenital (Figs. 26-14 and 26-15) disease with a variety of clinical manifestations in the skin, central nervous system, kidney, heart, and other organ systems. Congenital hypomelanotic macules have been found in up to 90% of patients with tuberous sclerosis. These lesions, typically located on the trunk and limbs, appear before any other skin findings. Their configuration can vary from small macules called "confetti" macules to ash-leaf macules, which are rounded at one end and pointed at the other. The shagreen patch, a connective tissue hamartoma, is a characteristic lesion most often found in the lumbosacral region. It is caused by subepidermal fibrosis and appears as a skin-colored, slightly elevated plaque with an "orange peel" appearance to its surface. The facial lesions, called adenoma sebaceum, are actually angiofibromas and are diagnostic of tuberous sclerosis. These red-to-pink nodules develop after 4 years of age. They tend to localize to the nasolabial folds, cheeks, and chin but can be seen on the forehead and scalp as well. Other sites of fibromatous involvement include the nail bed (Koenen's tumor) (see Fig. 26-15) and

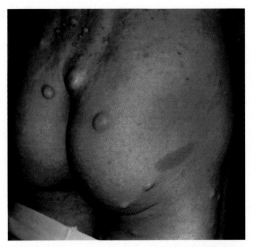

Figure 26-13.   **Neurofibromatosus.**

(*A*) Neurofibromatosis with cafe-au-lait lesion on buttocks.

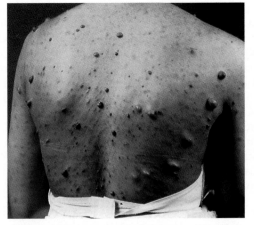

(*B*) Neurofibromatosis on the back. *(K.U.M.C.; Reed and Carnick)*

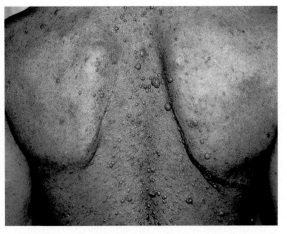

(*C*) Multiple neurofibromas in neurofibromatosus.

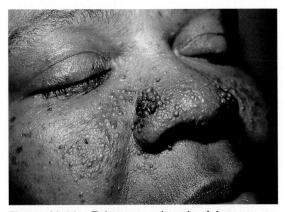

Figure 26-14. **Tuberous sclerosis Adenoma sebaceum (angiofibromas) in tuberous sclerosis.**

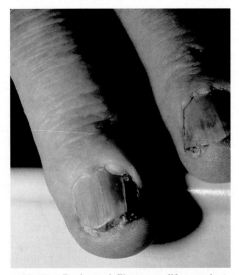

Figure 26-15.   **Periungal fibromas (Koenen's tumor) in tuberous sclerosis.**

the gingiva. Fibroepithelial tags, café-au-lait spots, and port wine hemangiomas are seen relatively commonly but are not, in themselves, diagnostic of tuberous sclerosis.

STURGE-WEBER SYNDROME. In Sturge-Weber syndrome, a port wine stain (nevus flammeus) covers a large part of the face and scalp in a unilateral distribution. The lesion lies in the territory of the ophthalmic division of the trigeminal nerve. In this syndrome, the cutaneous involvement precedes the cerebral involvement, which appears later in childhood as a contralateral spastic hemiparesis, unilateral seizures, hemisensory defects, and homonymous hemianopia.

SARCOIDOSIS. (See also Chap. 20.) Sarcoidosis (Fig. 26-16; see Fig. 20-1) is a granulomatous process affecting various organ systems. Lupus pernio, skin plaques, and maculopapular eruptions are relatively specific lesions for this disease. Lupus pernio is the most characteristic skin lesion in sarcoidosis. It consists of chronic, violaceous, indurated plaques with a predilection for the face, nose, ears and lips. Skin plaques are similar to lupus pernio, but they are located on the limbs, face, back, and buttocks. These plaques may have central atrophy or a hypopigmented appearance. Erythema nodosum is the most common nonspecific cutaneous manifestation of sarcoidosis and is a hallmark of acute disease with associated hilar adenopathy. Erythema nodosum is a hypersensitivity reaction that occurs with exposure to various antigens and appears clinically as tender, erythematous, subcutaneous nodules

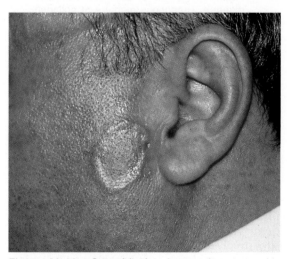

Figure 26-16. Sarcoidosis. A granulomatous skin plaque in sarcoidosis.

predominantly on the anterior shins. Other nonspecific skin changes include alopecia, erythroderma, erythema multiforme, pruritus, acquired ichthyosis, and dystrophic calcification.

ATOPIC DERMATITIS. (See also Chap. 9.) Allergic asthma, penicillin allergy, urticaria, marked reaction to insect bites, rhinitis, and conjunctivitis have all been associated with atopic dermatitis. These disorders may occur concomitantly or independently, and some patients may develop only one or two components of the atopic diathesis. Several genetically inherited disorders have atopic dermatitis as a part of the disorder. Netherton's syndrome is an autosomal recessive disease with hair abnormalities (trichorrhexis invaginata), a skin eruption termed ichthyosis linearis circumflexa, and atopic dermatitis. Other diseases associated with atopic dermatitis include ichthyosis vulgaris and Wiskott-Aldrich syndrome.

RHEUMATOLOGY
(see also Chap. 25)

DERMATOMYOSITIS. Dermatomyositis is an inflammatory myopathy with associated cutaneous manifestations. Progressive weakness is the major clinical finding and usually affects the muscles of the trunk and limb girdles more frequently than the peripheral muscles. There is an increased risk of internal malignancy. The cutaneous manifestations of dermatomyositis are pathognomonic and help one to make the diagnosis with confidence. Gottron's sign is the most specific skin finding. Macular or papular erythema develops on bony prominences such as the knuckles, elbows, and knees. Erythema may develop on sun-exposed areas, and chronic changes may include poikilodermatous lesions on the trunk and proximal extremities. The heliotrope rash, a subtle, erythematous or violaceous blush on the eyelids and periorbital region, is seen in approximately 60% of cases. Periungual telangiectasias and cuticular thromboses may also be noted along the nail fold.

SYSTEMIC LUPUS ERYTHEMATOSUS. Systemic lupus erythematosus (Fig. 26-17A–B; see Figs. 25-1–25-4 and 34-11) is a connective-tissue disease characterized by the presence of antibodies to nuclear antigens. The most frequent cutaneous finding is an erythematous rash of various types. The butterfly rash is an erythema-

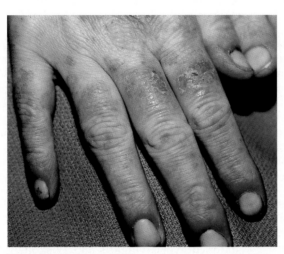

(A) Systemic lupus erythmatosus. Note sporing of knuckles (the opposite of dermatomyositis).

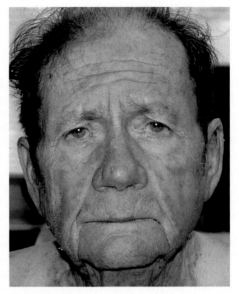

(B) Papulosquamous eruption of subacute cutaneous lupus.

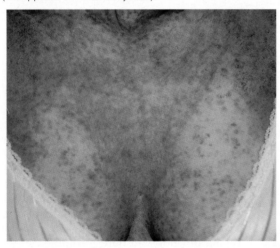

(C) Hypopigmentation with perifollicular pigment retention and skin tightening.

Figure 26-17. (A–C) **Collagen vascular disease.** Cutaneous markers of collagen vascular disease.

tous blush across the cheeks and nose appearing typically after sun exposure. A macular or papular rash, also following sun exposure, may develop anywhere on the body although sites of predilection are the "V" of the chest, extensor extremities, mid-upper back, and shoulders. On rare occasion, the atrophic, hyperpigmented, scarring lesions of chronic cutaneous lupus erythematosus (discoid lupus erythematosus) (see Figs. 25-1 and 25-3) may develop, while the annular or papulosquamous lesions of subacute cutaneous lupus erythematosus (see Figs. 25-2 and 26-17B) have a more frequent association with systemic disease. Panniculitis (lupus profundus), vasculitis, alopecia, livedo reticularis, and periungual telangiectasias are some of the

other skin findings that can be seen in systemic lupus erythematosus.

SCLERODERMA. (See Figs. 25-4–25-6 and 26-17C.) Scleroderma is a chronic systemic disease of unknown origin that affects the connective tissue and the vasculature. The disease is characterized by fibrosis and obliteration of the vessels in the skin, lungs, heart, gastrointestinal tract, and kidneys. The localized form of scleroderma, morphea, is confined to the skin. In systemic scleroderma, the clinical manifestations depend on the sites involved.

The skin shows induration and thickening. This may start as Raynaud's phenomenon (Fig. 26-18B) or nonpitting edema of the hands and fin-

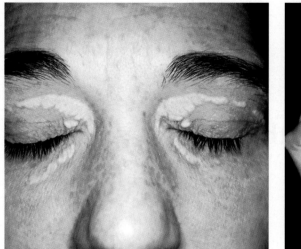

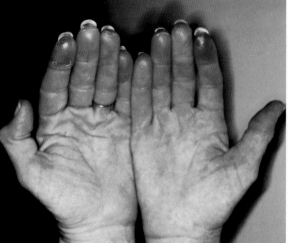

(*A*) Xanthelasma.

(*B*) Raynaud's disease with gangrene.

Figure 26-18. **Dermatosis due to internal disease.** (*Schering Corp.*)

gers. Flexion contractures and sclerodactyly may eventually evolve. The disease slowly extends to involve the upper extremities, face, trunk, and possibly the lower extremities. It begins as painless edema, which leads to tightening of the skin. In the final or atrophic stage, the skin becomes smooth, hard, tense, and bound down to underlying structures. This leads to the mask-like facies that consists of microstomia, radial furrowing around the mouth, and tightening of the skin over the nose, giving it a beak-like appearance. Mat-like telangiectasias of the face and upper trunk, as well as alopecia and anhidrosis, are also seen.

BIBLIOGRAPHY

Berger BW. Current aspects of Lyme disease and other Borrelia burgdorferi infections. Dermatol Clin 1997;15 : 247.

Callin J. Dermatological signs of internal disease, ed 2. Philadelphia, WB Saunders, 1995

Cohen PR. Cutaneous paraneoplastic syndromes. Am Fam Physician 1994;50:1273.

Danzi JT. Extraintestinal manifestations of idiopathic inflammatory bowel disease. Arch Intern Med 1988;148:297.

Feingold KR, Elias PM. Endocrine-skin interactions: Cutaneous manifestations of pituitary disease, thyroid disease, calcium disorders, and diabetes. JAAD 1987;17 : 921.

Goens JL, Janniger CK, De Wolf K. Dermatologic and systemic manifestations of syphilis. Am Fam Physician 1994;50:1013.

Hauck RM, Manders EK. Familial syndromes with skin tumor markers. Ann Plast Surg 1994;33:102.

Heymann WR. Cutaneous manifestations of thyroid disease. JAAD 1992;26:885.

Kirsner RS, Federman DG. Cutaneous clues to systemic disease. Postgrad Med 1997;101:137; 144:147.

Lebwohl M. Atlas of the skin and systemic disease. New York, Churchill Livingstone, 1995.

Loucas E, Russo G, Millikan LE. Genetic and acquired cutaneous disorders associated with internal malignancy. Int J Dermatol 1995:34:749.

Lucky AW. Pigmentary abnormalities in genetic disorders. Dermatol Clin 1988;6:193.

Mana J, Marcoval J, Graells J, et al. Cutaneous involvement in sarcoidosis: Relations to systemic disease. Arch Dermatol 1997;133:882.

Mannis, Mascal, Huntley. Eye and skin disease. Philadelphia, Lippincott–Raven Publishers, 1996.

Ostezan LB, Callen JP. Cutaneous manifestations of selected rheumatologic diseases. Am Fam Physician 1996; 53:1625.

Perez MI, Kohn SR. Cutaneous manifestations of diabetes mellitus. JAAD 1994;30:519.

Ross M, White GM. Hyperpigmentation, bullae, and keratotic papules in a renal dialysis patient: Pseudoporphyria cutanea tarda (PPCT), acquired perforating disorder of renal dialysis (APD). Arch Dermatol 1993;129:231.

Wechsler HL. Cutaneous disease in systemic lupus erythematosus. Clin Dermatol 1985;3:79.

27

Diseases Affecting the Hair

Thelda Kestenbaum, M.D.*

Hair is an extremely important part of an individual's appearance. Loss of hair on the scalp or an excessive amount of unwanted hair on other body parts causes great psychological distress. Our perception of femininity and masculinity is greatly affected by hair quantity, hair distribution, and hair styling.

GRAY HAIR

Graying of the hair is a normal process of aging and develops earlier in Caucasians than in African-Americans by about a decade. By age 50 years, half of whites are 50% gray. There are cases of repigmentation in senile white hair following electron-beam therapy, but these are rare, and loss of pigment is generally permanent. Premature graying may indicate underlying disease such as pernicious anemia. Patchy white hair may develop in areas of the scalp affected by alopecia areata. A frontal white patch of hair may be inherited as an autosomal dominant trait (piebaldism). Persons who are said to have "turned gray overnight" have probably had a diffuse form of alopecia areata in which the dark hairs were lost preferentially to gray hairs.

Elimination of gray hair is considered desirable by millions of persons, and there are a myriad of products on the market to help achieve this goal. Hair dyes color on a temporary or permanent basis. The most common chemical that causes hair-dye contact dermatitis is paraphenylenediamine, which is on a standard tray of patch test substances in a dermatologist's office and should be tested for in suspected cases so as to avoid repeated episodes.

HIRSUTISM AND HYPERTRICHOSIS

Hirsutism is the excessive growth of terminal hair in a male sexual growth pattern. Hypertrichosis is the excessive growth of hair that is not in a male sexual growth pattern. Drugs can induce hirsutism or hypertrichosis (Table 27-1).

Hirsutism

Hirsutism in women is often difficult to judge because there are major ethnic and racial variations. Women from Scandinavia and Asia are much less likely to have hirsutism than women from the Mediterranean regions.

Androgen excess and drug-induced hirsutism must be ruled out. Tests for dehydroepiandrosterone sulfate, testosterone, follicle-stimulating hormone/luteinizing hormone ratio, and prolactin help rule out endocrinologic causes.

*Assistant Professor, Department of Medicine, Division of Dermatology, University of Kansas Medical Center, Kansas City, Kansas

---

TABLE 27-1
DRUGS THAT CAN CAUSE
HIRSUTISM AND HYPERTRICHOSIS

Hirsutism

Androgens

Danazol

Progesterone

Hypertrichosis

Acetazolamide

Corticosteroids

Cyclosporine

Diazoxide

Interferon

Minoxidil

Penicillamine

Phenytoin

Psoralens

Streptomycin

Androstenedione, cortisol, sex hormone-binding proteins, and 17-hydroxyprogesterone levels may also be obtained, depending on clinical suspicion.

Among the diseases one needs to rule out in hirsutism are polycystic ovarian disease, adrenal hyperplasia, Cushing's syndrome, adrenal tumors, ovarian tumors, pituitary tumors, and hypothyroidism. Both hypothyroidism and obesity can reduce sex hormone-binding globulin, thus causing an increase in free testosterone and hirsutism. A first-line test to diagnose polycystic ovarian disease is a serum testosterone level.

Most women with hirsutism have no hormonal abnormalities, or only minor ones, and are placed in the familial or idiopathic group. As hormonal assays become more sophisticated, it is being appreciated that many patients in this group have subtle androgen "abnormalities." One should not let a familial history of hirsutism lull one into thinking a patient has "familial hirsutism." The congenital adrenal hyperplasias (21-hydroxylase defect and 11-hydroxylase defect) are inherited.

TREATMENT

Spironolactone (Aldactone) may be helpful in cases of idiopathic hirsutism by interfering with androgen biosynthesis, blocking the action of androgens at the receptor level, and decreasing 5α-reductase levels in the follicle. Oral flutamide and oral contraceptives have proved to be effec-

tive treatment in some patients. Oral finasteride may be helpful but is not approved for this use and may not be as efficacious as spironolactone.

Hypertrichosis

Hypertrichosis may be congenital or acquired. Congenital generalized types are very rare and have been described as being inherited and occurring sporadically. Some of the "dog-faced" or "monkey-faced" persons in circus sideshows probably had this condition. A host of rare syndromes may have congenital hypertrichosis as a feature. Congenital localized hypertrichosis has been noted on the margin of the pinna in infants of diabetic mothers. Localized congenital hypertrichosis over the base of the spine ("faun tail") may be a marker of underlying spinal abnormalities.

Acquired hypertrichosis may be generalized or localized also. Acquired hypertrichosis lanuginosa ("malignant down") is a rare but striking cutaneous manifestation of internal malignancy. Fairly generalized hypertrichosis may occur in patients with diverse diseases such as porphyrias, dermatomyositis, anorexia nervosa, mercury intoxication, insulin-resistant diabetes, Cushing's disease, hypothyroidism, postencephalitis, multiple sclerosis, head injuries, and POEMS syndrome [polyneuropathy (sensorimotor), organomegaly (heart, spleen, kidneys), endocrinopathy, skin changes (hyperpigmentation, hypertrichosis, hyperhidrosis, thick skin, clubbed nails, leukorychia, angiomas)]. Drugs can induce hypertrichosis (see Table 27-1). Localized acquired hypertrichosis may occur over areas of inflammatory dermatoses such as venous stasis or areas occluded by a plaster cast or may be a feature of a benign nevus. Acquired hypertrichosis of ears and eyebrows as well as long eyelashes may be seen in patients with acquired immunodeficiency syndrome (AIDS). Hairy pinnae may be an ethnic variant seen in men from India, or it may be a feature of XYY syndrome. Hairy elbows may be familial and unassociated with other problems.

TREATMENT

Treatment of excessive hair growth may include shaving, depilatories, bleaching, plucking, waxing (really a sort of plucking), laser, and electrolysis. Electrolysis is the only permanent method of hair removal and usually requires more than one treatment of each hair follicle that one wishes to ablate. It should be done by someone trained in the technique. Inquiry should be made whether the operator uses sterile needles to deliver the electrical current to the hair follicle to prevent any possibility of accidental transmission of blood-borne disease.

Shaving, contrary to popular belief, does not increase the amount of hair that regrows. Chemical depilatories and bleaching agents are available over the counter and frequently prove effective but may be irritating to the skin of some persons. Waxing and plucking have the advantage of removing the unwanted hair for longer periods without retreatment than does shaving. Plucking, waxing, and electrolysis may cause a folliculitis. Electrolysis also can cause scarring when done incorrectly, and is expensive. Laser treatment may offer some help.

SAUER NOTES

1. Shaving the hair does not increase growth.
2. Frequent shampooing does not damage normal scalp hair.
3. Dandruff does not cause hair loss unless the scalp becomes severely secondarily infected.
4. Excessive brushing of the hair can cause hair breakage and hair loss.
5. Hair length is genetically predetermined by the duration of the anagen phase.

ALOPECIA (HAIR LOSS)
(see Figs. 27-1–27-6)

Alopecia of the scalp is of considerable concern to both men and women. It is helpful in differentiating among the many causes of alopecia to examine the hair and scalp and observe whether the hair loss is diffuse or patchy and whether the scalp appears scarred. A careful history and physical examination of the hair and scalp is most important. Nonscarring hair loss is more common than scarring hair loss (Table 27-2).

Nonscarring Alopecia

DIFFUSE NONSCARRING ALOPECIA

Loss of up to one half of the scalp hair may occur without clinically obvious hair loss. Among the more common causes of nonscarring hair loss are

TABLE 27-2
TYPES OF NONSCARRING AND SCARRING HAIR LOSS

Nonscarring Hair Loss

Diffuse
Androgenetic (male pattern hair loss, female pattern hair loss)
Telogen effluvium (secondary to systemic disease, postpartum, weight loss)
Drugs and toxins
Endocrinopathy (hypothyroidism, hyperthyroidism)
Hair loss associated with skin disease (systemic lupus erythematosus, exfoliative dermatitis)
Congenital syndromes (many associated with hair shaft defects–rare)
Loose anagen syndrome

Patchy
Alopecia areata
Trichotillomania
Tinea
Secondary syphilis
Traumatic (traction) alopecia
Loose anagen syndrome

Scarring Hair Loss
Tinea
Severe folliculitis of the scalp
Hair loss associated with other skin disease (discoid lupus erythematosus, scleroderma, lichen planus, also called lichen planopilaris)
Trauma (chemical burns, radiation overdosage)
Scarring vertex alopecia in African-Americans
Idiopathic (pseudopelade of Brocq)
Congenital (aplasia cutis, epidermal nevi)
Tumors (metastatic/benign)

androgenic hair loss, telogen effluvium, alopecia areata, and tinea. An appropriate history and laboratory testing are necessary (Table 27-3).

One must exclude syphilis, thyroid disease, iron deficiency, drug-induced (Table 27-4) and toxin-induced (thallium, boric acid, heavy metal) causes, and systemic lupus erythematosus and dermatomyositis as etiologic factors. When acne and hirsutism or other reasons make one suspect an androgen excess, appropriate hormonal studies should be done. Careful questioning about current or recent illness, past medical history, weight loss, recent childbirth in women, drug in-

TABLE 27-3
LABORATORY STUDIES TO EVALUATE NONSCARRING ALOPECIA

Baseline

Complete blood cell count

Ferritin

VDRL with dilutions

Thyroid screening

Microscopic examination of hair

Fungal culture

Other

Scalp biopsy

Antinuclear antibody

Hormones (*e.g.* dehydroepiandrosterone sulfate, testosterone, androstenedione)

Borate and thallium levels

Heavy metal screens

gestion, hairdressing procedures, and family history of baldness is important.

Androgenetic hair loss (also called pattern baldness, hereditary baldness, androgenic baldness, male pattern hair loss, and female pattern hair loss) is diagnosed by most lay persons, and they do not consult a physician. It is defined as an alopecia induced by androgens in those genetically predisposed, and it occurs in both men and women. It is thought to be an autosomal dominant trait with partial variable penetrance for both men and women. The fact that it is probably the most common cause of nonscarring diffuse hair loss in women is underappreciated by both patients and physicians. Of course a work-up to exclude other causes of diffuse hair loss should be done (see Table 27-3). In women with this problem the thinning is usually on the crown, and its onset is usually in young adulthood. Telogen effluvium may be a feature.

Telogen effluvium is the shedding of an excessive number of hairs that are in the telogen (resting) phase. Normally about 13% of the scalp hairs are in telogen phase, 83% are in anagen (growth) phase, and the remainder are in a catagen phase. It may be that some persons with telogen effluvium have a shortening of the anagen phase and note not only increased shedding but also decreased hair length. It is normal to shed from 50 to 100 hairs daily from the scalp. Various events such as childbirth, high fever, rapid and

marked weight loss, drug use, and virtually any major insult to the body may increase the ratio of telogen to anagen hairs. Within 2 or 3 months after the triggering even, the patient notes an increase in hair shedding. It is usually reversible in 4 to 6 months.

There is a form of chronic telogen effluvium of unclear cause that occurs primarily in middle-aged women that affects the entire scalp, starts abruptly, and fluctuates over a prolonged period. This may be difficult at times to differentiate from androgenetic alopecia. Not only is there diffuse thinning but also a bitemporal recession. Certainly, if bitemporal recession is noted, other signs of virilization should be looked for and an androgen-secreting tumor should be ruled out. A wider frontal partline, retention of the normal frontal hair line, and many miniaturized hairs are characteristic of androgenetic alopecia and not of chronic telogen effluvium. Generally, chronic telogen effluvium is self-limiting, and total baldness is not a feature. This condition may be incorrectly diagnosed as androgenetic alopecia.

Loose anagen syndrome is a disorder usually presenting in young blond girls that is typically sporadic but may be familial, suggesting an autosomal dominant pattern of inheritance. It is

TABLE 27-4
SOME DRUGS THAT CAN CAUSE ALOPECIA

Allopurinol	Immunoglobulin
Amiodarone	Interferon
Amphetamine	Isoniazid
Anabolic steroid	Itraconazole
Anticoagulants	Levodopa
Anticonvulsants	Lithium
Antimalarials	Monoamine oxidase inhibitor
Antithyroid	Nicotinic acid
Benzimidazole	Nitrofurantoin
β-Blockers	Oral contraceptive
Bromocriptine	Progesterone
Captopril	Retinoids
Chemotherapeutic drugs	Salicylates
Cholesterol-lowering agents	Sulfasalazine
Cimetidine	Terfenadine
Colchicine	Testosterone
Corticosteroids	Tricyclics
Gentamicin	Vitamin A
Gold	

characterized by easily (and painlessly) pluck-able dystrophic anagen hairs. The plucked hairs when examined microscopically have mis-shapen, irregular, shrunken roots that may have a mousetail-like appearance. The proximal seg-ment of the hair shaft closest to the root often ap-pears distorted and twisted with ruffling of the cuticle. Normally with a gentle pull using the fin-gers anagen hairs are not dislodged. If a hair pluck is performed with a needleholder or hemo-stat at the base of the hairs and the extraction of hairs is not done with the proper quick, forceful pull, one may see distortion of the normal hair roots that may mimic loose anagen hairs. Clinically this condition presents as a diffuse hair loss, but there may be a patchy component. It has recently been appreciated that the onset may be in adults, so it is important to examine hair roots microscopically in patients with diffuse hair loss to make sure they are not misdiagnosed as hav-ing telogen effluvium. Usually this is an isolated phenomenon, but it has recently been noted that it may be associated with alopecia areata, Noonan's syndrome, and AIDS. The condition may improve with age.

Postpartum alopecia is a telogen effluvium of the delayed anagen-release form. In this form of telogen effluvium, some follicles remain in prolonged anagen rather than normally cycling into telogen during the latter part of pregnancy. When finally released from anagen, which occurs 1 to 5 months postpartum, increased hair shed-ding is noted. Hair shedding continues usually for no longer than 6 months, but sometimes for up to 1 year. Most women have a return of their prepregnancy hair density.

To estimate whether an excessive number of hairs are in a resting phase, one can grasp and lightly pull with the fingers 50 to 100 closely grouped hairs from six to eight separate areas of the scalp and expect to remove a total of two to five telogen hairs in a normal scalp. A more ac-curate method, but painful and not usually nec-essary, is the hair pluck, which involves putting rubber tubing around a needleholder or hemo-stat to pluck about 50 hairs out by the roots quickly. The hair bulbs are examined microscop-ically to determine whether there is a normal tel-ogen–anagen ratio. An increase in number of tel-ogen hair bulbs may be seen in androgenetic alopecia, for example, so an abnormally high tel-ogen–anagen ratio does not entirely rule out other entities. A negative pull test does not rule out resolved telogen effluvium or low-grade tel-ogen effluvium.

TREATMENT

ANDROGENETIC HAIR LOSS

1. Topical minoxidil (Rogaine and Rogaine Extra Strength 60-mL bottle) may be helpful for this problem. It is available in a 2% and a 5% con-centration. It has been studied in men more than in women. Younger men (under 40 years of age) with mild to moderate hair loss of less than 10 years' duration respond the best. It takes 12 months to see maximal response, and it is expensive. One milliliter is applied twice daily to the scalp with one of several different applicator types in the package. Slightly fewer than half of patients using it obtain significant improvement. The use of the drug must be maintained indefinitely to maintain the new hair growth.

2. Oral finasteride (Propecia), a 5α-reductase in-hibitor, taken orally at 1 mg per day has re-cently been approved by the Food and Drug Administration for treatment of androgenetic alopecia in men. This drug was previously used in a 5-mg tablet (Proscar) for treatment of benign prostatic hyperplasia. Finasteride is a specific inhibitor of type II 5α-reductase, which catalyzes conversion of testosterone to dihydrotestosterone. This drug causes a 50% decrease in prostate-specific antigen concen-trations.

Finasteride is not approved for use in women. It is teratogenic, and it is important that pregnant women not take the drug or handle crushed or broken tablets.

Four percent of men aged 18 to 41 years of age taking finasteride in clinical trials reported decreased libido, erectile dysfunction, or a de-creased volume of ejaculate. This drug must be taken indefinitely to maintain hair growth.

TELOGEN EFFLUVIUM

Treatment consists of pointing out the causative factor and reassuring the patient that he or she will not become bald. Usually the hair loss slowly ceases, and the normal hair pattern is reestablished. Tell the patient that regrowth takes at least 6 months.

PATCHY NONSCARRING ALOPECIA

Alopecia areata (Fig. 27-1) is said to account for between 1% and 3% of new patient visits to the offices of dermatologists. Prevalence is 0.1% to 0.2% of the population. It is a nonscarring, usu-ally patchy but sometimes diffuse, hair loss of

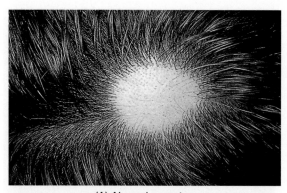

(A) Alopecia areata.

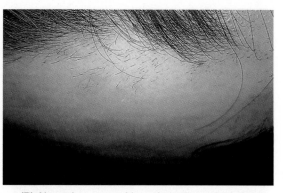

(B) Alopecia areata with exclamation point hairs.

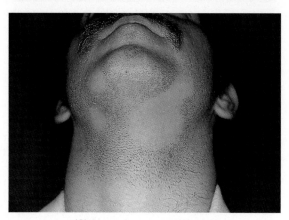

(C) Alopecia areata of beard.

Figure 27-1. Hair loss (alopecia) due to alopecia areata. (*Neutrogena Skin Care Institute*)

unclear cause. Many cases are familial, and it is believed that there may well be an autoimmune etiology. It is seen more commonly in patients with atopic dermatitis, thyroid disease, vitiligo, and Down syndrome.

Usually this disease presents as asymptomatic, totally bald areas. Exclamation-point hairs are often noted at the margin of the bald spots. These are broken-off hairs that are thicker distally and thinner proximally near the scalp like the top part of an exclamation point (!) and are considered pathognomonic of alopecia areata.

Typically the scalp is involved, but any hair-bearing area of the body may be affected, such as the eyelashes, eyebrows, and beard.

In the majority of cases in adults, in which only one or a few bald spots appear, regrowth usually occurs in 6 to 12 months, and reassurance is all that is needed. Factors that bode a bad prognosis are young age at onset, extensive early hair loss, and associated atopy. If all the scalp hair is lost, the term *alopecia totalis* (Fig. 27-2) is used; and if all body hair is lost, then the term *alopecia universalis* (Fig. 27-3) is used. These latter two se-

vere forms of alopecia areata have poor prognoses and are, fortunately, rare.

Trichotillomania (Fig. 27-4) is a disorder of self-inflicted hair pulling that may affect up to 8 million Americans. It is in the obsessive–compulsive spectrum of disease. Most patients are reluc-

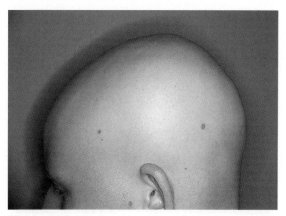

Figure 27-2. Hair loss (alopecia) due to alopecia areata totalis. (*Neutrogena Skin Care Institute*)

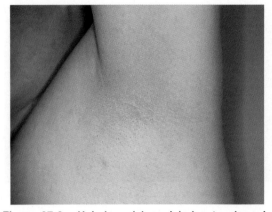

Figure 27-3. Hair loss (alopecia) due to alopecia areata universalis (axilla). (*Neutrogena Skin Care Institute*)

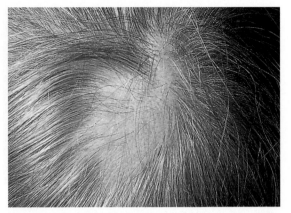

Figure 27-5. Hair loss (alopecia) due to traumatic alopecia from massager. (*Neutrogena Skin Care Institute*)

tant to admit to this behavior. Trichotillomania usually begins in childhood. Certainly in children suffering from this condition some attempt at evaluating the child's home situation is in order. A scalp biopsy with examination of multiple sections may help differentiate trichotillomania from alopecia areata, which it may mimic clinically. A fungal culture should be performed to rule out tinea capitis. A gentle hair pull helps rule out loose anagen syndrome.

Traumatic alopecia (Fig. 27-5) from cosmetic treatments to the hair may result in a patchy, nonscarring hair loss that is frequently especially marked around the periphery of the scalp. Frequent use of hair permanents, hair straighteners, and hair dyes can lead to patchy hair loss marked by broken off hairs. Tight ponytails and tight braiding (especially "corn-row" braiding) may lead to traction alopecia that is usually non-

scarring but in some persons can cause scarring if prolonged. Inquiry about hair care is always necessary in evaluating patients with alopecia.

Tinea capitis (see Fig. 19-10) is more commonly seen in children than in adults and can cause a patchy hair loss characterized by broken off hairs and scaling of the scalp. Currently in the United States the most common fungal organism causing this condition (*Trichophyton tonsurans*) does not cause fluorescence with a Wood's light. Usually tinea causes a nonscarring hair loss. A severely inflammatory tinea can result in scarring. A potassium hydroxide slide and fungal culture establish this diagnosis. A fungal culture is more likely than a KOH to be positive in tinea capitis. Therapy with an oral antifungal agent is indicated.

Secondary syphilis may cause patchy, nonscarring hair loss or, less frequently, diffuse, nonscarring hair loss. A serum VDRL or RPR test with dilutions should help make this diagnosis.

TREATMENT

ALOPECIA AREATA

Topical corticosteroids and topical anthralin may be helpful and are fairly safe treatments for alopecia areata. Intralesional corticosteroids and psoralens with ultraviolet light have been used. Generally the adverse effects of systemic corticosteroids do not warrant their use. Appropriate referrals for hairpieces and informing the patient of the existence of the National Alopecia Areata Foundation (P.O. Box 150760, San Rafael, CA 94915-0760; telephone: 415-456-4644) for education information and local support group information are often helpful in this frequently very

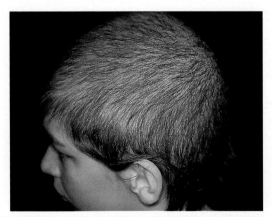

Figure 27-4. Hair loss (alopecia) due to trichotillomania. (*Neutrogena Skin Care Institute*)

stress-producing disorder that lacks an effective treatment.

TRICHOTILLOMANIA

1. Selective serotonin reuptake inhibitors may be effective.
2. Clomipramine (Anafranil) has been reported effective for some patients with trichotillomania.

Scarring (Cicatricial) Alopecia

As skin disorders that can lead to a scarring hair loss one should include discoid lupus erythematosus, scleroderma, lichen planus (lichen planopilaris), fungal infections, and prolonged inflammatory tinea. Metastatic carcinoma and trauma of various types can cause scarring hair loss. A skin biopsy and a fungal culture are indicated to help establish the diagnosis in cases of scarring alopecia (Fig. 27-6).

One particular type of trauma from the use of hot combs may cause scarring hair loss, but 10 African-American women recently diagnosed with "hot comb" alopecia may instead have an idiopathic follicular degeneration syndrome characterized by premature desquamation of the inner root sheath (Sperling and Sau, 1992).

Headington suggests (Headington, Dermatol Clin 1996) that the follicular degeneration syndrome may not be a true clinicopathologic entity and that various hair care practices including chemical straightening as well as hot combs and hair styles involving tight traction perhaps lead to a scarring alopecia. Perhaps the more nebulous term *scarring vertex alopecia* in African

Americans is a more appropriate umbrella under which to place "hot comb" alopecia and "follicular degeneration syndrome" for now.

Another "new" scarring hair loss reported in Australia termed *postmenopausal frontal fibrosing alopecia* may in fact be a frontal variant of lichen planopilaris (Kossard, 1997). This was described as progressive, asymptomatic, marginal scarring hair loss extending to temporal and parietal areas in menopausal women.

Lichen planopilaris usually presents as a patchy, scarring hair loss that is progressive and may be associated with lesions of lichen planus elsewhere on the skin. Early lesions of lichen planopilaris show lichenoid changes, but late lesions of lichen planopilaris may just show scarring and be fairly nondiagnostic. Antimalarials may show modest effectiveness; topical and intralesional steroids may be ineffective.

Folliculitis decalvans is a chronic folliculitis of unclear cause. It is characterized by recurrent, progressive pustules that gradually extend and destroy the hair follicle. Bacterial cultures may reveal *Staphylococcus aureus* but usually reveal nonpathogenic organisms. Fungal cultures should be done to exclude a scarring type of tinea capitis. Favus of the scalp caused by *Trichophyton schoenleinii* may mimic this disease. Therapy with oral antibiotics is occasionally effective.

Pseudopelade of Brocq (alopecia cicatrisata) is a scarring alopecia of unknown cause that presents with skin-colored areas of permanent hair loss without a clinically evident folliculitis. It may be a separate entity or the end stage of another skin disorder such as lichen planopilaris. There is no effective treatment.

MISCELLANEOUS DISORDERS AFFECTING THE HAIR

TRICHORRHEXIS NODOSA. This is probably the most common hair-shaft abnormality and is usually caused by traumatic hairdressing procedures. Clinically, one sees circumferential tiny white specks on the hair shaft. When viewed under the microscope these areas prove to be transverse fractures resembling the bristles of two brooms interlocked in appearance. These fracture points often lead to breaking off of the hairs and the complaint that the hair does not grow as long as it used to. There may be inherited causes of trichorrhexis nodosa, but these are much more rare. An association with hypothyroidism is of interest. Clinically, these fracture points on the

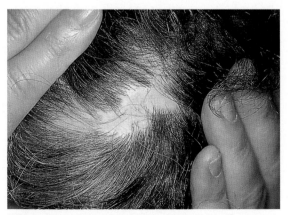

Figure 27-6. Hair loss (alopecia) due to alopecia cicatrisata (scarring). (*Neutrogena Skin Care Institute*)

hair shaft may be confused with nits of head lice or hair casts.

UNCOMBABLE HAIR SYNDROME ("SPUN GLASS HAIR"). This interesting hair-shaft abnormality is characterized by hair shafts that are triangular on cross-section. On electron microscopy, longitudinal grooves are seen. Clinically, onset is usually around 3 years of age, when the hair seems totally wild and unable to be combed or brushed. The hair is usually a silvery blond color. Although usually generalized, it can be localized. Eyebrows and eyelashes are normal. Spontaneous improvement may occur during childhood. Oral biotin may prove helpful. Some cases may be inherited.

The same triangular hair-shaft abnormality has been described in loose anagen syndrome and after spironolactone therapy.

ACQUIRED PROGRESSIVE KINKING OF THE HAIR. This odd and rare entity arises during the teens or early adult years in young men. Gradually and progressively in a Caucasian person the hair becomes kinky, dry, and more unmanageable. It is unassociated with internal disease. Unlike uncombable hair syndrome, the hair shaft in this disorder is not triangular but is elliptical with partial twists at irregular intervals. The duration of anagen (growth phase) is said to be reduced. Oral retinoids or local radiation may induce a clinically similar problem.

Interestingly, a seemingly converse clinical picture has been described in African-American patients with the acquired immunodeficiency syndrome, who develop softer, silkier hair that replaces the previously kinky hair. In addition, the color is said to become ashen and the hair is sparse.

TRICHOPTILOSIS ("SPLIT ENDS"). Longitudinal splitting of the distal hair shaft is usually a result of weathering and is seen with overuse of cosmetic hairstyling. Hair pulling and scratching may be causative. Hair-shaft defects that cause increased hair fragility are more likely to promote "split ends."

BUBBLE HAIR. Excessive heat from hair dryers and perhaps other chemical treatment of the hair may cause distinctive "bubbles" in the hair shaft. Clinically, these hairs may appear brittle and broken off.

PSEUDOFOLLICULITIS BARBAE. This problem is usually seen in the beard area of African American men. Close shaving in people with kinky or curly hair may cause the newly emerging hair shaft to grow back into the skin surface or pierce the follicular wall causing inflammation and a foreign body reaction. Clinically, it presents as papulopustules, which may lead to hyperpigmentation and scarring. Hair plucking and electrolysis can induce this same problem.

The best treatment is to avoid shaving; if that is not possible, avoid close shaving and clip the beard. Rubbing the area to be shaved with a course washcloth or sponge may be helpful prior to shaving. Topical retinoic acid may be of some benefit.

TRICHOSTASIS SPINULOSA. This is a common condition in adults that clinically resembles comedones ("blackheads") and occurs on the face or upper body. Retention of multiple vellus hairs (up to 50) is the cause of this problem. It may be treated with topical tretinoin (Retin-A) or waxing.

GREEN HAIR. The deposition of copper on the hair, from tap water used to wash the hair (or from swimming pool water), may cause a greenish hue in blond hair. Pretreating the hair with some types of conditioners may help prevent the discoloration. Shampooing with a penicillamine-containing mixture may reduce the green color.

BIBLIOGRAPHY

Abramowicz M. Propecia and Rogaine extra strength for alopecia. Med Lett 1998;40:25.

Barrett S. Commercial hair analysis: Science or scam? JAMA 1985;254:1041.

Camacho F, Montagna W. Trichology, diseases of the pilosebaceous follicle. S. Karger Publishers, 1998.

Dawber R. Disease of Hair and Scalp. Oxford, Blackwell Science, 1997.

Dawber R. Hair and scalp disorders: Common presenting signs, differential diagnosis and treatment. Philadelphia, Lippincott–Raven, 1995.

Drake LA, Dinehart SM, Farmer ER, et al. Guidelines of care for androgenetic alopecia. J Am Acad Dermatol 1996;35:465.

Elston DM, et al. Bubble hair. J Cutan Pathol 1992;19:439.

Headington JT. Telogen effluvium: New concepts and review. Arch Dermatol 1993;129:356.

Kossard S, Lee MS, Wilkinson B. Postmenopausal frontal fibrosing alopecia: a frontal variant of lichen planopilaris. J Am Acad Dermatol 1997;36:59.

Leonidas JR. Hair alteration in black patients with the acquired immunodeficiency syndrome. Cutis 1987;39:537.

Leung AKC, Robson WLM. Hirsutism. Int J Dermatol 1993; 32:773.

Olsen EA. Disorders of hair growth: Diagnosis and treatment. New York, McGraw-Hill, 1994.

Sawaya M. Clinical updates in hair. Dermatol Clin 1997; 15:37.

Sharma VK. Pulsed administration of corticosteroids in the treatment of alopecia areata. Int J Dermatol 1996:35.

Sommer S, Render C, Burd R, Sheehan-Dare R. Ruby laser treatment for hirsutism: Clinical response and patient tolerance. Br J Dermatol 1998;138:1009.

Sperling LC, Sau P. The follicular degeneration syndrome in black patients: hot comb alopecia revisited and revised. Arch Dermatol 1992;128:68.

Whiting D. Update on hair disorders. Dermatol Clin 1996;14.

Whiting DA. Male pattern hair loss: Current understanding. Int Dermatol 1998:37.

28

Diseases Affecting the Nails

Thelda Kestenbaum, M.D.*

The most common nail dystrophies are caused by fungal infection, psoriasis, trauma, impaired circulation, and aging. Nail disease may be divided into (1) primary nail diseases, (2) nail dystrophies associated with cutaneous disease, and (3) nail dystrophies that reflect internal disease. There is considerable overlap between some of these categories.

Growth of fingernails is approximately 0.1 mm/day. Nails grow more rapidly on the middle finger than they do on the thumb or fifth finger. Toenails grow at one half or one third of the rate of fingernails. Diseases such as psoriasis or nail biting hasten nail growth. Old age and decreased circulation may slow nail growth.

Nail anatomy is discussed in Chap. 1. The nail matrix is responsible primarily for the nail plate. Calcium only accounts for a small percent of the nail plate by weight, contrary to the opinon of many people.

PRIMARY NAIL DISEASES

Brittle Nails

Brittle nails may affect up to 20% of the population overall and affect about 35% of the elderly population. Repetitive use of harsh detergents,

nail-polish removers, and repeated wetting and drying are among the more common causes. Dry, cold environments lead to increased evaporation of water from the nail plate and cause brittleness. Normal water content of the nail is 18%, and when it is below 16% the nail is brittle. When the water content is above 25% the nail is soft. After soaking the hands in lukewarm water is an optimal time to apply an emollient (skin cream) to help prevent water evaporation. Topical emollients with mineral oil, α-hydroxy acids (*e.g.*, lactic acid), phospholipids, or urea may be especially helpful. Nail enamel may help seal in moisture, but overuse of nail-polish remover (more then once a week) can be dehydrating. A good time to trim the nails is when they are well hydrated and thus less likely to be frayed by trimming.

Brittle nails are not associated with low calcium content but are associated with low cystine content. Frequently, brittle nails also develop onychorrhexis (longitudinal striations) and onychoschizia (horizontal layering).

Biotin may be helpful in treatment of brittle nails. Several vitamin supplements and gelatin have been recommended, but it is difficult to objectively measure their efficacy.

Onychorrhexis

Onychorrhexis is an excessive longitudinal striation of the nail plate and may well be a normal

*Assistant Professor, Department of Medicine, Division of Dermatology, University of Kansas Medical Center, Kansas City, Kansas

sign of aging because it occurs in up to 85% of the elderly. Persons with rheumatoid arthritis or decreased peripheral circulation, as well as skin diseases such as psoriasis, alopecia areata, lichen planus, or Darier's disease, may also develop this nail dystrophy.

Onychoschizia (Lamellar Dystrophy)
(Fig. 28-1)

This is a horizontal layering of the nail plate. It is very common and more common in women than men. Frequently it is associated with brittle nails.

Although constant exposure to damaging environmental factors such as solvents, detergents, and trauma may be important, probably frequent and prolonged wetting and drying with water is the most important and frequent causative factor.

Melanonychia Striata

Longitudinal hyperpigmented bands are most common in African-Americans but also occur in Asians as a normal finding. A solitary longitudinal streak in a Caucasian patient is cause for worry because, although it may just be caused by a nevus involving the nail matrix, it may also be caused by a melanoma.

Factors that make one more suspicious of an underlying subungual melanoma when evaluating a longitudinal hyperpigmented band in the nail are involvement of one nail rather than multiple nails, appearance in the sixth decade of life or later, abrupt onset, enlarging size, irregular border, leaching of pigment from the nail to the nail folds (Hutchinson's sign), and accompanying nail dystrophy such as partial nail destruction. Although traumatic friction can cause linear hyperpigmentation too, it is important to remember that in many cases of subungual melanoma, previous trauma has been reported to occur. The thumbnail, great toenail, and index fingernail are most likely to be involved in subungual melanoma. Melanoma in African-Americans occurs subungually in 25% of cases.

Many drugs, especially the chemotherapeutic agents, can cause longitudinal nail hyperpigmentation. Sometimes systemic diseases such as pernicious anemia, Addison's disease, or AIDS may be responsible.

Nail Biting (Onychophagia)

The common "nervous" habit of nail biting of some children and fewer adults is very difficult to stop. About 50% of children at some time bite their nails, but usually it is a transient problem. Nail biting actually hastens the growth of nails. It is a good way to spread warts.

If nail biting or nail picking (onychotillomania, Fig. 28-2) are persistent or severe, one should consider that this may be a manifestation of obsessive–compulsive disorder or an obsessive–compulsive spectrum disorder.

Infections

Primary nail infections can occur from several causes. Bacterial and candidal infections (Fig. 28-3B) can cause paronychial reactions. Candidal infections are often chronic and cause inflamma-

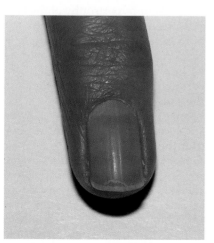

Figure 28-1. Onychoschizia.

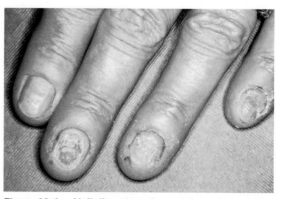

Figure 28-2. Nail disorders. Onychotillomania or picking of nail plate. *(Westwood Pharmaceuticals)*

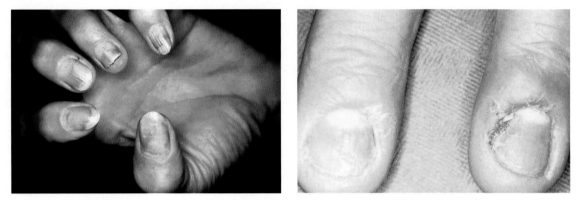

(*A*) Onycholysis contact reaction to nail hardener.   (*B*) Candidal paronychia.

Figure 28-3. **Nail disorders.** (*Westwood Pharmaceuticals*)

tion and swelling of the proximal and lateral nail folds. These infections are very resistant to therapy (see Chap. 19). Bacterial paronychias are more acute, are painful, require antibiotics, and may require surgical drainage of pus. Green nails (Fig. 28-4) are a unique and distinctive infection from which *Candida albicans* and *Pseudomonas aeruginosa* can be cultured.

Hangnails (Agnails)

Some patients are prone to develop small cutaneous tags from the lateral folds. Accidental or intentional pulling on these skin flaps tears into the deeper skin, with resultant bleeding and a painful raw area that is susceptible to bacterial infection. This can be prevented by removal of the hangnail with scissors. Nail biters and people with dry skin are more prone to this problem.

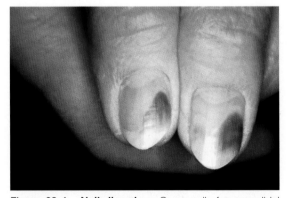

Figure 28-4. **Nail disorders.** Green nails from candidal and pseudomonal infection. (*Westwood Pharmaceuticals*)

Treatment of the infection, which may develop into a bacterial paronychia, is with hot soaks, local application of antiseptic tinctures or ointments, and, in severe cases, use of systemic antibiotics.

Ingrown Nails (Onychocryptosis)

The mechanism of this disorder is the growth of the lateral edge of the nail plate, usually of the big toes, into the adjacent lateral nail fold. Congenital malalignment of the great toenail is a condition in which the nail plate is deviated laterally with respect to the longitudinal axis of the distal phalanx and may play a causative role of ingrown nails in some children. External pressure from shoes that fit too tightly and improper cutting of the nails are among common causes of this condition. Some people have overcurvature of the nail plate or hypertrophy of the lateral nail fold predisposing them to this condition.

Prophylactic management is simple: The toenail, especially the big toenail, should never be trimmed in a semilunar manner but should be trimmed straight across, so that the corner lies above the skin groove.

Treatment of an acute process consists of hot soaks and local application of an antiseptic tincture. After the pain has lessened, the placement of a pledget of cotton gently under the lateral nail plate may be sufficient to raise the pointed corner above the skin surface. More resistant cases are treated by removing the overlying skin by excision, or by removing the lateral section of the nail back to the nail matrix with destruction of the nail matrix with phenol or surgery.

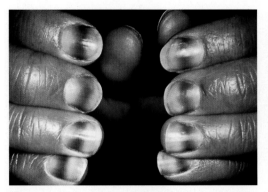

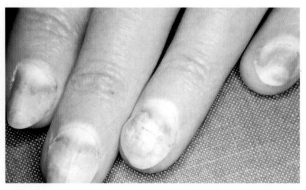

(*A*) Hyperpigmentation of nails in an African-American patient following x-irradiation of hands.

(*B*) Hereditary leukonychia totalis and partial onycholysis.

Figure 28-5. **Nail disorders.**

Leukonychia
(Fig. 28-5B)

The common "white spots" of the nail plate have been responsible for many interesting homespun etiologic labels such as "gift spots." Leukonychia is a whitening of the nail plate, may appear as white spots or white lines (horizontal or vertical), and may even involve the entire nail plate.

Leukonychia should be differentiated from pseudoleukonychia, which is a whiteness in the nail bed (like that seen in Muehrcke's lines). The most common type of leukonychia is small white spots that may be caused by trauma.

Total leukonychia is rare and may be seen following use of certain medications (*e.g.*, Trazodone). It can also be inherited with or without other associated abnormalities (see Fig. 28-5B). It has been noted in AIDS patients.

Mee's lines are really a type of leukonychia characterized by horizontal white lines that grow out with the nail plate. They were originally described with arsenic ingestion, but numerous other systemic problems can cause them.

Longitudinal white streaks may arise from nevoid changes of the nail matrix or Darier's disease (Fig. 28-6).

Allergic Contact Reactions
(see Fig. 28-3A)

It may be that up to 1.5 billion dollars is spent per year in the United States for nail products and nail services. Considering the number of nail cosmetics used, contact dermatitis is not common and allergic reactions to nail cosmetics probably account for only 8% to 13% of all cosmetic contact dermatitis.

The usual culprits for contact dermatitis in nail cosmetics are methacrylates in sculptured nails and cyanoacrylates in nail glues. These reactions usually cause onycholysis (lifting up of the nail plate from the nail bed distally) and paronychia, which can be quite painful and disfiguring. The pain in the nail may persist long after the nail dystrophy has healed. Sometimes an irritant reaction or a secondary yeast infection is responsible for the nail dystrophy rather than a true contact dermatitis.

Allergic sensitivity to chemicals in nail polish usually does not present as a nail dystrophy but instead as a contact dermatitis on the eyelids, face, or neck. The most common sensitizer in nail polish is toluene sulfonamide formaldehyde resin. Some manufacturers are replacing it with (hopefully) less sensitizing chemicals.

Overuse of liquid cuticle removers may cause an irritant rather than an allergic contact

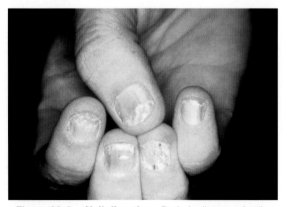

Figure 28-6. **Nail disorders.** Darier's disease of nails.

dermatitis. These products usually contain sodium or potassium hydroxide. Formaldehyde (found in nail hardeners) used to be a common sensitizer but has been removed in high concentration from American nail products.

Median Nail Dystrophy (Medial Canaliform Dystrophy)

Median nail dystrophy is a longitudinal splitting of the nail plate that is central or just off center typically on the thumbnails (Fig. 28-7). This may resolve and recur spontaneously. The cause is unknown.

Habit Tic Deformity

This is a self-induced nail dystrophy caused by the index fingernail or third fingernail picking at the proximal nail fold of the affected thumbnail on the same hand (Fig. 28-8). It consists of multiple, small, horizontal depressions in a longitudinal, linear distribution down the central nail plate. The lunula may be enlarged and the cuticle is usually absent in the affected nail.

NAIL DISEASE SECONDARY TO OTHER DERMATOSES

Any skin disease that involves the nail unit may cause nail disease. Resolution of a dermatosis involving the nail takes much longer than on the skin. Fingernails take about 6 months and toe-

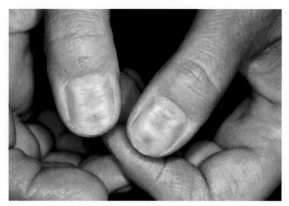

Figure 28-8. **Nail disorders.** Traumatic, habit-tic injury to plate. (*Westwood Pharmaceuticals*)

nails take about 1 year to grow out completely. Aging decreases the rate of nail growth, whereas psoriasis hastens nail growth.

Onychomycosis
(Fig. 28-9 and see Fig. 28-14)

Fungal infections of the nails account for at least half of all nail diseases. Prevalence increases with aging and in AIDS. Dermatophytes account for most fungal infections of the nail but *Candida* species and a host of saprophytes may also cause disease.

Newer oral antifungal agents have made this problem much more effectively and rapidly treatable. Tinea of the nails is covered in detail in Chap. 19.

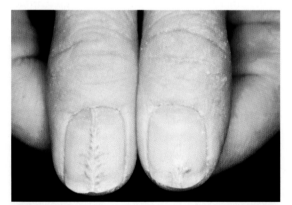

Figure 28-7. **Nail disorders.** Medial canaliform dystrophy.

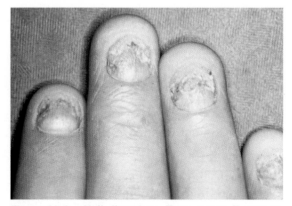

Figure 28-9. **Nail disorders.** Tinea due to *T. rubrum*. (*Westwood Pharmaceuticals*)

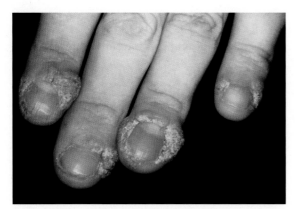

Figure 28-10. **Nail disorders.** Periungual warts in lymphoma patient. (*Westwood Pharmaceuticals*)

Warts
(Fig. 28-10)

Verrucae (warts) can occur anywhere on the body, but one of the most difficult warts to treat is the type that grows around the nail and under the nail plate. If a periungual wart is large and extends rather far under the nail, a deformed nail may result from the wart or its removal. One must be leery of cryotherapy or cautery of a wart on the proximal nail fold because the nail matrix is underneath this area and a permanent nail dystrophy may result. The patients should be told about this possibility in advance. The management of these problem warts is discussed in Chapter 17. Topical treatments are often helpful.

Squamous cell carcinoma may be the diagnosis of a "recalcitrant wart." It has been associated with some human papilloma viruses. Periungual fibromas and osteochondromas may mimic periungual warts. A squamous cell carcinoma of the nail bed, especially in a young person, should make the clinician consider an underlying HIV infection.

Eczematous Eruptions of the Nail Unit

The nail becomes involved when dermatitis affects the nail matrix. A multiplicity of nail changes including pitting, roughness, grooving, ridging, onycholysis, onychomadesis, and koilonychia may occur with any dermatitis (eczema) that involves the nail unit. When the dermatitis heals, the nail heals also, but the mark of the dermatitis on the nail takes much longer to resolve.

An unusual reaction of the nail is the development of highly polished nail surface in some patients with severe itching or itchy skin disorders. This is caused by constant rubbing of the skin with the flat dorsal nail surface instead of scratching with the distal end of the nail.

Psoriasis

The nails are involved in 10 to 50% of people with psoriasis and up to 86% of patients with psoriatic arthritis (Fig. 28-11). Psoriatic nails without other cutaneous involvement may occur in 1 to 5% of patients. Small indentations of the dorsal nail plate occur when psoriasis affects the proximal nail matrix (which produces the dorsal nail plate). This is called pitting of the nails. Nail pitting is probably the most common nail finding in psoriasis but is not pathognomonic. Pitting of the nails may be seen also with alopecia areata or eczema and without other skin disease or internal disease.

A reddish-brown discoloration of the nail bed called the "oil drop" sign, onycholysis, onychorrhexis, subungual hyperkeratosis, thinning

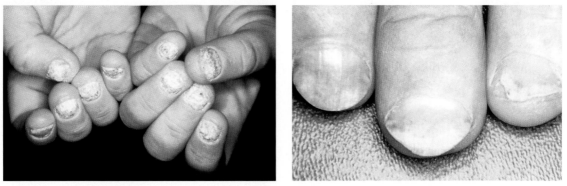

(*A,B*) Psoriasis of nails showing crumbling, pitting, and distal detachment of plates.

Figure 28-11. **Nail disorders.**

of the nail plate, spotted lunulae, Beau's lines, and leukonychia are among the plethora of nail changes associated with psoriasis.

Treatment includes topical steroids, intralesional steroids, Dermanail (with or without 2–10% LCD) and topical 5-fluorouracil. However, psoriasis involving the nails is typically more difficult to treat than psoriasis on the skin.

Lichen Planus
(Fig. 28-12)

About 1 to 10% of patients with lichen planus have nail involvement. Lichen planus is a papulosquamous disease that may cause a pterygium or wing-like deformity of the nail, longitudinal ridging, thinning of the nail plate, onycholysis, or even atrophy of the nails among other nail changes. As with psoriasis of the nails, treatment is not very effective.

Twenty-Nail Dystrophy

Twenty-nail dystrophy is characterized by lackluster appearance with longitudinal striations, roughness, and some pitting, which may be seen in all 20 nails, usually in children. This may improve spontaneously over some years. Although this problem was described as a primary nail disease, many authors believe these are the nail changes of psoriasis, lichen planus, or alopecia areata that are seen without other manifestations of the disorder. Less commonly, IgA deficiency and autoimmune hematologic abnormalities are associated. It may represent a subgroup of endogenous eczema with a predilection for the nail

matrix or an autoimmune response in the nail matrix.

Nonspecific and specific nail changes can occur along with alopecia areata, Darier's disease, epidermolysis bullosa, ichthyosis, and many other dermatoses.

NAIL DISEASE SECONDARY TO INTERNAL DISEASE

Changes in the nails can reflect internal disease (Fig. 28-13). The great majority of these changes are nonspecific. One recent survey (Jemec) of nondermatologic in-patients found that the most common fingernail findings were absent lunulae (23%), leukonychia (12%), and red lunulae (5%). The following significant associations were noted: pulmonary disease and clubbing; hematologic disease and brittle nails; hematologic disease and Terry's nails; gastrointestinal disease and pincer nails; and gastrointestinal disease and subjective complaints. Only 0.4% of patients had onycholysis. The mean age of the population was 73 years. As people age, the lunule may become smaller. Also, there may be apparent leukonychia when the white lunule loses its well-defined distal border and extends forward so it is sometimes difficult to correctly segregate absent lunulae and leukonychia.

Beau's Lines

Beau's lines, or transverse indentations of the nails, may develop with any of a large group of systemic and cutaneous disturbances.

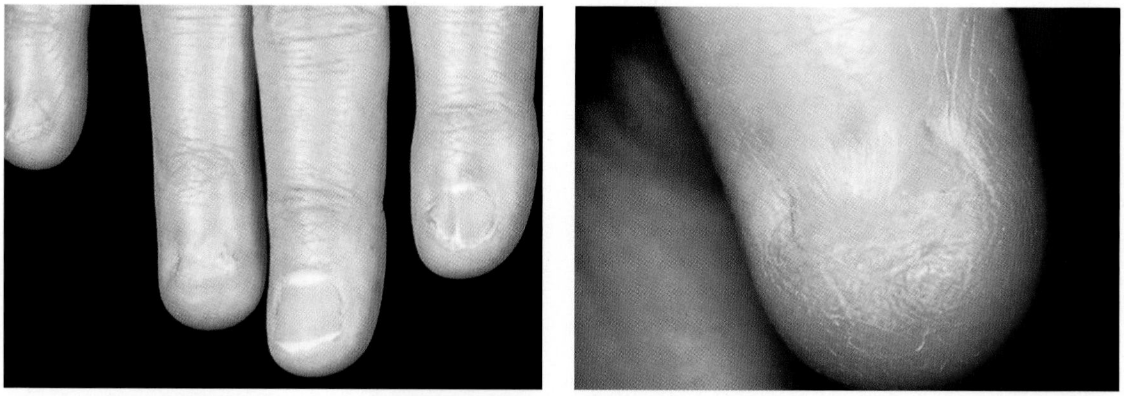

(*A,B*) Lichen planus showing pterygium and plate atrophy on close-up of fingernails

Figure 28-12. **Nail disorders.**

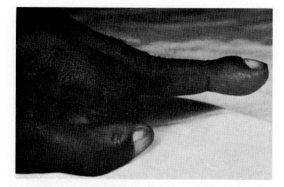

Figure 28-13. Nail disorders. Hippocratic or clubbed nails and fingers in an African-American male with cardiovascular syphilis.

Beau's lines are caused by a temporary growth disturbance in the nail plate. The width of Beau's lines varies directly with the duration of the internal disease. A temporary interference with growth in the nail matrix leads to a Beau's line, but a severe interference can lead to total cessation of nail growth and onychomadesis (nail shedding). Almost any severe systemic illness can lead to the development of Beau's lines. If one knows the rate of nail growth (about 0.1 mm/day for fingernails and half that or less for toenails), the approximate date of the illness can be estimated from examination of the nails. A Beau's line on one nail may be the result of a localized disease such as herpetic whitlow involving one nail matrix. Newborns may have transient Beau's lines.

Clubbed Nails (Hippocratic Nails)
(Fig. 28-13)

Clubbing of the nails may be acquired, idiopathic, or hereditary–congenital. About 80% of acquired bilateral clubbing is associated with respiratory ailments including pulmonary carcinoma and 10 to 15% is associated with cardiovascular and extrathoracic diseases. Multiple, diverse systemic diseases have been associated with clubbing including hepatic disease, thyroid disease, toxin exposure, and POEMS syndrome. Clubbing may be inherited as an autosomal dominant and not associated with other diseases.

These changes apparently are linked to the prolonged anoxemia that is present. Increased blood flow to the nail is seen in all acquired cases but is not seen in hereditary clubbing.

Koilonychia (Spoon Nails)

Koilonychia is a concavity of the nail plate classically associated with iron-deficiency anemia, but it may be seen in about half of the patients with hemochromatosis. Thyroid disease (hyperthyroidism and hypothyroidism), polycythemia, syphilis, and impaired circulation are among the many disease states that may be associated with koilonychia.

Koilonychia may be seen as part of many other skin diseases such as lichen planus or psoriasis. There is an autosomal dominant variety that has no associated internal disease but may be associated with total leukonychia. It may be seen in normal children within the first year or two of life. Injury to the nail may cause the koilonychia seen in the toenails of those who pull rickshas and fingernails of mechanics.

Terry's Nails and Half-and-Half Nails

A nail exhibiting a red, pink, or brown transverse distal band occupying 20% to 60% of the total nail length with the remaining proximal portion exhibiting a dull whitish ground-glass appearance may be a sign of renal disease and has been termed the half-and-half nail. If the distal band is less than 20% of the total nail length the patient has Terry's nails, classically seen with cirrhosis of the liver. However, 25% of some hospital patient populations have been shown to have this problem. These whitish nail discolorations are a type of pseudoleukonychia because they do not involve the nail plate but rather involve the nail bed.

Muehrcke's Lines

Double white horizontal lines in the nail bed can be seen in patients with chronic, severe hypoalbuminemia and therefore do not grow out with the nail plate as do Mees' lines. Any disease causing low albumin levels may give rise to this.

Syphilis
(see Fig. 28-13)

Of the three stages of syphilis, secondary syphilis is most likely to involve the nail. Fragile nails, onycholysis, onychorrhexis, koilonychia, pitting thinning of the nail, onychomadesis, clubbing, paronychia, and hypertrophic nails (onychauxis) may result. A peculiar, lilac-colored 0.5- to 1-mm discoloration behind and parallel to the free border of the nail was described by Milan in 1922 as very indicative. If not pathognomonic of syphilis this may just be a prominent onychodermal band. Ripple, wave-like deformities (probably a variation of Beau's lines) of the nail plate have been described. A chancre of primary syphilis may occur around the nail.

Nail signs of syphilis are as protean as are other skin lesions. Ordering a serum VDRL or RPR with dilutions is an important part of workup for most nail dystrophies.

Acquired Immunodeficiency Syndrome

Flagrant, recalcitrant fungal infections of the nails, a destructive, almost granulomatous-like psoriatic involvement of the nails, melanonychia striata (sometimes with a pseudo-Hutchinson's sign and seen with or without antiretroviral treatment), proximal or total leukonychia, Beau's lines, clubbing, onychoschizia, brittle nails, yellow nails, blue nails, small lunulae, periungual erythema, and squamous cell carcinoma of the nail bed have all been associated with HIV infection.

In particular, onychomycosis that involves the proximal nail plate, most nails (rather than a few nails), and infections with saprophytic fungi should make one suspicious of HIV infection.

OTHER CONDITIONS OF THE NAILS

The following conditions of the nails are defined briefly.

Drug Reactions

Ingested drugs or chemicals can affect the nails in many ways. The changes can include pigmentation (even a pseudo-Hutchinson's sign), Beau's lines, nail shedding, onycholysis, thickening of the plate, and vascular changes. Cancer chemotherapeutic agents can cause all of the above problems. Antimalarial agents and psoralens can cause pigmentary changes in particular.

Anonychia

Usually this is total congenital absence of the nail. Less drastic is partial presence of the nail or

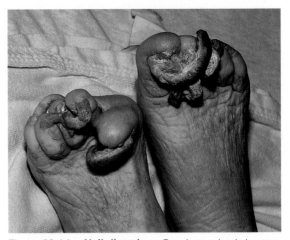

Figure 28-14. Nail disorders. Onychogryphosis in a patient with onychomycosis.

hypoplasia. These conditions may be hereditary or part of several congenital syndromes, including fetal hydantoin syndrome or fetal alcohol syndrome. Less commonly they may be seen as a variant of lichen planus involvement of the nails.

Onychauxis

Onychauxis is the thickening of the nail plate. Trauma, decreased circulation, psoriasis, and fungal infection are among the more common causes of onychauxis. If the hypertrophy of the nail is caused by one side of the nail matrix growing more rapidly than the other, one observes a claw-like appearance of the nail plate that is called onychogryphosis (Fig. 28-14).

Onycholysis
(see Fig. 28-5B)

Onycholysis is the distal or lateral separation of the nail plate from the nail bed. Probably psoriasis, fungal infection, and trauma (physical and chemical) from overly vigorous manicuring are among the more common causes. An allergic or irritant reaction to nail cosmetics may also be a culprit (see Fig. 28-3A).

Photosensitizing drug reactions (Fig. 28-15), hyperthyroidism, anemia, syphilis, and decreased circulation are among some of the systemic causes. Probably systemic causes are less common then local causes.

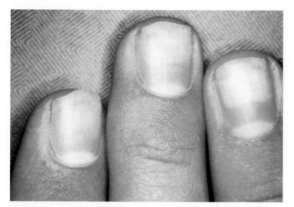

Figure 28-15. Nail disorders. Photosensitivity onycholysis from demeclocycline. (*Westwood Pharmaceuticals*)

Yellow-Nail Syndrome

Yellow nails may be associated with lymphedema, pulmonary disease, malignancy, and rarely AIDS. All the nails appear bright yellow, are thickened, and grow slowly.

Pincer Nails (Omega Nails)

Pincer nails have excessive curvature along the long axis of the nail and usually affect the great toenails. The nail plate in pincer nails arises from under the proximal nail fold normally but then distally it becomes laterally compressed to varying degrees. Tight shoes and osteoarthritis may play a role. Recently, it has been described as a nail sign of gastrointestinal disease.

BIBLIOGRAPHY

Baran R, Barth J, Dawber R. Nail disorders common presenting signs, differential diagnosis and treatment. New York, Churchill Livingstone, 1991.

Baran R, Dawber RPR. Disease of the nails and there management. Cambridge, Blackwell Scientific, 1994.

Belsito DV. Contact dermatitis to ethylcyanoacrylate-containing glue. Contact Dermatitis 1987;17:234.

Camacho F, Montagna W. Trichology, diseases of the pilosebaceous follicle. S. Karger Publishers, 1998.

Castello V, Pardo OA. Diseases of the nails, ed 3. Springfield, IL, Charles C. Thomas, 1960.

Cohen PR. The lunule. J Am Acad Dermatol 1996;34:943.

Cribier B, Mena ML, Rey D, et al. Nail changes in patients infected with human immunodeficiency virus. Arch Dermatol 1998;134:1216.

Daniel CR, et al. The spectrum of nail disease in patient with human immunodeficiency virus infection. J Am Acad Dermatol 1992;27:93.

Fenton D. New edition: Samman's the nails in disease, ed 5. Butterworth-Heineman, 1995.

Grossman M. Scher R. Leukonychia review and classification. Int J Dermatol 1990;29:535.

Hano R, Mathes BM, Krull EA. Longitudinal nail biopsy in evaluation of acquired nail dystrophies. J Am Acad Dermatol 1986;14:803.

Jemec GB, Kollerup G, Jensen LB, Mogensen S. Nail abnormalities in nondermatologic patients: Prevalence and possible role as diagnostic aids. J Am Acad Dermatol 1995;32:977.

Jerasutus S, et al. Twenty-nail dystrophy. Arch Dermatol 1989;126:1068.

Kechijian P. Onycholysis of the fingernails: Evaluation and management. J Am Acad Dermatol 1985;12:552.

Kestenbaum T. Nail diseases. Kans Med J 1982;83:302.

Pappert AS, Scher RK, Cohen JL. Nail disorders in children. Pediatr Clin North Am 1991;38:921.

Ralph DC. Diagnosis of onychomycosis and other nail disorders: A pictorial atlas. New York, Springer-Verlag, 1996.

Samman PD, Fenton DA. The nails in disease, ed. Chicago, Year Book Medical Publishers, 1986.

Scher RK, Daniel CR III. Nails, therapy, diagnosis, surgery, ed. 2. Philadelphia, WB Saunders, 1997.

Waills M, Bowen WR, Guin JD. Pathogenesis of onychoschizia (lamellar dystrophy). J Am Acad Dermatol 1991;24:44.

Walters DS, Scher RK. Nail terminology. Int J Dermatol 1995;34:9.

Zaias N. The nail in health and disease, ed. East Norwalk, CT, Appleton & Lange, 1988.

29

Diseases of the Mucous Membranes

The mucous membranes of the body adjoin the skin at the oral cavity, nose, conjunctiva, penis, vulva, and anus. Histologically, these membranes differ from the skin in that the horny layer and the hair follicles are absent. Disorders of the mucous membranes are usually associated with existing skin diseases or internal diseases.

Only the most common diseases of the mucous membranes are discussed here. At the end of the chapter is a listing of the uncommon conditions of these areas.

GEOGRAPHIC TONGUE
(Fig. 29-1)

Geographic tongue is an extremely common condition of the tongue that usually occurs without symptoms. When these lesions are noticed for the first time by the individual, they may initiate fears of cancer.

CLINICAL APPEARANCE. Irregularly shaped (map-like or geographic) pale red patches are seen on the tongue. Close examination reveals that the filiform papillae are flatter or denuded in these areas. The patches slowly migrate over the tongue surface and heal without scarring.

COURSE. The disorder may come and go but may be constantly present in some persons.

ETIOLOGY. The cause is unknown, but the lesions seem to be more extensive during a systemic illness.

SUBJECTIVE COMPLAINTS. Some patients complain of burning and tenderness, especially on eating sour or salty foods.

Differential Diagnosis

Syphilis, secondary mucous membrane lesions:
    Similar clinically, but acute in onset, usually

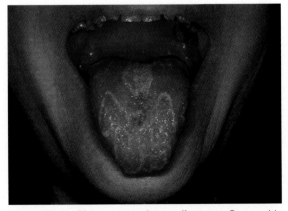

Figure 29-1. Mucous membrane diseases. Geographic tongue. *(Neutrogena Corp.)*

more inflammatory; other cutaneous signs of syphilis; darkfield examination and serology positive (see Chap. 16).

Treatment

1. Reassure patient that these are not cancerous lesions.
2. There is no effective or necessary therapy. However, if patient complains of burning and tenderness, prescribe:
Kenalog in Orabase 15.0
Sig: Apply locally t.i.d. 1/2 hour p.c.

APHTHOUS STOMATITIS
(Fig. 29-2)

Canker sores are extremely common, painful, superficial ulcerations of the mucous membranes of the mouth.

COURSE. One or more lesions develop at the same time and heal without scarring in 5 to 10 days. They can recur at irregular intervals.

ETIOLOGY. The cause is unknown, but certain foods, especially chocolate, nuts, and fruits, can precipitate the lesions or may even be causative. Trauma from biting or dental procedures can initiate lesions (pathergy). Some cases in women recur in relation to menstruation. A viral cause has not been proved. A pleomorphic, transitional L-form of an α-hemolytic *Streptococcus* species (*S. sanguis*) has also been implicated as causative.

Differential Diagnosis

Syphilis, secondary lesions: Clinically similar; less painful; other signs of syphilis; darkfield examination and serology positive (see Chap. 16).

Treatment

Most persons who get these lesions learn that very little can be done for them and that the ulcers heal in a few days.

1. Toothpaste swish therapy. Brush the teeth and swish the toothpaste around in the mouth after each meal and at bedtime. If done soon after the onset of ulcers, extension of the lesions can be prevented and early healing can be helpful in many cases.

SAUER NOTES

1. I wish to emphasize the value of the toothpaste swish therapy for aphthous stomatitis. It is especially valuable if begun soon after lesions appear.
2. The toothpaste swish also aids healing of self-inflicted tongue-bite sores.

2. Kenalog in Orabase (prescription needed) applied locally after meals will relieve some of the pain.
3. Tetracycline therapy. An oral suspension in a dosage of 250 mg per teaspoonful (or the pow-

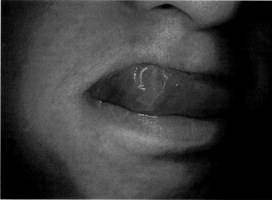

(*A*) Recurrent aphthous ulcer of tongue.

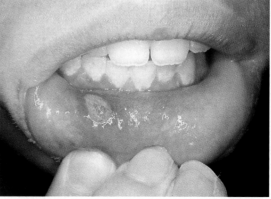

(*B*) Aphthous ulcer in patient with cyclic neutropenia.

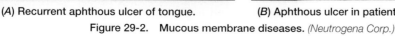

Figure 29-2.   Mucous membrane diseases. *(Neutrogena Corp.)*

dery contents of a 250-mg capsule in a tea-spoon of water) kept in the mouth for 2 min-utes and then swallowed, four times a day, is beneficial. This mixture can be applied with a piece of cotton soaked in this solution.
4. Systemic corticosteroids may occasionally be used for severe ulcers.

HERPES SIMPLEX

Herpes simplex virus infection can occur as a group of umbilicated vesicles on the mucous membranes of the lips, the conjunctiva, the penis, and the labia. Frequently recurring episodes of this disease can be quite disabling (see Chap. 17).

FORDYCE'S DISEASE

This is a physiologic variant of oral sebaceous glands in which more than the normal number exist. When they are suddenly noticed, the person becomes concerned as to the diagnosis.

The lesions are asymptomatic, yellowish-orange, 1- to 2-mm papules on the lips and labia minora.

OTHER MUCOSAL LESIONS AND CONDITIONS

Mucosal lesions can also be due to the following:

PHYSICAL CAUSES. Sucking of lips, pressure sores, burns, actinic or sunlight cheilitis, factitial disorders, tobacco, other chemicals, and allergens are causative.

INFECTIOUS DISEASES (FROM VIRUSES, BACTERIA, SPIROCHETES, FUNGI, AND ANIMAL PARASITES). Gangrenous bacterial infections are called *noma. Ludwig's angina* is an acute cellulitis of the floor of the mouth due to bacteria, abscesses, and sinuses and may be due to dental infection. *Trench mouth*, or *Plaut-Vincent's disease*, is an acute ulcerative infection of the mucous membranes caused by a combination of a spirochete and a fusiform bacillus.

SYSTEMIC DISEASES. (Fig. 29-3.) These include lesions seen with *hematologic diseases* (e.g., leukemia, agranulocytosis from drugs or other causes, thrombocytopenia, pernicious anemia, cyclic or periodic neutropenia), *immunocompromised conditions* (such as the acquired immuno-

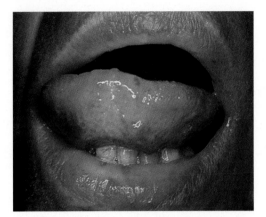

Figure 29-3. Mucous membrane diseases. Rendu-Osler-Weber disease of lips and tongue. (*Neutrogena Corp.*)

deficiency syndrome, organ transplants, lymphomas), *collagen diseases* (lupus erythematosus and scleroderma), *pigmentary diseases* (e.g., Addison's disease, Peutz-Jeghers syndrome), and *autoimmune diseases*, which cross over in several categories but include pemphigus and pemphigoid, and possibly benign mucosal pemphigoid.

DRUGS. *Phenytoin sodium* causes a hyperplastic gingivitis; *bismuth* orally and intramuscularly causes a bluish-black line at the edge of the dental gum (see Fig. 9-13); certain drugs cause hemorrhage and secondary infection of the mucous membranes.

METABOLIC DISEASES. Mucosal lesions are seen in primary systemic amyloidosis, lipoidosis, reticuloendothelioses, diabetes, and other disorders.

TUMORS, LOCAL OR SYSTEMIC. These include leukoplakia, squamous cell carcinoma, epulis, and cysts.

Rarer Conditions of Oral Mucous Membranes

HALITOSIS. Halitosis, or fetor oris, is a disagreeable odor of the breath.

PERIADENITIS MUCOSA NECROTICA RECURRENS. (Fig. 29-4.) Also known as Sutton's disease, this is a painful, recurrent, ulcerating disease of the mucous membranes of the oral cavity. The single or multiple deep ulcers exceed 10 mm and heal with scarring. Systemic corticosteroids may be indicated.

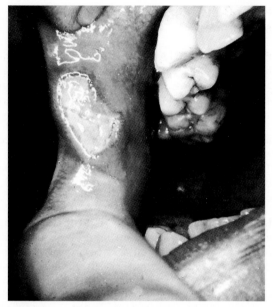

Figure 29-4. **Periadenitis mucosa necrotica recurrens.**

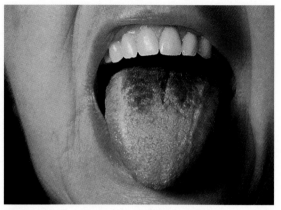

Figure 29-5. **Mucous membrane diseases.** Black tongue. (*Neutrogena Corp.*)

HAND-FOOT-AND-MOUTH DISEASE. A common vesicular eruption of the hands, feet, and mouth. Usually affecting children, it lasts up to 2 weeks. Most cases are caused by coxsackievirus A16.

KOPLIK'S SPOTS. Bright red, pinpoint-sized lesions on the mucous membranes of the cheek are seen in patients before the appearance of the rash of measles.

BURNING TONGUE (GLOSSODYNIA). This rather common complaint, particularly of middle-aged women, is usually accompanied by no visible pathology. The cause is unknown, and therapy is of little value, but the many diseases and local factors that cause painful tongue must be ruled out from a diagnostic viewpoint. The entire mouth can also burn. Tricyclic antidepressants have been used with some success.

BLACK TONGUE (HAIRY TONGUE, LINGUA NIGRA). (Fig. 29-5.) Overgrowth of the papillae of the tongue, apparently caused by an imbalance of bacterial flora, is due to the use of antibiotics and other agents.

HAIRY LEUKOPLAKIA OF THE TONGUE. (See Fig. 18-6.) A slightly raised, poorly demarcated lesion with a corrugated or "hairy" surface appears on the sides of the tongue. It is seen mainly

in immunosuppressed homosexual men infected with human immunodeficiency virus. Human papillomavirus and Epstein-Barr virus have been identified in biopsy specimens (see Chap. 18).

MOELLER'S GLOSSITIS. This painful, persistent, red eruption on the sides and the tip of the tongue persists for weeks or months, subsides, and then recurs. The cause is unknown.

FURROWED TONGUE (GROOVED TONGUE, SCROTAL TONGUE). The tongue is usually larger than normal, containing deep longitudinal and lateral grooves of congenital origin, due to syphilis, or as part of Melkersson-Rosenthal syndrome (see Dictionary–Index).

GLOSSITIS RHOMBOIDEA MEDIANA. (Fig. 29-6.) This rare disorder, characterized by a smooth reddish lesion, usually occurs in the center of the

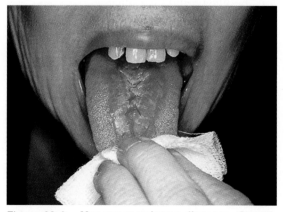

Figure 29-6. **Mucous membrane diseases.** Glossitis rhomboidea mediana. (*Neutrogena Corp.*)

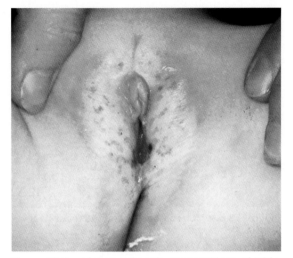

Figure 29-7. **Lichen sclerosis et atrophicus of labia, age 3 years.**

tongue. This term is poor because there is no inflammation and the reddish plaque may not always be in the center.

SJÖGREN'S SYNDROME. This rare entity is characterized by dryness of all of the mucous membranes and of the skin in middle-aged women. The primary form of this syndrome is in many cases associated with a cutaneous vasculitis. The secondary type of Sjögren's syndrome is associated with rheumatic and collagen diseases.

CHEILITIS GLANDULARIS. This chronic disorder of the lips is manifested by swelling and secondary inflammation, due to hypertrophy of the mucous glands and their ducts.

Rarer Conditions of Genital Mucous Membranes

FUSOSPIROCHETAL BALANITIS. This uncommon infection of the penis is characterized by superficial erosions. It must be differentiated from syphilis by a darkfield examination and blood serology.

BALANITIS XEROTICA OBLITERANS. (See *Atrophies of the Skin* in the Dictionary–Index.) This whitish atrophic lesion on the penis is to be differentiated from leukoplakia. The female counterpart is licheen sclerosus et atrophicus.

LICHEN SCLEROSUS ET ATROPHICUS. This is a rare atrophy of the skin (usually around the neck) and of the genital and perirectal mucous membranes. In children (Fig. 29-7) it is the most common chronic genital dermatitis. The prognosis is better in younger patients. In older patients there is a slight increase in the incidence of squamous cell cancer. (See *Atrophies of the Skin* in the Dictionary–Index.)

BIBLIOGRAPHY

Axell T. The oral mucosa as a mirror of general health or disease. Scand J Dent Res 1992;100:9.

Bell GF, Rogers RS III. Observations on the diagnosis of recurrent aphthous stomatitis. Mayo Clin Proc 1982;57:297.

Daley TD. Common acanthotic and keratotic lesions of the oral mucosa: A review. Can Dent Assoc J 1990;56:407

Eversole LR. Immunopathology of oral mucosal ulcerative, desquamative and bullous disease: selected review of the literature. Oral Surg Oral Med Oral Pathol 1994;77:555.

Novick NL. Diseases of the mucous membrane. Clin Dermatol 1987;5.

Van der Waal I. Diseases of the salivary glands and Sjögren's syndrome. 1997.

30

Dermatologic Reactions to Sun and Radiation

Physical agents such as heat, cold, pressure, and radiant energy (x-rays, lasers, ultraviolet rays, gamma rays) can produce both irritative reactions and allergic reactions on the skin. The two common physical irritations of the skin are sunburn, due to ultraviolet radiation, and radiodermatitis, due to ionizing radiation. Allergic reactions can also develop from these two physical agents and from the other agents listed previously.

SUNBURN

A sunburn can be mild and desired or severe and feared. The most severe reactions come from prolonged exposure at swimming areas or when the unfortunate person falls asleep under an ultraviolet lamp. The degree of reaction depends on several factors, including length and intensity of exposure, the patient's complexion, and previous conditioning of the skin.

Sun-reactive "skin typing" of white-skinned persons became necessary when psoralens and ultraviolet light therapy were developed for the treatment of psoriasis. Type I persons always burn, never tan; type II persons usually burn and tan with difficulty; type III persons sometimes have a mild sunburn and tan about average; and type IV persons rarely burn and tan with ease.

Dr. James Kalivas contributed material in this chapter in previous editions of the book.

The typing has been further expanded to type V for brown-skinned persons and type VI for black-skinned persons, both of whom never sunburn and do tan.

Certain drugs can increase the sensitivity of the skin to sunlight (Fig. 30-1). The reaction can vary in intensity from a simple erythema to a measles-like rash or to a severe bullous eruption. A list of these photosensitizing drugs is given in Chap. 9.

PRIMARY LESIONS. Varying degrees of redness develop within 2 to 12 hours after exposure to the ultraviolet radiation and reach maximum intensity within 24 hours. Vesiculation occurs, in severe cases, along with systemic weakness, chill, malaise, and local pain.

SECONDARY LESIONS OR REACTIONS. Scaling or peeling, although not desired by the sun devotee, is the aftermath of any overexposure. Vesiculation can be complicated by secondary infection. An increase in pigmentation is usually the desired end result, but this tanning is not accomplished by overzealous exposure.

LATE REACTIONS TO SUNLIGHT. Actinic or senile keratoses appear mainly after the age of 50 years but are seen in highly susceptible persons in their 30s. Chronic sun and wind exposure on the part of a light-complexioned farmer, sailor, or gardener leads to the development of these su-

293

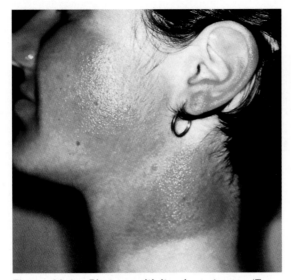

Figure 30-1. Photosensitivity dermatoses. (*Texas Pharmaceutical*) Photosensitivity dermatitis following demeclocycline therapy

perficial, red, scaling keratoses on exposed surfaces of the face, the lip (actinic cheilitis; Fig. 30-2), the ears, the neck, and the dorsa of the hands. They are precursors of squamous cell carcinoma.

Malignant melanomas, basal cell carcinomas, and squamous cell carcinomas can be the late result of excessive sun exposure. An increasing number of these cancers are being discovered. The light-complexioned person and those with dysplastic nevi are more susceptible. The genetic factor is important, as are other factors. Ultraviolet light induces malignancy by causing mutation of cellular DNA and suppressing the immune system's surveillance of malignant cells.

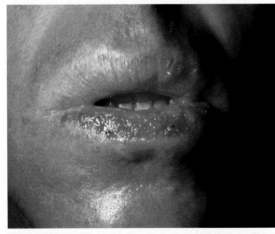

Figure 30-2. Dermatoses due to physical agents. Actinic cheilitis. (*Schering Corp.*)

Wrinkling, freckling, and aging of the skin are promoted by injudicious chronic sun exposure. These reactions may be worsened in future years by ozone depletion by chlorocarbons.

Treatment

PROPHYLACTIC

The ultraviolet rays from the sun or from other sources can be either completely blocked or partially blocked from the skin surface by sunscreens.

Most sunscreens contain *p*-aminobenzoic acid (PABA), either esterified or nonesterified, but some are PABA-free. Products with the higher sun protective factor (SPF) ratings screen out relatively more ultraviolet B, which comprises the wavelengths responsible for acute sun damage. Shade UVA Guard, Solbar, and other broad-spectrum sunscreens may be used when one also wants protection against ultraviolet A (the longer wavelengths are responsible for most exogenous photosensitizations and can accentuate the carcinogenicity of UVB and cause photoaging). Parsol 1789 (Umbrelle and others) is a newer broad-spectrum sunscreen. Zinc oxide microfine is a modification of an older sunscreen (zinc oxide) with very broad spectrum protection.

Sensible and gradual sun exposure of the skin is the best preventive measure for sunburn, but most persons learn this the hard way. Maximum sun protection does not normally lead to vitamin D deficiency.

Regular suntanning salon use has doubled in the past 10 years to 6% of the population in the United States. It is not safe and increases UVA (long-wavelength) radiation to potentially dangerous levels. Vitamin C (2 grams daily) combined with vitamin E (1000 IU daily) slightly reduces the sunburn reaction.

SAUER NOTES

1. The brand of sunscreen one uses is not as important as the fact that the sunscreen has an SPF of 15 or over and screens out UVA also.

2. The duration for which the sunscreen remains on the skin, especially after swimming or sweating, is also important.

3. Sunscreen preparations, especially for susceptible persons, should be applied every day, as if they were a cosmetic or shaving lotion.

4. For acne-prone persons it is best to avoid oily or greasy sunscreens.

5. The use of sunscreens on the skin of children is encouraged.

6. Sunscreening clothing, such as Solumbra or FrogWear, can be helpful.

7. If excessive sweating or water exposure occurs a sunscreen should be reapplied every 1 to 2 hours.

8. Suntanning salons give intense UVA exposure at varying wavelengths and cause skin cancer and photoaging. They should be avoided.

9. The ultraviolet light index was developed by the National Weather Service, the Center for Disease Control, the National Association of Physicians for the Environment, and the American Academy of Dermatology to indicate the sunlight intensity based on weather conditions. Minimal danger is indicated by 0 to 2, and 10+ indicates high risk of unprotected sun exposure.

ACTIVE

A young woman presents with a painful, erythematous, vesicular skin reaction on her face, back, and thighs of 24 hours' duration following a holiday trip to the beach (first- and second-degree burns).

1. Burow's solution wet dressing
   Sig: 1 packet of Domeboro to 1 quart of cool water. Apply cloths wet with the cool solution to the affected areas for as long a time as necessary to keep comfortable.
2. Calamine lotion or Pramosone lotion.
   Sig: Apply locally t.i.d. to affected areas.
3. Blisters can be drained but should not be débrided.
4. Systemic analgesics and even systemic corticosteroids may be used.
5. Ultraviolet injury to the cornea calls for expert ophthalmologic treatment.
6. Burns that are severe, with significant areas of débrided skin, can be treated with Silvadene cream.

SUBSEQUENT CARE.
A day or two later, to soften the scales and to prevent secondary infection, prescribe:

1. Polysporin ointment, Bactroban ointment, or Silvadene cream.
   Sig: Apply locally t.i.d. in thin coat.
2. Warn the patient to exercise caution in resuming sun exposure to the now very sensitive skin.

SAUER NOTES

1. Dermatologists are not "crying wolf" when they implore persons to avoid excessive sun exposure.
2. Basal cell cancer (the most common of cancers), squamous cell cancer, and malignant melanoma (the deadliest of skin cancers) are related to sun exposure in most cases.
3. Millions of dollars are spent for wrinkle creams, bleaches for "liver spots," and moisturizers, yet persons continue to abuse their skin in the sun.
4. Suntanning salons are not safe and should be avoided.
5. Dihydroxyacetone self-tanning lotions are safe for persons who insist on having a tanned look, but they provide little protection.

RADIODERMATITIS
(Fig. 30-3)

X-rays and other forms of radiation therapy are established as unique therapeutic modalities. As with all potent medicinal agents, they must be administered intelligently. When they are not so administered, the result is varying degrees of damage to the skin and the underlying organs. We are concerned here with the skin changes known as radiodermatitis.

Rarely, even diagnostic radiation procedures such as fluoroscopy can cause radiodermatitis.

CLINICAL LESIONS. Acute radiodermatitis is divided into three degrees of severity, similar to the reactions from thermal burns. The first degree is manifested by the slow development of erythema, hyperpigmentation, and usually hair loss. A single dose of x-rays necessary to produce

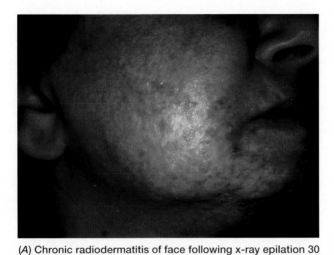

Figure 30-3. **Dermatoses due to radiation.** (*Schering Corp.*)

(*A*) Chronic radiodermatitis of face following x-ray epilation 30 years previous.

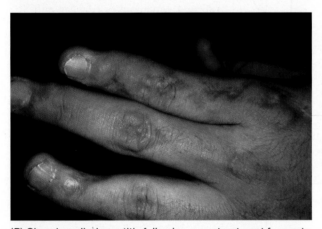

(*B*) Chronic radiodermatitis following x-ray treatment for warts at age of 3 years. Photograph taken at age 21 years.

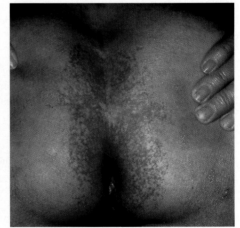

(*C*) Chronic radiodermatitis of anterior neck following x-ray epilation for hypertrichosis.

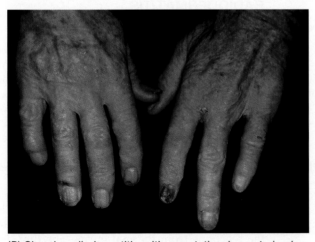

(*D*) Chronic radiodermatitis, with amputation, in a veterinarian.

(*E*) Chronic radiodermatitis following therapy for pruritus ani.

PHOTOSENSITIVITY DERMATOSES **297**

these changes is called an "erythema dose." All of the changes in the first degree are reversible.

The second degree is characterized by vesicle formation, erosions, hair loss secondary to infection, and delayed healing. Atrophy and telangiectasia are the end results.

The third degree of radiodermatitis includes ulceration, infection, and greatly delayed healing. Malignant changes, usually squamous cell carcinomas can occur in the chronic ulcer or scar.

Chronic radiodermatitis can follow acute radiation injury or develop slowly, following repeated small radiation exposures (see Fig. 30-3).

SAUER NOTE

The dosage of ionizing radiation on the skin is cumulative; the effect of previous radiation therapy is never erased by the passage of time.

ETIOLOGY. Many factors influence the development of radiodermatitis. These include the physical factors of kilovoltage, milliamperage, distance, filters, and the half-value layer; the individual factors of health, age, complexion, type of lesions, and size and depth of the area to be treated; and the treatment factors of dosage, number of treatments, and interval between treatments.

Treatment

PROPHYLACTIC

If all these etiologic factors are remembered, acute and chronic radiodermatitis will not develop following radiation therapy for benign skin conditions. However, certain degenerative changes are unavoidable when therapy must be directed toward the removal of a malignant condition. Ionizing therapy should be administered only by competently trained dermatologists or radiologists. It is most important for all concerned to remember that when a so-called complete course of radiation therapy has been given to a particular body area, no further radiation should be administered to this area at any future time.

ACTIVE

Acute cases of radiodermatitis can be treated symptomatically with bland local measures.

Therapy for chronic radiodermatitis should be carried out by a dermatologist, a surgeon, or a plastic surgeon. The damaged skin is markedly sensitive to other forms of irritation, such as wind, sunlight, harsh cosmetics, and local therapy. Changes indicative of squamous cell cancer transformation should be watched for carefully and treated aggressively.

PHOTOSENSITIVITY DERMATOSES

The most valuable clue to the diagnosis of photodermatitis, or "light eruption," is the characteristic sharp demarcation between normal covered and abnormal exposed skin. At times, airborne contact dermatitis (as from ragweed pollen) may mimic the distribution of photodermatitis, but the latter tends to spare key areas such as the submental region and the eyelid folds. Phototesting may be necessary in some cases to distinguish between the two conditions (Table 30-1). Often, the patient does not realize that sunlight (*i.e.*, ultraviolet light) is evoking or aggravating the eruption and may even deny the possibility.

Once a presumptive diagnosis of light eruption is reached, the next step is to determine whether it is secondary to exogenous factors, either external or internal, or whether it is primary (endogenous).

Exogenous Photosensitivity

INTERNAL AGENTS

Most systemic photosensitizers produce dose-proportionate, nonimmunologic phototoxic reactions (see Figs. 9-1 and 30-1). This means that virtually all, except possibly the most darkly pigmented persons, who take the drug will be potentially photosensitized. The most frequent offenders are demeclocycline (Declomycin HCL) (see Fig. 28-15), doxycycline (Vibramycin, Monodox), chlorpromazine (Thorazine), sulfonamides, thiazides, and sulfonylureas. (In the drug eruption section of Chapter 9 there is a more complete list of photosensitizers.)

Clinically, the eruption most often resembles an exaggerated sunburn but may take the form of itching (without a rash) in the exposed areas (*e.g.*, hydrochlorothiazide). It may present as large blisters (*e.g.*, nalidixic acid) or as nail detachment (*i.e.*, onycholysis) (see Chap. 28).

TABLE 30-1
INTERPRETATION OF RESULTS FROM PHOTOTESTING AND PHOTOPATCH TESTING

Disorder	Minimal Erythema Dose (MED)*	Delayed Erythema Dose (DED)*	Response to UVA	UVA + Photopatch
Polymorphous light eruption	Normal, except in eczematous form of disease	Reproduces the clinical lesion after several days	Normal or abnormal, as in some solar urticarias and purpuras	Normal
Other endogenous light-sensitive disorders	Often abnormal	Variable	Variable, depending on particular action spectrum	Normal
Drug-induced photodermatitis (usually are phototoxic)	Variable, depending on light source (may include UVA, in which case MED appears abnormal)	Usually normal	Usually abnormal	Usually normal (unless drug is related to test material)
Contact photodermatitis (usually are photoallergic)	Usually normal	Usually normal	Usually normal	Abnormal and specific
"Persistent light reactor"	Abnormal	Abnormal and proportional to MED	Normal or abnormal, as in actinic reticuloid	Variable

*MED and DED determinations made with UVB light; DED = $n \times$ MED, where n = 3–10.

TREATMENT

1. The patient should avoid prolonged exposure to sunlight, even through window glass because UVA is often the culprit and it passes through window glass. This precaution may have to be taken for many months after a severe photodermatitis.
2. The patient should avoid further exposure to the photosensitizers or to related compounds.

EXTERNAL AGENTS

Most topical photosensitizers produce photoallergic reactions with at least some element of phototoxicity as well.

Photoallergy is difficult to confirm without photopatch testing (see Table 30-1). Soap photoallergy (Fig. 30-4) is less common now than it once was, because halogenated salicylanilides were removed from the market. The fragrance

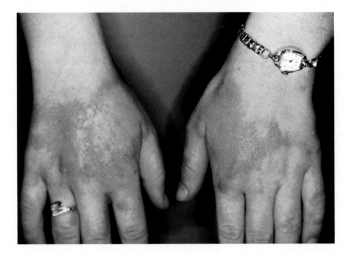

Figure 30-4. Photosensitivity dermatoses.
Photosensitivity with residual hyperpigmentation from soap. (*Texas Pharmaceutical*)

musk ambrette has become an important cause of photoallergic dermatitis.

Clinically, photoallergic contact dermatitis appears eczematous, whereas acute phototoxic contact dermatitis is edematous or bullous. Erythema is common to both. Occasionally, photoallergy lingers for months or even years without further exposure to the allergen ("persistent light reactor").

Topical phototoxic agents include tars and psoralens. Psoralens are found in many plants and a few colognes. Acute phototoxic dermatitis typically is followed by striking hyperpigmentation with bizarre configurations (*e.g.*, berlock dermatitis [see Fig. 24-5] and phytophotodermatitis). Phytophoto-dermatitis is due to oils from plants such as lime, celery, parsnip, corn, parsley, buttercup, and carrot.

Actinic reticuloid resembles the persistent light reactor state but gives different phototest results (see Table 30-1) and resembles cutaneous lymphoma histologically.

TREATMENT

1. The patient should avoid sunlight (even glass-filtered sunlight) and strong fluorescent lighting, if possible. Topical sunscreens as a rule are only partially effective, especially in chronic cases. The patient should select a sunscreen with the highest SPF that does not irritate, preferably one that also screens out ultraviolet A. Many sunscreens contain PABA or PABA ester (padimate). It should be noted that PABA itself occasionally causes photoallergic reactions.
2. Topical corticosteroids may give some symptomatic relief, and, if severe, systemic corticosteroids may be necessary.
3. The patient should avoid further exposure to the photosensitizer.

Endogenous Photosensitivity

After ruling out exogenous photosensitivity by means of the history, phototesting, or both (see Table 30-1), the clinician may then consider the so-called primary light-sensitive disorders. Most often, this means one of the porphyrias, polymorphous light eruption, or one of the collagen vascular disorders. (Photosensitivity caused by deficient melanin pigment, as in vitiligo and albinism, is discussed in Chap. 24, "Pigmentary Dermatoses.")

Porphyrias

PORPHYRIA CUTANEA TARDA
(Fig. 30-5)

The most common porphyria with cutaneous manifestations is symptomatic porphyria or porphyria cutanea tarda (PCT). Patients with this disorder usually are older than 40 years, drink heavily, and are unaware that they are sensitive to sunlight. Diabetes mellitus is found in 25% of cases of PCT; 90% or more have hepatic siderosis. Nearly all untreated patients with PCT show abnormal bromsulfophthalien retention. PCT is relatively uncommon in women who are not taking estrogens. A PCT-like illness has been observed in patients undergoing hemodialysis for chronic renal failure. PCT also has been linked to several toxins (*e.g.*, hexachlorobenzene and dioxin). Hepatitis C infection has been implicated as a possible etiologic agent in some patients and may be related to some of the associated liver disease. HIV-positive patients have an increased incidence of PCT associated with hepatitis C infection.

LESIONS. Cutaneous lesions are prominent in porphyria cutanea tarda and include facial plethora, hyperpigmentation of exposed areas, hypertrichosis (this may be the presenting complaint in women, who sometimes are then treated with estrogen!), blisters, erosions mainly over the dorsal hands (secondary to very fragile skin), milia, and localized areas of scleroderma

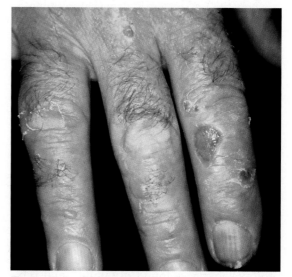

Figure 30-5. Photosensitivity dermatoses. Porphyria cutanea tarda with blisters and hyperpigmentation. (*Texas Pharmaceutical*)

(later may occur in nonexposed areas). Acute abdominal crises or other neurologic attacks do not occur in PCT, even after drugs such as barbiturates and sulfonamides. Such crises may occur, however, in the less common inherited disorder, variegate porphyria. The skin lesions in variegate porphyria are very similar to those in PCT.

DIAGNOSIS

The diagnosis of porphyria cutanea tarda is made by demonstrating greatly elevated urinary uroporphyrin excretion (over 500 μg/24 h). Urinary coproporphyrin levels are variable. A tentative diagnosis may be made by finding the characteristic orange-pink fluorescence of a freshly voided acidified urine sample under Wood's illumination (may be "negative" if the uroporphyrin excretion is less than 1000 μg/L).

TREATMENT

Phlebotomy: The treatment of choice for PCT is multiple phlebotomies over a period of months. The schedule is generally less aggressive than one would use for hemochromatosis. A lasting remission, both clinically and biochemically, is usually achieved by withdrawal of 1 pint of blood every few weeks until 10 to 30 pints have been withdrawn.

Chloroquine: An alternative treatment is low-dose chloroquine or hydroxychloroquine therapy (high doses may cause acute toxic hepatitis). A dose of hydroxychloroquine, 100 mg, is given twice weekly for several months. Caution: Deaths have been associated with this therapy.

Abstinence from alcohol (by the patient) is very important. Foreign chemicals such as estrogens, iron, and possibly phenytoin (Dilantin) may aggravate the disease. Patients with variegate porphyria may experience severe crises similar to acute intermittent porphyria (pain, paralysis) when given barbiturates, griseofulvin, and so on.

Alkalinization of the urine with sodium bicarbonate to increase porphyrin excretion in the kidney may be helpful in treatment.

PROTOPORPHYRIA

The second most common cutaneous porphyria, protoporphyria, is found in families and typically begins in childhood. It frequently is misdiagnosed as contact dermatitis, solar urticaria, or psychoneurosis. Patients complain bitterly of burning and stinging of the exposed areas after a very short time (minutes) in the sun. For several days after exposure, even through window glass, they may display erythema, edema, and purpura of the skin. Sometimes urticaria or vesicles occur. Photosensitivity may persist well into adult life, but between attacks there are usually few objective skin lesions. Cholelithiasis and hepatic failure occasionally occur as late complications.

DIAGNOSIS

The diagnosis of protoporphyria rests on demonstrating elevated free erythrocyte protoporphyrin levels (more than 100 μg/dL packed red blood cells). Fluorescence microscopy may be used to screen blood smears for the disease.

TREATMENT

1. Oral carotene (Solatene) in a dosage of from 60 to 180 mg daily is the treatment of choice. Foods high in beta carotene such as V-8 juice can be efficacious.
2. Topical sunscreens generally are not very effective.

Polymorphous Light Eruption

Polymorphous light eruption (PMLE) is included here, although opinion is divided as to whether it is in fact related to lupus erythematosus. PMLE is characteristically seasonal (spring or summer), implying a threshold or dose–response relation-

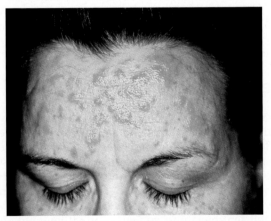

Figure 30-6. Photosensitivity dermatoses. Papular polymorphic light eruption off and on for 15 years. (*Texas Pharmaceutical*)

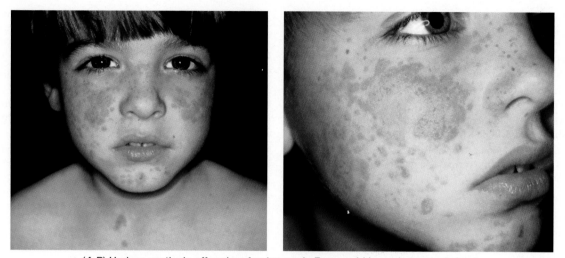

(*A,B*) Hydroa aestivale off and on for 4 years in 7-year-old boy; close-up of cheek.

Figure 30-7.   **Photosensitivity dermatoses.**(*Texas Pharmaceutical*)

ship. It most commonly affects children or young adults (Fig. 30-6).

The skin lesions, as the name implies, are variable, with papules and vesicles being most common. Plaques, wheals (solar urticaria may be related to PMLE), and petechiae sometimes occur (solar purpura also may be a related condition). Subjective symptoms are less severe than those of protoporphyria. When blisters are prominent, hydroa (aestival vacciniform) is the term often applied (Fig. 30-7).

TREATMENT

1. Topical broad-spectrum sunscreens and corticosteroids offer some relief.
2. Oral antimalarials are usually effective but should be given in short courses because of the ocular risks.

OTHER PHOTODERMATOSES

Examples of other photosensitive disorders are solar purpura, solar urticaria, pellagra, Hartnup disease, xeroderma pigmentosum, Bloom's syndrome, actinic reticuloid, actinic granuloma, and rosacea. Poikiloderma (which consists of reticulate hypopigmentation and hyperpigmentation, telangiectasia, and superficial or cigarette-paper wrinkling atrophy) approaching that seen in radiodermatitis may also be induced by ultraviolet light, both on an acquired basis (poikiloderma of Civatte) and, less commonly, on an inherited ba-

sis (poikiloderma congenitale of Rothmund-Thomson syndrome).

Except for rosacea and pellagra, effective treatment for all of these conditions is severely lacking.

Actinic Keratoses
(*see Figs. 32-8 and 32-9*)

Also known as solar keratoses or senile keratoses, actinic keratoses are dry, gritty, yellowish white (occasionally hyperpigmented) excrescences on a telangiectatic base typically located on the face, ears, and hands of patients with fair complexions who have spent years in the sun. Because a significant number evolve slowly into squamous cell carcinoma, they merit careful, thorough removal (see Chap. 32).

BIBLIOGRAPHY

Altmeyer P, Hoffmann K, Stucker M. Skin cancer and UV radiation. 1997.

Bleicher PA. Chronic UVA induces photodamage. Journal Watch for Dermatology 1996;4:2.

Caldiron B. Thinning of the ozone layer: Facts and consequences. J Am Acad Dermatol 1992;27:653.

DeLeo VA. Photoallergic contact dermatitis. Arch Dermatol 1992;128:1513.

Fitzpatrick TB. The validity and practicality of sunreactive skin types I through VI. Arch Dermatol 1988;124:869.

Gilchrest BA. Photodamage. Boston, Blackwell Science, 1995.

Gonzalez E, Gonzalez S. Drug photosensitivity, idiopathic photodermatoses, and sunscreens. J Am Acad Dermatol 1996;35:6.

Harber LC, Bickers DR. Photosensitivity diseases, ed 2. Boca Raton, FL, CRC Press, 1989.

Krutmann J. Photoimmunology, ed 1. Blackwell Science, 1995.

Morison. Phototherapy and photochemotherapy of skin disease, ed 2. Philadelphia, Lippincott–Raven, 1991.

Naylor MF, Farmer KC. The case for sunscreens, a review of their use in preventing actinic damage and neoplasia. Arch Dermatol 1997;133:1146.

Robinson JK, et al. Executive summary of the national "Sun Safety Protecting Our Future" conference: American Academy of Dermatology and Centers for Disease Control and Prevention. J Am Acad Dermatol 1998;38:5.

Stevens BR, et al. Porphyria cutanea tarda. Arch Dermatol 1993;129:337.

Taylor CR, Stern RS, Leyden JJ, et al. Photoaging/photodamage and photoprotection. J Am Acad Dermatol 1990;22:1.

Westerhof W, Nieuweboer-Krobotova L. Treatment of vitiligo with UV-B radiation vs topical psoralen plus UV-A. Arch Dermatol 1997;133:1525.

31

Genodermatoses

Virginia P. Sybert, M.D.*

The inherited skin disorders are individually rare, but in the aggregate comprise a significant proportion of dermatologic practice. Some are of minimal medical significance; others are life-threatening, life-shortening, or debilitating. For some, treatment is available. For others, there is no management beyond diagnosis. For a growing number of conditions, both the causal mutations and the specific perturbations in cellular function are known.

Genetic skin disorders are unique in that the diagnosis automatically invokes the issues of recurrence risk to relatives and prenatal diagnosis (Table 31-1). These are topics not usually in the domain of the dermatologist. Identification of a genodermatosis may require referral for medical genetics evaluation and counseling. The availability and applicability of molecular (DNA) testing changes daily. Medical genetics centers are most likely to be aware of these resources. On-line resources include:

HELIX: http://www.hslib.washington.edu/helix/ A listing of laboratories offering molecular testing for research and/or clinical purposes.

OMIM: http://www3.ncbi.nlm.nih.gov/omim/ A catalog of mendelian disorders in man with references, clinical synopses, and hyperlinks to other databases.

*Professor, Department of Medicine, University of Washington School of Medicine, Seattle, Washington

GENLINE: http://www.hslib.washington.edu/genline/ Similar to OMIM, but aimed at the clinician; includes information about treatment.

Many common skin disorders also have a significant genetic component. The risk for psoriasis, atopic dermatitis, vitiligo, alopecia areata, or systemic lupus erythematosus is much higher among close relatives of affected individuals than for the general population. Even acne and onychomycosis enjoy genetic contribution. These disorders are discussed elsewhere and are not further addressed here. This chapter deals with only a handful of many inherited skin disorders.

DISORDERS OF KERATINIZATION

Ichthyoses

The ichthyoses (Table 31-2, Fig. 31-1) share in common a thickened stratum corneum, which results in scaly skin. The distribution and severity of scaling, the presence of erythroderma, the mode of inheritance, and associated abnormalities differ among them. The degree to which life is impaired ranges from minimal to lethal. The genetic alterations responsible for some of these conditions are known. Treatment remains general and nonspecific. Use of keratolytics (α-hydroxy acids such as lactic acid, glycolic acid, and

303

TABLE 31-1
PATTERNS OF INHERITANCE

Mode of Inheritance	Risk to Relatives	Key Features
Autosomal dominant	50% to offspring born to affected parents	May be sporadic (new mutation) or inherited from affected parent
		Males and females equally affected
Autosomal recessive	25% to offspring born to carrier parents	Parents are heterozygote carriers
		Males and females equally affected
X-linked dominant	50% to inherit gene from affected mother	Usually lethal in males
X-linked recessive	50% to inherit gene from carrier mother	Males express condition
	Daughters of affected fathers = 100% risk to inherit gene	Females show condition to varying degrees, depending on X-inactivation. Ranges from no obvious features to full-blown expression.
	Sons of affected fathers = 0% risk to inherit gene	

urea-based emollients) can be helpful. The oral retinoids are effective and should be considered in the more severe forms of ichthyoses. Their long-term use is limited by significant side effects including dryness of the mucous membranes, alterations in serum lipids, musculoskeletal pain, bony alterations, and teratogenicity.

Palmar-plantar Keratodermas

Palmer-plantar keratodermas (PPK) (Fig. 31-2) are conditions in which thickening of the stratum corneum and scaling, with or without erythroderma, are limited primarily to the palms and soles. They are distinguished, as are the more generalized ichthyoses, by mode of inheritance and associated findings. One autosomal dominant form (Howell-Evans) is associated with esophageal carcinoma. Papillon-Lefèvre is an autosomal recessive PPK associated with gingivitis and premature tooth loss. The biochemical defect is known for one form of PPK: Unna-Thost/Voerner disease of PPK with epidermolytic hyperkeratosis results from mutations in either K9 or K1, type I acidic keratins.

DISORDERS OF ADHESION

Mechanobullous disorders, the epidermolysis bullosa syndromes, (Table 31-3, Fig. 31-3) share in common fragility of the skin and are distinguished, one from the next, by the histological level of blister formation, mode of inheritance, and associated cutaneous features. Most present at birth or soon thereafter. Scarring is primarily limited to the dystrophic forms, where the separation of the skin occurs below the basement membrane of the dermis. Extensive involvement in the newborn period can occur in epidermolysis bullosa simplex–Dowling–Meara, recessive epidermolysis bullosa dystrophica, and in junctional epidermolysis bullosa. Neonatal or infant death due to sepsis or intestinal protein loss and inanition is common in the most severe forms. Respiratory mucosa is often involved in the Herlitz form of junctional epidermolysis bullosa. Accurate diagnosis requires electron microscopy; in some instances, immunofluorescence studies can be utilized. Treatment consists of protection of skin surfaces and avoidance of trauma, lancing of small blisters to prevent lateral spread by the pressure of blister fluid, topical antibiotics, and nonadherent dressings. More severe forms may require a team approach to management of complications.

DISORDERS OF PIGMENTATION

There are many molecules that contribute to skin color. This discussion is limited to alterations in melanin, the major contributor. Perturbations in pigment production are due to alterations or defects anywhere along the pathway from the differentiation and migration of neural crest derivatives, through the enzymatic production of melanin, to the packaging and transport of melanosomes.

(Text continues on page 312)

TABLE 31-2
ICHTHYOSES

Disorder	Inheritance	Basic Defect	Major Dermatologic Findings	Associated Features	Miscellaneous
Ichthyosis vulgaris	AD	Unknown	Mild to moderate white scale Spares flexures and neck; involves face Keratosis pilaris Atopic dermatitis (50%)	None	Improves with age and warm weather
X-linked ichthyosis (sterol sulfatase deficiency)	XLR	Mutation/deletion of sterol sulfatase gene	Moderate to severe white-brown scale Spares face; involves neck	Corneal opacities Possible increased risk of testicular malignancy	Pregnancies with affected males have low to absent estriol levels; failure of spontaneous initiation of labor is common
Bullous congenital ichthyosiform erythroderma (epidermolytic hyperkeratosis)	AD	Mutations in K1 or K10 (suprabasal keratins)	Red skin with blisters and scale evident at birth Marked hyperkeratosis Face usually least affected Inter- and intrafamilial variability	Secondary skin infection bacterial and fungal common	Skin is tender; skin fragility improves with age
Lamellar ichthyosis/nonbullous congenital ichthyosiform erythroderma	AR	Heterogenous, some caused by mutations in transglutaminase 1	LI: mild erythroderma; brown, adherent, plate-like scale NCIE: erythroderma; fine, white scale; many cases with overlap in phenotype	Secondary tinea infection common	Collodion membrane common at birth, ectropion

(continued)

TABLE 31-2 *(Continued)*

Disorder	Inheritance	Basic Defect	Major Dermatologic Findings	Associated Features	Miscellaneous
Harlequin fetus	AR	Unknown; probably heterogenous	Severe, armor plate–like hyperkeratosis; in survivors, phenotype becomes similar to BCIE	Among survivors, mental retardation has been noted in a few	Rare spontaneous survival; handful of survivors treated with oral retinoids
Conradi Hunermann	XLD	Unknown; heterogenous	Feathery scale on erythrodermic base; follicular atrophoderma	Seizures; MR Chondrodysplasia punctata Cataracts	Asymmetry typical in XLD form
	AR	Thought to be peroxisomal disorders			
Sjogren-Larsson syndrome	AR	Fatty alcohol dehydrogenase deficiency	Mild to moderate fine, adherent scale; pruritus	Progressive spastic paraparesis Mild MR Glistening white dots on retina	
Netherton syndrome	AR	Unknown; Heterogenous	Variable erythroderma and scale; classic pattern of ichythyosis linearis circumflexa	Trichorrhexis invaginata (bamboo hair)	Failure to thrive; food allergies
Collodion baby	AR if isolated; otherwise, depends on underlying disorder	Heterogenous	Plastic wrap-like membrane peels within few weeks after birth, revealing underlying skin which may range from minimally xerotic to lamellar ichthyosis	This is a feature of many disorders including lamellar ichthyosis, hypohidrotic ectodermal dysplasia, Gaucher disease and lamellar exfoliation of the newborn	

AD, autosomal dominant; AR, autosomal recessive; XLR, X-linked recessive; K, keratin; MR, mental retardation.

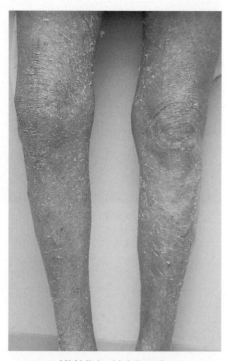

(*A*) X-linked ichthyosis.

Figure 31-1. **Ichthyosis.**

(*B*) Young girl with nonbullous congenital ichthyosiform erythroderma.

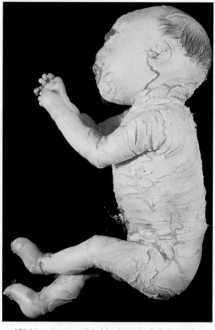

(*C*) Newborn with Harlequin ichthyosis.

(continued)

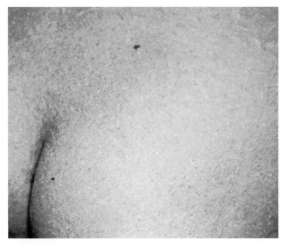

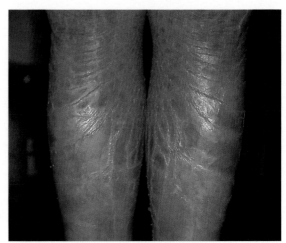

(D) Ichthyosis vulgaris, dominant type, of buttocks.

(E) Lamellar ichthyosis of legs.

Figure 31-1. *(continued)*

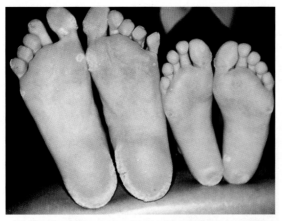

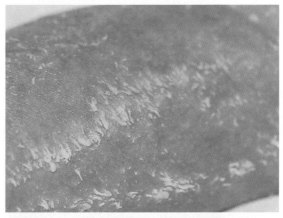

(A) Keratosis plantaris of feet of father and daughter.

(B) Feathery scale of X-LD conradi Hunermann disease.

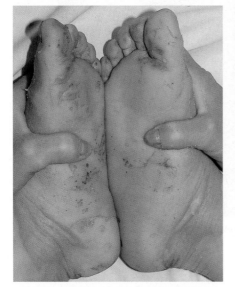

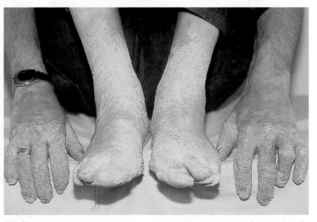

(D) Palmar-plantar hyperkeratosis with severe palm and sole involvement and extension onto wrists and shins. In this family, elbows, knees, and gluteal cleft are involved in some affected individuals.

(C) Palmar-plantar hyperkeratosis. The hands and soles are thickened, with erythroderma evident at margins. Young girl shares same condition as her father.

Figure 31-2. **Genodermatoses.** *(Westwood Pharmaceuticals)*

TABLE 31-3
EPIDERMOLYSIS BULLOSA

Disorder	Mode of Inheritance	Basic Defect Mutations	Major Dermatologic Findings	Associated Features	Electron Microscopy
EBS-WC (Weber-Cockayne; localized)	AD	Basal keratins (KRT 5) (KRT 14)	Blisters primarily limited to hands and feet. Onset can be at birth but usually thereafter. Occasionally delayed until adolescence. Palmar/plantar hyperkeratosis may occur.	None	Level of split within basal keratinocyte
EBS-K (Koebner; generalized)	AD	Basal keratins (KRT 5) (KRT 14)	Blisters soon after birth, generalized. May have oral involvement/nail involvement.	None	Level of split within basal keratinocyte
EBS-DM (Dowling-Meara; herpetiform)	AD	Basal keratins (KRT 5) (KRT 14)	Marked blistering at birth. With time clustering of small blisters in rosettes may occur. Oral involvement common. Nails often dystrophic. Progressive palmar/plantar hyperkeratosis common. Dyspigmentation common.	Can result in neonatal/infant death. Blistering tends to diminish with age.	Clumping of tonofilaments within basal cells with cytolysis
EBS with muscular dystrophy	AR/AD	Plectin (PLEC1)	Relatively severe simplex disease, may be mistaken for junctional EB.	Muscular dystrophy of various types has been described.	Split at hemidesmosomal attachment plate

(continued)

TABLE 31-3 (Continued)

Disorder	Mode of Inheritance	Basic Defect Mutations	Major Dermatologic Findings	Associated Features	Electron Microscopy
EBS with mottled hyperpigmentation	AD	Basal keratin (KRT 5)	Blisters similar to EBS-K. Development of hyper/hypopigmented spots.	None	Level of split within basal keratinocyte
JEB-Herlitz (gravis) (letalis)	AR	Various components of laminin (LAMA3) (LAMc2) (LAMB3)	Widespread severe. GI, respiratory, and GU mucosa often involved. Usually lethal.		Level of split within lamina lucida, decrease/absence of hemidesmosomes
JEB-mitis (GABEB)	AR	Type 17 collagen; Laminin (BPAG2/COL17A1) (LAMB3)	More mild, gradual atrophic appearance of healed skin	None	Similar to JEB-H; may have relatively more hemidesmosomes
JEB with PA	AR	Integrins (ITGB4) (ITGB6)	Similar to JEB-L, usually lethal.	Pyloric atresia, intestinal malabsorption	Same as JEB-H
EBD-C-T (Cockayne-Touraine)	AD	Type 7 collagen (COL7A1)	Blistering and scarring limited and localized to areas of greatest trauma. Mild oral involvement. Milia.	None	Split below basement membrane; decrease in anchoring fibrils
EBD-H-S (Hallopeau-Siemens)	AR	Type 7 collagen (COL7A1)	Widespread, severe blistering, progressive scarring. Pseudamputation of digits. Development of cutaneous malignancy common in adult life. Oral mucosa involved. Milia.	FTT, anemia, GI involvement is progressive	Same as EBD C-T; absence of anchoring fibrils

AD, autosomal dominant; AR, autosomal recessive; EBS, epidermolysis bullosa simplex; JEB, junctional epidermolysis bullosa; GI, gastrointestinal; GU, genitourinary

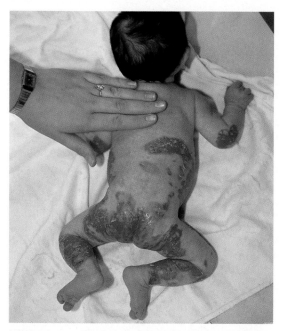

(A) Newborn with junctional epidermolysis bullosa–Herlitz.

Figure 31-3. **Epidermolysis bullosa.**

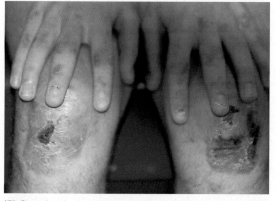

(B) Scarring in a patient with dystrophic epidermolysis bullosa.

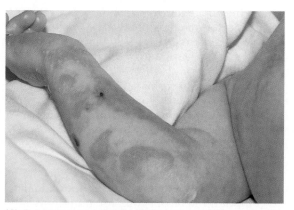

(C) Extensive superficial blistering in a patient with epidermolysis bullosa simplex–Dowling–Meara.

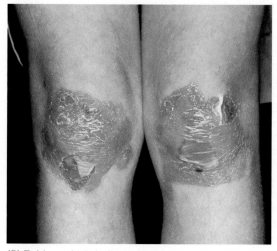

(D) Epidermolysis bullosa dystrophica, dominant type, of knees in 5-year-old girl.

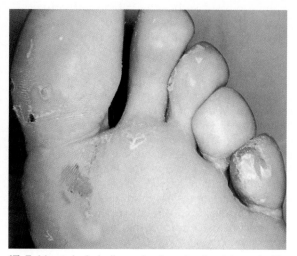

(E) Epidermolysis bullosa simplex, dominant type, in 23-year-old man.

Hypopigmentation

Waardenburg syndromes I and II and piebaldism (Fig. 31-4A) share in common white patches of skin, a white forelock, premature graying of the hair, and autosomal dominant inheritance. All are due to a failure of migration and invasion of melanocytes into the epidermis. Individuals with Waardenburg syndrome I also have dystrophia canthorum and heterochromia irides. Those with Waardenburg syndrome I or II may be deaf. Hirschsprung's disease occurs in approximately 10%. Waardenburg syndrome I and some instances of Waardenburg syndrome II are due to mutations in PAX3. Mutations in MITF have been found in some cases of Waardenburg syndrome II, confirming genetic heterogeneity within this group. Piebaldism, which is caused by mutations in the C-kit protooncogene, is usually characterized only by skin changes, although deafness has been reported in some patients. In all three of the disorders there are no melanocytes in the depigmented areas.

The oculocutaneous albinisms are a group of autosomal recessive disorders that are distinguished from each other by the degree of pigment production and whether they are "tyrosinase positive" or "tyrosinase negative." Affected individuals have pink skin, transillumination of the irises, white to light yellow hair, and often visual disturbances such as foveal hypoplasia and nystagmus. Many mutations in the tyrosinase gene have been identified in both tyrosinase-positive and tyrosinase-negative forms of oculocutaneous albinism, and many affected individuals are compound heterozygous for mutations at this locus. In addition, mutations in the P gene, located on chromosome 15, have been identified in some tyrosinase positive albino individuals. There is also an X-linked recessive form of oculocutaneous albinism, which is very rare.

Tuberous sclerosis (see Chap. 26) is an autosomal dominant disorder that results from mutations in genes at one of at least two loci: one on chromosome 9, the other at chromosome 16. It is characterized by a number of cutaneous changes including angiofibromas, connective tissue nevi (shagreen patches), periungual fibromas, and hypopigmented macules (ashleaf spots) (Fig. 31-5). Melanocytes and keratinocytes in these light-colored areas contain "effete" or poorly melanized small melanosomes. Mental retardation, seizures, and renal involvement are the other major features of this condition that has *very variable* expression.

Hypomelanosis of Ito is the term given to the presence of hypopigmentation or hyperpigmentation distributed along the lines of Blaschko (see Fig. 31-4B). The biologic basis for this phenomenon is not understood. Individuals with these skin changes often have structural malformations and mental retardation. Almost two thirds of patients are mosaic for detectable chromosomal aneuploidy. Mosaicism for X chromosome alterations, tetrasomy 12p, triploidy, trisomy 18, and chimerism are the more common abnormalities reported. It appears that it is the presence of two chromosomally distinct lines, rather than specific cytogenetic alterations, that confers this striking pigment anomaly.

Individuals with hypopigmentation due to any cause need to be protected from excessive sun exposure.

Hyperpigmentation

Neurofibromatosis (see Fig. 31-4C, Chap. 26), is a reactively common (1/3000) autosomal dominant disorder caused by mutations in the NF1 gene, which resides on chromosome 17.

It is a disorder of neural crest cells, including the melanocyte. Affected individuals manifest pigment abnormalities including café-au-lait spots (brown macules and patches), usually numbering more than five and larger than 5 mm in children and 1.5 cm in adults; axillary, inguinal, and inframammary freckling (Crowe's sign); and general increase in skin color (hypermelanosis). Pigment in these areas is packaged in giant melanosomes, a feature also common in café-au-lait spots not associated with neurofibromatosis. Over time, affected persons develop benign tumors, neurofibromas, which arise from Schwann cells and can occur along any myelinated nerve. These may be few or number in the thousands. Severe complications include: plexiform neurofibromas—which are large disfiguring growths—pseudoarthrosis, mental deficiency (5 to 10%), sarcomatous degeneration of benign growths, optic glioma, and leukemia (less than 1%). This is a progressive condition that is extremely variable in its expression.

The clinical features of McCune–Albright syndrome are giant café-au-lait spots, polyostotic fibrous dysplasia, and endocrine abnormalities (primarily precocious puberty). It results from a postzygotic mutation. Affected individuals who reproduce have no risk for affected offspring, as embryos with the abnormal gene present in all cells cannot develop.

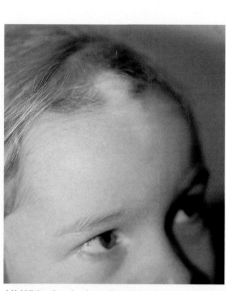

(A) White forelock and patch of unpigmented skin in young girl with piebaldism.

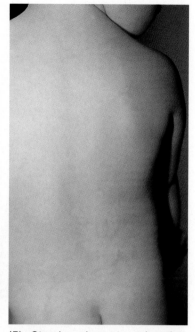

(B) Streaky pigment variegation, along the lines of Blaschko in patient with mosaicism for 46,XX/47,XX + rea (12).

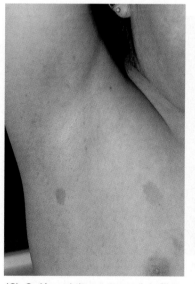

(C) Café-au-lait spots and axillary freckling in neurofibromatosis.

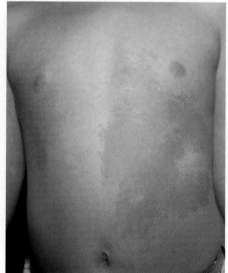

(D) Giant café-au-lait in a patient with McCune–Albright syndrome.

Figure 31-4. **Genodermatoses with pigmentary changes.**

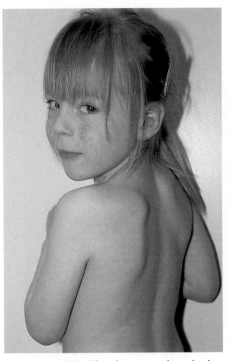

(A) Young girl with tuberous sclerosis; hypopigmented macules; angiofibromas on cheeks.

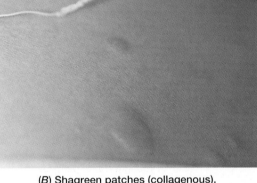

(B) Shagreen patches (collagenous).

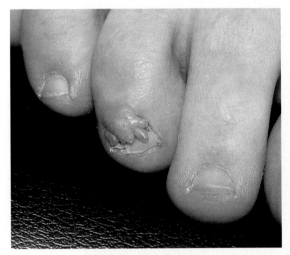

(C) Periungual fibroma.

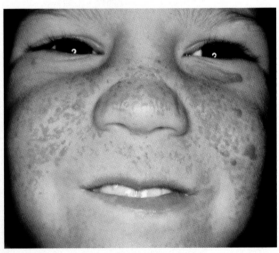

(D) Adenoma sebaceum in 4-year-old boy with epilepsy.

Figure 31-5.   **Cutaneous manifestations of tuberous sclerosis.**

Incontinentia pigmenti (Fig. 31-6) is an X-linked dominant condition affecting females almost exclusively and is usually lethal prenatally in affected males.

Newborns present with blistering distributed along the lines of Blaschko. Over weeks to months, these areas become hyperkeratotic and warty in appearance. This gradually subsides and hyperpigmentation develops, also along the lines of Blaschko, but not necessarily in or limited to the areas of blistering. This hyperpigmentation persists throughout childhood but may fade

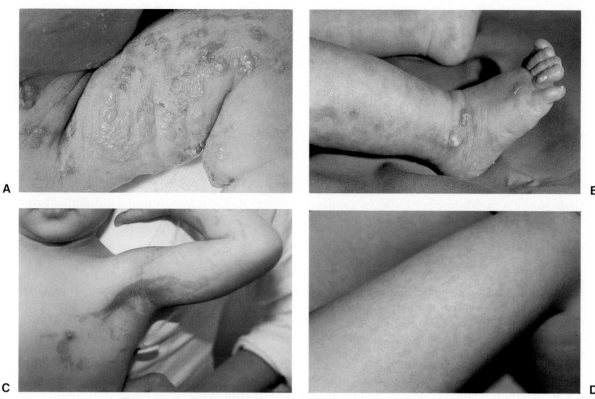

Figure 31-6.   Genodermatoses. (*A–D*) Stages I–IV of incontinentia pigmenti.

to hypopigmented hairless skin in adult life. The severity of associated problems varies. These include central nervous system abnormalities including seizures and mental retardation, retinal vascular dysplasia and visual defects, alopecia, hypodontia and peg-shaped teeth, nail dysplasia, and skeletal abnormalities.

DISORDERS OF ELASTICITY

Ehlers-Danlos syndrome (EDS) is the eponym given to a group of conditions, some of which share little in common. Recent efforts have been made to limit application of this eponym to those conditions in which fragility, thinness, or hyperelasticity of the skin is a primary finding.

EDSs I and II are similar, with II being more mild. EDS I is characterized by soft velvety hyperextensible skin that is fragile, tears easily, and heals poorly, with thin cigarette-paper scars. There is easy bruiseability. Over time, elastosis perforans serpiginosa can become a significant management problem. Patients have marked ligament laxity. Individuals with Ehlers-Danlos

syndrome type III have essentially normal skin, but marked hyperextensibility of large and small joints. Electromicroscopy of skin shows abnormal collagen bundles in these conditions. In some families, mutations in the α1 chain of type 5 collagen (COL5A1) have been identified. Ehlers-Danlos syndrome type IV, the arterial or Sack-Barabas type, is autosomal dominant, as are Ehlers-Danlos syndromes type I, II and III. The skin in type IV is thin and taut, rather than velvety and soft. This is a disorder of type III collagen (COL3A1) and affects the lining of vessels and viscera. Rupture of these is the major medical complication and death is common before age 50 years.

Cutis laxa is a heterogeneous group of autosomal recessive and X-linked recessive conditions, which share laxity, not elasticity, of the skin. The skin is soft and progressively loses tone. Affected individuals have a prematurely aged "hound dog" appearance to the face. X-linked cutis laxa, also referred to as Ehlers-Danlos syndrome type IX, is caused by a defect in the NMK gene, whose product transports copper. Thus, mutations in NMK result in secondary deficiency of copper-dependent enzymes. Internal involvement includes progressive hydronephrosis and bladder diverticuli, emphysema and pulmonary blebs, and hernias. Intellect ranges from mild mental retardation to normal. The NMK gene is also involved in Menkes syndrome, a much more severe disorder. Skin of affected males is thin and pale, with a prominent venous pattern. The hairs are fine, sparse, and fragile and demonstrate pili torti (twisting). Neurologic involvement is usually severe and progressive. Prenatal diagnosis is available for both X-linked cutis laxa and Menkes syndrome. Daily use of a dietary copper histidine supplementation when instituted shortly after birth may have some benefit in slowing progression of neurologic symptoms.

In pseudoxanthoma elasticum, there is progressive deterioration of elastic fibers in the dermis, choroid of the eye, and blood vessels. The skin becomes progressively involved by cobblestoned, yellowish plaques, especially at the nape of the neck and in the folds of the skin. These are clinically similar to solar elastosis. Progressive atherosclerotic disease, presumably due to calcified plaques developing on abnormal vessel walls, results in claudication, gastrointestinal bleeding, and stroke. Breaks in Bruch's membrane of the eye are seen as angioid streaks on eye examination. This is a feature typical of the disorder. The changes in pseudoxanthoma elasticum are progressive. Making the diagnosis is unusual in childhood unless there is a positive family history and a high index of suspicion. Pedigrees have been consistent with both autosomal dominant and autosomal recessive modes of inheritance. The condition is likely to be genetically heterogeneous.

DISORDERS OF APPENDAGES
(see Chap. 27)

Hair

Inherited defects in hair can affect the development of follicles, hair growth, and hair structure. Congenital alopecias are rare. They may be isolated or associated with other origin involvement. Most are autosomal recessive. The disorder of hair growth in childhood is the loose anagen syndrome, a condition in which the anagen roots are structurally abnormal, the hairs are poorly anchored and easily plucked, and the growth period is reduced. Affected children have thin, short hair that "never needs to be cut." It tends to improve with time and by adult life hair may appear normal although still relatively loosely anchored. Inheritance is uncertain. Structural hair-shaft abnormalities are listed in Table 31-4.

Nails

Isolated inherited disorders of nails are rare, and most abnormalities are part of syndromes. Pachyonychia congenital syndrome (Fig. 31-7) is a term used for two autosomal dominant conditions: type 1, Jadassohn-Lewandowski syndrome, and type 2, Jackson-Lawler syndrome. In pachyonychia congenital syndrome, the nail plates are thickened or may be small or absent. Nail changes may appear within the first few years of life or not until later. Not all nails are necessarily involved. Other physical findings include palmar plantar hyperkeratosis, leukokeratosis of the oral mucosa, and follicular keratosis at the elbows and knees. Epidermal cyst, steatocystoma multiplex, and natal teeth are typical of type 2. Mutations in keratins, keratin 16 in type 1 and keratin 17 in type 2, have been found.

Nail-patella syndrome (Fig. 31-8) is an autosomal dominant disorder marked by variable nail dystrophy with usually symmetric involvement. Skeletal abnormalities are also a feature and include hypoplasia to absence of the patellae, malformations of the elbows and scapulae, and iliac horns. Renal involvement ranges from glomerulonephritis to severe renal failure and occurs in up to a third of affected individuals. The gene is linked to the ABO blood group on the long arm of chromosome 9.

ECTODERMAL DYSPLASIAS

There are over 100 genetic conditions whose major findings involve alterations in two or more of the primary ectodermal derivatives: hair, teeth, sweat glands, and nails. Historically, the ectodermal dysplasias have been divided into those with relatively normal sweating—hidrotic—and those with heat intolerance—hypohidrotic or anhidrotic. The most common of the ectodermal dysplasias is X-linked recessive hypohidrotic ectodermal dysplasia (Christ-Siemens-Touraine syndrome) (Fig. 31-9A). Affected males may present with a collodion membrane at birth and have heat intolerance because of inability to

TABLE 31-4
HAIR DISORDERS

Name	Inheritance	Basic Defect	Microscopic Features	Associated Abnormalities
Monilethrix	AD	Mutations in type II hair keratin: hHb6 hHb1	Beaded hairs; regular or irregular narrowing and widening of hair shaft	None
Pili annulati	AD	Unknown; bands are due to air-filled cavities in cortex	Ringed hair; alternating bands of light and dark	None
Pili torti	X-LR	Mutations in MNK1 (ATP7A)	Twisting along longitudinal axis of hairshaft	Menkes syndrome
	AD	Unknown		
Pili trianguli et canaliculi (uncombable, spangled hair)	AD	Unknown	Grooved, triangular hair	None
Trichorrhexis invaginata	AR	Unknown	Nodal swelling of hairshaft—similar to bamboo	Netherton syndrome
Trichorrhexis nodosa	AD	Unknown	Fraying of medulla due to abnormal cuticle; appearance of opposing broomheads	Argininosuccinic aciduria
	AR	Unknown		Trauma
	Acquired	Argininosuccinate lycose deficiency		Can be seen in any fragile hair
Trichothiodystrophy	AR	Decrease in disulfide bonds; decrease in cysteine in hair	Thin fragile hairs with birefrigent regions in polarized microscopy	Heterogeneous—may be associated with any of: Ichthyosis Mental retardation Failure to thrive Short stature Infertility or maybe isolated

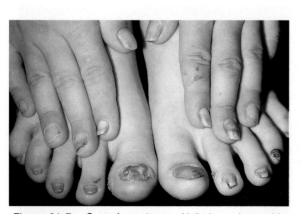

Figure 31-7. **Genodermatoses.** Nails in pachyonychia congenital syndrome.

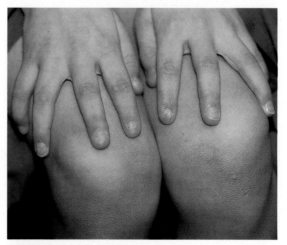

Figure 31-8. **Genodermatoses.** Nails in nail-patella syndrome.

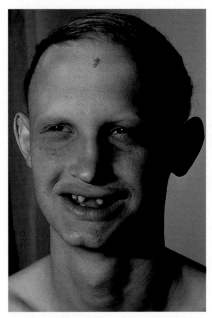

(A) Male with sparse hair; peg-shaped teeth and hypodontia, and typical facies of hypohidrotic ectodermal dysplasia.

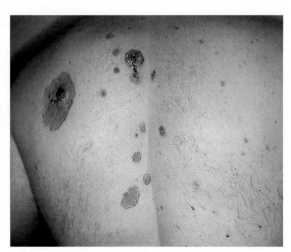

(B) Basal cell nevus syndrome of back.

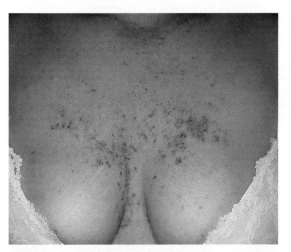

(C) Darier's disease of chest.

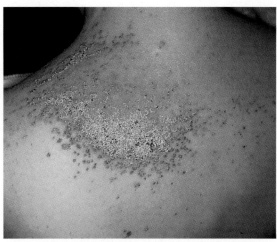

(D) Darier's disease of posterior shoulder.

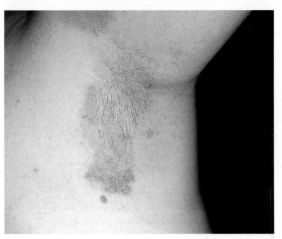

(E) Hailey-Hailey disease of axilla.

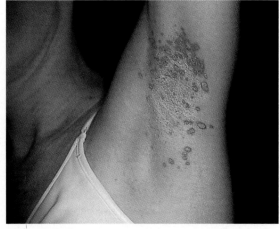

(F) Xanthoma disseminatum of axilla.

Figure 31-9. **Genodermatoses.** (*Ortho-Pharmaceutical Corp.*)

TABLE 31-5
DISORDERS ASSOCIATED WITH MALIGNANCY

Disorder	Mode of Inheritance	Gene	Major Dermatologic Findings	Associated Features	Typical Malignancy
Ataxia telangiectasia	AR	ATM	Progressive telangiectases on skin conjunctiva; premature graying of the hair	Ataxia; CNS degeneration; immunodeficiency	Lymphoreticular
Basal cell nevus syndrome	AD	PTC	Basal cell nevi; palmar/plantar pits/ epidermal cysts	Many, including odontogenic keratocysts and skeletal abnormalities	Basal cell carcinoma; medulloblastoma-ovary
Bloom syndrome	AR	BLM	Malar telangiectases	Immunodeficiency; growth failure; infertility in males	Many different organs
Cowden syndrome	AD	PTEN	Tricholemmomas; acral keratoses; palmar/plantar keratoses; oral papillomas	Thyroid abnormalities; fibrocystic breast disease; GI polyps	Breast; ovary; thyroid
Dyskeratosis congenita	XLR / ?AR	DKC1	Progressive reticular hyperpigmentation / Nail dystrophy; oral leukoplakia.	Bone-marrow failure	Squamous cell cancer
Fanconi syndrome	AR	FACA FACC	Café-au-lait spots; patchy hyperpigmentation; Sweet's syndrome	Bone-marrow failure; radial ray defects; short stature	Hematopoietic; hepatocellular
Gardner syndrome	AD	APC	Epidermal inclusion cysts; fibromas; desmoid tumors	Intestinal polyps; mandibular osteomas	GI malignancies
MEN 2A/2B	AD	RET	Mucosal neuromas	Marfanoid habitus / Ganglioneuromas of GI tract / Pheochromocytoma	Thyroid
Peutz-Jeghers	AD	STK11	Lentigines on lips, mucosa palms, soles, fingertips.	GI polyposis	GI malignancy; ovary; testicle; uterus; pancreas
Rothmund-Thomson syndrome	AR	Unknown	Facial telangiectases; Poikiloderma; alopecia	Short stature Radial ray defects; hypogonadism; cataracts	Squamous cell cancer
Xeroderma pigmentosa (many complementation groups)	AR	ERCC2 ERCC3 ERCC5 XPCC XPAC	Progressive dyspigmentation; telangiectases; atrophy; progressive actinic changes	Neurologic involvement in XPA, XPC, XPD	Squamous cell cancer; basal cell cancer; malignant melanoma

319

sweat, hypodontia and peg-shaped teeth, and sparse hair. Female carriers may have patchy hair loss and patchy distribution of sweat glands, with minimal to significant tooth involvement. The gene has been mapped to the proximal long arm of the X chromosome and mutations in it have been identified in approximately 10% of affected individuals studied to date.

HAMARTOMAS AND MALIGNANCIES

A number of genetic skin conditions are marked by development of cutaneous and extracutaneous malignancy. Table 31-5 lists some of these.

BIBLIOGRAPHY

General

Sybert VP. Genetic skin disorders. New York, Oxford University Press, 1997.

Ichthyosis Review

Traupe H. The ichthyoses: A guide to clinical diagnosis, genetic counseling, and therapy. New York, Springer-Verlag, 1989.

Epidermolysis Bullosa Review

Uitto J, Pulkkinen L, McLean WH. Epidermolysis bullosa: A spectrum of clinical phenotypes explained by molecular heterogeneity. Mol Med Today 1997;3:457.

Lin A, Carter DM (eds). Epidermolysis bullosa: Basic and clinical aspects. New York, Springer-Verlag, 1992.

Pigment Disorders

ALBINISMS

King RA, Hearing VJ, Creel DJ, Detting WS. Albinism. In: The metabolic and molecular bases of inherited disease, ed 7. Scriver CR, Beaudet AL, Sly WS, Valle ED, eds. New York, McGraw-Hill, 1997;4303.

HYPOMELANOSIS OF ITO

Sybert VP. Hypomelanosis of Ito: A description, not a diagnosis. J Invest Dermatol 1994;103:1415.

Elasticity Disorders

Neldner KH. Pseudoxanthoma elasticum. Clin Dermatol 1988;6:1.

Steinmann B, Royce PM, Superti-Furga A. The Ehlers-Danlos syndrome. In: Connective tissue and its heritable disorders. Royce PM, Steinmann B (eds). Wiley-Liss, New York, 1992:351.

Disorders of Appendages

HAIR

Birnbaum PS, Baden IH. Heritable disorders of hair. Dermatol Clin 1987;5:137.

NAILS

Juhlin L, Baran R. Hereditary and congenital nail disorders. In: Diseases of the nails and their management, ed 2. Baran R, Dawber RPR (eds). Oxford, Blackwell, 1994.

DYSPLASIAS ECTODERMAL

Freire-Maia N, Pinheiro M. Ectodermal dysplasias: A clinical and genetic study. New York, Alan R. Liss, 1984.

Neurofibromatosis

Eichenfield LF, Levy ML, et al. Guideliines of care for neurofibromatosis type 1. JAAD 1997;34:4.

Gutmann DH, Aylsworth A, et al. The diagnostic evaluation and multidisciplinary management of neurofibromatosis 1 and neurofibromatosis 2. JAMA 1997;278:1.

General Genetics

Khavari PA. Gene therapy for genetic skin disease. Dermatology Foundation 1997;31:3.

Motulsky AG. Screening for genetic diseases. N Engl J Med 1997;336:18.

Spitz JL. Genodermatoses. Baltimore, Williams & Wilkins, 1996.

Sybert VP. Principles of genetics in the molecular era. Arch Dermatol 1993;129:1409.

32

Tumors of the Skin

CLASSIFICATION

A patient comes into your office for care of a tumor on his skin. What kind is it? What is the best treatment? This complex process of diagnosing and managing skin tumors is not learned easily. As an aid to the establishment of the correct diagnosis, all skin tumors (excluding warts, which are due to a virus) are classified (1) as to their histologic origin, (2) according to the patient's age group, (3) by location, and (4) on the basis of clinical appearance.

A complete histologic classification is found at the end of this chapter, whereas only the more common tumors are classified and discussed here. This histologic classification is divided into epidermal tumors, mesodermal tumors, nevus cell tumors, lymphomas, and myeloses. In making a clinical diagnosis of any skin tumor, one should apply a histopathologic label. Whether the label is correct or not depends on the clinical acumen of the physician and whether the tumor, or a part of it, has been examined microscopically.

Histologic Classification*

EPIDERMAL TUMORS

Tumors of the Surface Epidermis
1. Benign tumors: defined as neoplasms that probably arise from arrested embryonal cells
   a. Seborrheic keratosis
   b. Pedunculated fibroma (skin tag, fibroepithelial polyp, acrochordon)
   c. Cysts
      - Epidermal cyst
      - Trichilemmal (pilar or sebaceous cyst)
      - Milium
      - Dermoid cyst
      - Mucous cyst
2. Precancerous tumors
   a. Actinic keratosis and cutaneous horn
   b. Arsenical keratosis
   c. Leukoplakia
3. Carcinoma: squamous cell carcinoma

---

*This partial classification and the complete one at the end of this chapter are modified from the one listed by Walter F. Lever and Gundula Schaumberg-Lever. Histopathology of the skin, ed 8. Philadelphia, JB Lippincott, 1997.

321

Tumors of the Epidermal Appendages

1. Basal cell carcinoma
2. Sebaceous gland hyperplasia
3. Numerous other types both benign and malignant, usually classified by appendage of origin

MESODERMAL TUMORS

Tumors of Fibrous Tissue

1. Histiocytoma and dermatofibroma
2. Keloid

Tumors of Vascular Tissue

1. Hemangiomas

NEVUS CELL TUMORS

Nevi

1. Junctional (active) nevus
2. Intradermal (resting) nevus
3. Dysplastic nevus syndrome (familial atypical mole–melanoma syndrome or sporadic atypical mole–melanoma syndrome)

Malignant Melanoma

LYMPHOMA AND MYELOSIS

Monomorphous Group

Polymorphous Group

1. Mycosis fungoides (cutaneous T-cell lymphoma)

SAUER NOTES

1. A histologic examination should be performed on every malignant skin tumor.
2. Similarly, a biopsy should be performed on any tumor when a malignancy cannot be definitely ruled out clinically.

Classification by Age Groups

An age-group classification is helpful from a differential diagnostic viewpoint. Viral warts are considered in this classification because of the frequent necessity of differentiating them from other skin tumors. The most common tumors are listed first.

TUMORS OF CHILDREN

1. Warts (viral), very common
2. Nevi, junctional type, common
3. Molluscum contagiosum (viral)
4. Hemangiomas

5. Café-au-lait spot
6. Granuloma pyogenicum
7. Mongolian spot
8. Xanthogranulomas

TUMORS OF ADULTS

1. Warts (viral), plantar type common
2. Nevi
3. Cysts
4. Pedunculated fibromas (skin tags, acrochordons)
5. Sebaceous gland hyperplasias
6. Histiocytomas (dermatofibromas, sclerosing hemangiomas)
7. Keloids
8. Lipomas
9. Granuloma pyogenicum

ADDITIONAL TUMORS OF OLDER ADULTS

1. Seborrheic keratoses
2. Actinic keratoses
3. Capillary hemangiomas
4. Basal cell carcinomas
5. Squamous cell carcinomas
6. Leukoplakia

Classification of Tumors Based on Location

Scalp: seborrheic keratosis, epidermal cyst (pilar cyst), nevus, actinic keratosis (bald males), wart, trichilemmal cyst, basal cell carcinoma, squamous cell carcinoma, nevus sebaceous, proliferating trichilemmal tumor, cylindroma, syringocystadenoma papilliferum.

Ear: seborrheic keratosis, actinic keratoses, basal cell carcinoma, nevus, squamous cell carcinoma, keloid, epidermal cyst, chondrodermatitis nodularis helicis, venous lakes (varix), gouty tophus.

Face: seborrheic keratosis, sebaceous gland, hyperplasia, actinic keratosis, lentigo, milium, nevi, basal cell cancer, squamous cell cancer, lentigo maligna melanoma, flat wart, trichoepithelioma, dermatosis papulosa nigra (black females), fibrous papule of the face, colloid milium, dilated pore of Winer, keratoacanthoma, pyogenic granuloma, Spitz nevus, ephelides, hemangioma, adenoma sebaceum, apocrine hidrocystoma, eccrine hidrocystoma, trichilemmoma, trichofolliculoma, Merkel cell carcinoma, angiosarcoma (elderly males), nevus of Ota, warty dyskeratoma, atypical fibroxanthoma, angiolymphoid hyperplasia with eosinophilia, blue nevus.

Eyelids: pedunculated fibroma, seborrheic keratosis, milium, syringoma, basal cell carcinoma, xanthoma.

Neck: pedunculated fibroma, seborrheic keratosis, epidermal cyst, keloid.

Lip and mouth: Fordyce's disease, lentigo, venous lake (varix), mucous retention cyst, leukoplakia, pyogenic granuloma, squamous cell carcinoma, granular cell tumor (tongue), giant cell epulis (gingivae), verrucous carcinoma, white sponge nevus, acral lentiginous melanoma.

Axilla: pedunculated fibroma, epidermal cyst, molluscum contagiosum, lentigo (multiple lentigo in neurofibromatosis called Crowe's sign).

Chest and back: seborrheic keratosis, angioma, nevi, ephelides, actinic keratosis, lipoma, basal cell carcinoma, epidermal cyst, keloid, lentigo, café-au-lait spot, squamous cell carcinoma, melanoma, hemangioma, histiocytoma, steatocystoma multiplex, eruptive vellus hair cyst, blue nevus, nevus of Ito, Becker's nevus.

Groin and crural areas: pedunculated fibroma, seborrheic keratosis, molluscum contagiosum, wart, Bowen's disease, extramammary Paget's disease.

Genitalia: wart, molluscum contagiosum, squamous intraepithelial lesions, epidermal cyst, angiokeratoma (scrotum), pearly penile papules (around edge of glans), squamous cell carcinoma, seborrheic keratosis, erythroplasia of Queyrat, Bowen's disease, median raphe cyst of penis, verrucous carcinoma, hidradenoma papilliferum (labia majora).

Hands: wart, seborrheic keratosis, actinic keratosis, lentigo, myxoid cyst (proximal nail fold), squamous cell carcinoma, glomus tumor (nail bed), ganglion, common blue nevus, acral lentiginous melanoma, giant cell tumor of tendon sheath, pyogenic granuloma, acquired digital fibrokeratoma, recurrent infantile digital fibroma, traumatic fibroma, xanthoma, Dupytren's contracture.

Feet: wart, nevi, blue nevus, acral lentiginous melanoma, seborrheic keratosis, verrucous carcinoma, eccrine poroma

Arms and Legs: seborrheic keratosis, lentigo, wart, histiocytoma, actinic keratosis, squamous cell carcinoma, melanoma, lipoma, xanthoma, clear cell acanthoma (legs), Kaposi's sarcoma (legs, classic type).

Classification Based on Clinical Appearance

The clinical appearance of any tumor is a most important diagnostic factor. Some tumors have a characteristic color and growth that is readily distinguishable from any other tumor, but a large number, unfortunately, have clinical characteristics common to several similar tumors. A further hindrance to making a correct diagnosis is that the same histopathologic lesion may vary in clinical appearance. The following generalizing classification should be helpful, but, if in doubt, the lesion should be examined histologically.

FLAT, SKIN-COLORED TUMORS

1. Flat warts (viral)
2. Histiocytomas
3. Leukoplakia

FLAT, PIGMENTED TUMORS

1. Nevi, usually junctional type
2. Lentigo
3. Café-au-lait spot
4. Histiocytomas
5. Mongolian spot
6. Melanoma (superficial spreading type)

RAISED, SKIN-COLORED TUMORS

1. Warts (viral)
2. Pedunculated fibromas (skin tags)
3. Nevi, usually intradermal type
4. Cysts
5. Lipomas
6. Keloids
7. Basal cell carcinomas
8. Squamous cell carcinoma
9. Molluscum contagiosum (viral)
10. Xanthogranuloma (yellowish, usually children)

RAISED, BROWNISH TUMORS

1. Warts (viral)
2. Nevi, usually compound type
3. Actinic keratoses
4. Seborrheic keratoses
5. Pedunculated fibromas (skin tags)
6. Basal cell epitheliomas
7. Squamous cell carcinoma
8. Malignant melanoma
9. Granuloma pyogenicum
10. Keratoacanthomas

RAISED, REDDISH TUMORS

1. Hemangiomas
2. Actinic keratoses
3. Granuloma pyogenicum
4. Glomus tumors
5. Senile or cherry angiomas

RAISED, BLACKISH TUMORS

1. Seborrheic keratoses
2. Nevi
3. Granuloma pyogenicum
4. Malignant melanomas

5. Blue nevi
6. Thrombosed angiomas or hemangiomas

SEBORRHEIC KERATOSES
(Fig. 32-1 and see Fig. 34-4)

It is a rare elderly patient who does not have any seborrheic keratoses. These are the unattractive "moles" or "warts" that perturb the elderly patient, occasionally become irritated, but are benign.

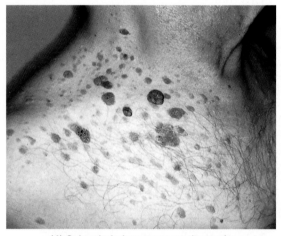

(A) Seborrheic keratoses on the neck.

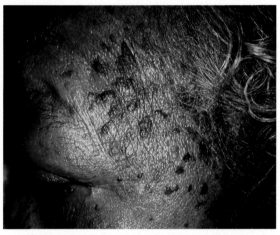

(B) Dermatosis papulosa nigra on temple area.

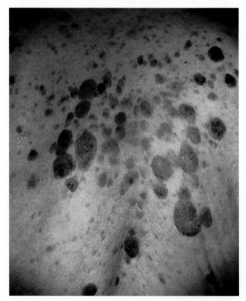

(C) Seborrheic keratoses on back.

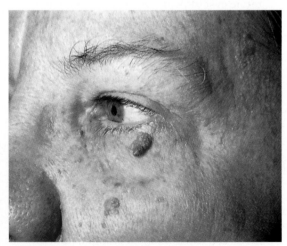

(D) Pedunculated seborrheic keratosis of eyelid.

Figure 32-1.   **Epidermal tumors.** *(Stiefel Laboratories, Inc.)*

Dermatosis papulosa nigra is a form of seborrheic keratosis of African-Americans that occurs on the face, mainly in women. These small, multiple tumors can be removed, but there is the possibility of causing keloids or hypopigmentation.

Stucco keratoses are numerous white 1- to 3-mm seborrheic keratoses mainly over feet, ankles, and lower legs.

DESCRIPTION. The size of seborrheic keratoses varies up to 3 cm for the largest, but the average diameter is 1 cm. The color may be flesh-colored, tan, brown, or coal black. They are usually oval in shape, elevated, and have a greasy, warty sensation to touch. White, brown, or black pinhead-sized keratotic areas called pseudohorned cysts are commonly seen within this tumor. There is an appearance of being superficial and "stuck on" the skin. Pruritus is common and sudden appearance may occur. Numerous lesions coming on rapidly can be a marker of underlying cancer (sign of Leser-Trélat).

DISTRIBUTION. The lesions appear on the face, neck, scalp, back, and upper chest, and less frequently on arms, legs, and the lower part of the trunk.

COURSE. Lesions become darker and enlarge slowly. Trauma from clothing occasionally results in infection and bleeding, and this prompts the patient to seek medical care. Any inflammatory dermatitis around these lesions causes them to enlarge temporarily and become more evident, so much so that many patients suddenly note them for the first time. Malignant degeneration of seborrheic keratoses is doubted.

ETIOLOGY. Heredity is the biggest factor, along with old age. They are seen more commonly in patients with an oily, acne–seborrhea type of skin.

Differential Diagnosis

Actinic keratoses: See Table 32-1.
Pigmented nevi: Longer duration, smoother surface, softer to touch; may not be able to differentiate clinically (see later in this chapter).
Flat warts: In younger patients; acute onset, with rapid development of new lesions (see Chap. 17).
Malignant melanoma: Less common, usually with rapid growth, indurated; examine histologically (see later).

Treatment

A 58-year-old woman requests the removal of a warty, tannish, slightly elevated 2×2-cm lesion of the right side of her forehead.

1. The lesion should be examined carefully. The diagnosis usually can be made clinically, but if there is any question, a scissors biopsy (see Chap. 2) can be performed. It would be ideal if all of these seborrheic keratoses could be examined histologically, but this is not economically feasible or necessary.
2. An adequate form of therapy is curettement, with or without local anesthesia, followed by a light application of trichloroacetic acid. The resulting fine atrophic scar will hardly be noticeable in several months.

TABLE 32-1
DIFFERENTIAL DIAGNOSIS

Parameter	Actinic or Senile Keratosis	Seborrheic Keratosis
Appearance	Flat, brownish, reddish, or tan scale firmly attached to skin, poorly demarcated	Greasy, elevated, brown or black; scale is warty and can be easily scratched away at times, "stuck on," well demarcated
Location	Sun-exposed areas	Face, back, and chest
Complexion	Blue eyes, light hair, dry skin	Brown eyes, dark hair, oily skin
Subjective complaints	Some burning and stinging	Occasional itching
Precancerous	Yes	No

SAUER NOTES

1. For many benign lesions it often is best cosmetically to err on the side of surgical undertreatment rather than overtreatment. You can always remove any remaining growth later, but you cannot put back what you took off.

2. Scarring should be kept to a minimum.
3. After any surgical procedure, I hand out the "Surgical Notes" sheet. Skin-surgery sites usually heal without any complication. However, there are always questions and concerns from the patient about aftercare.

SURGICAL NOTES

Minor surgery has been performed for the removal or biopsy of a skin lesion.

If liquid nitrogen was used to remove the growth, a blister or peeling at the growth site will develop in 24 hours; or

If electrosurgery or burning was used, a crust and scab will form; or if a biopsy was made, there will be a crust or suture(s).

The sites treated heal better if they are uncovered. Do not pick at the spot and try to avoid accidentally hitting the area. One or more scabs will form in the course of healing.

You can wash over the area lightly. Do not apply any creams to the lesions until the scabs have fallen off completely. If for cosmetic reasons you feel you must cover the site with a bandage, then apply alcohol, Polysporin ointment, or Betadine solution to the site twice a day.

A certain amount of redness and swelling around the surgery site is to be expected. Also you might have a small amount of drainage and crusting. A mild amount of redness and infection can be treated with Polysporin ointment locally three times a day.

If more drainage or infection develops, apply a wet dressing with sheeting, or soak the area. Use a solution made with 1 teaspoon of salt to 1 pint of cool water and apply for 20 minutes three times a day. Make a fresh solution every day.

If the infection becomes excessive, call the office or go to a hospital emergency department. This action should be necessary only very rarely.

If the scab is knocked off prematurely, bleeding may occur. This can be stopped by applying firm pressure with gauze or cotton for 10 minutes by the clock, and then releasing pressure gradually. The 10-minute pressure can be repeated as needed.

Depending on the size of the surgery site, healing takes from 1 to 8 weeks. Some scarring or loss of pigment at the surgery site is possible. A few individuals have a tendency to form thick or keloidal scars, which is not predictable.

If a biopsy was done, you will be receiving a bill for the pathology study from the laboratory. Call the office in 7 days for this report.

Return to the office for further care or follow-up as directed.

Electrosurgery can be used, but this usually requires anesthesia.

Liquid nitrogen freezing therapy works well, if available. It is the therapy of choice of most dermatologists. *Do not freeze excessively.*

Surgical excision is an unnecessary and more expensive form of removal.

PEDUNCULATED FIBROMAS (SKIN TAGS, ACROCHORDONS)
(Fig. 32-2)

Multiple skin tags are common on the neck and the axillae of middle-aged, usually obese, men and women. The indications for removal are two-fold: cosmetic, as desired and requested by the patient, and to prevent the irritation and the secondary infection of the pedicle that frequently develops from trauma of a collar, necklace, or other article of clothing.

DESCRIPTION. Pedunculated pinhead-sized to pea-sized soft tumors of normal skin color or darker are seen. The base may be inflamed from injury and the lesion may thrombose and turn black if twisted. This can cause alarm in the patient.

DISTRIBUTION. The lesions occur on the neck, axillae, or groin, or less frequently on any area.

COURSE. These fibromas grow very slowly. They may increase in size during pregnancy. Some become infected or thrombosed and drop off.

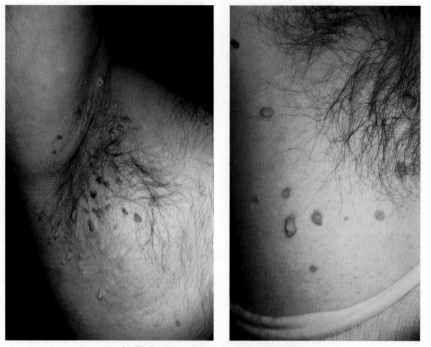

(*A,B*) Pedunculated fibromas in axilla.

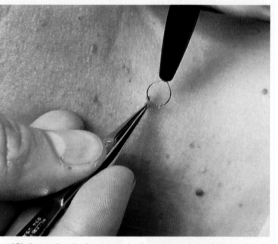

(*C*) A method of removal of pedunculated fibroma.

Figure 32-2. **Epidermal tumors.** (*Stiefel Laboratories, Inc.*)

Differential Diagnosis

Filiform wart: Digitate projections, more horny; also seen on chin area (see Chap. 17).

Pedunculated seborrheic keratosis: Larger lesion, darker color, warty or velvety appearance (see preceding section).

Neurofibromatosis: Lesions seen elsewhere; larger; can be pushed back into skin; also café-au-lait spots; hereditary; single lesions do not indicate systemic disease (see Chaps. 26 and 31).

Treatment

A 42-year-old woman has 20 small pedunculated fibromas on her neck and axillae that she wants removed. This should be done by electrosurgery. Without anesthesia, gently grab the

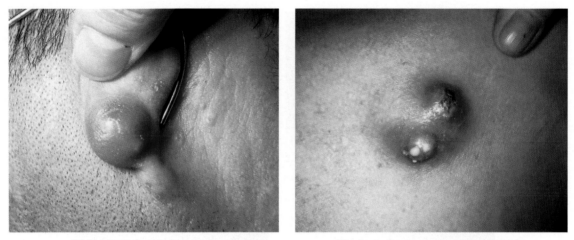

(*A*) Epidermal cyst of earlobe.   (*B*) Infected epidermal cyst on shoulder.

Figure 32-3. **Cysts of the skin.** (*Texas Pharmacal*).

small tumor in a thumb forceps and stretch the pedicle. Touch this pedicle with the electrosurgery needle and turn on the current for a split second. The tumor separates from the skin, and no bleeding occurs. The site heals in 4 to 7 days.

For very small lesions, a short spark with the electrosurgical needle suffices. Scissor excision with or without local anesthetic is commonly done.

CYSTS
(Figs. 32-3–32-5)

The three types are epidermal cyst; trichilemmal, pilar, or sebaceous cyst; and milium.

An *epidermal cyst* (Fig. 32-3) has a wall composed of true epidermis and probably originates from an invagination of the epidermis into the dermis and subsequent detachment from the epidermis, or it can originate spontaneously. The most common locations for epidermal cysts are the face, ears, neck, back, and scalp, where tumors of varying size can be found.

Trichilemmal cysts are also formerly known as wens and pilar or sebaceous cysts (Fig. 32-4). They are less common than epidermal cysts, occur mainly on the scalp, usually are multiple, and show an autosomal dominant inheritance. The sac wall is thick, smooth, and whitish and can be quite easily enucleated.

Milia (Fig. 32-5) are very common, white, pinhead-sized, firm lesions that are seen on the

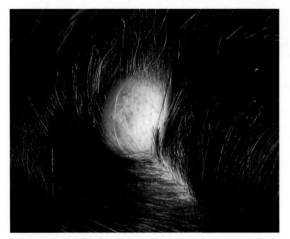

Figure 32-4. **Cysts of the skin.** Pilar or sebaceous cyst of scalp. (*Texas Pharmacal*)

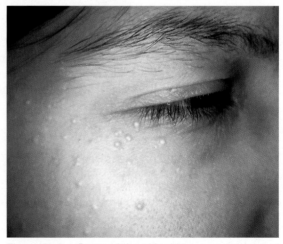

Figure 32-5. **Cysts of the skin.** Milia on upper cheek of 21-year-old woman. (*Texas Pharmacal*)

face. They are formed by proliferation of epithelial buds following trauma to the skin (dermabrasion for acne scars), following certain dermatoses (pemphigus, epidermolysis bullosa, and acute contact dermatitis), or from no apparent cause.

Differential Diagnosis of Epidermal and Trichilemmal Cysts

Lipoma: Difficult to differentiate clinically; more firm, lobulated; no cheesy material extrudes on incision; removal is by complete excision or by liposuction; clinically similar to hibernoma.

Dermoid cyst: Clinically similar; can also be found internally; usually a solitary skin tumor; histologically, contains hairs, eccrine glands, and sebaceous glands.

Mucous cysts (Fig. 32-6): Translucent pea-sized or smaller lesions on the lips, treated by cutting off top of the lesion and carefully lightly cauterizing the base with a silver nitrate stick or light electrosurgery.

Synovial cysts (mytoid cysts) of the skin (Fig. 32-7): Globoid, translucent, pea-sized swellings around the joints of fingers and toes.

Treatment of Epidermal and Trichilemmal Cysts

Several methods can be used with success. The choice depends on the ability of the operator and the site and the number of cysts. Cysts can regrow after even the best surgical care, because of incomplete removal of the sac.

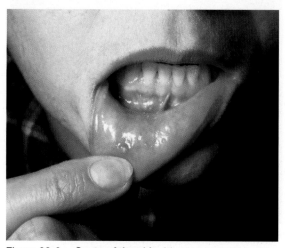

Figure 32-6.   Cysts of the skin. Mucous cyst on lower lip. (*Texas Pharmacal*)

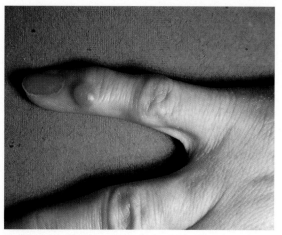

Figure 32-7.   Cysts of the skin. Synovial cyst on finger. (*Texas Pharmacal*)

1. A single 3-cm cyst on the back should be removed by surgical excision and suturing. This can be done in two ways: either by incising the skin and skillfully removing the intact cyst sac or by cutting straight into the sac with a small incision, shelling out the evacuated lining by applying strong pressure to the sides of the incision, and suturing the skin. The latter procedure is simpler, requires a smaller incision, and is quite successful.

2. A patient with several cysts in the scalp can be treated in another simple way. A 3- to 4-mm incision can be made directly over and into the cyst. The cheesy, foul-smelling contents can be evacuated by pressure and the use of a small curette. The sac can then be popped out of the hole with very firm pressure, or the sac can be grasped with a small hemostat and pulled out of the opening. No suturing or only a single suture is necessary. The resulting scar will be imperceptible in a short time.

3. If, during incision by any technique, a solid tumor is found instead of a cyst, the lesion should be excised completely and the material studied histologically. This diagnostic error is common because of the clinical similarity of cysts, lipomas, and other related tumors.

Treatment of Milia

1. Simple incision of the small tumors with a scalpel or a Hagedorn needle and expression of the contents by a comedone extractor is sufficient.

2. Another procedure is to remove the top of the milia lightly with electrodesiccation.

PRECANCEROUS TUMORS

Precancerous types of tumors include actinic keratosis and cutaneous horn, arsenical keratosis, and leukoplakia.

Actinic Keratosis
(Fig. 32-8)

Actinic keratosis is a common skin lesion of light-complexioned older persons that occurs on the skin surfaces exposed to sunlight. A small percentage of these lesions develop into squamous cell carcinomas. Because of the popularity of sunbathing, these lesions (probably 5–10%) are seen also in persons in the 30- to 50-year-old age group.

DESCRIPTION. Lesions are usually multiple, flat or slightly elevated, brownish or tan colored, scaly and adherent, measuring up to 1.5 cm in diameter, and often arising on an ill-defined base (Fig. 32-9). Individual lesions may become confluent. A *cutaneous horn* may be a proliferative, hyperkeratotic form of actinic keratosis that resembles a horn (Fig. 32-10). A cutaneous horn can also originate from a seborrheic keratosis, wart, squamous cell carcinoma, basal cell carcinoma, or keratoacanthoma. If a biopsy is done, enough of the base of the lesion must be removed to obtain an accurate histologic diagnosis.

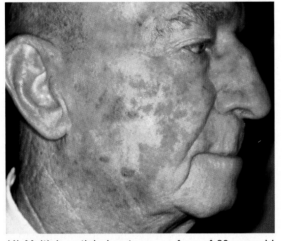

(A) Multiple actinic keratoses on face of 80-year-old, fair-complexioned farmer.

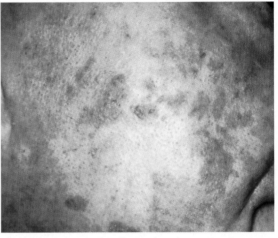

(B) Close-up.

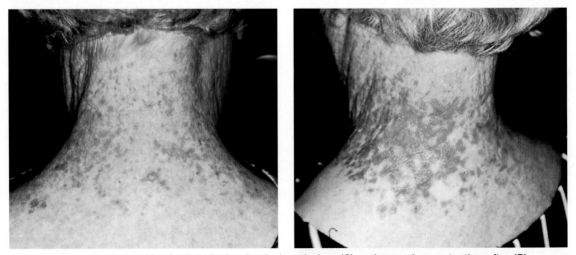

Actinic keratoses of back of neck showing lesions before (C) and normal accentuation after (D) therapy with 5-fluorouracil for 2 weeks.

Figure 32-8. **Actinic keratoses.** (*Dermik Laboratories, Inc.; Owen Laboratories, Inc.*)

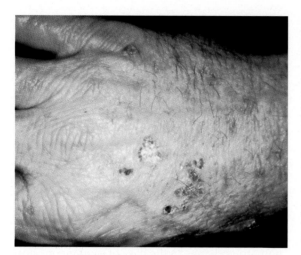 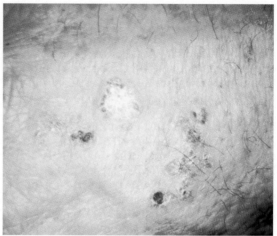

(A) Lesions on dorsum of hands. (B) Close-up in 44-year-old, blue-eyed outdoor worker.

Figure 32-9. **Actinic keratoses.** (*Dermik Laboratories, Inc.; Owen Laboratories, Inc.*)

DISTRIBUTION. Areas of skin exposed to sunlight, such as face, ears, neck, and dorsum of hands, are involved.

COURSE. The lesion begins as a faint red, slightly scaly patch that enlarges slowly, peripherally and deeply, over many years. A sudden spurt of growth could indicate a change to a squamous cell carcinoma.

SUBJECTIVE COMPLAINTS. Patients often complain that these lesions are sensitive or they burn and sting.

ETIOLOGY. Heredity and sun exposure are the two main causative factors. The blue-eyed, thin-skinned, light-haired person with a family his-

tory of such lesions is the best subject for multiple actinic keratoses.

SEX INCIDENCE. The disorder is most commonly seen in men.

DIFFERENTIAL DIAGNOSIS

Seborrheic keratosis: see Table 32-1.
Squamous cell carcinoma: Any thickened lesion that has grown rapidly should undergo biopsy (see later in this chapter).
Arsenical keratosis: Mainly on palms and soles; history of arsenic ingestion.

TREATMENT

A 60-year-old farmer has three small actinic keratoses on his face. The lesions should be exam-

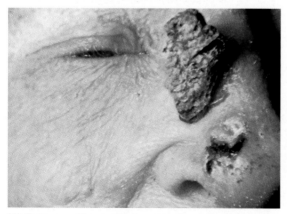 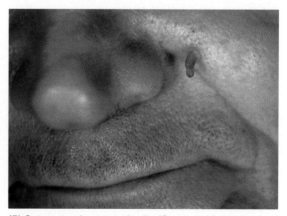

(A) Cutaneous horn with basal cell carcinomatous degeneration of the base. (*Texas Pharmacal*).

(B) Cutaneous horn, on cheek. (*Syntex Laboratories, Inc.*)

Figure 32-10. **Cutaneous horn.**

ined carefully. *If there is any evidence of induration or marked inflammation, the lesion should undergo biopsy* (see Chap. 2.) There are two methods of removal of these keratoses. For a single lesion, or only three or four lesions, a one-visit surgical treatment is usually preferable, especially if the lesion is relatively thick.

SURGICAL METHOD. Liquid nitrogen, if available, applied very lightly to the lesion is an effective and rapid method of removal. This is the therapy of choice of dermatologists.

Curettement, followed by destruction of the base by acid or electrosurgery, is satisfactory. Local anesthesia is usually necessary. Firmly scrape the lesion with the dermal curette, which removes the mushy, scaly keratosis and exposes the more fibrous normal skin. Experience provides the necessary "feel" of the abnormal versus the normal tissue. Some of the bleeding can be controlled by pressure or use of either one of the two following procedures: (1) application with a cotton-tipped applicator of a saturated solution of trichloroacetic acid, aluminum chloride solution, or Monsel solution cautiously to the bleeding site; or (2) electrocoagulation of the bleeding base. Small lesions heal in 7 to 14 days. No bandage is required.

FLUOROURACIL METHOD. For the patient with multiple superficial actinic keratoses, fluorouracil therapy is effective and eliminates for some months or years the early damaged epidermal cells. Thus, this fluorouracil therapy is really a cancer-prevention routine.

Several preparations and strengths of solutions and creams are available, but the two most commonly indicated are as follows:

Fluoroplex 1% solution, or cream   30.0
Efudex 2% solution or Efudex 5% cream   10.0
    Sig: Apply with fingers to area to be treated twice a day.
    Comment: It is wise to treat only a small area on the face at a time. Give instructions carefully and warn the patient that it is natural for the skin to get quite red and irritated and sore after 4 to 5 days. Most commonly the course of therapy is for 2 weeks. Some patients must stop therapy sooner, and some need more time to get the desired effect.

After completion of the course of therapy, the skin usually heals rapidly. A corticosteroid cream may be prescribed to hasten healing.

Another form of administration of fluorouracil is the pulse method. Here the medication is applied twice a day for only 2 to 4 consecutive days of each week, for a total duration of 3 or 4 months of therapy.

This therapy may have to be repeated in several months or years. If some keratoses are too thick to be removed by this fluorouracil method, then the liquid nitrogen or surgical method, as described first, is indicated for these lesions.

TREATMENT OF A CUTANEOUS HORN
(Fig. 32-10)

The same surgical technique as for actinic keratosis is used. *To rule out cancer, most cutaneous horns should be sent with intact base for histopathologic examination.* The incidence of squamous cell carcinomatous change in the base of a cutaneous horn is appreciable.

Arsenical Keratosis

Prolonged ingestion of inorganic arsenic (*e.g.,* Fowler's solution, Asiatic pills) can result in the formation many years later of small, punctate keratotic lesions, mainly seen on the palms and the soles. Progression to a squamous cell carcinoma can occur but is unusual.

SAUER NOTES

1. Patients with actinic keratoses should be requested to return every 6 to 12 months for examination; this is especially important if they have extensive actinic damage.

2. All patients with actinic keratoses should be told to use a sunscreen lotion or cream to lessen the occurrence of future keratoses.

TREATMENT

Small arsenical keratoses can be removed by electrosurgery; larger lesions can be excised and skin grafted if necessary.

Leukoplakia
(Fig. 32-11)

Leukoplakia is an actinic keratosis of the mucous membrane.

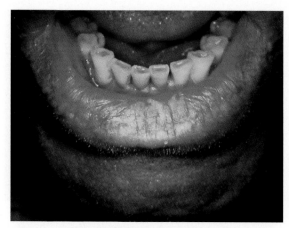

(*A*) Leukoplakia on lower lip, mild.

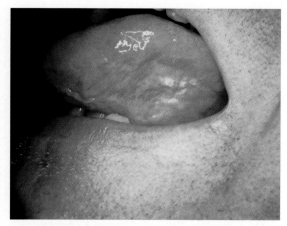

(*B*) Leukoplakia on tongue, from chronic biting. (*Westwood Pharmaceuticals*)

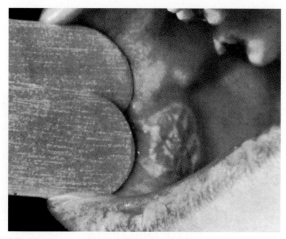

(*C*) Biopsy-proved leukoplakia on the mucous membrane of the cheek. This was erroneously diagnosed, clinically, as lichen planus.

Figure 32-11.   **Leukoplakia.**

DESCRIPTION. A flat, whitish plaque occurs localized to the mucous membranes of lips, mouth, vulva, and vagina. Single or multiple lesions may be present.

COURSE. Progression to squamous cell carcinoma occurs in 20% to 30% of chronic cases.

ETIOLOGY. Smoking, sunlight, and chronic irritation are the important factors in the development of leukoplakia. *Recurrent actinic cheilitis* may precede leukoplakia of the lips. The vulvar form may develop from *presenile* or *senile atrophy* of this area.

DIFFERENTIAL DIAGNOSIS

Lichen planus: A lacy network of whitish lesions, mainly on the sides of the buccal cavity; when on lips, it may clinically resemble leukoplakia; lichen planus elsewhere on body (see Chap. 14). Biopsy is often indicated.

Pressure calluses from teeth or dentures: Evidence of irritation; differentiation may be possible only by biopsy.

On the vulva, *lichen sclerosus et atrophicus* or *kraurosis vulvae*: No induration, as in leukoplakia of this area; can extend onto skin of

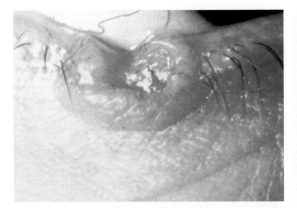

(*A*) Of the lower eyelid. Note telangiectasia on the rolled edge of the ulcer. *(Drs L. Calkins and A. Lemoine)*

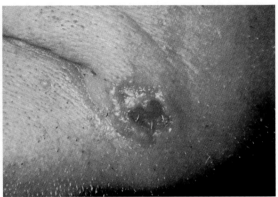

(*B*) Ulcerated lesion on chin. (*K.U.M.C.*)

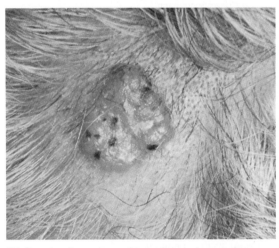

(*C*) Basal cell carcinomatous change in a syringocys-tadenoma papilliferum nevus on the scalp.

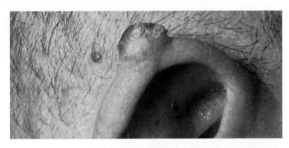

(*D*) On helix of the ear.

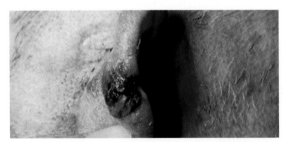

(*E*) Hemorrhagic lesion on helix of ear.

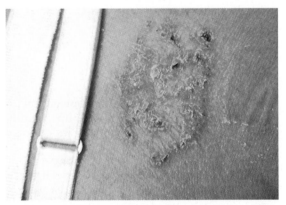

(*F*) Superficial basal cell carcinoma on posterior aspect of shoulder. Patient took arsenic (Fowler's solution) for 3 months (30 years previously) for psoriasis.

Figure 32-12.   **Basal cell carcinomas.** (*Texas Pharmacal*)

inguinal folds and perianal region; pruritus may or may not be present. Biopsy is helpful.

TREATMENT

Small patch of leukoplakia is seen on lower lip of man who smokes considerably.

1. The lesion should be examined carefully. *Perform a biopsy on any questionable area that shows inflammation and induration.* If a squamous cell carcinoma is present, the patient should receive surgical or radiation therapy by a physician who is an expert in this form of treatment.
2. Advise against use of tobacco products. The seriousness of continued smoking or other use of tobacco must be pointed out to the patient. Many early cases of leukoplakia disappear when smoking is stopped.
3. Eliminate any chronic irritation from teeth or dentures.
4. Protect the lips from sunlight with a sunscreen stick.
5. Electrosurgery, preceded by local anesthesia, is excellent for small, persistent areas of leukoplakia. The coagulating current is effective. Healing is usually rapid.
6. Liquid-nitrogen freezing is also quite effective.

EPITHELIOMAS AND CARCINOMAS

Basal Cell Carcinoma
(see Figs. 3-1C, 3-3A, 32-10, 32-12, and 34-15)

Basal cell carcinoma is the most common malignancy of the skin. Fortunately, a basal cell epithelioma or carcinoma is almost never a metastasizing tumor, and the cure rate can be close to 100% if these lesions are treated early and adequately.

DESCRIPTION. There are four clinical types of basal cell carcinoma: (1) noduloulcerative, (2) pigmented, (3) fibrosing (sclerosing, morphealike), and (4) superficial.

The *noduloulcerative basal cell carcinoma* is the most common type. It begins as a small waxy nodule that enlarges slowly over the years. A central depression usually forms that eventually progresses into an ulcer surrounded by a pearly or waxy border. The surface of the nodular component has a few telangiectatic vessels, which are highly characteristic.

The *pigmented type* is similar to the noduloulcerative form, with the addition of brown or black pigmentation.

The *fibrosing type* is extremely slow growing, is usually seen on the face, and consists of a whitish, scarred plaque with an ill-defined border, which rarely becomes ulcerated. This type is difficult to treat.

The *superficial form* may be single or multiple, is usually seen on the back and the chest, and is characterized by slowly enlarging red, scaly areas that, on careful examination, reveal a nodular border with telangiectatic vessels. A healed atrophic center may be present. Ulceration is superficial when it develops.

DISTRIBUTION. Over 90% of the basal cell carcinomas occur on the head and the neck, with the trunk next in frequency. These tumors are rarely found on the palms or the soles.

COURSE. The tumor is very slow growing, but sudden rapid growth periods do occur. Bleeding is common. Destructive forms of this tumor can invade cartilage, bone, blood vessels, or large areas of skin surface and result in death. There are rare reports of metastasizing basal cell carcinomas; these are usually very large tumors.

ETIOLOGY. Basal cell carcinomas develop most frequently on the areas of the skin exposed to sunlight and in blond or red-haired persons. Trauma and overexposure to radium and x-radiation can cause basal cell carcinomas. Long-term ingestion of inorganic arsenic can lead to formation of superficial basal cell carcinomas. Most authors believe that a basal cell tumor is a carcinoma of the basal cells of the epidermis. Lever and Schaumberg-Lever (see Bibliography) and others believe it not to be a carcinoma but a nevoid tumor (epithelioma) derived from incompletely differentiated embryonal cells.

AGE GROUP. This tumor can occur from childhood to old age but is seen most frequently in men older than age 50 years.

DIFFERENTIAL DIAGNOSIS

SAUER NOTE

Whenever the clinical appearance of a skin tumor suggests a basal cell carcinoma, the lesion should be studied histologically.

Squamous cell carcinoma: More rapid growth, firm, scaly papule or nodule, more inflammation, no pearly telangiectatic border; biopsy is necessary.

Other lesions that can mimic a basal cell carcinoma are *sebaceous hyperplasias* (very common, have a central dell), *keratoacanthomas, sebaceous adenomas, large comedones, warts, nevi, small cysts,* and *scarring from injury or radiation.*

Superficial basal cell carcinomas can resemble lesions of *psoriasis, seborrheic dermatitis, lupus vulgaris,* and *Bowen's disease.*

If multiple basal cell carcinomas are found, one should consider the *basal cell nevus syndrome.* This is a rare hereditary condition characterized by multiple genetically determined basal cell carcinomas, cysts of the jaws, peculiar pits of the hands and feet, and developmental anomalies of the ribs, the spine, and the skull.

TREATMENT

A 48-year-old woman has an 8×8-mm basal cell carcinoma on her forehead.

1. Inform the patient that she has a cancer of the skin that needs to be removed. Tell the patient that this tumor usually does not spread into the body, but if it is not treated it can spread on the skin. State that removal of the lesion is almost 100% effective but periodic examinations are necessary to check for any regrowth. If this tumor recurs, it will regrow only at its previous site. Tell the patient that a scar will result from the treatment.
2. If the diagnosis of the lesion is not definite clinically, a biopsy, as described in Chap. 7, can be done safely. Further treatment depends on the laboratory report.
3. Surgical excision of a basal cell carcinoma is the only method of treatment that should be attempted by the physician who only occasionally is confronted with these tumors. (Some criticism will arise from this statement, but it is our belief that a great amount of experience is necessary to remove these tumors adequately by curettement, chemocautery, electrosurgery, cryosurgery, radiation, or any combination of these methods. If the operator believes that he or she is qualified in these procedures, then this statement is not meant for him or her.) To excise the lesion, the area is anesthetized, an elliptical incision is made with a scalpel to include a border of 3 to 4 mm

around the tumor, one side of the excised skin is tagged with a piece of suture, the incision is closed, and the specimen is submitted for careful histologic examination (see Chap. 7). If the pathologist states that the tumor extends up to the edge of the excision, a further, more radical excision should be performed.
4. The patient should return for a checkup on a definite schedule, such as in 4 months, then every 6 months for four visits, then yearly, for a total of 5 years. Ten-year follow-up is being suggested by some authors.

Treatment of recurrent, deeply ulcerated, fibrosing or large superficial basal cell carcinomas should be in the domain of the competent dermatologist, surgeon, or radiologist. Mohs'-type surgery for these more difficult lesions is microscopically controlled and, unless the tumor is massive, results in a high cure rate.

Squamous Cell Carcinoma
(Figs. 32-13 and 34-14)

This rather common skin malignancy can arise primarily or from an actinic keratosis or leukoplakia. The grade of malignancy and metastasizing ability varies from grade I (low) to grade IV (high). Other terms for this tumor include *prickle cell epithelioma* and *epidermoid carcinoma.* The incidence has increased significantly in the last decade.

DESCRIPTION. The most common clinical picture is a rapidly growing nodule that soon develops a central ulcer and an indurated raised border with some surrounding redness. This type of lesion is the most malignant. The least malignant form has the clinical appearance of a warty, piled-up growth, which may not ulcerate. However, it is important to realize that the grade of malignancy can vary in the same tumor from one section to another, particularly in the larger lesions. This variation demonstrates the value of multiple histologic sections.

DISTRIBUTION. The lesion can occur on any area of the skin and mucous membrane but most commonly on the face, particularly the lower lip and ears, tongue, and dorsa of the hands. Chronic trauma associated with certain occupations can lead to formation of this cancer on unusual sites.

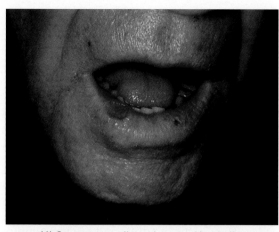

(A) Squamous cell carcinoma of lower lip.

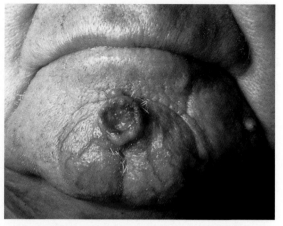

(B) Squamous cell carcinoma of chin.

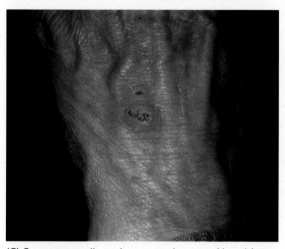

(C) Squamous cell carcinoma on dorsum of hand (compare with Fig. 1)

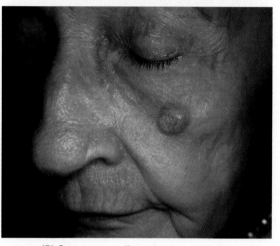

(D) Squamous cell carcinoma on cheek.

Figure 32-13. **Squamous cell carcinoma.** *(Westwood Pharmaceuticals)*

COURSE. The course varies with the grade of malignancy of the tumor. Lymph-node metastases (4 to 5% incidence) may occur early in the development of the tumor or may never occur. The cure rate can be very high when the lesions are treated early and with the best indicated modality.

ETIOLOGY. As in basal cell carcinomas, many factors contribute to provide the soil for growth of a squamous cell carcinoma. A simple listing of factors is sufficient: hereditarily determined type of skin; age of patient (elderly); trauma from chemicals (tars, oils), heat, wind, sunlight, x-radiation, PUVA therapy (psoralen plus long wave ultraviolet light), and severe burns; skin diseases that form scars, such as discoid lupus erythematosus, lupus vulgaris, and chronic ulcers; ingestion of inorganic arsenic; and in the natural course of xeroderma pigmentosum. Immunosuppressed patients, such as organ-transplant patients and patients with the acquired immunodeficiency syndrome, have an increased incidence of basal cell and squamous cell carcinoma.

> **SAUER NOTE**
>
> Whenever the clinical appearance of a skin tumor suggests a squamous cell carcinoma, the lesion should be studied histologically.

AGE AND SEX INCIDENCE. Most tumors are seen in elderly men, but exceptions are not rare.

Differential Diagnosis

Basal cell carcinoma: Slower growth, pearly border with telangiectasis, less inflammation; biopsy may be necessary to differentiate (see preceding section).
Actinic keratosis: Slow-growing, flat, scaly lesions; no induration; little surrounding erythema (see preceding section).
Pseudoepitheliomatous hyperplasia: Primary chronic lesion, such as old stasis ulcer, bromoderma, deep mycotic infection, syphilitic gumma, lupus vulgaris, basal cell carcinoma, and pyoderma gangrenosum; differentiation is often impossible clinically and very difficult histologically.
Keratoacanthoma (Fig. 32-14): Very fast-growing single or, more rarely, multiple lesions; clinically, this is a firm, raised nodule with a central crater; it should be studied histologically; it may disappear spontaneously. On the other hand, a few keratoacanthomas can be highly destructive locally. Histologically, a keratoacanthoma can be difficult to distinguish from a squamous cell carcinoma.

Treatment

Because of the rapid locally invasive nature of squamous cell carcinomas, intensive surgical or radiation therapy, or both, is indicated. A discus-

sion of such procedures is beyond the scope of this text, but consult Chap. 7 for an overview.

HISTIOCYTOMA AND DERMATOFIBROMA
(Fig. 32-15)

Histiocytomas and dermatofibromas are common, usually single, flat or only slightly elevated, tannish, reddish, or brownish nodules, less than 1 cm in size, that occur mainly on the anterior tibial area of the leg. These tumors have a characteristic clinical appearance and firm button-like feel that establishes the diagnosis. They often dimple when firm pressure is applied from both sides. They occur in adults and are nonsymptomatic and unchanging.

The histologic picture varies with the age of the lesion. The younger lesions are called histiocytomas, and the older ones dermatofibromas. If the nodule contains many blood vessels it is histologically labeled a sclerosing hemangioma.

Differential Diagnosis

Fibrosarcoma: Active growth with invasion of subcutaneous fat; any questionable lesions should be excised and examined histologically.

Treatment

No treatment is indicated. If there is any doubt as to the diagnosis, surgical excision and histologic examination are indicated.

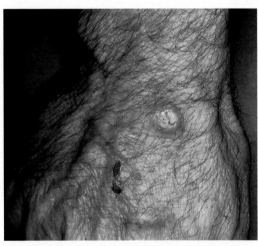
(*A*) Keratoacanthoma on dorsum of hand.

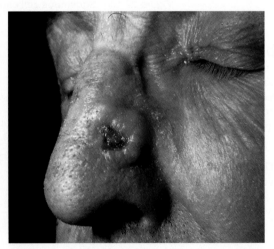
(*B*) Keratoacanthoma, on nose that healed without therapy, except for biopsy.

Figure 32-14. Keratoacanthoma. (*Syntex Laboratories*)

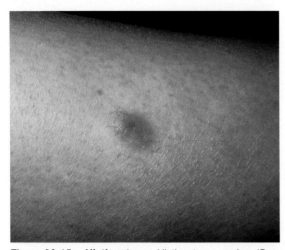

Figure 32-15. **Histiocytoma.** Histiocytoma, on leg. (*Syntex Laboratories, Inc.*)

For the female patient who shaves her legs and hits this lesion, liquid nitrogen applied lightly to the papule will flatten it.

KELOID
(Fig. 32-16)

A keloid is a tumor resulting from an abnormal overgrowth of fibrous tissue following injury in certain predisposed persons. Unusual configurations can occur, depending on the site, the extent, and the variety of the trauma. This tendency occurs so commonly in African-Americans that one should think twice before attempting a cosmetic procedure on a dark-skinned person or on any other person with a history of keloids. The back and the upper chest areas are especially prone to this proliferation.

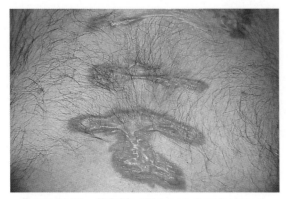

Figure 32-16. **Keloids.** Keloids on chest (common).

> ## SAUER NOTE
>
> Before any surgical procedure, the patient should be warned that a hypertrophic scar or keloid could follow the procedure. This is especially frequent following surgery on the chest or upper back.

Differential Diagnosis

Hypertrophic scar: Initially same clinically and histologically as a keloid; flattens spontaneously in most cases after one or several years and does not extend beyond the original site of trauma.

Treatment

Therapy is unsatisfactory. Intralesional corticosteroids after cryospray or massaging with a corticosteroid ointment for 60 seconds daily after bath or shower. Occasionally combined procedures using excision and intralesional corticosteroid injections or interferon α-2b (Intron A) injections have been successful. Silicone sheeting therapy has its advocates.

HEMANGIOMAS
(Fig. 32-17)

Hemangiomas are vascular abnormalities of the skin. Heredity is not a factor in the development of these lesions. There are nine types of hemangiomas, which vary as to depth, clinical appearance, and location:

- Superficial hemangioma
- Cavernous hemangioma
- Mixed hemangioma (when both superficial and cavernous elements are present)
- Spider hemangioma
- Port wine hemangioma
- Nuchal hemangioma
- Capillary hemangioma
- Venous lake
- Angiokeratoma

Superficial and Cavernous Hemangiomas
(see Figs. 3-1D and 33-11)

The familiar bright-red, raised "strawberry" tumor has been seen by all physicians. Strawberries

(*A*) Two spider hemangiomas on the arm of a pregnant woman.

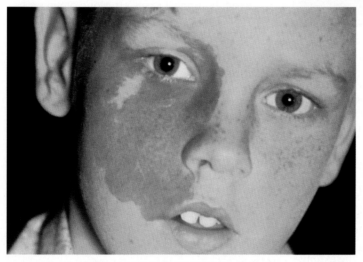

(*B*) Port wine stain on the face of a boy.

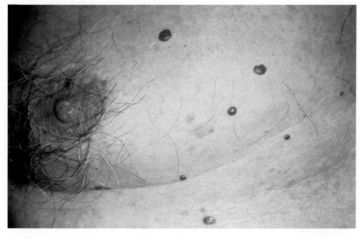

(*C*) Capillary (cherry, senile) angiomas on the chest near the nipple.

Figure 32-17. Hemangiomas. (*Ortho Pharmaceutical Corp.*)

have to grow, and they start from a small beginning. The parents are usually the first to notice the small, red, pinhead-sized, flat lesions. They are noticed at, or soon after, birth. These red tumors can occur on any area of the body and can begin as small lesions and stay that way, remaining as *superficial hemangiomas*, or they can enlarge and extend into the subcutaneous tissue, forming a *cavernous type*. The enlargement can occur rapidly or slowly. Occasionally there can be multiple lesions.

Two aspects of the larger hemangiomas can be disturbing. First, the mere presence of the lesion or lesions causes concern to parents. If the lesion is on an exposed area of the body, this causes additional concern and comment by relatives, neighbors, and other well-meaning persons, which can be most disconcerting.

Second, if the lesion is large and near an eye, the urogenital area, the neck, the rectum, the nose, or the mouth, it can, by its physical size, cause an obstructive problem. Systemic corticosteroids, arterial embolization, cryosurgery, laser surgery, compression, and interferon have been used successfully. Surgery may be indicated. However, even some massive hemangiomas in these areas can be left alone and resolve amazingly over a period of several months.

TREATMENT

The treatment of hemangiomas that are not of the obstructive type has been the subject of considerable discussion. To begin with, the size, the depth, and the location of the hemangiomas, and the pressure on the physician from parents and relatives are factors that must be considered for every case.

There are those who favor treating almost every superficial or cavernous hemangioma, and there are others who believe that all hemangiomas should be left alone to involute spontaneously. The latter group stand behind the studies of our English colleagues, Bowers, Simpson, and others, who showed that around 85% of hemangiomas disappeared without any appreciable scar by the age of 7 years. They also found that the hemangiomas usually stopped growing by the age of 1 year. We advocate the treatment of some hemangiomas, and we leave others alone. Let us illustrate with two case histories.

CASE 1

A 6-week-old child is brought in by her parents. She has a 4×4-mm slightly raised red lesion on her cheek. The parents first noticed it when she was 3 weeks of age, when it was of pinhead size.

1. Reassure the parents that this birthmark is not hereditary and that it will not turn into a cancer.
2. Inform them that this lesion should be treated because it probably will enlarge and could become a significant deformity. If one wishes, one can explain that the lesion, if left alone, might or might not enlarge, and if it does enlarge it will probably disappear without much of a mark in 5 to 7 years. However, treatment at this time is suggested to possibly abort any further growth.
3. A simple form of therapy is cryosurgery with liquid nitrogen.

CASE 2

An 8-month-old girl is brought in by her parents. They state that she has a birthmark on her cheek that began at the age of 3 weeks. Their physician was consulted and stated that the lesion should be watched, because "a lot of them just go away."

At the age of 3 months, the lesion had grown further, but the physician still advised them to wait and watch.

Now at the age of 8 months the red hemangioma measures 12×12×5 mm and has a bluish mass at the base. It is a mixed hemangioma.

1. Reassure the parents that the lesion is not hereditary and that it will not turn into a cancer.
2. Because the child is now 8 months of age, and the lesion has in all probability reached its maximum growth, no treatment is indicated. The parents must be told in no uncertain terms why no treatment is necessary. They are told that you believe it will not enlarge further and that you know from your experience, and that of others, that it will probably be gone by the age of 2 or 3 years and almost certainly by the age of 5 to 7. You can almost predict that the residual mark will be insignificant. However, if it does not disappear completely by that age, the remaining, usually insignificant lesion can be excised.

To *summarize,* the advantages of *early* treatment of *small* superficial or cavernous hemangiomas are as follows: (1) The lesion is eliminated completely, or almost completely; (2) it is not left to chance the fact that it might or might not enlarge considerably; (3) apprehension on the part of the parents and relatives regarding the course of the lesion is alleviated; and (4) with properly applied cryotherapy no mark is left, or only a slight one that would be no worse than that resulting from leaving the hemangioma alone. Other treatments that may be beneficial are high dose systemic or intralesional corticosteroids, surgery, interferon α-2b, embolization, lasers, and pentoxifylline.

The advantages of *not* treating one of these hemangiomas are as follows: (1) The residuum after 5 to 7 years may be better cosmetically than if the lesion had been treated; and (2) the cost of therapy and trauma to the patient is saved.

Spider Hemangioma
(see Fig. 32-17A)

A spider hemangioma consists of a small pinpoint- to pinhead-sized central red arteriole with radiating smaller vessels like the spokes of a wheel or the legs of a spider. These lesions develop for no apparent reason or may develop in association with pregnancy or chronic liver disease. The most common location is on the face. The reason for removal is cosmetic.

DIFFERENTIAL DIAGNOSIS

Venous stars: Small, bluish, telangiectatic veins, usually seen on the legs and the face but may appear anywhere on the body; these can be removed, if desired, by the same method as for spider hemangioma.

Hereditary hemorrhagic telangiectasis (Rendu-Osler-Weber disease) (see Fig. 29-3): Small, red lesions on any organ of the body that can hemorrhage and are numerous on lips and oral mucous membranes as well as far into the gastrointestinal tract; get family history.

TREATMENT

A spider hemangioma is present on the cheek of a young woman who is 6 months postpartum. This lesion developed during her pregnancy and has persisted unchanged.

Electrosurgery is the treatment of choice. The fine epilating needle is used with either a very low coagulating sparking current or a low cutting current. The needle is stuck into the central vessel and the current turned on for 1 or 2 seconds until the vessel blanches. No anesthetic is necessary in most patients. The area will form a scab and heal in about 4 days, leaving an im-

perceptible scar. Rarely, a second treatment is necessary to eliminate the central vessel. If the radiating vessels are large and persistent, they can be treated in the same manner as the central vessel.

> ### SAUER NOTE
> It is advisable to tell the patient that it will be difficult to remove every vessel in a spider hemangioma. To attempt to do so might cause a scar.

Port Wine Hemangioma
(Fig. 32-17B)

The port wine hemangioma is commonly seen on the face as a reddish purple, flat, disfiguring facial mark. It can occur elsewhere in a less extensive form. Faint reddish lesions are often found on infants on the sides of the face, the forehead, the eyelids, and the extremities. The color increases with crying and alarms the mother, but most of these faint lesions disappear shortly after birth. When located above the palpebral tissue it can be associated with underlying hemangioma at the meninges occasionally in association with seizures (Sturge–Weber syndrome).

TREATMENT

An extensive port wine hemangioma is present on the left side of the face of a man.

1. Laser-beam (flash lamp–pulse dye laser) is an effective form of therapy.
2. Cosmetics, such as Dermablend or Covermark, or any good pancake type of makeup, are effective to a certain degree.

Nuchal Hemangioma

Nuchal hemangioma is a common, persistent, faint red patch on the posterior neck region, at or below the scalp margin. It does not disappear with aging, and treatment is not effective or necessary. Because the posterior neck area is also the site of the common lichen simplex chronicus, it is well to remember that following the cure of the lichen simplex a redness that persists could be a nuchal hemangioma that was present for years and not noticed previously.

Capillary Hemangioma
(Fig. 32-17C)

Capillary or cherry hemangiomas are also called senile hemangiomas, but this term obviously should not be used in discussing the lesion with the patient who is in the 30- to 60-year-old age group. These pinhead-sized or slightly larger, bright red, flat or raised tumors are present in many young adults and in practically all elderly persons. They cause no disability except when they are injured and bleed.

Treatment is usually not desired, but if it is, light electrosurgery is effective.

Venous Lake (Varix)

Another vascular lesion that occurs in older persons is a *venous lake*. Clinically, it is a soft, compressible, flat or slightly elevated, bluish-red, 3- to 6-mm lesion, usually located on the lips or the ears. Lack of induration and rapid growth distinguish it from a *melanoma*. Lack of pulsation distinguishes a venous lake on the lower lip from a *tortuous segment of the inferior labial artery*.

Treatment is usually not desired, only reassurance concerning its nonmalignant nature.

Angiokeratomas

Three forms of angiokeratoma are known. *Mibelli's form* occurs on the dorsa of the fingers, the toes, and the knees; *Fabry's form* occurs over the entire trunk in an extensive pattern; and the *Fordyce form* occurs on the scrotum. The lesions are dark-red, pinhead-sized papules with a somewhat warty appearance.

Treatment is not indicated for Mibelli's form and the Fordyce form.

The Fabry form (angiokeratoma corporis diffusum), however, is the cutaneous manifestation of a systemic phospholipid storage disease in which phospholipids are deposited in the skin, as well as in various internal organs. Death usually occurs in the fifth decade from the result of such deposits in the smooth muscles of the blood vessels, in the heart, and in the kidneys (see Chap. 26).

NEVUS CELL TUMORS

Classification

MELANOCYTIC NEVI

1. Junctional or active nevus

2. Intradermal or resting nevus
3. Dysplastic nevus syndrome

MALIGNANT MELANOMA

Melanocytic Nevi
(Figs. 32-18A–E and 34-16)

Nevi are pigmented or nonpigmented tumors of the skin that contain nevus cells. Nevi are present on every adult, but some persons have more than others. There are two main questions concerning nevi or moles: When and how should they be removed? What is the relationship between nevi and malignant melanomas?

Histologically, it is possible to divide benign nevi into *junctional* or *active nevi* and *intradermal* or *resting nevi*. Combinations of these two forms commonly exist and are labeled compound nevi.

In the *dysplastic nevus syndrome (familial atypical mole–melanoma syndrome)*, the nevi are more numerous and larger than ordinary (usually 5 to 15 mm in size), have an irregular border, and show a haphazard mixture of tan, brown, pink, and black. There is a propensity for this type of nevus, especially when familial, to develop into malignant melanomas.

Clinically, one never can be positive with which histopathologic type of nevus one is dealing, but certain criteria are helpful in establishing a differentiation between the forms.

DESCRIPTION. Clinically, nevi can be pigmented or nonpigmented, flat or elevated, hairy or nonhairy, warty, papillomatous, or pedunculated. They can have a small or a wide base. The brown- or black-pigmented, flat or slightly elevated, nonhairy nevi are usually junctional nevi. The nonpigmented or pigmented, elevated, hairy nevi are more likely to be the intradermal nevi.

A nevus with a depigmented area surrounding it is called a *halo nevus* or *leukoderma acquisitum centrifugum* (see Fig. 32-18D). The nevus in the center of the halo that histologically has an inflammatory infiltrate usually involutes in several months in contradistinction to the rarer noninflammatory halo nevus. Excision of the halo nevus is usually not indicated unless the central nevus has the appearance of melanoma.

DISTRIBUTION. Nevi are very prevalent on the head and the neck but may be on any part of the body. The nevi on the palms, the soles, and the genitalia are usually junctional nevi.

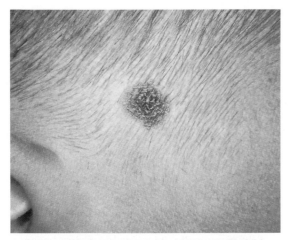

(*A*) Junctional nevus in scalp of 12-year-old child.

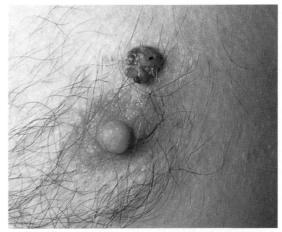

(*B*) Compound nevus, on chest above nipple.

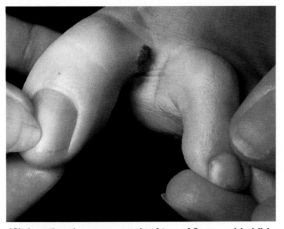

(*C*) Junctional nevus on web of toe of 8-year-old child.

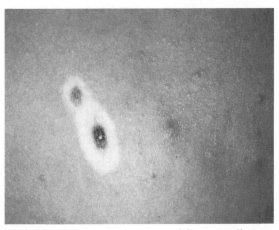

(*D*) Halo nevus, or leukoderma acquisitum centrifugum, on the back.

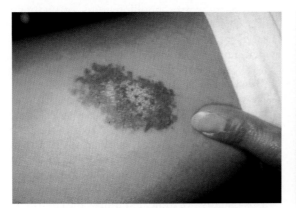

(*E*) Giant pigmented nevus on thigh.

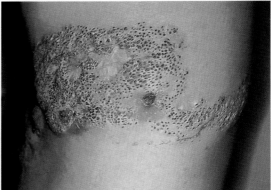

(*F*) Nevus comedonicus on abdomen.

Figure 32-18. **Nevus cell tumors.** (*The Upjohn Company*)

COURSE. A child is born with no, or relatively few, nevi, but with increasing age, particularly after puberty, nevi slowly become larger, can remain flat or become elevated, and may become hairy and darker. A change is also seen histologically with age. A junctional-type active nevus, although it may remain as such throughout the life of the person, more commonly changes slowly into an intradermal or resting nevus. Some nevi do not become evident until adult or later life, but the precursor cells for the nevus were present at birth. A malignant melanoma can originate from a junctional nevus, compound nevus, very rarely an intradermal nevus, and from dysplastic nevi, particularly in relationship to ultraviolet exposure. Most melanomas arise *de novo*. A benign junctional nevus in a child can histologically look like a malignant melanoma. Known as a *Spitz nevus*, this poses a difficult diagnostic and management problem. It is usually a dome-shaped reddish-brown tumor and rarely can occur in adults.

HISTOGENESIS. The origin of the nevus cell is disputed, but the most commonly accepted theory is that it originates from melanocytes.

Differential Diagnosis

IN CHILDHOOD

Warts: Flat or common warts not on the hands or the feet may be difficult to differentiate clinically; should see warty growth with black "seeds" (the capillary loops), rather acute onset, and rapid growth (see Chap. 17).
Freckles: On exposed areas of the body; many lesions; fade in winter; not raised.
Blue nevus: Flat or elevated, soft, dark bluish or black nodule.
Granuloma pyogenicum: Rapid onset of reddish or blackish vascular tumor, usually at site of injury and often with history of bleeding.
Molluscum contagiosum: One, or usually more, crater-shaped, waxy tumors (see Chap. 17).
Urticaria pigmentosa: Single, or multiple slightly elevated, yellowish to brown papules that urticate with trauma (see Chap. 26).

IN ADULTHOOD

Warts: Usually rather obvious; black "seeds" (see Chap. 17).
Pedunculated fibromas: On neck and axillae (see earlier in this chapter).

Histiocytoma (see Fig. 32-15): On anterior tibial area of leg; flat, button-like in consistency (see earlier in this chapter).

Other epidermal and mesodermal tumors are differentiated histologically.

IN OLDER ADULTS

Actinic or senile keratosis: On exposed areas; scaly surrounding skin usually thin and dry; not a sharply demarcated lesion (see earlier in this chapter).
Seborrheic keratosis: Greasy, waxy, warty tumor, "stuck on" the skin; however, some are difficult to differentiate clinically from nevus or malignant melanoma (see earlier in this chapter).
Lentigo: Flat, tan or brown spot, usually on exposed skin surface, sometimes appears as a small splotchy, splash of flat black color (solar ink-spot lentigo).
Malignant melanoma (Fig. 32-19 and see Fig. 34-2C): Seen at site of junction nevus or can arise from skin that appears normal, shows a change in pigmentation either by spreading, becoming spotty, or turning darker; may bleed, form a crust, or ulcerate (see following section).
Basal cell carcinomas and squamous cell carcinomas: If there is any question of malignancy, a biopsy is indicated (see earlier in this chapter).

Treatment

CASE 1

A mother comes into your office with her 5-year-old son, who has an 8x8-mm flat, brown nevus on the forehead. She wants to know if this "mole" is dangerous and if it should be removed.

1. Examine the lesion carefully. This lesion shows no sign of recent growth or change in pigmentation. (If it did, it should be excised and examined histologically.)
2. Reassure the mother that this mole does not appear to be dangerous and that it would be unusual for it to become dangerous. If any change in the color or growth appears, the lesion should be examined again.
3. Tell the mother that it is best to leave this nevus alone at this time. The only treatment would be surgical excision, and you are quite sure that her boy would not sit tight for this

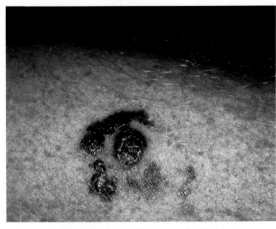

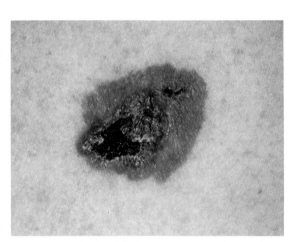

(*A*) Malignant melanoma, on arm.

(*B*) Malignant melanoma in a nevus present since birth, on the scapular area.

Figure 32-19.   **Malignant melanomas.** (*The Upjohn Company*)

procedure unless he was given a general anesthetic. When the boy is 16 years of age or older, the lesion can be examined again and possibly removed at that time by a simpler method under local anesthesia.

CASE 2

A 25-year-old woman desires a brown, raised, hairy nevus on her upper lip removed. There has been no recent change in the tumor.

1. Examine the lesion carefully for induration, scaling, ulceration, and bleeding. None of these signs is present. (If the diagnosis is not definite, a scissor biopsy may be performed safely and the base gently coagulated by electrosurgery or Monsel solution applied. Further treatment depends on the biopsy report.)
2. Tell the patient that you can perform a biopsy and remove the mole safely but that there will be a residual, very slightly depressed scar and that probably the hairs will have to be removed separately after the first surgery has healed.
3. Surgical excision with tissue examination is the best method of removal. However, hairy, raised, pigmented nevi have been removed by shave excision with biopsy for years with no proof that this form of removal has caused a malignant melanoma.
4. First, following local anesthesia, perform a shave biopsy. Then electrosurgery can be

done with the coagulating or cutting current or with cautery or applying aluminum chloride or Monsel solution. The site should not be covered and will heal in 7 to 14 days, depending on the size. If the hairs regrow, they can be removed later by electrosurgical epilation (see Chap. 6).

SAUER NOTES: DO'S AND DON'TS REGARDING NEVI

1. Don't remove a nevus in a child by electrosurgery or laser; remove only by surgical excision and submit nevus for histopathologic examination.
2. Do remember that in a child a benign junctional nevus may resemble a malignant melanoma histologically (Spitz nevus). Don't alarm the parents unnecessarily, because these nevi are no threat to life.
3. Don't remove a flat pigmented nevus, particularly on the palm, the sole, or the genitalia, by electrosurgery or laser. These should be excised surgically, if indicated, and should be examined histologically.
4. Don't remove any suspicious nevus by electrosurgery or laser. Excise it and examine it histologically.

5. Don't perform a radical deforming surgical procedure on a possible malignant melanoma until the biopsy report has been returned. Many of these tumors can turn out to be seborrheic keratoses, granuloma pyogenicum, and so on.

MALIGNANT MELANOMA
(Fig. 32-19)

The incidence of malignant melanoma has increased considerably in the past 2 decades. Predisposing factors for the development of malignant melanoma include heredity, complexion (fair skin, red or blonde hair, blue eyes), ultraviolet exposure (the incidence of melanoma in the United States is increased in those states nearer the equator or with milder winters so people are outside more with less clothing), and the presence of large *bathing-trunk congenital nevi* (greater than 20 cm). The person with hereditary dysplastic nevi is more prone to develop a malignant melanoma. An appreciable percentage of melanomas arise from preexisting nevi. Although melanomas make up only 1% of all skin cancers, they account for over 60% of the deaths due to skin cancer in the United States. The incidence of malignant melanoma is increasing faster than any other cancer. The best chance for a cure lies in early diagnosis and prompt, adequate treatment of the primary lesion.

There are four major types of malignant melanomas. They differ in terms of mode of onset, course, prognosis, and incidence.

1. The most common melanoma is the *superficial spreading melanoma*, which develops from an *in situ* lesion. It grows slowly with a resulting good prognosis.
2. *Nodular melanomas* grow quite rapidly and have a poorer prognosis.
3. *Acral lentiginous melanoma*, the least frequent type, occurs, as the title signifies, on the palms, soles, and around the nails as well as perioral and perirectal; is the most common type seen in African-Americans or dark skinned Caucasians; ulcerates; and metastasizes rapidly, so that it has a poor prognosis.
4. *Lentigo maligna melanoma* develops from a lentigo maligna, occurs on the exposed areas of the body in the elderly, mainly on the fore-

arms and face, grows slowly peripherally, and has a high survival rate.

DESCRIPTION. The classic malignant melanoma is a black or purple nodule, but it may be flat or pedunculated and may be pink, red, tan, brown, or black or have no color (amelanotic).

The changes in a recent or longstanding skin lesion that should arouse suspicion include change in the size or shape, change in pigmentation (particularly the development of pseudopodia or areas of satellite pigmentation or leakage of pigment into surrounding skin), erythema surrounding the lesion, induration, friability with easy bleeding tendency, and ulceration.

DISTRIBUTION. The site of predilection for a melanoma varies with the type of lesion. The superficial spreading melanoma is seen most commonly on the backs of males and the legs of women, in areas of sunburns. The nodular melanoma is seen in any location, more frequently in males. The acral type is seen, as indicated, on the palms and soles, and the lentigo maligna melanoma occurs mainly on face and arms in areas of chronic sun exposure.

COURSE. The greater the depth of involvement of the growth, the worse the prognosis. Clark has defined five levels of invasion; Breslow measured the tumor thickness with a micrometer placed in the eyepiece of the microscope. Risk groups have been defined using these measurements (Table 32-2). For instance, a melanoma less than 0.76 mm thick and not invading the reticular dermis is in a low-risk group. Regional lymph-node involvement or distant metastases

TABLE 32-2
MALIGNANT MELANOMA STAGES ACCORDING TO THE AMERICAN JOINT COMMITTEE ON CANCER (AJCC)

Stage 1a	Disease localized to skin with thickness ≤ 0.75 mm
Stage 1b	Disease localized to skin with thickness 0.75 to 1.5 mm
Stage IIa	Disease localized to skin with thickness 1.5 to 4.0 mm
Stage IIb	Disease localized to skin with thickness ≥ 4.0 mm
Stage III	In transit metastasis or regional lymph node involvement
Stage IV	Distant involvement

gravely affect the prognosis. The most common sites of distant metastases to other organs are the lung, liver, brain, and bowel.

HISTOPATHOLOGY. The histopathologic diagnosis of melanoma can be difficult at times. An adequate biopsy or, better yet, an initial complete excisional biopsy provides the most information.

Differential Diagnosis

Benign nevus: No recent change in lesion, not black, border smooth, single color, symmetrical, no bleeding; hairy nevi are most frequently benign, but if there is any question as to the diagnosis, a biopsy, preferably by complete excision, is indicated.

The other lesions to be thought of in the differential diagnosis are the same as under nevi (see earlier section), with the addition of a pigmented basal cell epithelioma (biopsy indicated for diagnosis) and a subungual hematoma (history of recent injury; if in doubt, perform a biopsy).

Treatment

Rapid and adequate therapy is indicated after the diagnosis and staging are completed. The procedures include wide surgical excision, lymph node dissection (often involving sentinel lymph node biopsy involving gamma probe guidance as the initial step), chemotherapy, and immunotherapy.

LYMPHOMAS
(Table 32-3)

Mycosis Fungoides (Cutaneous T-Cell Lymphoma)
(see Fig 26-8A-C)

This polymorphous lymphoma involves the skin only, except in some rare cases that terminally invade the lymph nodes and the visceral organs. As is true with most lymphomas, the histology may change gradually to another form of lymphoma, with progression of the disease. However, most cases of mycosis fungoides begin as such and terminate unchanged.

Mycosis fungoides is a T (thymus-derived) helper cell lymphocyte malignancy. The name *cutaneous T-cell lymphoma* is preferred by many.

Monoclonal antibodies and gene rearrangement studies may help in the histologic diagnosis of this disease.

Associations with human T-cell lymphotrophic virus types I and II and Epstein-Barr virus are found in some patients with mycosis fungoides.

DESCRIPTION. The clinical picture of this disease is classic and is divided into three stages: the erythematous stage, the plaque stage, and the tu-

TABLE 32-3
LYMPHOMAS OF SKIN

	T-cell Lymphoma	B-cell Lymphoma
Indolent	Mycosis fungoides	Follicle center cell lymphoma
	Mycosis fungoides-associated follicular mucinosis	Immunocytoma (marginal zone B-cell lymphoma)
	Pagetoid reticulosis	
	CD30+ cutaneous large T-cell (anaplastic; immunoblastic; pleomorphic)	
	Lymphomatoid papulosis	
Intermediate	—	Large B-cell lymphoma of the leg
Aggressive	Sézary syndrome	—
	CD30-negative cutaneous large T-cell lymphoma (immunoblastic; pleomorphic)	
Provisional	Granulomatous slack skin	Intravascular large B-cell lymphoma
	Cutaneous T-cell lymphoma, small/medium-sized	Plasmacytoma
	Subcutaneous panniculitis-like T-cell lymphoma	

Chan JKC. Is the REAL Classification for Real? Do We Need a Separate Classification for Cutaneous Lymphomas? Advances in Anatomic Pathology 1997; 4:6.

mor stage. The course usually proceeds in order, but all stages may be evident at the same time, or the first two stages may be bypassed (the d'emblée type of tumor stage mycosis fungoides).

Erythematous stage: Commonly seen are scaly, red, rather sharply defined patches that resemble atopic eczema, psoriasis, or parapsoriasis. The eruption may become diffuse as an *exfoliative dermatitis*. Itching is usually quite severe.

Plaque stage: The red scaly patches develop induration and some elevation, with central healing that results in ring-shaped lesions. This stage is to be differentiated from tertiary syphilis, psoriasis, erythema multiforme perstans, mycotic infections, and other lymphomas.

Tumor stage: This terminal stage is characterized by nodular and tumor growths of the plaques, often with ulceration and secondary bacterial infection. These tumors are to be differentiated from any of the granulomas (see Chap. 20). Prognosis is poor.

COURSE. The early stages may progress slowly, with exacerbations and remissions over many years, or the disease may be rapidly fulminating. Once the tumor stage is reached, the eventual fatal outcome is more imminent. Gene rearrangement studies may help make the diagnosis in skin lesions and may help predict the prognosis of positive lymphadenopathy.

TREATMENT

The combined services of a dermatologist, an oncologist, a radiologist, and an internist or a hematologist are required for the management of this sometimes fatal disease.

Locally, for early cases, a tar cream (LCD 5% in a water-washable base or in a corticosteroid cream) plus ultraviolet B therapy is quite beneficial. PUVA therapy (see Chap. 6) is also temporarily effective in resolving lesions. Local nitrogen mustard solution or ointment on the erythematous- and plaque-stage lesions has proved to be effective for some cases.

Use of systemic therapy depends on the stage and extent of the disease. Most therapists believe that one should treat the symptoms and signs only as they appear. Corticosteroids are quite helpful, especially for the first two stages. Radiation therapy for the superficial type is effective for plaque and small tumor lesions; electron-beam radiation therapy can be administered

to the total body, either early or late in the disease.

Systemic chemotherapeutic agents enter into the therapy routine in the plaque and tumor stages of mycosis fungoides but are usually unsuccessful. These include the alkylating agents cyclophosphamide (Cytoxan), chlorambucil (Leukeran), and nitrogen mustard; the plant alkaloid vincristine (Oncovin); the antimetabolite methotrexate; the antibiotic doxorubicin (Adriamycin); and the antibiotic derivative bleomycin (Blenoxane). Monoclonal antibodies are also being used for therapy, as is interferon α-2a. Extracorporeal photophoresis therapy and systemic retinoids are other recent therapeutic modalities. A specific retinoid (LGD 1069, Tegretin) acting on RXR retinoid receptors is currently being tested.

COMPLETE HISTOLOGIC CLASSIFICATION

A histologic classification of tumors of the skin is listed here. Those tumors discussed in the first part of this chapter are marked with an asterisk. The rarer tumors listed are defined. This classification is modified from Lever and Schaumberg-Lever (1997).

SAUER NOTE

A histologic examination of tissue is indicated for a definite diagnosis of most growths of the skin.

I. EPIDERMAL TUMORS

A. Tumors of the Surface Epidermis
1. Benign tumors
   a. Linear epidermal nevus (Fig. 32-20): a rather common tumor usually present at birth, consisting of single or multiple lesions in various forms that give rise to several clinical designations, such as hard nevus, nevus verrucous, nevus unius lateris, papilloma, and, when systematized (more generalized), ichthyosis hystrix. No nevus cells are present.
   *b. Seborrheic keratosis and dermatosis papulosa nigra
   *c. fibroma
   d. Cysts
      *1) Epidermal cyst

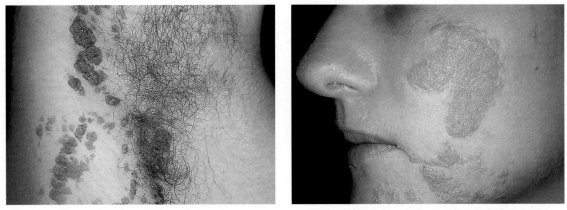

(*A*) Linear epidermal nevus in axilla. (*B*) Nevus unius lateris of face.

Figure 32-20. **Rarer tumors of the skin.** (*Owen/ Galderma*)

*2) Trichilemmal, pilar, or sebaceous cyst
3) Steatocystoma multiplex: a dominantly inherited condition with small, moderately firm, cystic nodules adherent to the overlying skin, which on incision yield an oily fluid
*4) Milium
*5) Dermoid cyst
*6) Mucous retention cyst
e. Clear cell acanthoma: a rare, usually single, slightly elevated, flat, pale red, scaling nodule less than 2 cm in diameter, nearly always located on the lower extremities.
f. Warty dyskeratoma: a solitary warty lesion with a central keratotic plug, most commonly seen on the scalp, face, and neck.
*g. Keratoacanthoma
2. Precancerous tumors
*a. Senile or actinic keratosis and cutaneous horn
*b. Arsenical keratosis
*c. Leukoplakia
3. Epitheliomas and carcinomas
*a. Basal cell carcinoma
*b. Squamous cell carcinoma
c. Bowen's disease and erythroplasia of Queyrat: Bowen's disease is a single red scaly lesion with a sharp but irregular border that grows slowly by peripheral extension. Histologically, it is an intraepidermal squamous cell carcinoma (Fig. 32-21). Erythroplasia of Queyrat (see Fig. 34-14D) represents Bowen's disease of the mucous membranes and occurs on the glans penis and rarely on the vulva. The lesion has a bright red, velvety surface.
d. Paget's disease (see Fig. 34-14C): a unilat-

eral scaly red lesion resembling a dermatitis, usually present on the female nipple, but the lesion can be extramammary. The early lesion on the nipple is an intraductal carcinoma that also involves the mammary ducts and deeper connective tissue. In the perirectal area it can be associated with underlying bowel cancer.

B. Tumors of the Epidermal Appendages
1. Nevoid tumors
a. Organic nevi or hamartomas
1) Sebaceous nevi
a) Nevus sebaceous (Jadassohn) (Fig. 32-22): seen on the scalp or face as a single lesion present from birth, slightly raised, firm, hairless, yellowish, with furrowed surface. Large examples may be associated

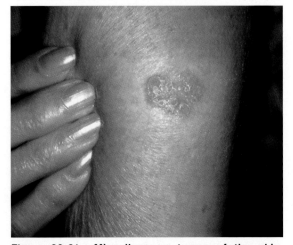

Figure 32-21. **Miscellaneous tumor of the skin.** Bowen's disease, on arm. (*Syntex Laboratories, Inc.*)

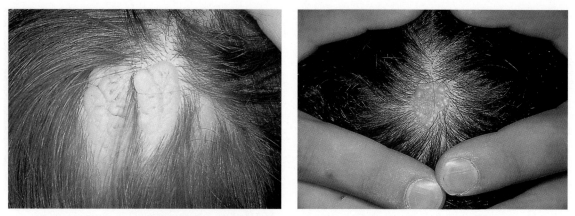

(*A*) Nevus sebaceous of Jadassohn on scalp. (*B*) Nevus sebaceous on scalp.

Figure 32-22.   **Rarer tumors of the skin.** (*Owen/ Galderma*)

with a "neurocutaneous syndrome" of epilepsy and mental retardation. Basal cell and squamous cell carcinomas can develop within these growths in approximately 10% of cases.

b) Adenoma sebaceum (Pringle's disease): part of a triad of epilepsy, mental deficiency, and the skin lesions of adenoma sebaceum. This is called tuberous sclerosis. The skin lesions occur on the face and consist of yellowish brown, papular, nodular lesions with telangiectases. Histopathology shows an angiofibroma (see Chap. 26).

c) Sebaceous hyperplasia (Fig. 32-23): very common on the face in older persons and consists of one or several small, yellowish, translucent, slightly umbilicated nodules

d) Fordyce's disease (see Chap. 29): a rather common condition of pinpoint-sized yellowish lesions of the vermilion border of the lips or the oral mucosa

b. Adenomas or organoid hamartomas

1) Sebaceous Adenoma: a very rare solitary tumor of the face or the scalp, smooth, firm, elevated, often slightly pedunculated, and measuring less than 1 cm in diameter; may be associated with an adenocarcinoma of the bowel (Muir-Torre syndrome)

2) Apocrine adenomas

a) Syringocystadenoma Papilliferum (Fig. 32-24): This adenoma of the apocrine ducts appears as a single verrucous plaque, usually seen on the scalp. Basal cell epitheliomatous change occasionally does occur. May arise in sebaceous nevi.

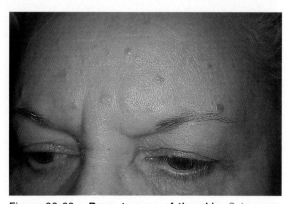

Figure 32-23.   **Rarer tumors of the skin.** Sebaceous gland hyperplasia (common).

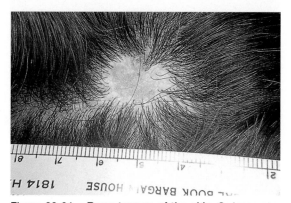

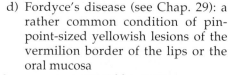

Figure 32-24.   **Rarer tumors of the skin.** Syringocystadenoma papilliferum. (*Owen/Galderma*)

b) Hidradenoma papilliferum: This adenoma of the apocrine glands occurs almost exclusively on the labia majora and the perineum of women as a single, intracutaneous, benign tumor covered by normal epidermis.

c. Benign epitheliomas or suborganoid hamartomas
  1) Apocrine epitheliomas
    a) Syringoma: This is characterized by the appearance of pinhead-sized soft, yellowish nodules at the age of puberty in women, developing around the eyelids, the chest, the abdomen, and the anterior aspects of the thighs.
    b) Cylindroma (Fig. 32-25): These appear as numerous smooth, rounded tumors of various size on the scalp in adults and resemble bunches of grapes or tomatoes. These tumors may cover the entire scalp like a turban and are then referred to as turban tumors.
  2) Hair epitheliomas
    a) Trichoepithelioma (Fig. 32-26): also known as epithelioma adenoides cysticum and multiple benign cystic epithelioma when multiple. This begins at the age of puberty, frequently on a hereditary basis, and is characterized by the presence of numerous pinhead- to pea-sized, rounded, yellowish or pink nodules on the face and occasionally on the upper trunk. May also appear as a single lesion that can be confused with a basal cell cancer histologically.

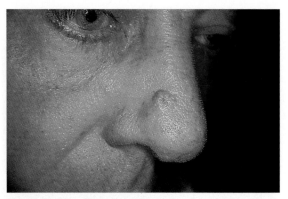

Figure 32-26. **Rarer tumors of the skin.** Trichoepithelioma on nose. (*Owen/Galderma*)

    b) Calcifying epithelioma (Malherbe) (Fig. 32-27) or pilomatrixoma (see Fig. 29-6): Malignant degeneration is very rare. There is a perforating form.
  3) Eccrine epitheliomas
    a) Eccrine spiradenoma (Fig. 32-28): a rare, usually solitary, intradermal, firm, tender nodule
    b) Clear cell hidradenoma: a rare, well-circumscribed, often encapsulated tumor of dermis and subcutaneous tissue
    c) Eccrine poroma (Fig. 32-29): This occurs as an asymptomatic solitary tumor on the soles and the palms.

2. Carcinomas of sebaceous glands and eccrine and apocrine sweat glands (rare)

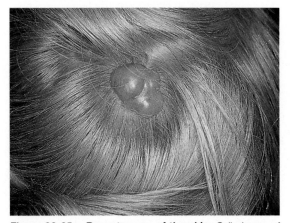

Figure 32-25. **Rarer tumors of the skin.** Cylindroma of the scalp.

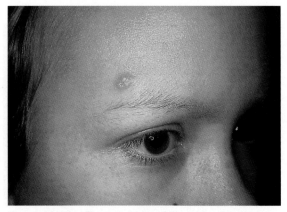

Figure 32-27. **Rarer tumors of the skin.** Calcifying epithelioma of Malherbe on forehead. (*Owen/Galderma*)

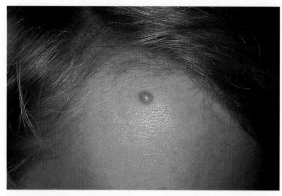

Figure 32-28. **Rarer tumors of the skin.** Eccrine spiro-adenoma of forehead.

C. Metastatic Carcinoma of the Skin

This occurs frequently from carcinoma of the breast and melanoma but rarely from other internal carcinomas. Metastatic carcinoid nodules may appear in the skin, as well as in lymph nodes and the liver. The primary tumor and the metastases produce excess 5-hydroxytryptamine (serotonin), which in turn produces attacks of flushing of the skin.

II. MESODERMAL TUMORS

A. Tumors of Fibrous Tissue
*1. Histiocytoma and dermatofibroma
*2. Keloid
3. Fibrosarcomas
   a. True fibrosarcoma: a rare tumor that starts most commonly in the subcutaneous fat, grows rapidly, causes the overlying skin to appear purplish, and finally ulcerates
   b. Dermatofibrosarcoma protuberans: a tumor that grows slowly in the corium and

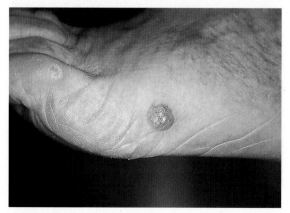

Figure 32-29. **Rarer tumors of the skin.** Eccrine poroma on foot.

spreads by the development of adjoining reddish or bluish nodules that may coalesce to form a plaque that can eventually ulcerate. Margins are very difficult to evaluate making recurrence common. Mohs' surgery and positive CD34 immunohistochemical staining are helpful.

B. Tumors of Mucoid Tissue
1. Myxoma: clinically seen as fairly well circumscribed, rather soft intracutaneous tumors with normal overlying epidermis
2. Myxosarcoma: subcutaneous tumors that eventually ulcerate the skin
*3. Synovial cyst of the skin

C. Tumors of Fatty Tissue
1. Nevus lipomatosus superficialis: a rare, circumscribed nodular lesion, usually in the gluteal area
2. Lipoma: a rather common tumor that can be multiple or single, lobulated, of varying size, and in the subcutaneous tissue
3. Hibernoma: a form of lipoma composed of embryonic type of fat cells
4. Liposarcoma
5. Malignant hibernoma

D. Tumors of Nerve Tissue and Mesodermal-Nerve Sheath Cells
1. Neuroma: rare, single or multiple small reddish or brown nodules that are usually tender as well as painful.
2. Neurofibroma: benign flesh-colored soft tumor that is frequently single, but when multiple it is associated with neurofibromatosis; when very large it is called a plexiform neuroma. Can have sarcomatous degeneration.
3. Neurofibromatosis (see Figs. 26-13, 31-4C, and 33-6). Also known as von Recklinghausen's disease, this hereditary disease classically consists of pigmented patches (café-au-lait spots), pedunculated skin tumors, and nerve tumors. All of these lesions may not be present in a particular case.
4. Neurilemoma
5. Granular cell schwannoma or myoblastoma. From neural sheath cells, this appears usually as a solitary tumor of the tongue, the skin, or the subcutaneous tissue.
6. Malignant granular cell schwannoma or myoblastoma

E. Tumors of Vascular Tissue
*1. Hemangioma
2. Granuloma pyogenicum (Fig. 32-30): Also known as "proud flesh," this is a rather com-

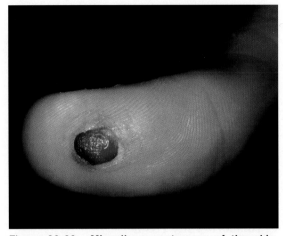

Figure 32-30. Miscellaneous tumors of the skin.
Granuloma pyogenicum on thumb. (*Syntex Laboratories, Inc.*)

mon end result of an injury to the skin that may or may not have been apparent. Vascular proliferation, with or without infection, produces a small red tumor that bleeds easily. It is to be differentiated from a malignant melanoma. Biopsy and mild electrocoagulation are curative.

3. Osler's disease: See Rendu-Osler-Weber disease in the Dictionary–Index.
4. Lymphangioma: A superficial form, lymphangioma circumscriptum, appears as a group of thin-walled vesicles on the skin surface, whereas the deeper variety, lymphangioma cavernosum, causes a poorly defined enlargement of the affected area, such as the lip or the tongue. Large lymphatic cisternae may underlie apparently superficial tumors.
5. Glomus tumor: a rather unusual small, deep-seated, red or purplish nodule that is tender and may produce severe paroxysmal pains. The solitary lesion is usually seen under a nail plate, on the fingertips, or elsewhere on the body and may erode underlying bone.
6. Hemangiopericytoma
7. Kaposi's sarcoma (multiple idiopathic hemorrhagic sarcoma) (Fig. 32-31 and see Figs. 18-6 and 18-11): most commonly seen on the feet and the ankles as multiple bluish red or dark brown nodules and plaques associated with visceral lesions. Sarcomatous malignant degeneration can occur.

   Kaposi's sarcoma is also seen as part of the acquired immunodeficiency syndrome (see Chap. 18). In this complex, the sarcoma lesions are small, oval, red or pink papules that occur on any area of the body.

   Both AIDS-related and non–AIDS-related Kaposi's sarcoma have been associated with human herpesvirus simplex type 8, which is also called Kaposi's sarcoma herpesvirus.
8. Hemangioendothelioma
9. Postmastectomy lymphangiosarcoma (Stewart–Treves syndrome)

F. Tumors of Muscular Tissue

1. Leiomyoma: solitary leiomyomas may be found on the extremities and on the scrotum, whereas multiple leiomyomas occur on the back and elsewhere as pinhead- to pea-sized, brown or bluish, firm, elevated nodules. Both forms are painful and sensitive to pressure, particularly as they enlarge.
2. Leiomyosarcoma: very rare

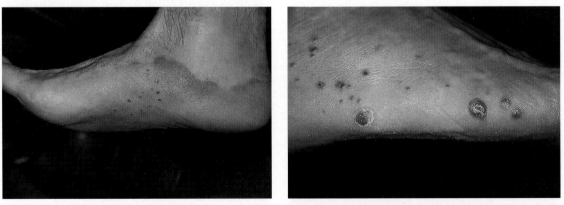

(*A*) Kaposi's sarcoma of foot. (*B*) Kaposi's sarcoma of foot.
Figure 32-31. Rarer tumors of the skin. (*Owen/ Galderma*)

G. Tumors of Osseous Tissue
1. Osteoma cutis
   a. Primary: The primary form of osteoma cutis develops from embryonal cell rests; these may be single or multiple.
   b. Secondary: Secondary bone formation may occur as a form of tissue degeneration in tumors, in scar tissue (such as acne), in scleroderma lesions, and in various granulomas.

H. Tumors of Cartilaginous Tissue
1. Nodular chondrodermatitis of the ear: a painful, hyperkeratotic nodule, usually on the inner rim of the helix of the ear of elderly males

III. NEVUS CELL TUMORS

A. Melanocytic Nevi
*1. Junctional (active) nevus
*2. Intradermal (resting) nevus
*3. Dysplastic nevus syndrome
4. Lentigines. These are to be differentiated from freckles (ephelides). A freckle histologically shows hyperpigmentation of the basal layer but no elongation of the rete pegs and no increase in the number of clear cells and dendritic cells. Juvenile lentigines (lentigo simplex) begin to appear in childhood and occur on all parts of the body. Senile lentigines (see Fig. 34-2), also known as "liver spots," occur in elderly persons on the dorsa of the hands, the forearms, and the face. Solar ink-spot lentigo is commonly seen on sun-exposed areas and has a characteristic black, splotchy, reticulated pattern. Lentigo maligna melanoma (see Fig. 33-8) is a dark brown or black macular, malignant lesion, usually on the face or arms of elderly persons, that has a slow peripheral growth (see under Malignant Melanoma earlier). Lentigines can be caused by ionizing radiation, a tanning bed, a sunlamp, PUVA therapy, and, most commonly, from sun exposure.
5. Mongolian spots (see Fig. 33-8). These are seen chiefly in Asian or African-American infants, usually around the buttocks. They disappear spontaneously during childhood.
   Related bluish patchy lesions are the nevus of Ota, seen on the side of the face, and the nevus of Ito, located in the supraclavicular, scapular, and deltoid regions. Laser therapy may be beneficial.
6. Blue nevus. Clinically, the blue nevus appears as a slate blue or bluish black, sharply circumscribed, flat or slightly elevated nodule, occurring on any area of the body. It originates from mesodermal cells.

*B. Malignant Melanoma

IV. LYMPHOMAS (SEE CHAP. 24)

A. Monomorphous Group
The non-Hodgkin's lymphomas are referred to as monomorphous lymphomas because, in contrast to Hodgkin's disease, they lack a significant admixture of inflammatory cells and are composed almost entirely of lymphoma cells largely derived from B lymphocytes or T lymphocytes. A classification of cutaneous lymphomas follows:

Lymphomas may have specific skin lesions containing the lymphomatous infiltrate, or nonspecific lesions may be seen. These latter consist of macules, papules, tumors, purpuric lesions, blisters, eczematous lesions, exfoliative dermatitis, and secondarily infected excoriations.

B. Polymorphous Group
1. Hodgkin's disease. Specific lesions are very rare, but nonspecific dermatoses are rather commonly seen.
*2. Mycosis fungoides
   a. Sézary's syndrome: This is a very rare form of exfoliative dermatitis (see Chap. 23) that occurs at an early stage of a lymphoma. It is diagnosed by finding unusually large monocytoid cells (so-called Sézary cells) in the blood and in the skin. This cell is indistinguishable from the mycosis cell, both of which are derived from the T cell.

V. MYELOSIS (SEE FIG. 26-2)

1. Leukemia: refers to circulating abnormal blood cells; may be seen along with lymphomas, but it is almost always associated with myelosis, such as myeloid leukemia. Cutaneous lesions are quite uncommon but may be specific or nonspecific.

VI. PSEUDOLYMPHOMA OF SPIEGLER-FENDT (SEE DICTIONARY–INDEX, FIG. 2C)

A benign, localized erythematous, nodular dermatosis usually on the face, with clinical and histologic features that make a distinction from lymphoma difficult. Some cases may eventually be diagnosed as a lymphoma.

BIBLIOGRAPHY

Abel EA, Wood GS, Hoppe RT. Mycosis fungoides: Clinical and histologic features, staging, evaluation, and approach to treatment. Cancer 1993;43:93.

Barnes LM, Nordlun JJ. The natural history of dysplastic nevi. Arch Dermatol 1987;123:1059.

Barnhill RL. Color atlas and synopsis of pigmented lesions. New York, McGraw-Hill, 1995.

Bernstein SC, Lim KK, Brodland DG, Heidelberg KA. The many faces of squamous cell carcinoma. Dermatol Surg 1996;22:243.

Bowers RE, Graham EA, Tomlinson KM. The natural history of the strawberry nevus. Arch Dermatol 1960;82:667.

Dalton JA, et al. Cutaneous T-cell lymphoma. Int J Dermatol 1997;36:801.

Drake LA, Ceilley RI, et al. Guidelines of care for actinic keratoses. J Am Acad Dermatol 1995;32:1.

Drake LA, Salasche SJ, Ceilley RI, et al. Guidelines of care for basal cell carcinoma. J Am Acad Dermatol 1992;26:117.

Drake LA, Ceilley RI, et al. Guideleines of care for nevi: II. Nonmelanocytic nevi, hamartomas, neoplasms, and potentially malignant lesions. J Am Acad Dermatol 1995;32:1.

Drake LA, Chanco Turner ML, Ceilley RI, et al. Guidelines of care for malignant melanoma. J Am Acad Dermatol 1993;28:638.

Drake LA, Salasche S, Ceilley RI, et al. Guidelines of care for cutaneous squamous cell carcinoma. J Am Acad Dermatol 1993;28:628.

Frieden IJ, et al. Guidelines of care of hemangiomas of infancy. J Am Acad Dermatol 1997;37:4.

Friedman RJ, Rigel DS, Kopf AW, Harris MN, Baker D. Cancer of the skin. Philadelphia, Harcourt Brace Jovanovich, 1990.

Johnson TM, Rowe DE, Nelson BR, et al. Squamous cell carcinoma of the skin (excluding lip and oral mucosa). J Am Acad Dermatol 1992;26:467.

Lever WF, Schaumburg-Lever G. Histopathology of the skin, ed 8. Philadelphia, JB Lippincott, 1997.

MacKie RM. Nevi as risk factors for melanoma. Pediatr Dermatol 1992;9:340.

Moy RL. Practical management of skin cancer. Philadelphia, Lippincott–Raven Publishers, 1998.

Preston DS. Nonmelanoma cancers of the skin. N Engl J Med 1992;327:1649.

Rigel DS, Friedman RJ, Kopf AW. The incidence of malignant melanoma in the United States: Issues as we approach the 21st century. J Am Acad Dermatol 1996;34:5.

Schwartz RA. Premalignant keratinocytic neoplasms. J Am Acad Dermatol 1996;35:2.

Stern RS, Boudreaux C, Arndt KA. Diagnostic accuracy and appropriateness of care for seborrheic keratoses. JAMA 1991;265:74.

33

Pediatric Dermatology

Vidya Sharma, M.B.B.S., M.P.H., M.D.*

Skin disorders in infants and children may be different from the same diseases in older children or adults. (Figs. 33-1 and 33-2) Certain skin conditions such as diaper dermatitis are only seen in infants; other conditions such as atopic dermatitis may appear different in children compared with adults. Pediatric dermatology can be divided into neonatal dermatoses and dermatoses of infants and children.

NEONATAL DERMATOSES (BIRTH TO 1 MONTH)
(Figs. 33-3 and 33-4, Table 33-1)

A few lesions may be noted at birth or shortly thereafter. It is useful to describe a lesion by its morphology in order to develop a differential diagnosis of what the disorder might be.

Blistering (Vesiculobullous) Lesions

Blistering lesions can be mechanically induced or caused by infections.

1. *Sucking blisters*: These are usually seen as oval bullae on the hands or forearm thought to be caused by sucking in utero. They resolve rapidly.

2. *Epidermolysis bullosa* (Fig. 33-3) (see Chap. 31): This refers to a group of inherited disorders with bullous lesions developing spontaneously or as a result of trauma.

3. *Infections* (Fig. 33-4): Herpes simplex, congenital varicella, and candidiasis present as blisters in the newborn. Herpes simplex lesions are important to recognize because disseminated herpes can be fatal in the newborn. Intravenous acyclovir must be started early.

Pustular Lesions

Some are self-limited and require no treatment; others may be a result of an infection.

1. *Erythema toxicum*: This is a characteristic benign condition of the newborn. Lesions occur anywhere with erythematous macules, papules, and pustules. It is self-limited.

2. *Transient neonatal pustular melanosis* (Fig 33-5): This is a benign self-limited disorder characterized by vesiculopustular lesions that rupture and evolve into hyperpigmented macules.

3. *Neonatal acne*: This may be pustular or papular with comedones. It is self-limited and very rarely scars. Topical erythromycin products are safe and may be helpful.

4. *Milia*: This is a self-limited common occurrence on the cheeks, nose, chin, and forehead. It presents as 1–2-mm white or yellow papules, which frequently are grouped. They usually dissipate without therapy.

*Associate Professor, Department of Pediatrics, University of Missouri; Staff Physician, Department of Dermatology, Children's Mercy Hospital, Kansas City, Missouri

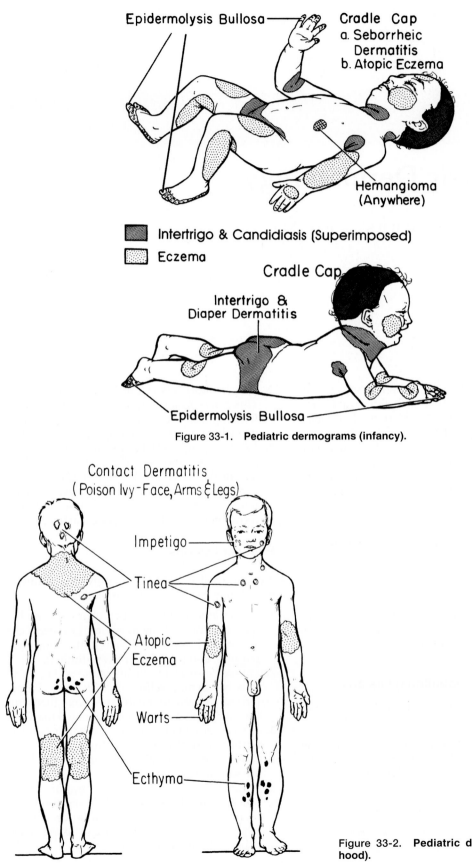

Epidermolysis Bullosa

Cradle Cap
a. Seborrheic Dermatitis
b. Atopic Eczema

Hemangioma (Anywhere)

■ Intertrigo & Candidiasis (Superimposed)

▨ Eczema

Cradle Cap

Intertrigo & Diaper Dermatitis

Epidermolysis Bullosa

Figure 33-1. **Pediatric dermograms (infancy).**

Contact Dermatitis
(Poison Ivy-Face, Arms & Legs)

Impetigo

Tinea

Atopic Eczema

Warts

Ecthyma

Figure 33-2. **Pediatric dermograms (child-hood).**

358

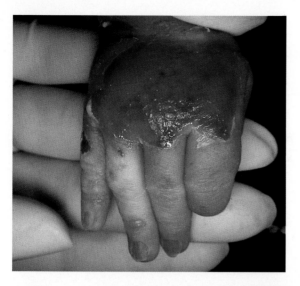

Figure 33-3.   **Epidermolysis bullosa.** Junctional type.

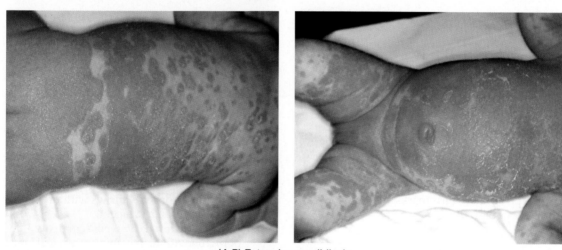

(*A,B*) Extensive candidiasis.

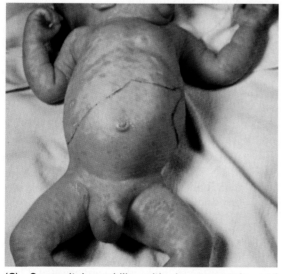

(*C*) Congenital syphilis with hepatomegaly and splenomegaly.

Figure 33-4.   **Candidiasis and syphilis.**

TABLE 33-1
NEONATAL DERMATOSES (BIRTH–1 MONTH)

Blistering (Vesiculobullous) Lesions	Pustular Lesions	Birthmarks	Papulosquamous Lesions
Mechanical	Erythema toxicum	White	Ichthyosis
Sucking blisters	Transient neonatal pustular melanosis	Albinism	Neonatal lupus erythematosus
Epidermolysis Bullosa		Piebaldism	Epidermal nevus
Bullous ichthyosiform	Acne	Ash-leaf macules	
Erythroderma	Milia	Brown	
Infectious		Café au lait spots	
Herpes simplex		Congenital pigmented nevus	
Varicella		Mongolian spots	
Candidiasis		Vascular	
		Nevus simplex (Salmon patch)	
		Nevus flammeus (Port wine stain)	
		Hemangioma—superficial, deep	

Birthmarks

Newborns may have many types of lesions that are grouped under "birthmarks" and may be categorized by color.

1. White
   a. *Albinism*: an uncommon inherited disorder with lack of pigment in the skin, hair, and eyes. A partial lack of pigmentation is termed *piebaldism* or *partial albinism*.
   b. *Ash leaf macules*: partially depigmented white macules in the shape of lance "ash

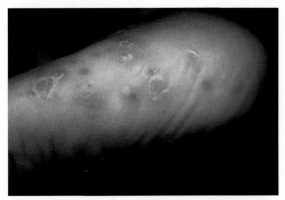

Figure 33-5. **Transient neonatal pustular melanosis.**

leaf" noted on the trunk, arms, or legs, usually associated with tuberous sclerosis
   c. *Nevus anemicus*: well-demarcated, hypopigmentation, border blanches with pressure, a localized vascular reaction
   d. *Nevus depigmentosus*: well-demarcated, hypopigmentation, may mimic "ash leaf" macule but shape less regular, not associated with underlying illness
2. Brown
   a. *Café-au-lait spots* (Fig. 33-6): light brown round or oval macules, may be a normal finding but may be seen in association with neurofibromatosis type 1. This condition should be suspected if more than six café-au-lait spots of greater than 0.5 cm are present in association with other findings.
   b. *Congenital pigmented nevus* (Fig. 33-7): usually flat tan to dark brown well-circumscribed lesions, may be small to large and hairy. They have a potential for developing malignant melanoma depending on the size (especially > 20 cm), location, border (irregular), color (especially black or multicolored), and texture.
   c. *Mongolian spots* (Fig. 33-8): flat deep brown to slate gray or blue-black in color found mostly over the lumbosacral areas and but-

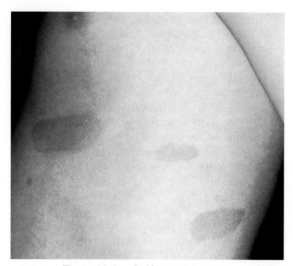

Figure 33-6.   **Café-au-lait lesions.**

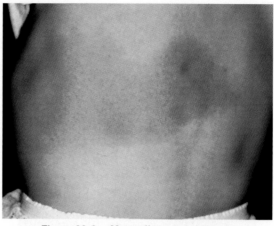

Figure 33-8.   **Mongolian spot on back.**

tocks, may be single or multiple, benign and self-limited

3. Vascular
   a. *Nevus simplex (Salmon patch)* (Fig. 33-9): These represent persistence of fetal circulation. Commonly referred to as "stork bite," these dull pink, flat, macular lesions are seen on the nape of the neck ("devil's bite"), glabella, upper eyelids, and nasolabial re-

gions. Ninety-five percent of these lesions fade in the first year, especially when on the face ("angel kisses").
   b. *Nevus flammeus (port-wine stain)* (Fig. 33-10): congenital vascular malformations composed of dilated capillaries. They usually do not involute, and laser therapy is an option. When above the palpebral fissure on the face they can be associated with the central nervous system vascular malformation (Sturge-Weber syndrome).
   c. *Hemangiomas* (Fig. 33-11): benign tumors of infancy consisting of proliferation of the vascular endothelium. They grow rapidly in infancy, stabilize, and involute in childhood, most resolving by 9 years of age. They may be superficial or deep. Management may consist of observation alone, oral

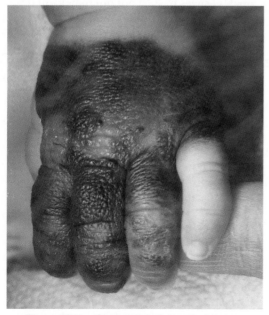

Figure 33-7.   **Congenital pigmented nevus.**

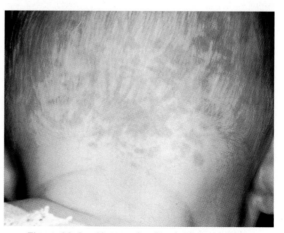

Figure 33-9.   **Nevus simplex (salmon patch).**

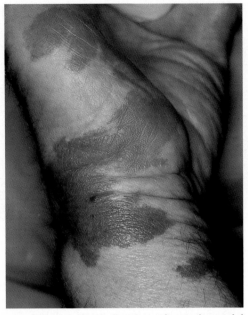

Figure 33-10. **Nevus flammeus (port wine stain).**

Prednisone, laser treatment, or surgery, including cryosurgery. When numerous they can be associated with hemangiomas in viscera (multiple hemangiomatosis syndrome).

Papulosquamous Lesions

1. *Ichthyosis* (Fig. 33-12): associated with dry, fish-like, adherent scaling. The rarer lamellar

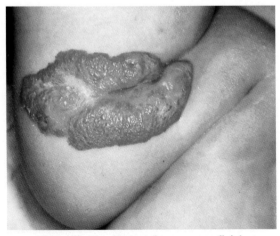

Figure 33-11. **Hemangioma—superficial.**

form and congenital ichthyosiform erythroderma, both bullous and nonbullous types, are present at birth. Ichthyosis vulgaris types are not present at birth.

2. *Neonatal lupus erythematosus* (Fig. 33-13): characterized by heart block and annular papulosquamous skin lesions on forehead and cheeks. Skin lesions usually fade by 6 to 7 months of age, while the heart block persists. This is the most common cause of neonatal heart block. Because this is maternally transmitted the mother needs to be checked for lupus. Anti-Ro or SSA antibodies may be present in mother or newborn.

3. *Epidermal nevus* (Fig. 33-14): linear warty surface lesions noted at birth, appearing anywhere on the body. They may rarely have other associated neurologic or skeletal abnormalities or have very rare malignant degeneration.

DERMATOSES OF INFANTS AND CHILDREN

(Tables 33-2 and 33-3; see Figs. 33-15–33-32)

Blistering Lesions (Vesiculobullous)

1. *Impetigo* (Fig. 33-15): present as erosions covered by a honey colored crust that may be small vesicles to start out but may form fragile bullous lesions commonly in exposed areas; caused by *Staphylococcus aureus* and less commonly by *Streptococcus pyogenes*

2. *Burns*: may be partial thickness with erythema or blisters or full thickness with loss of skin and scar formation

3. *Viral blisters* (Fig. 33-16): herpes simplex, varicella (chicken pox) and coxsackie (hand, foot, mouth disease) can present with blisters.

4. *Candida* (Fig. 33-17): can present with blisters in the diaper and intertriginous areas.

5. *Bullous disease of childhood (linear IgA dermatoses)*: sausage-shaped bullae noted on the buttocks, groin, and lower extremities in a "string of pearls" configuration. Usually a self-limited disease, which responds well to dapsone or sulfapyridine. Direct immunofluorescence is positive for IgA noted at the dermal–epidermal junction.

6. *Dermatitis herpetiformis*: benign disease with recurrent crops of severely pruritic grouped

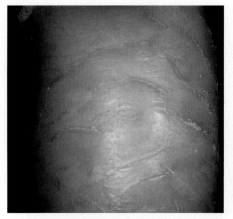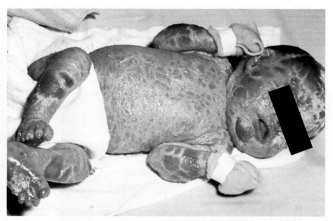

(A) Lamellar ichthyosis.   (B) Ichthyosiform erythroderma or harlequin fetus, fatal.

Figure 33-12. **Ichthyosis.**

TABLE 33-2
DERMATOSES OF INFANTS AND CHILDREN

Blistering Lesions	Pustular Lesions	Papules/Nodules	Vascular Lesions
Impetigo	Pustular Lesions	Skin color	Blanching
Burns	Infantile acropustulosis	Warts	Spider angioma
Viral blisters	Acne	Molluscum contagiosum	Drug eruptions
Candida		Keratosis pilaris	Nonblanching
Bullous disease of childhood		Granuloma annulare	Idiopathic thrombocytopenic purpura
Dermatitis herpetiformis		Angiofibroma	Henoch-Schönlein purpura
Incontinentia pigmenti		Brown	Meningococcemia
		Pigmented nevi	
		Urticaria pigmentosa	
		Yellow papules	
		Sebaceous nevus	
		Juvenile xanthogranuloma	
		Red papules	
		Papular acrodermatitis	
		Urticaria, papular urticaria	
		Erythema multiforme	
		Pyogenic granuloma	
		Viral exanthems	

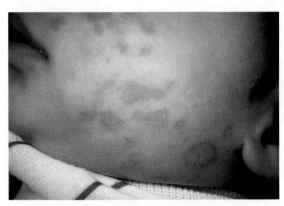

Figure 33-13. **Neonatal lupus erythematosus.**

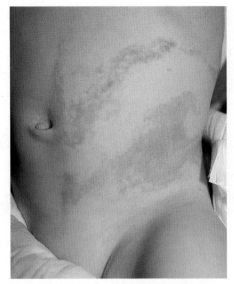

Figure 33-14. **Epidermal nevus.**

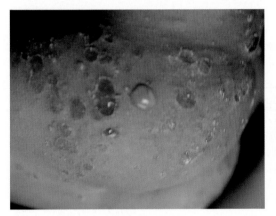

(*A*) Impetigo.

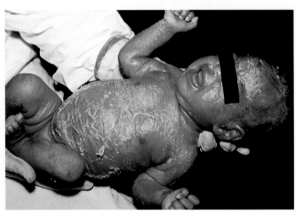

(*B*) Bullous impetigo or Ritter's disease; no thymus on autopsy.

Figure 33-15. **Impetigo.**

TABLE 33-3
DERMATOSES OF INFANTS AND CHILDREN

Papulosquamous Lesions	Eczematous Lesions	Diseases Affecting the Hair	Diseases Affecting the Nails	Dermatoses due to Physical Agents and Photosensitivity Dermatoses
Psoriasis	Atopic dermatitis	Congenital/Hereditary hair defects	Congenital nail defects	Sunburn
Pityriasis rosea	Seborrheic dermatitis	Alopecia areata	Twenty nail dystrophy	Polymorphous light eruption
Tinea versicolor	Immunodeficiency	Tinea capitas	Psoriasis/Atopic dermatitis	
	Contact dermatitis	Trichotillomania	Warts	
	Diaper Rash		Paronychia	

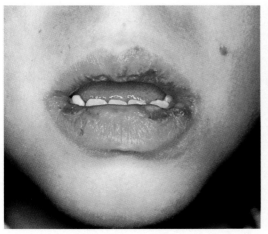

(*A*) Erosions of lips.

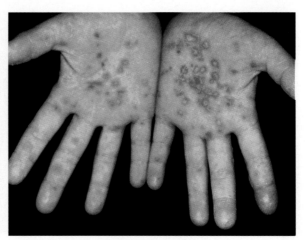

(*B*) Blisters on palms.

Figure 33-16. **Viral exanthem.**

vesicles or bullous lesions on the extensor surfaces of the limbs, shoulders, and buttocks; rare in infants and children and associated with nontropical sprue

7. *Incontinentia pigmenti* (Fig. 33-18): Rows of blisters are noted in the first few months of life or in utero, replaced by a warty stage followed by a pigmented stage.

Pustular Lesions

1. *Acropustulosis of infancy*: noted between birth and two years of age predominantly in African American infants. Recurrent crops of

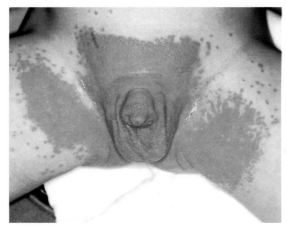

Figure 33-17. **Candidal rash.**

pruritic papulopustules or vesiculopustular lesions are seen on the palms, soles, and dorsum of hands and feet. It is self-limited.
2. *Impetigo* (see earlier) may also be pustular.

Papules/Nodules

1. Skin color
   a. *Warts*: caused by the human papilloma virus are transmitted by contact. They may dissipate without therapy. When they are noted in the genitalia sexual abuse should be considered.
   b. *Molluscum contagiosum*: a viral disease caused by a member of the pox virus group. Discrete single or multiple dome-shaped umbilicated papules may be found all over the body. It is contagious with a tendency for auto inoculation and may dissipate without therapy.
   c. *Keratosis pilaris*: an autosomal dominant disorder characterized by minute keratotic, follicular papules on the outer aspects of arms, thighs, and cheeks; seen in association with atopy and dry skin; may dissipate at puberty especially on face
   d. *Granuloma annular* (Fig. 33-19): skin-colored or dull red papules spread peripherally with a normal appearing center; usually found on the dorsum of hands and feet. The cause is unknown, and spontaneous

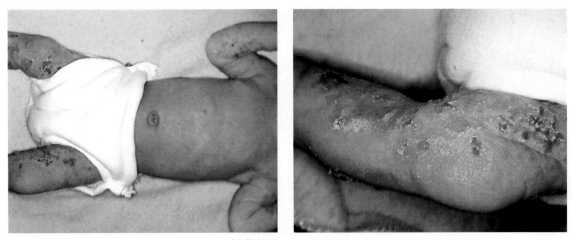

(*A,B*) Verrucous stage.

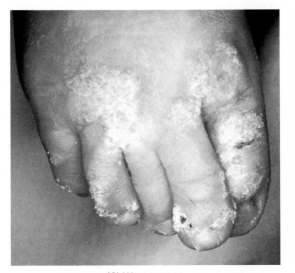

(*C*) Warty stage.

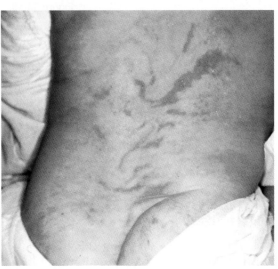

(*D*) Pigmented stage.

Figure 33-18. **Incontinentia pigmenti.**

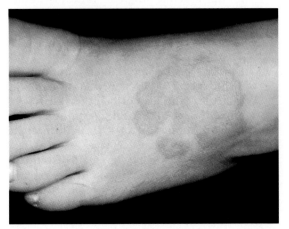

Figure 33-19. **Granuloma annular.** Dorsum of foot.

resolution in months to years is common. Intralesional corticosteroid injections and cryosurgery are helpful but painful.

    e. *Angiofibroma*: firm papules. When multiple and seen in a symmetrical distribution on the face they are associated with tuberous sclerosis.

2. Brown
    a. *Pigmented nevi* (Fig. 33-20): Depending on the basis of the location of the nevus cells, these may be called *junctional* (at the border of the epidermis and dermis, usually flat and black or dark brown), *intradermal* (within the dermis, usually flesh-colored and elevated) or *compound nevi* (both at the

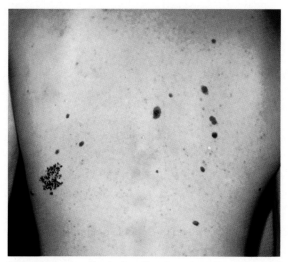

Figure 33-20. Nevi. Junctional nevi on the back and speckled lentiginous nevus far left midback.

junction of the epidermis and dermis and intradermal, usually elevated and brown). They occur anywhere on the body and may be flat, elevated, verrucous, or papillomatous. If they are black, multicolored, large ($\geq$ 6 mm), or irregular in border, an excisional biopsy should be considered.

b. *Urticaria pigmentosa* (Fig. 33-21): part of the mastocytosis syndrome, seen as tan brown macules and papules that urticate when stroked (Darier's sign); usually has an ex-

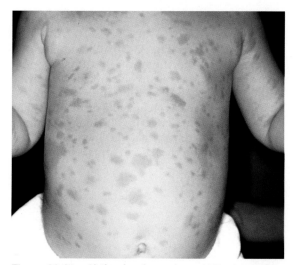

Figure 33-21. Urticaria pigmentosa. Urticaria pigmentosa of chest, in 2-year-old patient (note the red, urticating lesion below left nipple indicating a positive Darier's sign).

cellent prognosis if there is not systemic involvement and few lesions.

3. Yellow Papules
   a. *Xanthogranuloma (nevoxanthoendothelioma)*: usually develop in the first year of life and disappear around 5 years of age. They present as small yellow single or multiple papules on the scalp or body. Rarely there is eye involvement.
   b. *Nevus sebaceous (see Chap. 32)*: noted at birth as an orange oval or linear area on the scalp. At puberty they become raised and warty. Basal cell carcinomas develop in approximately 10 to 15% of children with nevus sebaceous. Nevus sebaceous may occur in conjunction with a benign, appendageal, warty tumor callled *syringocystadenoma papilliferum*.

4. Red Papules
   a. *Papular acrodermatitis (Gianotti-Crosti syndrome)*: nonpruritic flat-topped papules occur in the acral areas especially elbows and knees; originally associated with the hepatitis B virus, but recently many other viruses implicated; benign and self-limited
   b. *Papular urticaria*: lesions caused by a delayed hypersensitivity to a variety of arthropod bites; present as pruritic erythematous papules with surrounding urticaria. Recurrent crops are seen in the summer and can be quite extensive.
   c. *Erythema multiforme (see Chap. 12)*: an acute hypersensitivity syndrome presenting with macular, urticarial, or vesiculobullous lesions, especially on the palms, soles, hands, and feet. Target or "bull's eye" lesions with concentric alternating rings of red and white are a hallmark of this condition. It is commonly divided into erythema multiforme minor, which is a more benign, recurrent, and self-limited condition with one mucous-membrane surface involved and commonly associated with herpes simples virus; and erythema multiforme major, which presents with at least two mucous-membrane surfaces involved, widespread bullous lesions, and more systemic symptoms and is associated with mycoplasma pneumoniae or drugs.
   d. *Pyogenic granuloma*: An easily bleeding bright red papule may arise at sites of trauma or spontaneously.
   e. *Viral exanthems (see Fig. 33-16)*: Roseola, rubeolla, echo-viruses, coxsackieviruses, and rubella may present as erythematous macules and papules.

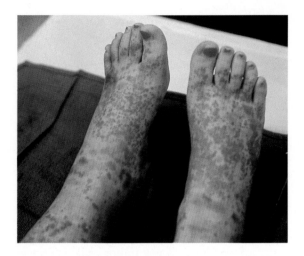

Figure 33-22. **Henoch–Schönlein purpura.**

Vascular Lesions

1. Blanching
   a. *Spider angioma*: small benign telangiectatic lesion usually on cheeks, nose, dorsum of hands and other sun-exposed areas that may disappear spontaneously
2. Nonblanching (purpura)
   a. *Idiopathic thrombocytopenic purpura*: a low-platelet disorder, usually presenting with nonblanching petechial lesions and bruises especially on areas of trauma
   b. *Henoch–Schönlein purpura* (Fig. 33-22): a vasculitis presenting with nonblanching erythematous papules followed by palpable, purpuric lesions usually on buttocks and lower extremities. Abdominal pain, joint swelling, and renal involvement may occur.
   c. *Meningococcemia*: presents with nonblanching petechial and purpuric lesions along with fever and signs of meningitis. Early diagnosis and treatment is life-saving.

Papulosquamous

1. *Psoriasis* (Fig. 33-23): seen fairly frequently, especially "guttate psoriasis," which is seen as a superantigen syndrome associated with streptococcal infections
2. *Pityriasis rosea*: commonly seen in the spring and fall, usually on the trunk, usually proceeded by 1 to 2 weeks by a herald patch. An unusual form is called *inverse pityriasis rosea*, with lesions located more in the groin and axilla.
3. *Tinea versicolor*: caused by a superficial fungal infection (*Pityrosporum orbiculare*), presents as a hypopigmented, asymptomatic disorder mainly on upper chest and back, occasionally on the neck and face. Fine, dry, adherent scale is revealed upon scratching.

Eczematous Lesions

1. *Atopic dermatitis* (Fig. 33-24): a hereditary disorder usually beginning around 1 to 4 months of age. In infants the involvement is usually of the face, scalp, trunk, and extremities. Toddlers have involvemennt of flexural skin and adolescents have involvement of hands and feet. There may also be hypopigmented scaly lesions on cheeks and arms referred to as *pityriasis alba*.

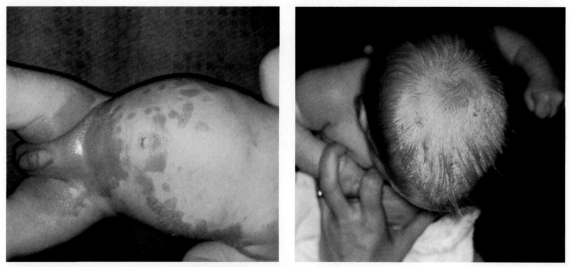

(*A,B*) Psoriasis in a 2.5-month-old child.

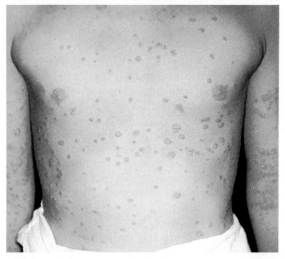

(*C*) Guttate psoriasis following streptococcal throat infection.

Figure 33-23.   **Psoriasis.**

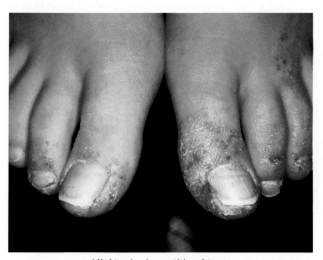

(*A*) Atopic dermatitis of toes.

Figure 33-24.   **Atopic dermatitis.**   *(continued)*

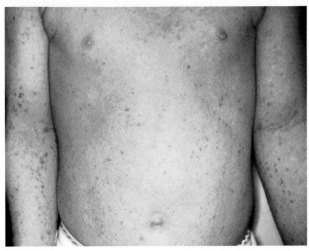

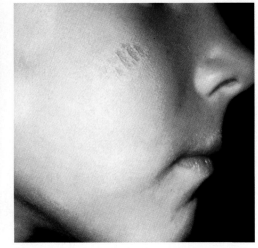

(*B*) Atopic dermatitis of chest and cubital fossae in a 9-year-old child.

(*C*) Hypopigmented atopic eczema of cheeks (pityriasis alba).

Figure 33-24.   *(Continued)*

2. *Seborrheic dermatitis* (Fig. 33-25): a scaly, crusting eruption noted in the "seborrheic areas" of the scalp ("cradle cap"), face, posterior auricular and intertriginous areas. It appears in infancy and usually clears spontaneously. It is also seen in adolescents and adults. Rarely it is mimicked by histiocytosis.

3. *Immunodeficiency*: Severe combined immunodeficiency, Omen's syndrome (familial reticuloendotheliosis with eosinophilia), and HIV infections can present as erythematous scaly eruptions in the intertriginous areas and be associated with yeast infections.

4. *Contact dermatitis* (Fig. 33-26): Generalized reactions to poison ivy or oak are common in children. An eczematoid, hyperpigmented

rash in the infraumbilical area may be seen in association with "nickel" sensitivity due to the metal snap on pants.

5. *Diaper rash* (Fig. 33-27): "Punched out" erosions are seen in Jacquet's dermatitis. Vesicular eruptions are seen secondary to candida albicans. Irritant or contact dermatitis is usually confined to the buttocks and perineal areas. Atopic dermatitis spares the diaper area.

Disease Affecting the Hair
(see Chap. 27)

1. *Congenital and hereditary hair defects* (Fig. 33-28): Many congenital hair-shaft defects pre-

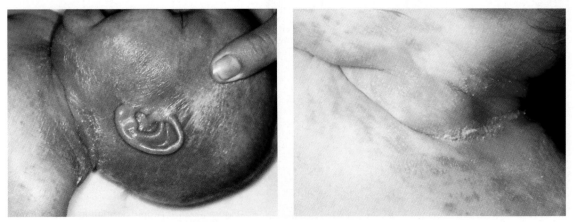

Figure 33-25.   **Seborrheic dermatitis.**

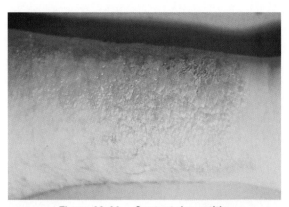

Figure 33-26.   **Contact dermatitis.**

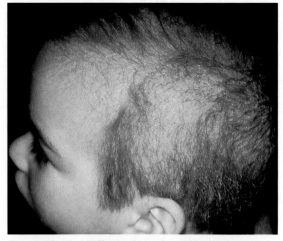

Figure 33-28.   **Diffuse alopecia with ectodermal defect in 3-year-old child.**

sent with broken-off, twisted, or spun glass-appearing hair. There is no satisfactory treatment for these conditions. They may be signs of underlying diseases. (See Chaps. 7 and 31).

2. *Alopecia areata* (Fig. 33-29) (see Chap. 27): a common disorder presenting with a sudden appearance of patches of smooth, sharply defined areas of hair loss. Short, tapering, "exclamation point" hairs tend to narrow as they enter the scalp. It is considered to be an autoimmune process involving the hair and has been associated with thyroiditis. The prognosis depends on the extent of the hair loss (the less the better), the area involved, and chronicity. The most commonly prescribed therapy is topical or intralesional corticosteroids.

3. *Tinea capitis* (Fig. 33-30A–B): Common organisms are *Trichophyton tonsurans, Microsporum canis* and *Microsporum audouinii.* "Black dot"

tinea (especially *T. tonsurans*) shows broken-off hairs and minimal inflammation making the diagnosis difficult. Fungal culture and potassium hydroxide mount can be diagnostic. The infection may be asymptomatic or present as seborrhea or inflammatory lesions of the scalp. A kerion (especially *M. canis*) is an inflammatory lesion with a pus-filled, boggy mass with hair loss. Treatment is with oral griseofulvin for at least 2 months. Newer antifungal agents (itraconazole, terbinafine) are also showing promise and may replace griseofulvin.

4. *Trichotillomania* (Fig. 33-31): commonly seen between 4 and 10 years of age in both sexes. Patients pluck, twirl, or rub hair-bearing areas

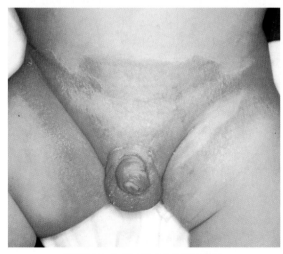

(*A*) Seborrheic diaper dermatitis.

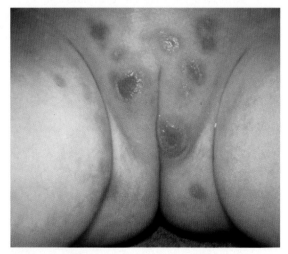

(*B*) Jacquet's diaper dermatitis.

Figure 33-27.   **Daiper dermatitis.**

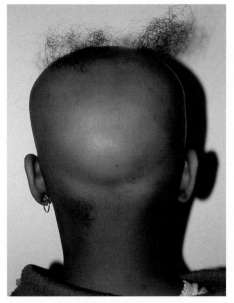

Figure 33-29. **Alopecia areata.** Note completely smooth bald area.

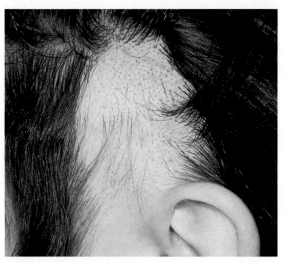

Figure 33-31. **Trichotillomania of the scalp.** Note: There is not complete baldness in area.

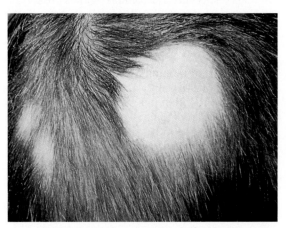

(A) Tinea of the scalp due to *M. audouinii*.

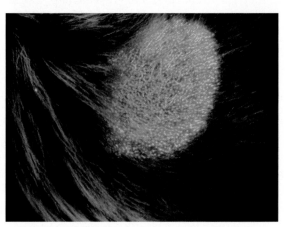

(B) Tinea hairs fluorescing under Wood's light.

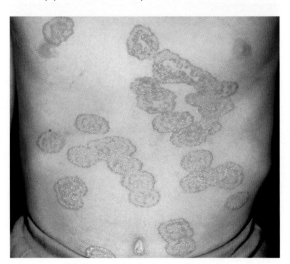

(C) Tinea of body due to *M. canis*.

Figure 33-30. **Tinea.**

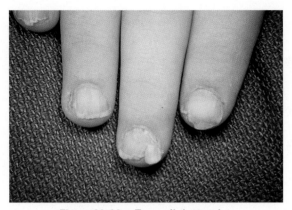

Figure 33-32.   **Ten-nail dystrophy.**

either consciously or subconsciously as a result of a habit. It usually affects the scalp but may also involve eyebrows and eyelashes. It is usually self-limited.

Disease Affecting the Nails
(see Chap. 28)

1. *Congenital nail defects*: Absent or poorly developed nails are associated with many syndromes, usually representing nail-matrix disorders. Ectodermal dysplasia is one syndrome associated with narrow nails with thin and fragile nail plates.
2. *Twenty nail dystrophy*: presents as thickened nails with exaggerated longitudinal ridges, noted in all nails of the hand [10-nail dystrophy (Fig. 33-32)] or hands and feet (20-nail dystrophy); self-limited and resolves over years
3. *Psoriasis/atopic dermatitis*: Nails may be thickened or shiny or contain ridges or pitting in these conditions. Alopecia areata can also be associated with nail pitting.
4. *Warts*: Children frequently develop warts around (periungual) and under (subungual) the nail. This can pose a therapeutic challenge.
5. *Paronychia*: usually presents as red, painful, inflamed lesion around the nail fold. It may be acute or chronic. The most common organism in the acute infection is *Staphylococcus aureus*. The chronic form is more often seen in thumb suckers, nail biters, and nail pickers and is commonly associated with *Candida albicans*.

Dermatoses due to Physical Agents and Photosensitivity Dermatoses

1. *Sunburn*: On the first sunny days, parents tend to underestimate the effects of the rays of the sun and overexpose their children. Parents should be taught the ABCs of sun exposure. Always stay out of the sun between 11 a.m. and 3 p.m. Block the sun with sunscreens for UVA and UVB protection with a sun protection factor of at least 30. Clothes, especially a hat and t-shirt, should be worn when outside. Solumbra or Frogwear sun-protective clothing offers especially good protection.
2. *Polymorphous light eruption*: a phototoxic reaction to UV rays characterized by a delayed response to light. It is very common in Native Americans and suggests a genetic inheritance. It begins in children with eczematous, papulovesicular, or plaque-like eruptions on cheeks, ears, nose, and dorsum of hands. If no additional sunlight exposure occurs lesions involute spontaneously in 1 to 2 weeks. Sunscreens need to screen out ultraviolet A (UVA, 310 to 400 nm) to be effective in most cases. Antimalarial drugs have also been used.

BIBLIOGRAPHY

Chapel KL, Rasmussen JE. Pediatric dermatology advances in therapy. JAAD 1997;36:513.

Freiden IJ. Which hemangiomas to treat and how. Arch Dermatol 1997;133:1593.

Hurwitz S. Clinical pediatric dermatology, ed 2. Philadelphia, WB Saunders, 1993.

Knowles S, Sharpiro L, Shean NH. Serious dermatologic reactions in children. Curr Opin Pediatr 1997;9:388.

Leung DY, Hanifin JM, Charlesworth EN, et al. Disease management of atopic dermatitis: A practice parameter. Ann Allergy Asthma Immunol 1997;79:197.

Ruiz-Maldonado R, Orozco-Covarrubias ML. Malignant melanoma in children: A review. Arch Dermatol 1997; 133:363.

Treadwell PA. Dermatoses in newborns. Am Fam Physician 1997;56:443.

Schachner LA, Hansen RC. Pediatric dermatology, ed 2. Philadelphia, WB Saunders, 1995.

Weston WL, Lane AT. Color textbook of pediatric dermatology, ed 1. St. Louis, Mosby–Year Book, 1991.

34

Geriatric Dermatology

LIFE STAGES AND THE SKIN

A brief review of important life stages and their influence on the skin is as follows:

PUBERTY. In males, at puberty, the beard, the pubic hair, and other body hair begin to grow in characteristic patterns that differ from the hair growth in females. Both sexes at this time notice increased activity of the apocrine glands, with axillary perspiration and body odor and increased development of the sebaceous glands, with the formation of varying degrees of *seborrhea* and the comedones, papules, and pustules of *acne*. Certain skin diseases tend to disappear around the onset of puberty, such as the infantile form of *atopic eczema*, *tinea of the scalp*, and *urticaria pigmentosa*.

PREGNANCY. Certain physiologic skin changes occur. Perspiration is increased. Hyper-pigmentation of the abdominal midline, nipples, vulva, and face (chloasma) is seen, and, in some brunettes, nevi and freckles also become more prominent and more pigmented. Malignant melanoma is not more common in pregnancy. Hypertrichosis of the scalp may be unnoticed until the excess hair begins to be shed after delivery. Striae of breasts, abdomen, and thighs appear. The skin diseases of pregnancy are *herpes gestationis* (see Fig. 26-11D–E), *impetigo herpetiformis*, *vulvar pruritus* (often due to candidal infection),

palmar erythema, *spider hemangiomas*, pyogenic granulomas, rarely erythema multiforme, and *pedunculated fibromas*. The following dermatoses are usually better, or disappear, during pregnancy: *psoriasis*, *acne* (can be worse), *alopecia areata*, and, possibly, *systemic scleroderma*.

MENOPAUSE. Common physiologic changes in the skin of women during menopause include hot flashes, increased perspiration, increased hair growth on the face, and varying degrees of scalp hair loss. Other skin conditions associated with menopause are *chloasma*, *pedunculated fibromas* (skin tags), *lichen simplex chronicus*, *vulvar pruritus*, *keratoderma climacterium* (palmar psoriasis), and *rosacea*.

GERIATRIC STATE. The diffuse atrophy of the skin that occurs in the aged person is partially responsible for the dryness that results in *senile pruritus* and *winter itch*. Other changes include excessive wrinkling and hyperpigmentation of the skin. Specific dermatoses noted with increased frequency are *seborrheic* and *actinic keratoses*, *basal cell* and *squamous cell carcinomas*, *senile purpura*, *pedunculated fibromas*, and *capillary senile hemangiomas*.

GERIATRIC DERMATOLOGY

Humans age gradually. Although the entire body changes slowly with advancing years, aging of the skin is readily visible and readily noticed by both

374

men and women. If the sale of cosmetics (*e.g.,* moisturizing creams, "age spot" removers, wrinkle creams, wigs, hair dyes for men and women) is any sign, it would seem obvious that the constant search for the "elixir of youth" is mainly directed toward maintaining a youthful-looking skin. Consider the interest in retinoic acid (Retin-A, Renova), α-hydroxy acids, chemical peels, botulism toxin, microdermabrasion, and laser skin resurfacing for wrinkles and aging skin. The two most important skin-care strategies to avoid signs of aging are to protect the skin from ultraviolet light and avoid exposure to tobacco smoke.

For the trained and careful observer, the elderly patient with even "normal skin" presents a wealth of skin changes, some obvious and others less obvious (Fig. 34-1).

Some of the earliest signs of aging of the skin are the development of the hyperpigmented macular lesions known as *freckles* and *lentigines* (Fig. 34-2). These can begin in persons in their 40s. They develop most commonly on the dorsa of the hands and on the face, in direct proportion to the genetically determined fair complexion of the person and the dosage of sun gained through the earlier years of life.

On the face, and to a lesser extent on the rest of the body, *wrinkling* of the skin also progresses with age. This is much more apparent in fair-skinned individuals.

Diffuse hyperpigmentation of the face and hands, again in the sun-exposed areas, becomes more definite with age. The quite common hyperpigmentation on the side of the neck, which is a combination of brown and red discoloration, seen particularly in women, is called *poikiloderma of Civatte* (Fig. 34-3).

Actinic keratoses (see Fig. 32-8) obviously have a definite predilection for the sun-exposed area of the body and also are related to the genetically determined complexion of the person and the environmental sun exposure.

The very common *seborrheic keratoses* (Fig. 34-4; see Fig. 32-1) can also be on the face but are most commonly seen on the neck, back, chest, and even in the crural area. These lesions can be so black and angry looking as to make one believe that one is dealing with a *malignant melanoma*. A biopsy may be necessary.

Another manifestation of aging is the development of *comedones* on the face lateral to the orbicular area (Fig. 34-5). This is called *Favre-Racouchot syndrome*.

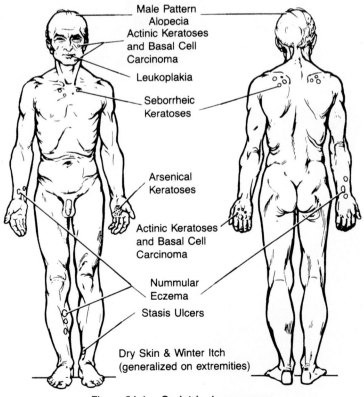

Male Pattern
Alopecia
Actinic Keratoses
and Basal Cell
Carcinoma

Leukoplakia

Seborrheic
Keratoses

Arsenical
Keratoses

Actinic Keratoses
and Basal Cell
Carcinoma

Nummular
Eczema

Stasis Ulcers

Dry Skin & Winter Itch
(generalized on extremities)

Figure 34-1. **Geriatric dermograms.**

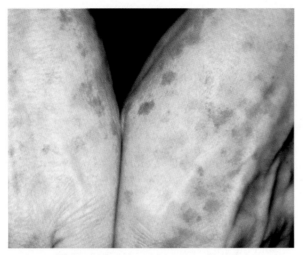

(*A*) Senile freckles on dorsum of hands.

Figure 34-2. **Freckles and lentigines.** (*Syntex Laboratories, Inc.*)

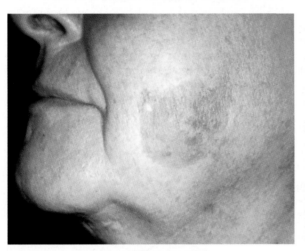

(*B*) Lentigo on cheek.

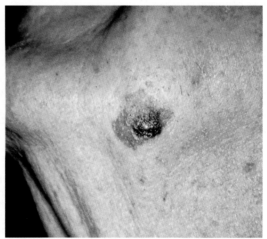

(*C*) Malignant melanoma in lentigo, on jaw area.

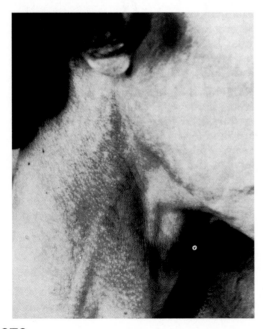

Figure 34-3. **Poikiloderma of Civatte.** Very common reddish brown discoloration on sides of neck seen mainly in women.

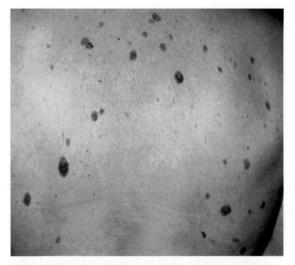

(*A*) Seborrheic keratoses over back of 71-year-old man.

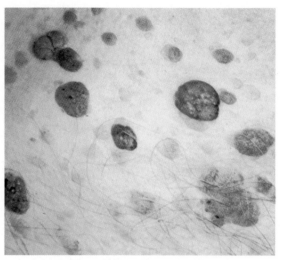

(*B*) Seborrheic keratoses, close-up.

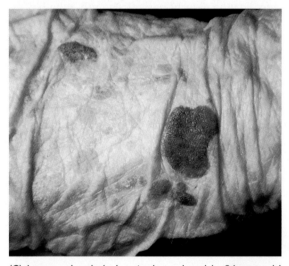

(*C*) Large seborrheic keratosis on hand in 84-year-old woman.

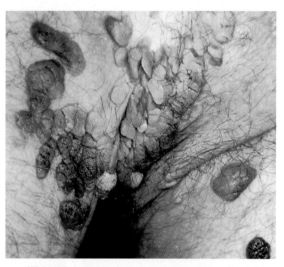

(*D*) Multiple seborrheic keratoses of crural area.

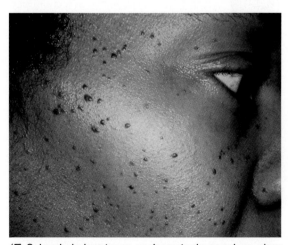

(*E*) Seborrheic keratoses or dermatosis papulosa nigra on face.

Figure 34-4. **Seborrheic keratoses.**

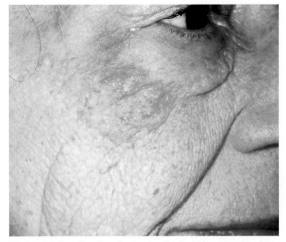

Figure 34-5. **Senile elastosis.** Senile elastosis with cysts and comedones of cheek (Favre-Racouchat syndrome). (*Syntex Laboratories, Inc.*)

Pedunculated fibromas and *pedunculated seborrheic keratoses* are extremely common on the neck and axilla. These can begin in the 40s and 50s.

Moving down to the trunk, practically every elderly person has small, bright red *capillary hemangiomas* (see Fig. 32-17). These are of no clinical significance but can sometimes be disturbing for vain persons.

On the legs, and to a lesser extent on the arms and body, it is common to see *dry skin* and *xerosis* (Fig. 34-6). Most persons are not aware of the fact that as they age, they need to decrease their frequency of bathing, or, more importantly, increase skin lubrication immediately after bathing, especially in the winter. *Winter itch* is quite common on the legs and can make the patient miserable, yet the treatment is simple, involving less frequent bathing and a corticosteroid ointment or lubricant.

Bruising occurs much more frequently in the aged skin and is most commonly seen on the extremities. This is referred to as *senile purpura*. Ecchymoses occur at sites where the patient often does not even remember any trauma.

In general, the color of the entire skin becomes pale and opaque.

The appendages of the skin change also. The most obvious and common changes are in the scalp, where the hair develops varying shades, from *grayness* to *pure white color* in certain persons.

Male-pattern alopecia, which can begin in the late teens, becomes more progressive through life. For the elderly patient, though, who has not had this hereditary balding problem, another form of hair loss, manifested as a diffuse thinning of the scalp hair, can develop. This *senile alopecia* can occur in both males and in females. Diffuse hair loss is also obvious in the axillae and the pubic area.

Excess facial hair is quite commonly seen in the elderly woman and can require shaving.

The nails do not change tremendously with age, but there is an increase in the longitudinal ridging. The toenails commonly become discolored, usually yellowish or brownish and often accompanied by onychomycosis (see Chap. 19).

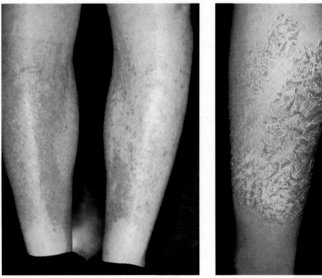

(*A*) Redness of winter itch on legs.

(*B*) Xerosis with secondary infection on legs.

Figure 34-6. **Xerosis.** (*Johnson & Johnson*)

The sebaceous glands and sweat glands become less active in the older person. For the unfortunate persons who have had acne for years, age can be pleasant for them, with a clearing of this problem. If a patient does present with a complaint of the recent development of acne, the patient should be asked carefully about the administration of *testosterone*, either orally or by injection.

The decrease in the secretion of oil and sweat glands contributes directly to the development of the dry skin or xerosis mentioned earlier.

The mucous membranes become drier. Patients complain of dry lips and tongue. The mucous membranes of the vaginal orifice also become dry, atrophic, and fragile.

Thus, essentially every elderly person has some evidence, however mild, of a skin problem.

INCIDENCE OF GERIATRIC SKIN DISEASES

For a study of the incidence of true skin diseases in a group of geriatric patients, here is a summary of a report in a classic study by Gip and Molin (see Bibliography).

These investigators studied 286 patients older than the age of 60 years who were hospitalized in a Swedish geriatric clinic. The skin of each patient was examined carefully. Histopathologic, bacteriologic, or mycologic examinations were undertaken in some cases.

In the 107 men there were 231 skin diagnoses (2.2 per person), and in the 179 women 372 skin diagnoses were made (2.1 per person). The number of skin diagnoses per person ranged from 1 to 5. No skin diagnoses were registered in 22 cases (only 8%) (5 men and 17 women).

All of the skin diagnoses were recorded. The following list contains the 10 most frequent dermatologic disorders registered (the numbers refer to the total number of dermatologic disorders found in the 286 men and women examined):

Pigmented nevus	143
Discoloration of the toenails	133
Seborrheic keratosis	84
Plantar hyperkeratosis	36
Stasis dermatitis of the legs	31
Seborrheic dermatitis	27
Dermatitis of the legs (unspecified)	23
Marked atrophy of the skin	19
Xanthelasma	12
Capillary hemangiomas	10

They attributed most of the cases of discoloration of the nails to (1) bacterial and fungal infections, related to air content of the nail plate, or (2) hemorrhage.

MANAGEMENT OF GERIATRIC SKIN PROBLEMS

SAUER NOTES

1. Nowhere is the broadness of the term *management* more meaningful than when it is used in reference to the handling of the skin problem for an elderly patient.
2. Management implies the imparting of much more information and instruction than the simple prescribing of "treatment."

The dermatologic management of an elderly patient is considerably complicated, however, by the patient's physical and mental inability to understand and carry out instructions. Writing out instructions carefully and legible can be very helpful. The correct application of wet dressings, coping with tub bathing, and even the simple application of creams and ointments are more complex processes for the elderly. And as age progresses and debility increases, this care is further complicated by having to be administered by another person, such as a family member or nurse; this, additionally, has aesthetic and economic limitations.

Most elderly patients can be treated at home, but some of the more severe skin problems are seen in institutionalized persons. Depending on the care available and the extent of the dermatosis, hospitalization may be necessary. The role of both corticosteroids and antibiotics in decreasing the number of elderly patients needing hospitalization is enormous and is most fortuitous.

CLASSIFICATION OF GERIATRIC DERMATOSES

The elderly patient is subject to the regular skin ills. However, as with the other age extreme, the child, there can be a different reaction by the aged skin to a given skin problem by virtue of the presence of fragility, dryness, and atrophy.

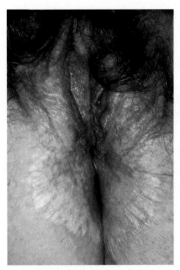 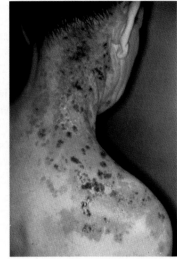 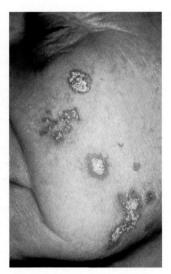

(*A*) Lichen sclerosus et atrophicus of vulva (not leukoplakia).

(*B*) Herpes zoster of shoulder and neck.

(*C*) Discoid lupus erythematosus of cheek in 77-year-old woman.

Figure 34-7. **Geriatric dermatoses.**

It is unusual to see certain skin problems in the aged, such as atopic eczema, acne, pityriasis rosea, impetigo, primary and secondary syphilis, herpes simplex, warts, exanthems, chloasma, and sunburn (Fig. 34-7).

A compilation of the more common problems of the geriatric patient is as follows, listed according to chapter groupings:

DERMATOLOGIC ALLERGY
(see Chap. 9).

Contact Dermatitis (see Figs. 9-1–9-4). For the geriatric patient this commonly is a dermatitis caused by the use of too harsh a local medication. This is seen quite frequently where too strong a salve is used in the treatment of itching legs.

Nummular Eczema (Fig. 34-8; see Figs. 9-12, 32-3, 32-5–32-7). This is quite a common problem, seen particularly in the winter and characterized clinically by coin-shaped vesicular areas on the arms, the legs, and, less frequently, the buttocks.

Drug Eruptions (Figs. 34-9 and 34-10; see Fig. 9-13). Drug eruptions are not too common but can be seen as a photosensitivity-type dermatitis when the patient is on a diuretic or a phenothiazine-type tranquilizer, or as an acne-like picture, due to the administration of testosterone.

PRURITIC DERMATOSES
(see Chap. 11)

Generalized Pruritus (Fig. 34-11). This is quite common and can defy adequate therapy. Careful examination of the patient is necessary to rule out any internal cause of the generalized pruritus. Rather frequently, and rather unfortunately, no apparent cause is ascertainable. Scalp and face itching can be a real problem.

Xerosis (see Fig. 34-6B). As a cause of the generalized itching in the winter this is rather easily managed by decreasing bathing and applying an emollient lotion or even a mild corticosteroid cream or ointment immediately after bathing. See Chapter 11 for a more detailed discussion of this problem in the elderly patient.

Localized Pruritic Dermatoses. These are not as common as the more generalized pruritic dermatoses.

VASCULAR DERMATOSES
(see Chap. 12)

Urticaria. This is not commonly seen.

Stasis Dermatitis (Fig. 34-12). This is rather common in elderly patients and is almost always associated with venous insufficiency due to varicose veins or other circulatory problems. It is important to stress that circulatory support

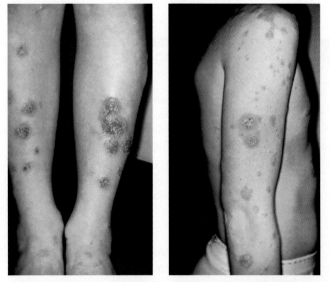

Nummular eczema of legs (*A*) and of arm (*B*) of same patient.

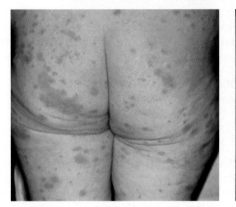

(*C*) Nummular eczema of buttocks.

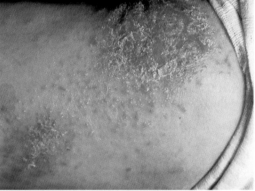

(*D*) Close-up showing oozing in nummular eczema of leg.

Figure 34-8.   **Nummular eczema.** (*Johnson & Johnson*)

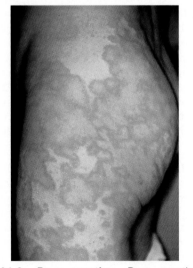

Figure 34-9. Drug eruption. Drug eruption from phenacetin. (*Johnson & Johnson*)

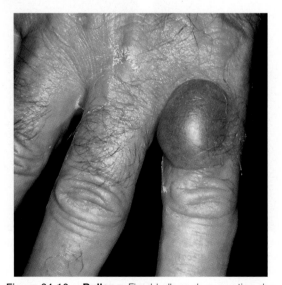

Figure 34-10.   Bullous. Fixed bullous drug eruption due to tetracycline.

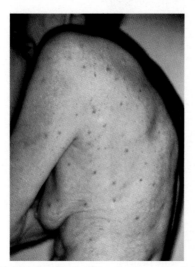

Figure 34-11. Senile pruritus. Senile pruritus in 74-year-old woman. (*Johnson & Johnson*)

dressings (Ace wrap) or garments (Jobst or Compass) are indicated on a continuing basis after the dermatitis has responded to therapy. This can prevent the development of stasis ulcers.

Atrophie Blanche. Arterial insufficiency of the legs from several causes can produce redness, scaling, ulcers, and, eventually, stellate scars. It occurs mainly over the ankles.

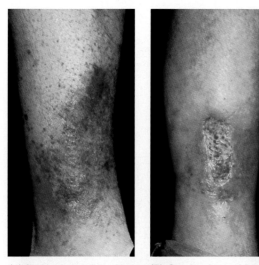

(*A*) Stasis dermatitis of leg aggravated by contact allergy to neomycin.

(*B*) Stasis ulcer of leg with varicose veins.

Figure 34-12. **Stasis dermatitis.**

SEBORRHEIC DERMATITIS, ACNE, AND ROSACEA
(see Chap. 13)

Seborrheic Dermatitis (see Figs. 13-1–13-3). This becomes less bothersome with age but can recur following a cerebrovascular accident, stroke, or Parkinson's disease.

Acne. This is rarely seen in the elderly patient. If it is present, the patient should be asked about intake of testosterone and corticosteroid drugs (especially if used more than 1 month), which can produce acne.

PAPULOSQUAMOUS DERMATOSES
(see Chap. 14)

Psoriasis (see Figs. 14-1–14-4 and 33-23). It is rare to see psoriasis develop as a new problem in an elderly person. Thus, most elderly persons who have psoriasis have learned to live with the disease.

DERMATOLOGIC BACTERIOLOGY
(see Chap. 15)

Furuncles and Carbuncles. These lesions are not too common.

Decubital Ulcers. The alternate term bedsore describes the pathogenesis of these chronic, painful, and debilitating ulcerations. They occur on pressure sites, mainly the buttocks and posterior aspect of heels. The patient is usually bedridden. Prophylactic measures are extremely important. Good nursing care can prevent some of these ulcers. The care should include turning the patient frequently, keeping the patient clean and dry, and applying powder to the bed. Once an ulcer has developed, the care is compounded. Donut-type sponge-cushion supports and special mattresses are indicated, with local application of povidone–iodine (Betadine) solution and continued good nursing care. Surgical dressings such as Opsite, Duoderm, Tegaderm, and Polymem may be helpful. Plastic surgery may be necessary.

Stasis Ulcers. These (see Fig. 34-12B) are the cause of marked disability in the elderly patient. The ulcers heal slowly and can be quite painful. The care required to heal these ulcers, or even prevent them from spreading, can be considerable. More often than not, other members of the family or nursing personnel must take over the management of these chronic sores.

SYPHILOLOGY
(see Chap. 16)

Tertiary syphilis of the skin or other organs is now rarely seen. The most common problem seen in the elderly patient in relation to syphilis is the persistently positive serology that occurs after adequate therapy. Some syphilologists are alarmed that dormant but persistent spirochetal infections can become clinically significant, with involvement of the eye and central nervous system.

DERMATOLOGIC MYCOLOGY
(see Chap. 19)

Candidal Infections. These are the most common mycologic infections seen in the elderly patient, particularly if the patient is obese. Lack of bathing and cleansing is a major factor. Prolonged antibiotic therapy may also be contributory as well as prolonged bedrest and incontinence of urine and feces.

DERMATOLOGIC PARASITOLOGY
(see Chap. 21)

Scabies. As an epidemic in a nursing home, scabies can be a difficult management problem. The elderly, especially if mentally confused, present a challenge for basic hygiene. When they itch, this itch is usually attributed to dry skin or senile pruritus. Only when several residents in the nursing home, and the personnel, begin to itch does one think of scabies as a cause. Then the therapy is difficult because so many persons are affected (and for personnel, possibly their families) that a basic simple therapy becomes a major management problem. All persons affected must be treated at the same time.

BULLOUS DERMATOSES
(see Chap. 22)

Pemphigoid (see Fig. 33-15). This is probably the most common bullous condition seen in elderly patients. Unfortunately the potent medications needed to treat this disease are often a major problem. Bullous pemphigoid (Fig. 34-13A) in the elderly should prompt a careful work-up to rule out an internal malignancy.

EXFOLIATIVE DERMATITIS
(see Chap. 23 and Fig. 23-1)

This is a miserable disease, and the cause can be difficult to determine. An axiom is that half of the patients older than age 50 years with exfoliative dermatitis have a lymphoma.

PIGMENTARY DERMATOSES.
(see Chap. 24)

Hyperpigmentation or hypopigmentation of the skin can occur in the elderly from many causes. Aside from a simple change in pigmentation of the skin due to age, other pigmentary problems are uncommon.

COLLAGEN DISEASES
(see Chap. 25)

Discoid lupus erythematosus can begin in old age (see Figs. 25-1, 25-3, and 34-7C).

THE SKIN AND INTERNAL DISEASE
(see Chap. 26)

Diabetes Mellitus. This causes a degeneration of the vascular supply, and skin changes in the diabetic are progressive with age. Ulcers, gangrene of the digits, and ulcerations of the mal perforans type (see Fig. 26-3) are most commonly seen.

DISEASES AFFECTING THE HAIR
(see Chap. 27)

Graying of the Hair and Thinning of the Hair. These were discussed earlier.

Hypertrichosis. This excessive growth of hair is common on the face of women.

DISEASES AFFECTING THE NAILS
(see Chap. 28).

Other than the development of increased ridging of the nail plates and the discoloration of the toenails, mentioned earlier, there are no major nail changes in the aged individual, except for onychomycosis (fungal infections of nails) of the toenails.

DISEASES OF THE MUCOUS MEMBRANES
(see Chap. 29)

The mucous membranes become dry and fragile with age.

DERMATOSES DUE TO PHYSICAL AGENTS
(see Chap. 30)

Effects of sunlight on the skin are extremely common and can result in simple hyperpigmentation

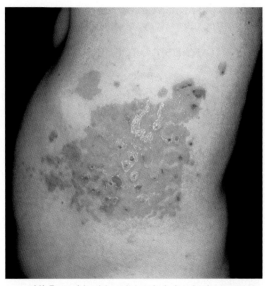

(A) Pemphigoid on lateral abdominal area.

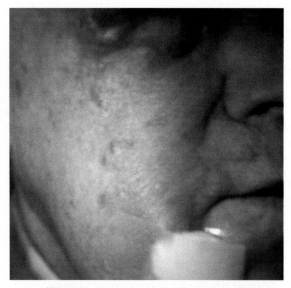

(B) Angiosarcoma on face of elderly male.

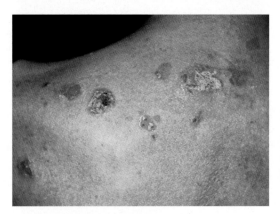

(C) Pemphigus vulgaris of upper back area.

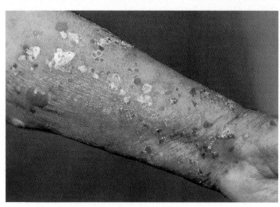

(D) Pemphigus vulgaris of forearm.

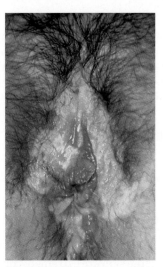

(E) Benign mucosal pemphigoid of vulva showing erosions.

Figure 34-13.   **Bullous diseases.**

and atrophy of the skin or can produce actinic keratoses (see Figs. 32-8, 32-9) that can occasionally eventuate as squamous cell carcinomas (Fig. 34-14; see Fig. 32-13).

PHOTOSENSITIVITY DERMATOSES
(see Chap. 30)

Photosensitivity problems are rarely seen unless triggered by drugs.

GENODERMATOSES
(see Chap. 31)

The genetic inheritance of the person has considerable influence on the aging of the skin, includ-

ing wrinkling, the effect of sunlight, the activity of the oil and sweat glands, and hair changes.

TUMORS OF THE SKIN
(see Chap. 32)

Seborrheic Keratoses (see Figs. 32-1, 34-4). As mentioned earlier, these are common, seen in almost every elderly person. The number of these lesions is genetically determined.

Pedunculated Fibromas. Such fibromas of the neck and axilla are quite common, and, again, there is a familial tendency for these to develop.

Precancerous Tumors. Tumors such as senile or actinic keratoses (see Figs. 32-8 and 32-9) develop

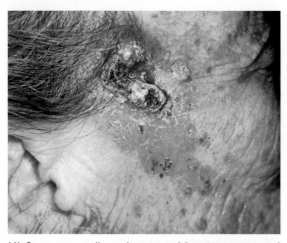

(*A*) Squamous cell carcinoma and keratoses on aged skin.

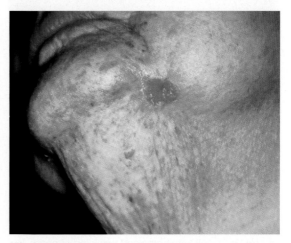

(*B*) Squamous cell carcinoma in area of chronic radiodermatitis for hypertrichosis of skin.

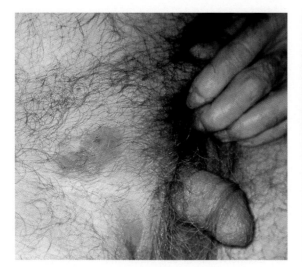

(*C*) Paget's disease of crural area.

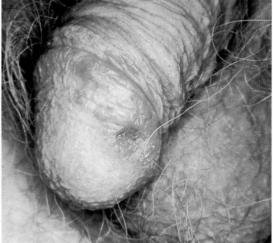

(*D*) Erythroplasia of Queyrat on penis.

Figure 34-14.   **Squamous cell carcinoma.** *(Syntex Laboratories, Inc.)*

in relation to earlier sun exposure and the genetic makeup of the skin complexion.

Squamous Cell Carcinoma *(see Figs. 32-12, 32-13, 34-14).* This can develop by itself or from degeneration of actinic keratoses.

Basal Cell Carcinomas *(Fig. 34-15; see Figs. 3-1C, 3-3, 32-11).* These are the most common malignancies of the skin in the elderly patient. These are characterized by waxy nodular lesions, with or without ulceration in the center.

Venous Lake or Varix. Occurring on the lips and ears, these are common and can frighten the patient into thinking that he or she has a melanoma.

Capillary Hemangiomas *(see Fig. 32-17).* These are present on the chest and back of almost every elderly person.

Nevi *(Fig. 34-16; see Fig. 32-18).* These mature with age, and many seem to disappear. Junctional elements are rarely seen in nevi in the geriatric patient.

Malignant Melanoma *(see Fig. 32-19).* This is an uncommon malignancy, but it can develop from a brownish-black, flat lesion known as a lentigo, which is usually seen on the face and arms. The result is a *lentigo maligna melanoma* (see Fig. 34-3C).

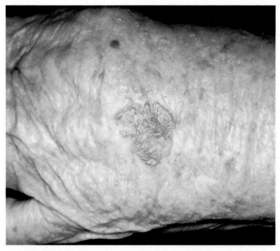

(A) Basal cell carcinoma and wrinkling of hand.

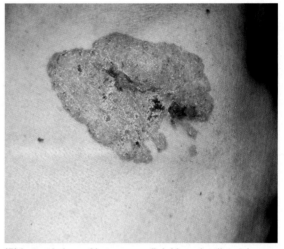

(B) Lateral view of large superficial basal cell carcinoma on back.

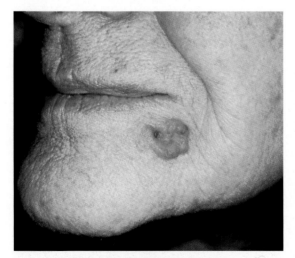

(C) Basal cell carcinoma on chin.

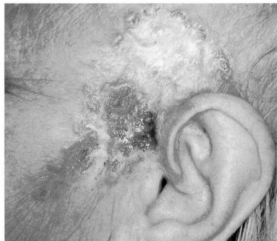

(D) Extensive basal cell carcinoma in a 79-year-old patient.

Figure 34-15.   **Basal cell carcinoma.** *(Syntex Laboratories, Inc.)*

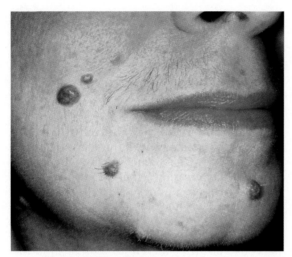

Figure 34-16. Compound nevi on face.

VITAMIN DEFICIENCIES. As the aged population continues to become a higher percentage of the total population and life expectancy increases, the nutritional status of this elderly population becomes increasingly important. The vitamin deficiencies are therefore discussed as follows.

Dermatoses due to lack of vitamins are rare in the United States. However, a common question asked by many patients is, "Doctor, don't you think my trouble is due to lack of vitamins?" The answer in 99% of cases is "No!"

Vitamin A. Phrynoderma is the name for generalized dry hyperkeratoses of the skin due to chronic and significant lack of vitamin A. Clinically, the texture of the skin resembles the surface of a nutmeg grater. Eye changes are often present, including night blindness and dryness of the eyeball.

Large doses of vitamin A (25,000 to 50,000 international units t.i.d.) are used in the treatment of patients with *Darier's disease, pityriasis rubra pilaris, comedone acne,* and *xerosis* (dry skin). The value of this therapy has not been proved. Vitamin A therapy in high doses should be for only 4 to 6 months at a time, with cessation of therapy for 6 to 8 weeks before resuming it again due to hepatotoxicity.

Hypervitaminosis A, due to excessively high and persistent intake of vitamin A in drug or food form, causes hair loss, dry skin, irritability, weight loss, and enlargement of the liver and spleen.

Isotretinoin (Accutane) is a vitamin A acid preparation that is beneficial for severe cystic acne and a few other rarer conditions.

Acitretin (Soriatane), another synthetic derivative of vitamin A, is useful for pustular and exfoliative psoriasis. *Both Accutane and Soriatane have severe side effects, including fetal abnormalities. They should never be prescribed unless the physician and patient thoroughly understand the potential dangers of these vitamin A derivatives.*

Vitamin B Group. Clinically, a patient with a true vitamin B deficiency is deficient in all of the vitamins of this group. Thus the classic diseases of this group, *beriberi* and *pellagra,* have overlapping clinical signs and symptoms.

Vitamin B1 (Thiamine). This deficiency is clinically manifested by beriberi. The cutaneous lesions consist of edema and redness of the soles of the feet.

Vitamin B2 (Riboflavin). A deficiency of this vitamin has been linked with red fissures at the corners of the mouth (perlèche) and glossitis. This can occur in marked vitamin B2 deficiency, but most cases with these clinical lesions are due to *contact dermatitis* or *malocclusion* of the lips from faulty dentures.

Nicotinic Acid. This deficiency leads to pellagra, but other vitamins of the B group are contributory. The skin lesions are a prominent part of pellagra and include redness of the exposed areas of hands, face, neck, and feet, which can go on to a fissured, scaling, infected dermatitis. Local trauma may spread the disease to other areas of the body. The disease is worse in the summer and heals with hyperpigmentation and mild scarring. Gastrointestinal and neurologic complications are serious. Dementia, dermatitis, and diarrhea are the "three Ds" of pellagra.

Vitamin C (Ascorbic Acid). Scurvy is now a rare disease, and the skin lesions are not specific. They include a follicular papular eruption, petechiae, and purpura.

Vitamin D. No skin lesions have been attributed to lack of this vitamin. Vitamin D and vitamin D2 (calciferol) have been used orally in the treatment of *lupus vulgaris.* Vitamin D3 (Dovonex ointment) is used topically for psoriasis.

Vitamin E. It has been reported that vitamin E is effective in treating *yellow nail syndrome.*

Vitamin K. Hypoprothrombinemia with purpura from various causes responds to vitamin K therapy.

The manifestations of fat deposition in the skin are seen often in the elderly population, and that is why it is included in this chapter.

LIPIDOSES
(see Fig. 26-18A)

This complex group of metabolic diseases causes varying skin lesions, depending somewhat on the basic metabolic fault. The most common skin lesions are xanthomas, which are characterized by yellowish plaques or nodules readily seen on the skin surface. Xanthomatous lesions are either due to *primary hyperlipidemia* or the secondary result of a primary disease such as *alcoholism, diabetes mellitus, hypothyroidism*, or, less commonly, *obstructive jaundice, nephrotic syndrome*, and *dysproteinemia*.

The diagnosis of a patient with a xanthoma would begin with tests for fasting plasma cholesterol and triglycerides. These tests should uncover 95% of the patients with hyperlipidemia. If these tests are abnormal, then plasma turbidity studies and plasma lipoprotein electrophoresis should be performed. On the basis of abnormal lipoprotein patterns, five types of familial hyperlipidemia can be recognized.

Clinically there are five general types of xanthomas. They are tendinous xanthomas, planar xanthomas (most common form is *xanthelasma* or *xanthelasma palpebrarum*), tuberous xanthomas, eruptive xanthomas, and xanthoma disseminatum. These can usually be correlated with specific lipoproteins.

For secondary hyperlipidemia, therapy would be aimed at the primary disease. For familial hyperlipidemia, diet therapy and drug therapy must be considered, based on the type of disease.

Xanthoma-like deposits in the skin occur in several other diseases, namely, the histiocytosis group of diseases, which are *Schüller-Christian syndrome, Letterer-Siwe disease*, and *eosinophilic granuloma*. Vesicular lesions can be seen in cases of Schüller-Christian syndrome, and a seborrheic dermatitis–like picture is evident in Letterer-Siwe disease (see Dictionary–Index, Fig. 2A).

Extracellular lipid accumulations occur in lipoid proteinosis, extracellular cholesterosis, and necrobiosis lipoidica diabeticorum. Skin lesions of the latter occur mostly in women, on the anterior tibial area of the leg, and are characterized by sharply circumscribed, yellowish plaques with a bluish border. Diabetes is present in the majority of patients. Disturbances of phospholipid metabolism include Niemann-Pick disease and Gaucher's disease. Patients with both disorders develop a yellowish discoloration of the skin.

NEUROSES AND PSYCHOSES

The aging population frequently falls victim to psychiatrically induced skin diseases. We have, therefore, put this review in this chapter.

A common belief among many members of the medical profession is that the majority of skin diseases are due to "nerves" or are a neurotic manifestation. This old idea is undoubtedly based on the familiar sight of the scratching skin patient; he just looks "nervous," and it makes one nervous and itchy merely to look at him. It is hard to know which came first for most patients, the itching or the nervousness. In practice, it is good to deemphasize the nervous element but not ignore it. An answer to patients and physicians who question the role of nerves in a particular case is to say that they play a definite role in many skin eruptions, but rarely are nerves the precipitating cause of a dermatosis. If a patient has an emotional problem and also has an itching dermatitis, a flare-up of the problem will intensify the itch, as it would aggravate another patient's duodenal ulcer or migraine headache.

Therapy for patients with skin disease in which "nerves" are believed to play a dominant part can be handled well by the calm, receptive, attentive, interested general physician. Simple local therapy prescribed with the confidence of a competent physician often establishes in the patient the necessary faith to cure the complaint. Occasionally, these patients do not respond to such therapy, and in rare cases the patient might benefit from special psychiatric care.

The following list divides the psychocutaneous diseases into those believed to be (1) related to psychoses, (2) related to neuroses, and (3) of questionable psychic relationship.

Dermatoses Related to Psychoses

Factitial dermatitis: The patient denies that he or she is producing the skin disease. This is not to be confused with neurotic excoriations.

Skin lesions due to compulsive movements: An example is the chronic biting of an arm in a feeble-minded patient.

Delusions: Of parasitism, cancer, syphilis, and so on (see Fig. 26-1B); various "proofs" are often presented by the patient to substantiate his or her existing belief. Pimozide (Orap) therapy is useful in some cases.

Dysmorphic syndrome: Patients have symptoms of cutaneous pain, burning, or other dysesthesias or, alternatively, have concerns about the structure and function of the skin (see Fig. 26-1B) or body contour. This is also called *cutaneous nondisease*. Symptoms most commonly involve the face, scalp, and genitals (*vulvodynia*). Do not confuse with lichen sclerosis et atrophicus (see Fig. 34-7A). This is a psychotic problem. Haloperidol (Haldol) in a low dosage of 1 to 2 mg twice daily can be helpful.

Trichotillomania in adults: This is a rare cause of hair loss.

Dermatoses Related to Neuroses

Neurotic excoriations (see Fig. 26-1): The patient admits picking or scratching the lesions.

Phobias: The patient fears contraction of a disease (*e.g.*, syphilophobia, acarophobia, cancerophobia, bacteriophobia).

Trichotillomania of children: This is not as serious as it is in adults. The physician's index of suspicion must be high to diagnose this disease (see Chap. 27).

Lichen simplex chronicus (see Figs. 11-1 and 11-2): The primary cause can be an insect bite, contact dermatitis due to a permanent wave, psoriasis, stasis dermatitis, or one of many other conditions that can initiate the scratching habit. The habit then outlives the disease, and the lichen simplex cycle develops.

Dermatoses of Questionable Psychic Causes

Hyperhidrosis of palms and soles
Dyshidrosis
Alopecia areata
Lichen planus
Chronic urticaria
Rosacea
Atopic eczema
Psoriasis
Aphthous stomatitis
Primary pruritus, local or generalized

INTERNAL CANCER
(see Figs. 26-2 and 26-8)

A final word on the geriatric population concerns the association of internal cancer and skin disease. Skin lesions may develop from internal malignancies either by metastatic spread or by the occurrence of nonspecific eruptions. The most interesting of the *nonspecific dermatoses* is the rare entity acanthosis nigricans. The presence of the velvety, papillary, pigmented hypertrophies of this disease in the axillae, the groin, and other moist areas of an adult indicates an internal cancer, usually of the abdominal viscera, in over 50% of cases. A benign form of acanthosis nigricans exists in children and becomes most manifest at the age of puberty. This benign form is not associated with cancer. Herpes zoster (see Fig. 34-7B) can be severe, painful, and at times, especially when severe, associated with underlying cancer.

A *dermatitis herpetiformis-like* eruption with vesicles and intense pruritus is seen occasionally in patients with an internal malignancy or lymphoma.

Purpuric lesions and pyodermas also occur as nonspecific changes in patients with malignancies (see Fig. 26-2).

Specific skin lesions showing the malignancy or lymphoma on biopsy occur in *mycosis fungoides*, *leukemia*, *lymphomas*, and *metastatic skin lesions* from internal malignancies.

BIBLIOGRAPHY

Arlian LG, Estes SA, Vyszenski-Moher DL. Prevalence of Sarcoptes scabiei in the homes and nursing homes of scabietic patients. J Am Acad Dermatol 1988;19:806.

Barthelemy H, Chouvet B, Cambazard F. Skin and mucosal manifestations in vitamin deficiency. J Am Acad Dermatol 1986;15:1263.

Castanet J, Ortonne J. Pigmentary changes in aged and photoaged skin. Arch Dermatol 1997;133:1296.

Cohen PR, Scher RK. Nail changes in the elderly. J Geriatr Dermatol 1993;1:45.

Cook JL, Dzubow LM. Aging of the skin. Arch Dermatol 1997;133:1273.

Drake LA, et al. Guidelines of care for photoaging/photodamage. J Am Acad Dermatol 1996;35:3.

Fleischer AB, Feldman SR, Bradham DD. Office-based dermatologic services provided to the elderly by physicians in the United States in 1990. J Geriatr Dermatol 1993;1:146.

Fleischer AB. Pruritus in the elderly: Management by senior dermatologists. J Am Acad Dermatol 1993;28:603.

Fosko SW. Management of photoaging in the elderly. J Geriatr Dermatol 1993;1:38.

Gip L, Molin L. Skin diseases in geriatrics. Cutis 1970;6:771.

Hurley HJ. Skin in senescence: A summation. J Geriatr Dermatol 1993;1:55.

Kantor GR. Investigation of the elderly patient with pruritus. J Geriatr Dermatol 1995;3:1.

Kligman AM. Psychologic aspects of skin disorders in the elderly. J Geriatr Dermatol 1993;1:15.

Kligman AM. An overview of cutaneous geriatrics. J Geriatr Dermatol 1994;2:6.

Newcomer VD, Young EM. Geriatric dermatology: Clinical diagnosis and practical therapy. New York, Igaku-Shoin, 1989.

Rousseau P. Pressure sores in the elderly. Geriatr Med Today 1988;7:28.

Warren R, Gartstein V, Kligman AM, et al. Age, sunlight, and facial skin. J Am Acad Dermatol 1991;25:751.

Young SJ. Drug Interactions. J Clin Psychiatry 1996;57:177.

Tropical Diseases of the Skin

Francisco G. Bravo, M.D.,* and Alejandro Morales, M.D.†

With the recent surge in popularity of eco-tourism, there has been an increase in exposure of people to the exotic areas of the planet. Uncommon diseases are now being transported via the airways to the "first world" quickly. The absence of basic modern needs of life, such as roads, electricity, and water, has caused dermatology in many areas to be years behind the rest of the world. Malnutrition, high humidity, insect bites, and lack of education all contribute to cause a variety of skin diseases in a manner and to a degree that is not observed in the developed world.

BACTERIAL INFECTIONS

BARTONELLA AND VERRUGA PERUANA. *(Fig. 35-1).* Until the AIDS era, bartonellosis was one of those exotic diseases that may have only been studied for board examinations. The first descriptions of the disease were at the beginning of this century and came from endemic areas in the

Peruvian Andes under two different names: *Carrión's disease* and *verruga peruana*; it was caused by *Bartonella bacilliformis*. The bacteria, a gram-negative rod, was transmitted from the natural reservoirs to humans by mosquitoes belonging to the *Lutzomya* family. The disease has two characteristic phases. At first, it produces an impressive bacteremia and parasitism of the reticuloendothelial system (Carrión's disease), in which microorganisms may be seen inside red blood cells on peripheral smears. The clinical picture is a systemic disease with fever, malaise, and high susceptibility to other bacterial infections, such as salmonellosis. The most distinct and relevant phase for dermatology is the eruptive phase, known as verruga peruana. It may follow the bacteremia or it may present *de novo*. Characteristically, an eruption of multiple papules, nodules, and tumors appears over a period of weeks. The more superficial lesions have an angiomatous appearance resembling pyogenic granulomas. No systemic symptoms are seen during this phase. Histologically, the lesion consists of a confluent proliferation of histiocytes and newly formed capillary vessels with focal areas of neutrophiles and nuclear dust. The natural course of the disease is toward spontaneous involution, although antibiotic treatment may induce a more prompt remission.

At the beginning of the 1980s some patients with AIDS presented with a clinical picture very similar to the eruptive phase of verruga peruana.

*Assistant Professor, Department of Dermatology, Universidad Peruana Cayetano Heredia; Attending Physician, Dermatology Service, Instituto de Enfermedades Infecciosas y Tropicales Alexander von Humboldt, Hospital Nacional Cayetano Heredia, Lima, Peru

†Associate Professor, Department of Dermatology, Universidad Peruana Cayetano Heredia; Chief, Instituto Dermatologica, Lima, Peru

391

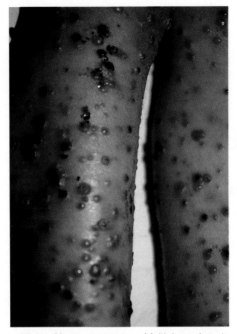

Figure 35-1. Verruga peruana. Multiple angiomatous lesions of verruga peruana.

This new disease was named *bacillary angiomatosis*. The histological descriptions of the eruptive lesions of bacillary angiomatosis (histiocytes and newly formed vessels) were identical to those described in verruga peruana, the only bartonellosis known at that time. The initial thought was to associate this new entity with cat-scratch disease, and with what was supposed to be its etiology, a new bacteria called *Afipia felis*. At a later time, isolation of a gram-negative rod from the lesions led to classifying it under a new family of bacteria called *Rochalimaea*. When genetic studies were made comparing the genes of *Bartonella bacilliformi* and the new *Rochalimaea* family, it became evident that they were closely related, and they were renamed under the *Bartonella* family. The new *Bartonella* species include *B. henselae*, *B. quintana* (both cause bacillary angiomatosis, cat-scratch fever, and systemic disease associated with fever), and *B. elizabethan*, which causes septicemia and endocarditis in alcoholics. Bacillary angiomatosis is now recognized as a disease characteristic in immunosuppressed patients of all kinds, although it has been reported in immunocompetent patients. The most likely natural reservoirs are domestic animals such as cats. It is cosmopolitan, as opposed to verruga peruana, which is still endemic to Andean areas of Peru and Ecuador.

ANTHRAX. *(Fig. 35-2). Anthrax* is an infection caused by *Bacillus anthraces*, an encapsulated gram-positive bacteria that can survive for up to 20 years in dry grass. It is a disease that occurs in people who work with cattle. Its contagiousness is favored by a preexisting lesion on the skin and can even be caused by the simple inhalation of spores. The cutaneous lesion is also called a malignant pustule; occurs in exposed areas of the skin, especially the face, neck, arms, or hands; and is usually a solitary lesion. One to five days after the inoculation a papule grows. A blister then forms on the edematous base that eventually breaks, leaving a hemorrhagic crust. Redness and edema may be very marked. General symptoms appear on the 3rd or 4th day. The conditions can be very toxic and even lead to death. Treatment is with intramuscular penicillin G, although *Bacillus anthraces* is also sensitive to tetracycline.

RHINOSCLEROMA. *Rhinoscleroma*, also known as *chloroma*, is a chronic disease of very slow progression that is potentially fatal. It is caused by *Klebsiella rhinoscleroma* (Frish bacillus). The first symptoms are generally nasopharyngeal. The lesions are slow growers, and often the patient does not seek medical attention for years. The initial stage is that of rhinitis. This is an exudating stage, with symptoms similar to a common cold including headache and difficulty breathing. There is a very purulent, fetid secretion with

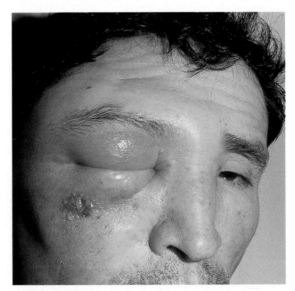

Figure 35-2. Anthrax. 48 hours after infection.

crusts and occasional epistaxis. The second stage has a proliferating pattern with improvement of the cold-like symptoms; however, obstruction and infiltration of nasal tissues by friable granulomatous tissue may extend into the pharynx and the larynx causing a change in the tone of voice with hoarseness. Later during a nodular period the nose takes on the size and shape similar to that of a "tapir." Respiration becomes difficult and it may be necessary to do a tracheotomy. The third stage is fibrotic sclerosis, and, although there may be clinical improvement and occasionally a spontaneous cure, usually there is very heavy distortion of the anatomic structures. Invasion and opacification of the bone of the nasal sinuses with eventual destruction may occur. The diagnosis is based on the clinical and histological picture and the presence of bacillus of Frish. Treatment includes antibiotics such as tetracycline, azithromycin, cephalosporin, and trimethoprim. It does not respond to sulfa preparations or penicillin. The best medication is tetracycline, 2 grams daily, in divided doses for a period of 6 months.

PINTA. *(Fig. 35-3). Pinta* is a treponemal disease of endemic behavior caused by *Treponema carateum.* Its occurrence has been restricted to lowland tropical areas of Central and South America, especially in the Amazon region. It is still reported in some aboriginal populations of the Brazilian Amazon. It shares some similarities with syphilis but, aside from an occasional juxta-articular lymph node, it is a purely cutaneous disease. Pinta is transmitted during childhood by direct contact with lesions from infected individ-

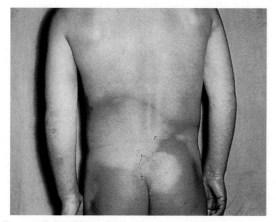

Figure 35-3. Pinta. Pinta showing early hyperpigmentation and depigmented patches on the back.

uals but not by sexual contact. Patients go through three different stages with early, secondary, and late lesions. The early or primary lesion is an erythematous papule that becomes scaly, psoriasiform, and even lichenified. It is usually located on lower extremities and becomes dyschromic with time. Secondary lesions appear about 2 months after the primary lesions. They are multiple, with morphology similar to the primary lesion, although smaller in size. They are bilateral and symmetrical and rarely located on the palms and soles. The most prominent change is, again, dyschromia with hyper- and hypopigmentation mixed in single lesion. They are mostly located over bony prominences. Spirochetes can be easily detected on deep scraping of lesions at any stage. All serological tests for syphilis are positive, and distinction from *T. palladium* infection is impossible. The diagnosis should be suspected in patients from endemic areas with extensive dyschromia. Treatment is based on penicillin therapy. The changes in color do not reverse with antibiotic therapy.

YAWS AND BEJEL. These two treponematoses are related to syphilis, although epidemiologically behave in an endemic fashion. *Yaws,* also called *pian* or *frambesia,* is a disease caused by *T. pertenue* with identical morphology to *T. pallidum.* It is endemic to all tropical areas around the world from Central and South American to Africa, Asia, Australia, and the Pacific islands. It is also acquired during childhood. The clinical manifestations go through the three classical stages of early, secondary, and late lesions. The primary lesion is chancroid in appearance, whereas the secondary lesions are papillomatous verrucous and similar to condylomas. In skin they resemble raspberries, giving origin to its French name, *frambesia.* Bone involvement can be rather destructive, ending in severe deformities and mutilations. Tertiary lesions can be gumma-like and achromic, as in pinta, and can produce palmoplantar hyperkeratosis. Treatment is again based on the use of penicillin.

Bejel is an endemic from of syphilis, produced by a variant of *T. pallidum.* At present, it is still reported in the Middle East, the African Sahara, and some areas of the tropical belt. Like the other endemic treponematoses, it is a disease of infants and children. The clinical manifestations are similar to the mucosal lesions of secondary syphilis with a condylomatous appearance. Tertiary lesions are similar to yaws.

INFECTIONS CAUSED BY MYCOBACTERIA

TUBERCULOSIS
(see Chap. 15).

LEPROSY
(see Chap. 15 and Fig. 15-14).

Infections Caused by Atypical Mycobacteria

SWIMMING POOL GRANULOMA. This is an infection caused by *Mycobacterium balnei* (Fig. 35-4). It produces an indolent verrucous nodule that may progress to ulcerations. It usually occurs in the extremities, especially at points of trauma. The incubation period ranges from approximately 2 to 6 weeks. The lesions are usually solitary, and there is no systemic reaction. Satellite lesions may appear and may simulate sporotrichosis. Minocycline seems to be the drug of choice, although rifampin, tetracycline, and doxycycline are alternative choices. Surgical excision or thermal therapy has been employed with relative therapeutic success.

MYCOBACTERIUM ULCERANS (BURULI ULCER). This mycobacterial infection was first described in southern Australia as *Bairnsdale ulcer*, and, later, endemic areas were also reported in Africa (from the Buruli valley) and South America. In west and central Africa it is considered to be a public health problem. This is, in fact, the third most common worldwide mycobacte-

riosis in immunocompetent patients, only after tuberculosis and leprosy. The bacteria lives in the environment and is acquired by humans through contamination of traumatic wounds. The classic clinical presentation is an ulcer, located most commonly on extremities. The cavity extends laterally, undermining the edges of the lesions, so the defect is always larger than what is seen at first glance. The ulceration continues to enlarge, producing marked destruction and mutilation of the affected areas. The morbidity of the disease is directly related to the skin lesions, with no systemic symptoms. The histologic findings consist of marked necrosis of the subcutaneous tissue with a paucity of inflammatory infiltrate. There is not granuloma formation, as opposed to other common mycobacteriosis. On special stains such as Ziehl–Neelsen, a huge amount of bacteria is seen in the necrotic areas in quantities only comparable to lepromatous leprosy. The necrosis is a direct effect of bacterial toxins. The diagnosis is made on the basis of the clinical and histologic findings. The bacteria is difficult to isolate, although it can be done on special mycobacterium media. New diagnostic techniques, including polymerase chain reaction (PCR) techniques, will allow early diagnosis in smaller lesions that are more susceptible to surgical excision, which is the definitive treatment.

PARASITIC DISEASE

Protozoal Dermatosis

LEISHMANIASIS. *Leishmaniasis* (Fig. 35-5) is an infectious process caused by intracellular parasites of the *Leishmania* family. The disease is transmitted from natural reservoirs to humans by mosquito bites. The different forms of cutaneous disease are produced by *Leishmania* species specific to certain regions in the world, such as those seen in the Middle East (*L. tropic*), Central America (*L. mexican*), and South America (*L. peruviana* and *L. braziliensis*). There is even an endemic area for leishmaniasis in the state of Texas. Different names are given to the disease depending on the geographical location: *Oriental sore* in Asia, *chiclero ulcer* in Mexico, *uta* in the Andes, and *espundia* in the Amazon basin. The classic cutaneous lesion consists of a round, isolated ulceration with slightly elevated and indurated borders, which is asymptomatic. The classic location is on areas of the body not covered by clothing and exposed to mosquito bites such as the face, neck, and extremities. The lesion itself is painless

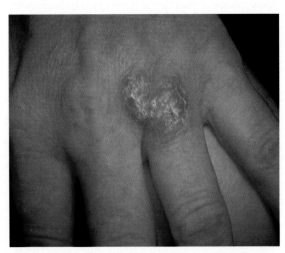
Figure 35-4. **Granuloma.** Swimming pool granuloma.

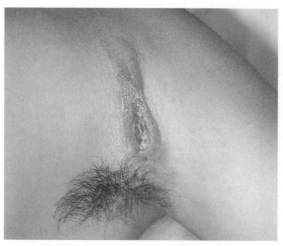

(*A*) Unusual location after recent visit to endemic area.

(*B*) Mucocutaneous form. The septum is involved.

Figure 35-5.   **Leichmaniasis.**

and tends to regress spontaneously. The variety known as *mucocutaneous leishmaniasis*, which is produced by *L. braziliensis*, is characterized by its ability to produce, after a dormant period, an ulceration on the mucosae of the nasal septum that can progress externally, mutilating the whole nose and nasolabial area. When the progression is on the mucosal side it may destroy the palate, producing a granulomatous infiltration of the pharynx, the larynx, and even the upper respiratory airway. The tissue destruction seen in leishmaniasis is, in fact, a result of the intense inflammatory reaction induced by the parasite, rather than the virulence of the microorganism itself. This sort of damaging mechanism is similar to what happens in leprosy. In an early lesion a heavy infiltration of histiocytes, many of them engulfing the leishmania organisms, is mixed with lymphocytes and plasma cells. The more organized the infiltrate becomes (clear-cut granulomas) the less likely that leishmanias will be seen on the biopsy specimens. This last detail makes the diagnosis rather difficult, unless one has a high degree of suspicion. Additional methods of diagnosis include direct examination of aspirate from the ulcer, culture in specific media, and PCR techniques. The leishmania test, an intradermal reaction to fragments of the parasite, is useful when working up a diagnosis in someone who is just an occasional visitor to endemic areas. The high sensitivity of the test makes it very useful to rule out rather than to confirm the diagnosis. Treatment, when indicated, is based on use of antimonial preparations and, in difficult cases, of

amphotericin B. Always consider leishmaniasis in the differential diagnosis of chronic cutaneous ulcerations, especially when there is a history of living in or traveling to endemic areas, some of them very popular among ecotourists.

SOUTH AMERICAN TRYPANOSOMIASIS (CHAGAS' DISEASE). Trypanosomiasis (South American) is caused by *Trypanosome cruzi* and is transmitted by a reduviid triatomine infection (kissing bug). In most cases, the port of entry is the conjunctiva, causing unilateral edema of the eyelids and inflammation of the lacrimal gland (Romaña sign). There are general manifestations such as headache, fever, myalgia, and hepatosplenomegaly. Fatal cases occur due to meningoencephalitis or myocarditis.

AMEBIASIS (INCLUDING FREE LIVING AMEBAS AND *ENTAMOEBA HISTOLYTICA*). Free living amebas are usually associated with disease of the central nervous system (Fig. 35-6). The infection is acquired by swimming in ponds and streams with still water. There are two types of meningoencephalitis produced by these organisms. The *Naegleria* species cause an acute form, with no skin manifestions. The subacute, granulomatous form is produced by two families, *Acanthamoeba* and *Balamuthia*. Infection by *Acanthamoeba* species is known to induce chronic ulcerative lesions in AIDS patients and, rarely, isolated, centrofacial plaques in immunocompetent hosts. In the 1990s, a new variety named *Balamuthia mandrillaris* has been recognized as the causative

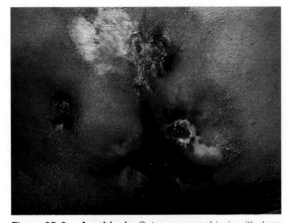

Figure 35-6. **Amebiasis.** Cutaneous amebiasis with deep ulcers of the buttocks caused by direct extension following amebic dysentery. (*Dr. A. Gonzalez-Ochoa*)

agent in many of the cases of free living ameba granulomatous meningoencephalitis in South America and Australia. Many of those cases have a primary skin lesion with a centrofacial plaque of granulomatous appearance, usually located on the nose. In the months following the cutaneous involvement, all patients develop focal central nervous system symptoms, with progressive deterioration resulting in death.

Entamoeba histolytica can produce a cutaneous lesion, most commonly in the anal margin and genital region, but also in skin that is not periorificial. The elementary lesions are large cutaneous ulcerations, vegetative lesions, and even abscesses.

Helminthic Dermatosis (Roundworm)

CUTANEOUS LARVA MIGRANS. (*Fig. 35-7*). This is a disease caused by hookworms, usually parasites of dogs and cats. The ova are excreted through the feces, and they remain viable in sandy, moist ground. The larva then penetrate the skin of bathers or people who walk on the contaminated ground. Usually the "culprits" are *Ancylostoma duodenal*, *Necator americanus*, and other hookworms. Clinically, the parasite causes a serpentine, erythematous, papular, pruritic skin eruption. The parasite is usually ahead of the tract. Vesicles, excoriation, and crusts are present. Treatment includes topical thiabendazole and albendazole 200 mg by mouth twice daily for three days.

LARVA CURRENS. As opposed to cutaneous larva migrans, in which lesions move over a period of days, the cutaneous form of strongyloidiasis moves over a period of hours, which is the reason for the "currens" denomination. It is more common in immunosuppressed patients in whom multiple tracts can be seen. At the present time, ivermectin is the treatment of choice, 200 micrograms per kilogram, and in immunosuppressed patients it can actually be life-saving.

GNATHOSTOMIASIS. This condition was first diagnosed in South America in Ecuador in 1979 and extensively studied by Oyague. It is caused by *Gnathostoma spinigerum*. Clinically, it produces a nodular migratory eosinophilic panniculitis. This parasite normally inhabits the stomach of domestic animals such as dogs and cats.

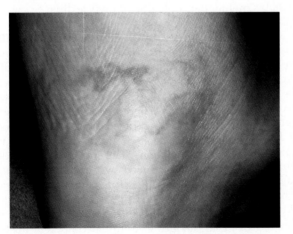

(*A*) Creeping eruption on plantar surface of heel.

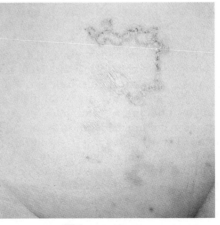

(*B*) Larva migrans.

Figure 35-7. **Larva migrans.**

The eggs are excreted in the stools of these animals. They then reach the rivers and hatch in the water and are ingested by organisms of a *Cyclops* species, developing into the second larval stage. This is later ingested by fish, forming a third larval stage in their muscular tissue which in turn is eaten by a definitive host. Humans, who are not the definitive hosts, could develop the characteristic panniculitis of this disease from eating raw fish such as in cebiche or sushi. The parasite migrates through the tissues, most commonly to the skin, but it may go to any of the internal organs. Clinically, after a variable incubation period of 4 weeks to 3 years, patients develop the classic symptom of pruritic edematous migrating cutaneous plaque, which on biopsy occasionally shows the parasite. More commonly, only a very intense eosinophilia through the dermis and subcutaneous tissue occurs. Treatment alternatives include albendazole 200 mg twice daily for 5 days or ivermectin 200 micrograms per kilogram in a single dose.

FILARIASIS. *Filariasis* is a systemic infection due to one of several different species of nematode, all transmitted by mosquito bites, with hematogenous (rather that cutaneous as in onchocerciasis) spreading of microfilaria. The symptoms are related to chronic inflammation of the lymphatic system. They commonly occur in tropical areas of the world. Loa loa infections are reported in West Africa. *Wuchereria bancrofti* and *Brugia malayi* are more common in Asia and tropical Africa. The symptoms are related to the stage of disease. During the hematogenous spread, microfilariae are abundant in blood, producing temporary migratory swelling in extremities that is self-limited and recurrent. Acute lymphangitis and lymphadenitis may affect the groin and axillae. Genital involvement includes acute orchitis, epididymitis, and funiculitis, which are very painful. They can also be recurrent and evolve into fibrosis. Urticaria may be part of the clinical presentation. Late changes are due to obstruction of lymphatics, giving origin to different forms of elephantiasis affecting the extremities and scrotum with massive edema. Diagnosis is reached by the presence of microfilaria in blood smears and by serological testing. Treatment is based on the use of diethylcarbamazine. Recent reports on the use of ivermectin seem very promising.

ONCHOCERCIASIS. *Onchocerciasis* is a chronic infestation of the skin by *Onchocerca volvulus*. This is a microfilarial nematode whose natural hosts are humans and fleas from the genus *Simulium*. The disease was first described in Africa and later in Central America. Recently, the reports extend the disease to the northern countries of South America. The transmission occurs when flies become infected by biting sick people. After a short period of maturation, the microfilariae move to the buccal apparatus of the insect and enter the skin of a noninfected human with the next blood meal. The infective forms become adults in 6 to 8 months inside cutaneous nodules, where they begin producing microfilariae. From there on the infection propagates to all the tegumentary system. Cutaneous involvement includes the characteristic nodules containing adult forms. They tend to locate in the scalp in Central American patients and on extensor surfaces in African patients. Other clinical presentations include facial erythema, facial livedoid discoloration, and prurigo-like eruption on buttocks and extremities. Later signs are extensive lichenification, dyschromia, elephantiasis of extremities and scrotum, and the so-called hanging groin. Ocular involvement is related to the direct invasion of eye structures by the microfilariae, resulting in complete and permanent loss of vision; this is the reason the disease was called *river blindness*. Diagnosis is easy to confirm either by direct scraping or by histologic analysis of skin lesions in which the adult form and microfilaria are identified. This disease is particularly worthy of mention because we can now count on a specific treatment which consists of the oral administration of ivermectin. It is extremely effective even as a single-dose therapy.

Trematodes Dermatosis (Flukes)

CERCARIA DERMATITIS. *Cercaria dermatitis* or *swimmer's itch* is caused by the penetration of the skin by schistosoma of birds or mammals. The cercaria are found in bodies of water. They can penetrate the skin of mammal and, if the host is receptive, reach the bloodstream and spread to other organs. In humans, who are not the definitive host, the cercaria are unsuccessful in reaching the blood; they are retained in the epithelial layers of skin and finally destroyed, resulting in dermatitis. Clinically, pruritic macules, papules, hemorrhages, and excoriations develop in the exposed areas. This resulting dermatitis is a product of the sensitization to the cercaria proteins. In massive or repeated infestations the signs and symptoms are consequently more severe.

Seabather's eruption (Fig. 35-8) is an eruption that generally occurs in the areas under swimwear after bathing in the ocean; however, it may also be seen in the axilla, neck, and flexor areas. It is pruritic and papular and occurs within hours after leaving affected waters. Occasionally, the skin eruption is complicated by fatigue, malaise, fever, chills, nausea, and gastrointestinal complaints. These episodes appear to be more severe after repeated attacks. This condition is caused by the schneiderian larvae of *Linuche unguiculata* (thimble jellyfish). This larva has been found in water samples, and in affected patients there have been demonstrated high IgG levels specific to *L. unguiculata*. Symptomatic treatment is accomplished with antihistamines, topical corticosteroids, and even oral corticosteroid therapy. It is a self-limiting condition that lasts about 12 days even without therapy.

SCHISTOSOMIASIS OR BILHARZIASIS. In South America, schistosomiasis is caused by *Schistosoma mansoni*. The reservoir is usually water contaminated with feces from infected people containing ova and free-swimming cercaria capable of penetrating human skin. The organisms pass rapidly through the epidermis and are carried by the blood and eventually mature into flukes in the intrahepatic portion of the portal system. The mature flukes migrate to the pelvic veins where eggs are laid. In the skin one may see a papular eruption identical to swimmer's itch or even urticarial reactions on occasion. In areas of high endemicity, there is granulomatous inflammation of the skin of the perineum with nodular masses, fistulae, and sinus tracts.

DERMATOSIS CAUSED BY ARTHROPODS

HUMAN SCABIES. *(Fig. 35-9; see Fig. 22-1).* This disease is usually transmitted through prolonged personal contact with infected people and less often by clothing and bed linens. The mite's location is in a "burrow" in the stratum corneum where it deposits its eggs. An allergic sensitization to the mite and or its products causes the clinical picture. Itching appears 2 to 4 weeks after the infestation and is classically more severe at night. As a clinical finding the burrow is pathognomonic and diagnostic. The remaining lesions are secondary to scratching, secondary infections, and allergic reaction.

The burrow is a skin-colored, tortuous, elevated line of 1 to 1.5 cm in length. They are usually found in the finger webs, flexor surface of the wrist, nipples, and elbows. In children, they are common in the palms and soles. The diagnosis is confirmed by a potassium hydroxide (KOH) preparation of the skin and the identification of the parasite. For treatment, permethrin 5% solution, one 8-hour application at night, is considered the standard treatment today. The gamma isomer of hexachlorobenzene (Lindane), 1% in a vanishing cream, was used for years, but it is used less commonly today because of its toxicity and should not be used in pregnant women and infants. With both medications a second application is made after 1 week. Note that this application should cover the entire body very thoroughly. A 6% sulfur precipitate in Vaseline for three consecutive days is employed in infants and pregnant women. Recently, ivermectin 200 micrograms per kilo, in a single dose, has been found to be very effective, but its safety is questioned by some authors. The nails should be cut short and scrubbed vigorously. Clothing and bed linen should be washed thoroughly. Norwegian scabies is the same disease but in an immunosuppressed individual. Typically, extensive, crusted, hyperkeratotic plaques are seen and itching may not be as prominent. The KOH examination shows a very severe infestation, and the patient is much more contagious. Treatment should include exfoliatives such as 20% urea or 20% salicylic acid in an ointment form.

Nodular scabies consists of brown or red

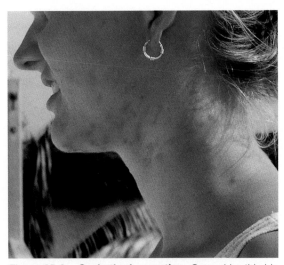

Figure 35-8. Seabather's eruption. Caused by thimble jellyfish off coast of Belize. (*Dr. Katy Schafer*)

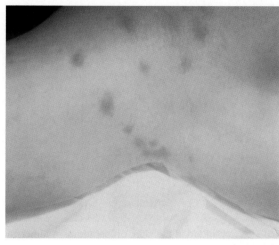 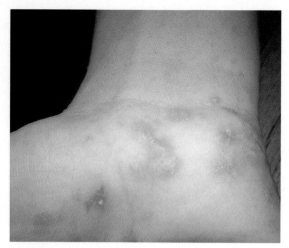

Figure 35-9. **Scabies.**

firm nodules on the penis, scrotum, or buttocks and may persist for months despite specific antimite treatment. It is a delayed allergic reaction with no mite present.

ANIMAL SCABIES. In this disease, very similar to papular urticaria, the mites invade human skin, but they do not become established in it. There are varieties from dogs, sheep, birds, and so forth. Excoriated, crusted papules can be seen and pruritus can be very severe especially in the evening.

Arachnidism

LATRODACTISM. *Latrodectus mactans* are small, dark spiders also called "black widows." They have a black or brown underside with a red, orange, or white hourglass marking on the back. They are commonly found in fields, under stones, and in outhouses. Their venom is neurotoxic, and they bite usually on the genitalia or buttocks. Pain develops within about an hour, with accompanying reddening and swelling. Systemic symptoms include muscle cramping, rigidity, and later weakness, sweating, bradycardia, hypothermia, and hypotension. The mortality rate is about 5% in children. Treatment alternatives include intravenous 10% calcium gluconate and corticosteroids; however, the most effective therapy is systemic antivenom.

LOXOSCELISM. *(Figs. 35-10C–D, 35-11). Loxosceles reclusus* is found in the United States, and *Loxosceles laeta* is found in Central and South America. The *Loxosceles* spiders are light-brown to chocolate in color, with nocturnal habits, and are commonly found seeking warmth in discarded clothing. Usually the affected areas include the arm and thigh in adults or the face in children. Pain develops 2 to 8 hours after the bite. The lesion becomes indurated and red, showing a central blister and necrosis that can be quite large. The necrotic area eventually becomes mummified; around the 14th day the resulting eschar may slough off. Rare symptoms include fever, chills, vomiting, and petechiae on skin, as well as thrombocytopenia and hemolytic anemia, especially in children. Treatment is with corticosteroids and dapsone, which may be effective in limiting the size and extension of the necrosis.

Disease Caused by Chiggers
(Fig. 35-12)

These mites, also known as *harvest mites*, are the cause of the infestation known as trombiculiasis. It is seen worldwide, although most frequently in tropical areas. The disease is acquired while walking through vegetation, and the affected area is usually on exposed skin depending on the clothing used. The offending chigger is the larval stage of the mite, 0.25 to 0.4 mm in diameter, orange to red in color, with three pairs of legs. It gets fixed to the skin by its buccal apparatus and starts a process of liquefying and sucking the skin elements. As a consequence it produces a type of papular urticaria: multiple red, itchy papules which are extremely pruritic. Topical treatment is with steroids and antipruritic lotions; occasionally this condition requires systemic antibiotic and steroid therapy.

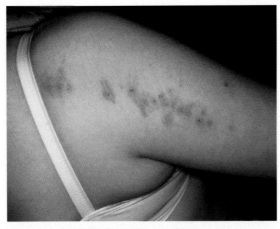

(A) Bedbug bites on the arm.

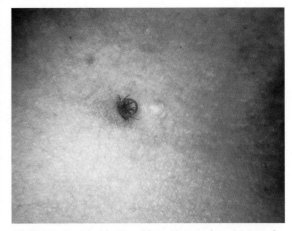

(B) Tick imbedded in the skin, presented as a tumor by patient.

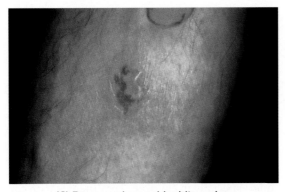

(C) Brown recluse spider bite on leg.

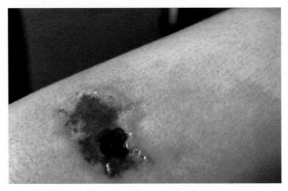

(D) Severe brown recluse spider bite on thigh.

Figure 35-10. **Anthropod bites.**

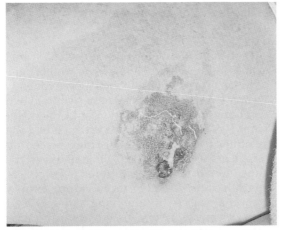

(A) Spider bite (*Loxosceles laeta*), erythema, central necrosis and blister formation.

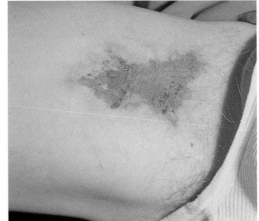

(B) Spider bite (*Loxosceles laeta*), vertical extension of necrosis due to gravity.

Figure 35-11. **Loxoceles.**

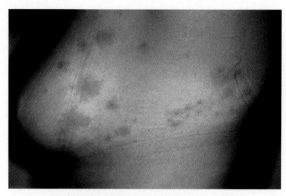

(*A*) Chigger bites collected under a bra.

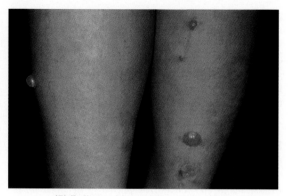

(*B*) Bullous chigger bites on the legs.

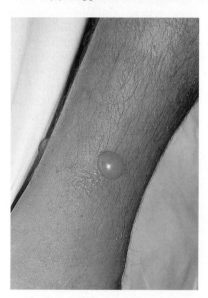

(*C*) Chigger bite, blister formation.

Figure 35-12.   Chigger bites.

Disease Caused by Nigua
(Fig. 35-13)

Tungiasis is a human infestation produced by *Tunga penetrans*, a sand flea that thrives in moist sandy ground near pigsties and cow sheds. It is widely distributed in tropical and subtropical areas of South America and Africa. It is known by various names (*pique*, *nigua*, *bicho dos pes*). It is commonly fertilized with cattle manure. The infection is produced by the female flea, which burrows into the skin of toeweb spaces and near the nail. The flea inserts her body full of eggs, to die at a later time. The initial clinical manifestation is a black dot, which is the burrow full of eggs that can later be seen on top of a papule or vesicle. Its walls are horny tissue from the epidermis itself. The lesion becomes infected or simply produces

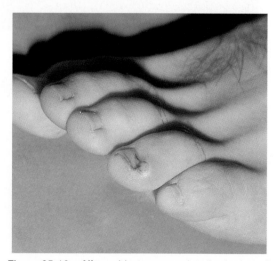

Figure 35-13.   **Nigua.** Most common location by toenail.

a foreign-body reaction that terminates in suppuration and opening of the cavity coalescing to form a honeycomb plaque. It may serve as a port of entry for a more severe infection and even gangrene. The best treatment is the extraction of all the insect parts, and, of course, the best prevention is to wear closed shoes.

Beetle Dermatitis
(Fig. 35-14)

Blister beetle dermatitis, or *paederus dermatitis*, is caused by contact with the body fluids of the paederus or "blistering" beetle. An increase in the incidence was seen in Peru and Ecuador with the El Niño phenomenon of 1997 and 1998. Clinically, an initial burning is felt with erythema and, later, the appearance of a blister usually in a linear fashion ("latigazo") in exposed parts of the body. Treatment includes compresses, topical corticosteroids, and, in some serious cases, oral prednisone and antibiotics.

FUNGAL INFECTIONS

HISTOPLASMOSIS. *(Fig. 35-15).* This disease is caused by *Histoplasma capsulatum*. Found throughout the world in temperate areas, *Histoplasma capsulatum* is a saprophytic fungus that grows in the soil, prevalently in soil of caves inhabited by bats. The disease is transmitted by the inadvertent inhalation of the spores. Epidemics have occurred through exploring infested caves or cleaning sites where chicken excrement (guano) may be present. A benign clinical form that may leave a calcified nodule in the lung similar to that of tuberculosis mimics the common cold. Primary infection, the most severe form of the disease, can disseminate and involve the reticuloendothelial system. Mucocutaneous nod-

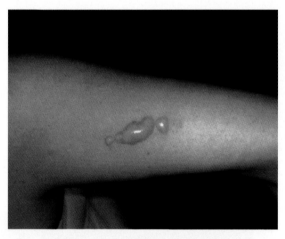

(*A*) Blister beetle bullous reaction on arm.

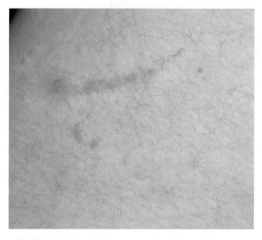

(*B*) Beetle dermatitis, whiplash effect (latigazo).

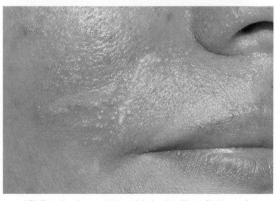

(*C*) Beetle dermatitis, whiplash effect (latigazo).

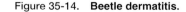

Figure 35-14. **Beetle dermatitis.**

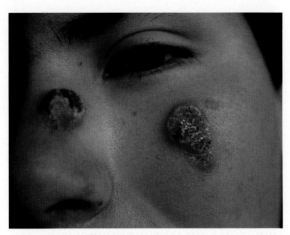

Figure 35-15. Histoplasmosis. Ulceration due to histoplasmosis.

COCCIDIOIDOMYCOSIS OR SAN JOAQUIN VALLEY FEVER. This disease is caused by *Coccidioides immitis*, a soil inhabitant. Infection in both humans and animals is acquired by the inhalation of fungus-laden dust particles or, rarely, through a primary infection of the skin. The severity of coccidioidomycosis can range from very mild, simulating a common cold, to an acute disseminated fatal disease, especially in patients with AIDS. An allergic reaction with erythema multiforme or erythema nodosum occurs in some cases. The basic symptoms of malaise and fever may suggest coccidioidomycosis if the patient has traveled through an endemic area. Diagnosis is made by KOH mounts of sputum or isolation of the fungus in a culture. Colonies of the coccidioidomycosis fast-growing phase are dangerous to handle, and the greatest care should be implemented while manipulating cultures. Treatment includes amphotericin B, ketoconazole, and itraconazole.

CHROMOBLASTOMYCOSIS. *(Figs. 35-16 and 35-17).* Chromoblastomycosis is a chronic cutaneous mycosis, characterized by a distinct clinical presentation and the presence of the so-called sclerotic bodies on tissue cuts. A great variety of fungi are able to cause the disease, including *Phialophora verrucosa*, *Fonsecaea pedrosoi*, *Fonsecaea compacta*, *Cladosporium carrionii*, *Rhinocladiella aquaspersa*, and *Botryomyces caespitosus*. The disease has been reported worldwide, with most

ules and granulomas may be seen. In AIDS the disease is seen in its most severe form. Primary cutaneous histoplasmosis occurs and is caused by direct inoculation. It is a nodular or indurated ulcer with accompanying lymphadenopathy. Occasionally an allergic response has been seen appearing as urticaria or as erythema annulare centrifugum. The diagnosis is accomplished by demonstrating the small intracellular histoplasma in sputum, bone marrow, or biopsy specimens. Treatment is done with ketoconazole or itraconazole.

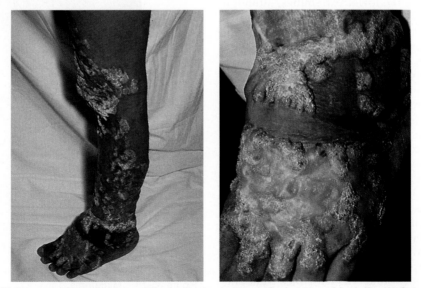

(A,B) Chromobastomycosis cauliflower-like leg lesion, with close-up of foot. *(Dr. W. Schorr)*

Figure 35-16. Chromoblastomycosis.

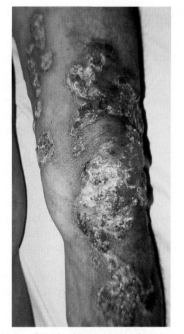

Figure 35-17. **Chromoblastomycosis.** Note the verrucous surface.

cases coming from the tropical and subtropical areas of South America and Africa. Some fungi have a preference for certain climates. *Fonsecaea pedrosoi* is most common in wet and humid areas within the torrid zones, whereas *C. carrionii* prefers dry and semidesert regions of the tropical–intertropical zones. The most commonly affected areas are the lower extremities, although in some arid geographic locations such as Venezuela, the upper girdle (shoulder, arm, back) is the prevalent site of infection. The primary process occurs at the site of inoculation, most probably through traumatized skin. The fungus is acquired from the environment, where it lives as saprophytes of wood, vegetable debris, or soil. The disease is not transmitted from person to person. The primary lesion is exophytic and either a papule, a nodule, or a tumor. The lesions multiply and tend to coalesce, forming plaques with a verrucous surface. Ulceration may develop, but there is no fistula formation, as in mycetoma, and the bone and muscle are spared. The affected limbs may end up in elephantiasis. The diagnosis is easily made by direct examination with KOH of scrapings from the lesion. The morphology adopted by the fungus is a cluster of oblong round cells with thick walls and flattened abutting surface, divided by septation

in more that one plane, and is known as *sclerotic bodies* or *muriform cells*. The histopathology shows pseudocarcinomatous hyperplasia with a granulomatous suppurative reaction in the dermis. The sclerotic bodies have a brown color and are easily identified by their size (4 to 12 microns) and look like copper pennies. Species identification is only possible after culture isolation on Sabouraud media for 4 to 6 weeks. Treatment options include surgical excision when the lesion is small. Pharmacologic agents that are reported to be useful, but probably not curative by themselves, include 5-flucytosine, itraconazole, and saperconazole.

MYCETOMA OR MADUROMYCOSIS. *(Fig. 35-18).* This disease is caused by at least 20 different fungi and actinomyces. The organisms gain entry into the body by trauma. It is more common in adult males who work outdoors barefoot or who expose large areas of the skin, as would stevedores. The clinical picture manifests over 10 or 15 years as nodules that later evolve into edematous areas with even larger nodules, and fistula that drain or expel "grains." Black grains are usually due to fungi, and red grains are usually due to actinomyces. Final diagnosis requires a culture

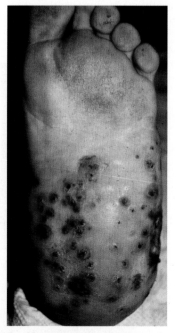

Figure 35-18. **Mycetoma.** The black granules are indicative of a fungal rather than an actinomycotic etiology.

study and treatment depends on the organism isolated.

SPOROTRICHOSIS. *(see Chap. 19).* Sporotrichosis (Fig. 35-19; see Fig. 19-16) is a mycotic infection produced by the environmental fungus, *Sporothrix schenckii*. It has worldwide distribution, although endemic areas do exist, for example, in the Peruvian Andes. It is commonly associated with trauma from rose thorns and is an occupational hazard for florists and gardeners. The classical picture (about 70% of the cases) is the so-called lymphocutaneous or sporotricoid pattern characterized by primary lesion, mostly an ulcerated plaque, followed by several satellite lesions either papular, nodular, or crusted, in a linear lymphatic distribution. It is commonly located on an extremity. There is a second type of presentation with only one isolated lesion as either a plaque, a nodule, or an ulcer. This is known as the fixed cutaneous form of sporotrichosis. Rarely, the infection can disseminate to involve multiple sites and organs. On histology, the findings are those of a granulomatous reaction, often with a suppurative component. The fungus is rarely seen on direct examination or on tissue cuts even with special stains. When visible, it has a levaduriform morphology. Fortunately, the fungus grows easily on Sabouraud media, which is the most reliable way to make the diag-

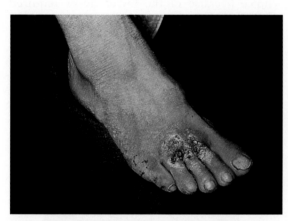

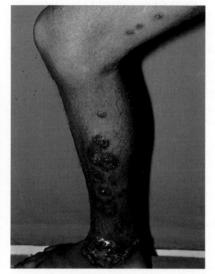

(A) Verrucous sporotrichosis on dorsum of foot. *(Dr. A. Gonzalez-Ochoa)*

(B) Sporotrichosis with lymphtic spread on leg. *(Dr. A. Gonzalez-Ochoa)*

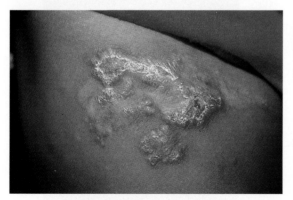

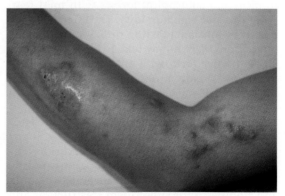

(C) Sporotrichosis, fixed lesion.

(D) Sporotrichosis with classic pattern.

Figure 35-19.

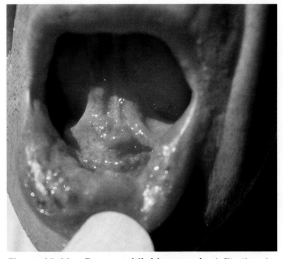

Figure 35-20. **Paracoccidioidomycosis.** Infiltrative deforming lesion of paracoccidioidomycosis.

nosis. The intradermal reaction known as the *sporotriquin test* is also of great help to exclude the diagnosis. Treatment options include the use of potassium iodide solution and itraconazole, both given for a period of four weeks after achieving total remission.

PARACOCCIDIOIDOMYCOSIS. *(Fig. 35-20).* As opposed to sporotrichosis and chromoblastomycosis, in which the disease is located at the inoculation site, paracoccidioidomycosis is a systemic disease with hematogenous spreading from a primary pulmonary focus. The infection has a specific geographic distribution through Central and South America. In some countries, such as Brazil, it reaches the status of a public health problem. The agent, *Paracoccidioides brasiliensis*, is a dimorphic fungus with special preference for tropical and subtropical forests with mild temperatures and high humidity. The infection is acquired by inhalation, with a primary lesion in the lung. From there it may take two courses: one is an aggressive form with an acute severe pneumonia and rapidly progressive systemic disease; the second form has a relentless course with chronic pulmonary disease. The typical patient is a middle-aged male agricultural worker. They may present themselves to the dermatologist with involvement of the mucosae and skin. The lesions on lips, buccal mucosae, gums, palate, and pharynx are infiltrating ulcerated plaques and nodules with subsequent destruction and scarring deformities of those structures. On the skin the lesions vary widely. They may begin as small acneiform pustules 2 to 3 mm in size that

later ulcerate, or they can adopt a pattern related to affected lymph nodes. Cold abscess may develop and in some instances multiple symmetric papules with verrucous surfaces may be present on the soles, easily misinterpreted as warts. The size of the fungus and its characteristic morphology allows easy identification on sputum preparations and scraping from the mucosa and cutaneous lesions. It is easy to recognize the yeast with multiple gemmations, giving the "pilot wheel" appearance. Identical structures are seen on histologic examination of the affected tissues. The reaction pattern seen on biopsy is a granulomatous reaction with multiple giant cells, some of them engulfing the budding elements. The fungus grows on Sabouraud medium in 4 or more weeks, as a mold at 20 to 26° C and as a yeast at 34 to 37° C. Treatment choices have evolved from sulfonamides to ketoconazole up to the new triazoles (itraconazole and fluconazole). At present, itraconazole is considered the drug of choice because of the lower doses required, shorter period of treatment, and fewer side effects.

LOBOMYCOSIS. *(Fig. 35-21).* This chronic skin infection is produced by *Loboa loboi*, a large fungus with levaduriform morphology. The disease is endemic in rural areas of the Brazilian Amazon. The same organism is able to cause dis-

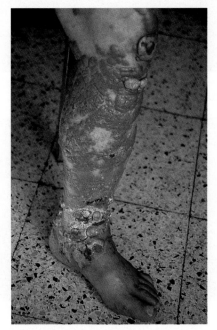

Figure 35-21. **Lobomycosis.** Note the smooth surface and compare to chromoblastomycosis (Fig. 35-17).

ease in dolphins in North America and Europe. The condition is acquired by primary inoculation from the environment through traumatized skin. The clinical lesions take years to develop. The classic clinical manifestation is the formation of nodules with a keloid appearance usually located on extremities, ears, face, and neck, with the scalp being spared in most cases. Other elementary lesions include infiltrated plaques, gummas, ulcers, and varicoid nodules. The histology consists of a massive histiocytic infiltrate without the pseudocarcinomatous hyperplasia commonly seen in chromoblastomycosis. This explains why in lobomycosis the nodules tend to have a smooth surface, as opposed to the verrucous surface of chromomycosis. The morphology of the fungus is quite distinctive, with globose, lemon-shaped buds 9 to 10 meters in diameter organized in short and long chains of uniform beads. The organism is easily seen in KOH preparations from lesions. The fungus has not been grown in culture media. The only effective treatment is wide surgical excision. Recurrence is very common.

NONINFECTIOUS MISCELLANEOUS DERMATOSES

PITYRIASIS ALBA. This is very common in children and consists of hypopigmented, poorly defined, scaly macules and plaques found on the face and upper outer arms. It is believed to be a mild form of atopic eczema. Lesions are first noticed after exposure to sunshine, where the surrounding sun-affected skin appears quite tan. Treatment consists of topical 1% hydrocortisone cream at night and sunscreens during the day.

PAPULAR URTICARIA. (*Fig. 35-22; see Fig. 35-10*). This term defines an exuberant reaction to arthropod bites. Initially there is an irritated weal and, later, an intensely pruritic papule develops at the site of the bite. There may be a central hemorrhagic puncture, a vesicle, or even a blister, especially in children. The number and localization of the lesions depend on the type of exposure and feeding habits of the arthropod. New bites may exacerbate quiescent old bites. Because of scratching, lesions can become infected and crusted. Localization of the affected areas help reveal the causative arthropod: Involvement of the legs suggests fleas, of the waist and thighs suggests chiggers, of the abdomen and arms suggests sarcoptic mange of dogs, and a generalized

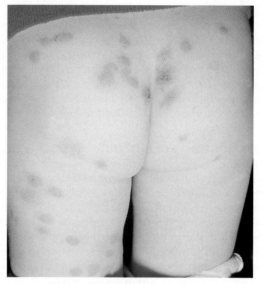

Figure 35-22.   **Papular urticaria.**

eruption suggests bird mites. Treatment consists of oral antihistamines, topical corticosteroids, and fumigation of the dwelling.

MILIARIA. (Fig. 35-23). Also known as *prickly heat*, *sudamina*, or *lichen tropicus*, this condition results from the obstruction of the sweat ducts caused by a combination of extreme heat and humidity. Depending on the level of obstruction, different clinical pictures can be seen. In the so-called *miliaria crystallina*, obstruction is very superficial; in *miliaria rubra*, the obstruction is deeper and clinically more pruritic. The lesions

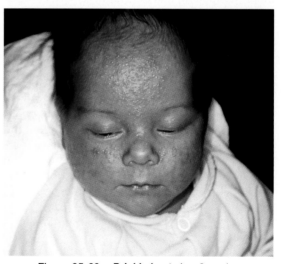

Figure 35-23.   **Prickly heat.** Age 3 weeks.

have an erythematous base and consist of tiny, follicular, red papules. In *miliaria profunda*, there can be associated anhydrosis, compensatory hyperhidrosis, and so-called tropical asthenia. Secondary infections are common. Treatment consists of seeking a cooler environment, loose clothing, fluids by mouth, and antibiotics where indicated for secondary infection.

PEMPHIGUS FOLIACEOUS (FOGO SELVAGEM). Fogo selvagem is an endemic type of pemphigus foliaceous, described in the Amazon regions of Brazil, and to a lesser degree in other countries in South America. It is clinically identical to the common type of pemphigus foliaceous, except for the young age of the population affected, and for its common presentation in families. An infectious agent has been postulated as the possible cause. The roles of viruses, streptococcus variants, and transmission of the disease by a *Simulium* species of fly have been subject of debate. The areas of prevalence are located in regions of wild jungle that have become agricultural. The disease may take a self-limiting course or, most likely, progress to a generalized form that is otherwise identical to the cosmopolitan forms of pemphigus. It is chronic, and treatment is based on high-dose corticosteroid therapy, as well as other forms of immunosuppressive therapy.

A FINAL WORD

Tropical dermatology is not exotic medicine anymore. The patient that one might see in a clinic in a Midwestern city may have just returned from a trip to the Amazon—less than a 23-hour flight—and the lithe ulceration he has on his right arm may not be just a simple impetigo, but a cutaneous from of leishmaniasis or another heretofore remote condition. A global world means global patients and, thus, requires global thinking. A sufficient history for the dermatology patient perhaps should include questions about the faraway places to which he or she may have traveled and the surroundings to which he or she may have been exposed. In jet-age dermatology, just looking may no longer be enough.

ACKNOWLEDGMENTS

We are grateful to Dr. Beatriz Bustamante and the Leishmania Group of the Instituto De Medicina Tropical Alexander Von Humboldt of the Universidad Peruana Cayetano Heredia for allowing us to use some of their clinical photos.

BIBLIOGRAPHY

Canizares O, Harman R. Clinical tropical dermatology, ed 2. Boston, Blackwell Scientific, 1992.

Chron. Derm A. XIV N 2183 Atti XXI Congr. Naz. A.D.0.1. Reggio Emilia, 1982. Editor Rino Cavalieri.

Cockerell CJ. The causative agent of bacillary angiomatosis. Int J Dermatol 1992;31:615.

Demis J. Clinical dermatology. Harper & Row, 1987.

Fisher AA. Atlas of aquatic dermatology. Orlando, FL, Grune & Stratton, 1978.

Grevelink SA, Lerner EA. Leishmaniasis. J Am Acad Dermatol 1996;34:257.

Lotti T, Hautmann G. Atypical mycobacterial infections: A difficult and emerging group of infectious dermatoses. 1993;321:499.

Lucchina LC, Wilson ME, Drake LA. Dermatology and the recently returned traveler: Infectious diseases with dermatologic manifestations. Int J Dermatol 1997;36:167.

Muelder K. Wounds that will not heal: the Buruli ulcer. Int J Dermatol 1992;31:25.

Negroni R. Paracoccidioidomycosis. Int J Dermatol 1993; 32:847.

Rook, Wilkinson, Ebling. Textbook of dermatology. Boston, Blackwell Scientific, 1992.

Schaller KF. Colour atlas of tropical dermatology and venerology. New York, Springer-Verlag, 1994.

Spach DH. Bacillary angiomatosis. Int J Dermatol 1992;31:19.

VII Monografia Del Colegio Ibero-Latinoamericano de Dermatologia: Gnathostomiasis. Ed. Wencesiao Ollague, Guayaquil, Ecuador, 1985.

Vargas-Ocampo F. Pityriasis alba: A histologic study. Int J Dermatol 1993:32:870.

Vetter RS, Visscher PK. Bites and stings of medically important venomous arthropods. Int J Dermatol 1998;37:481.

Werner AH, Werner BE. Sporotrichosis in man and animal. Int J Dermatol 1994:33:692.

Wong DE, Meinking BA, et al. Seabather's eruption: Clinical, histologic and immunologic features. J Am Acad Dermatol 1994;30:399.

36

Where to Look for More Information About a Skin Disease

"Doctor, I saw a patient yesterday who was diagnosed as having epidermolysis bullosa. I understand this is quite a rare condition. Where can I find the latest information on this subject?"

This is a question frequently asked of any teaching dermatologist. A computer will give you references, and some data bases will provide information about a dermatosis. But, assuming these are not readily available, there are other sources.

First, the inquiring physician or student should check out the Dictionary–Index of this book. Even for rare conditions there is at least a definition of the disease. The bibliography at the end of each chapter can also point one in the right direction for books or papers on a given subject.

Second, there are several comprehensive general texts on dermatology that include rare diseases. The following are suggested:

Arndt KA, LeBoit DE, Robinson JK, Wintraub BU. *Cutaneous Medicine and Surgery*. Philadelphia, WB Saunders, 1995.

Arnold HL Jr, Odum RB, James W. *Andrew's Diseases of the Skin*, ed 8. Philadelphia, WB Saunders, 1990.

Demis DJ, Dahl M, Smith EB, Thiers BH. *Clinical Dermatology*, 4 vols, loose-leaf. Philadelphia, JB Lippincott, revised annually.

Freedberg IM, Eisen AZ, Wolff K, et al. *Fitzpatrick's Dermatology in General Medicine*, ed 5, 2 vols. New York, McGraw-Hill, 1998.

Moschella SL, Hurley HJ. *Dermatology*, ed 3, 2 vols. Philadelphia, WB Saunders, 1992.

Champion RH, Burton JL, Burns DA, Breathnach SM. *Rook/Wilkinson/Ebling Textbook of Dermatology*, ed 6, 4 vols. Cambridge, MA, Blackwell, 1998.

These books fall into the category of color atlases:

McDonald CJ, Scott DA. *Dermatology in Black Patients*. Philadelphia, WB Saunders, 1988.

Schaumburg-Lever G, Lever WF. *Color Atlas of Histopathology of the Skin*. Philadelphia, JB Lippincott, 1989.

After these larger texts are consulted, a computer search could be done. A computer search on MEDLARS, or through other data bases, would direct one to pertinent references. MEDLARS (*MED*ical *L*iterature *A*nalysis and *R*etrieval *S*ystem) provides computer-produced literature searches, using *Index Medicus* from 1966 to present. Available from the National Library of Medicine is a *Guide to MEDLARS Services* (Assistant to the Director, National Library of Medicine, 8600 Rockville Pike, Bethesda, MD 20014). Additional computer sources include GRATEFUL MED and MEDLINE (on CD-ROM). A good listing of dermatology internet sites is given in the following journal article:

Sitaur C. Dermatology resources on the Internet: A practical guide for dermatologists. *International Journal of Dermatology* 1998;37 : 641.

These journals are highly pertinent:

Archives of Dermatology, a monthly journal published by the American Medical Association, Chicago. It is indexed in both the June and December issues.
Cutis, a monthly magazine for the general practitioner, published by Reed Medical Publishers, Danville, NJ 07834.
Fitzpatrick's Journal of Clinical Dermatology, published bimonthly by Kenet Publishing, Weston, MA.
Index Medicus, published monthly by the National Library of Medicine, and the *Cumulated Index Medicus*, published annually by the American Medical Association, Chicago. These contain current references to published papers and books, listed according to subject.
International Journal of Dermatology, a monthly journal, is the organ of the Society of Tropical Dermatology, published by Decker Publishing Co., Hamilton, Ontario, Canada L8N 3K7.
Journal of the American Academy of Dermatology, a monthly journal, published by the American Academy of Dermatology, Schaumberg, IL 60168.
Journal of Investigative Dermatology, a monthly journal published by the Society of Investigative Dermatology, Baltimore, MD 21202.
Year Book of Dermatology, published annually by Year Book Medical Publishers, Chicago. The *Year Book* contains abstracts of the majority of important articles related to the field of dermatology.

There are also many excellent foreign journals. Those in English include *Acta Dermato-Venereologica*, Stockholm, and the *British Journal of Dermatology*, London.

Specialized journals include:

American Journal of Contact Dermatitis. Philadelphia, Harcourt Brace Jovanovich.
American Journal of Cosmetic Surgery, quarterly, Los Angeles, American Board of Cosmetic Surgery.
American Journal of Dermatopathology, quarterly, Philadelphia, Lippincott Williams & Wilkins.
Clinics in Dermatology, quarterly, Philadelphia, Lippincott Williams & Wilkins.
Journal of Dermatologic Surgery and Oncology, monthly. New York, Elsevier.
Pediatric Dermatology, quarterly, Boston, Blackwell.
Seminars in Dermatology, quarterly, New York, Thieme-Stratton.
Sexually Transmitted Diseases, quarterly, Philadelphia, Lippincott Williams & Wilkins.

Reviews of dermatology include:

Arndt KA, Stern RS. *Medical and Surgical Dermatology*. New York, Springer International.
Callen JP, et al, eds. *Current Issues in Dermatology*. Boston, GK Hall.
Diepgen TL, et al. *Atlas of Dermatology*. 1998.
DuVivier A. *Dermatology Imagebank* [CD-ROM]. 1998.
Epstein E, ed. *Controversies in Dermatology*. Philadelphia, WB Saunders.
Fleischmajer R, ed. *Progress in Diseases of the Skin*. New York, Grune & Stratton.
Hurley HJ, et al. *Skin and Aging Journal*. February, 1998.
Olbricht, Bigby, Arndt. Manual of Clinical Problems in Dermatology. 1992.
Parish LC, Crissey JT, eds. *Clinics in Dermatology*. New York, Elsevier.
Rook AJ, Maibach HI, eds. *Recent Advances in Dermatology*. New York, Churchill Livingstone, issued occasionally.
Thiers BH. *Dermatologic Clinics*. Philadelphia, WB Saunders.

For further specialized information on a subject the bibliography at the end of the appropriate chapters in this book should be helpful.
Here are a few additional books that cannot be readily classified:

Ackerman AB, Ragaz A. *The Lives of Lesions*. Chicago, Year Book Medical Publishers, 1983.
Draelos ZD. *Cosmetics in Dermatology*, ed 2. Churchill Livingston, 1995.
Fitzpatrick TB. *Color Atlas Synopsis of Clinical Dermatology: Common and Serious Diseases*, ed 3. New York, McGraw-Hill, 1997.
Korting G. *Practical Dermatology of the Genital Region*. Philadelphia, WB Saunders, 1981.
Krusinski PA, Flowers FP. *Life-Threatening*

Dermatoses. Boca Raton, FL, CRC Press, 1987.

Litt JZ, Pawlar WA. *Drug Eruption Reference Manual*, ed 4. Cleveland, Wal-Zac Enterprises, 1995.

Lookingbill D. *Principles of Dermatology*, ed 2. WB Saunders, 1993.

Lynch PL, Edwards L. *Genital Dermatology*. Churchill Livingstone, 1994.

Sams WM, Lynch PJ. *Principles and Practice of Dermatology*, ed 2. Churchill Livingstone, 1996.

Shelley WB, Shelley ED. *Advanced Dermatologic Diagnosis*. Philadelphia, WB Saunders, 1992.

Shelley WB, Shelley ED. *Advanced Dermatologic Therapy*. Philadelphia, WB Saunders, 1987.

Tovell HMM. *Diseases of the Vulva in Clinical Practice*. New York, Elsevier, 1990.

Finally, a unique older publication is *A Dictionary of Dermatological Words, Terms and Phrases*, by Leider and Rosenblum. It was published by McGraw-Hill, New York, in 1968. Any interested student or physician will enjoy this dictionary and profit by perusing it.

For a list of dermatologic lay organizations and registries, consult volume 17 (1987), page 280 of the *Journal of the American Academy of Dermatology*.

Dictionary–Index

The purpose of the dictionary portion of this index is to define and classify some of the rarer dermatologic terms not covered in the text. Some very rare or unimportant terms have purposely been omitted, but undoubtedly some terms that are *not* rare and *are* important have also been omitted. Most of the histopathologic terms have been defined. Suggestions or corrections from the reader will be appreciated.

Page numbes followed by an "f" refer to figures.

413

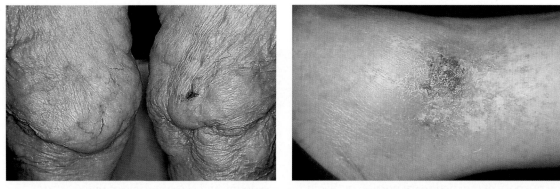

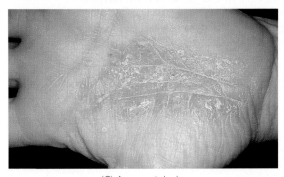

(A) Acrodermatitis chronica atrophicans on legs.

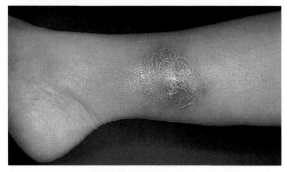

(B) Atrophie blanche on ankle.

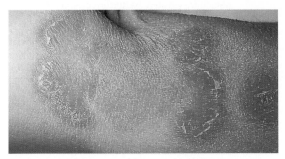

(C) Acropustulosis.

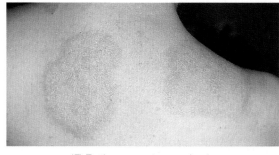

(D) Erythema induratum.

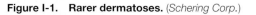

Figure I-1. Rarer dermatoses. (*Schering Corp.*)

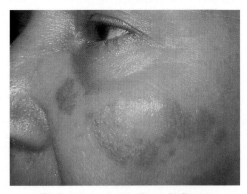

(E) Erythema perstans on elbow (*Drs. H. Shair and L. Grayson*).

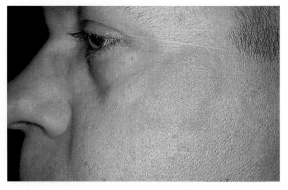

(F) Erythema perstans on back.

(G) Granuloma faciale (Dr. J. DeSpain).

(H) Jessner's benign lymphocytic infiltration of the skin.

Inflammatory

Acrodermatitis chronica atrophicans. A moderately rare idiopathic atrophy in older adults, particularly women, characterized by the presence of thickened skin at the onset, with ulnar bands on the forearm, changing into atrophy of the legs below the knee and of the forearms. In the early stages this is to be differentiated from scleroderma. High doses of penicillin may be effective. Late stage of Lyme disease.

Folliculitis ulerythematosa reticulata. A very rare reticulated atrophic condition localized to the cheeks of the face; seen mainly in young adults.

Ulerythema ophryogenes. A rare atrophic dermatitis that affects the outer part of the eyebrows, resulting in redness, scaling, and permanent loss of the involved hair.

Macular atrophy (anetoderma of Jadassohn). A very rare condition characterized by the appearance of circumscribed reddish macules that develop an atrophic center that progresses toward the edge of the lesion, seen mainly on the extremities. May be seen after acne, varicella, and other inflammatory skin diseases.

Lichen sclerosus et atrophicus (kraurosis vulvae, kraurosis penis, and *balanitis xerotica obliterans).* An uncommon atrophic process, mainly of women, which begins as a small whitish lesion that contains a central hyperkeratotic pinpoint-sized dell. These 0.5-cm or less whitish macules commonly coalesce to form whitish atrophic plaques. The most common localizations are on the neck, shoulders, arms, axillae, vulva, and perineum. Many consider kraurosis vulvae, kraurosis penis, and balanitis xerotica obliterans to be variants of this condition.

Poikiloderma atrophicans vasculare (Jacobi). This rare atrophic process of adults is characterized by the development of patches of telangiectasis, atrophy, and mottled pigmentation on any area of the body. This resembles chronic radiodermatitis clinically and may be associated with dermatomyositis or scleroderma. May precede the development of a lymphoma.

Hemiatrophy. May be localized to one side of the face or may cover the entire half of the body. Vascular and neurogenic etiologies have been proposed, but most cases appear to be a form of *localized scleroderma.*

Atrophoderma, idiopathic, of Pasini and Pierini. Similar to morphea (localized scleroderma) but without induration. The round or irregular depressed atrophic areas are asymptomatic and appear mainly on the trunk of young females.

Atrophie blanche. 382. A form of cutaneous atrophy characterized by scar-like plaques with a border of telangiectasis and hyperpigmentation that cover large areas of the legs and the ankles, mainly of middle-aged or older women.

Secondary atrophy. From inflammatory diseases such as syphilis, chronic discoid lupus erythematosus, leprosy, tuberculosis, scleroderma, etc.

Autoeczematization. *See* Id reaction

Autoerythrocyte sensitization syndrome (Gardner-Diamond syndrome, psychogenic purpura). Bizarre, tender ecchymotic lesions mainly in young females. May be associated with psychological disturbance. Skin lesions reproduced with intradermal injection of whole blood or red blood cell fractions.

Autohemotherapy. A form of nonspecific protein therapy, administered by removing 10 mL of venous blood from the arm and then immediately injecting that blood intramuscularly into the buttocks. It has been shown to produce a fall in circulating eosinophils, presumably due to a mild increase in the adrenal steroid hormones.

Canities. Gray or white hair.
Carney Complex. Myxomas (heart, skin, breast), spotty
pigmentation (lentigines, blue nevi), endocrinopathies (Cushing's syndrome,
acromegaly, sexual precocity) and schwanno-
mas.
Carcinoid syndrome, A potentially malignant tumor of
the argentaffin chromaffin cells of the appendix
or the ileum. Some of these tumors or their
metastases produce large amounts of serotonin
(5-hydroxytryptamine), which causes transient
flushing of the skin accompanied by weakness,
nausea, abdominal pain, diarrhea, and sweating. The redness usually begins on the head and
the neck and then extends down on the body.
These episodes last from several minutes to a
few hours. Repeated attacks of the erythema
lead to the formation of permanent telangiectasias and a diffuse reddish purple hue to the
skin. The diagnosis can be made by the finding
of over 25 mg of 5-hydroxyindoleacetic acid in a
24-hour urine sample.
Carotenemia. Buildup of carotene or similar yellow-or-
ange pigment in the blood and keratin layer of
the skin. Stains skin a characteristic yellow.
Harmless condition due to eating large amounts
of foods such as carrots and tomatoes (lycopene-
mia due to similar pigment called lycopene).
Caseation necrosis. Histologically, this is a form of tissue
death with loss of structural detail leaving pale
eosinophilic, amorphous, finely granular material. It is seen especially in tuberculosis, syphilis,
granuloma annulare, and beryllium granuloma.
Cat-scratch disease, 195, 223. Manifested by inflammation at the site of a cat scratch or bite obtained a few days previously. Malaise,
headache, low-grade fever, chills, generalized
lymphadenopathy, and splenomegaly occur. A
maculopapular rash or erythema nodosum-like
eruption occurs occasionally. Caused by
Bartonella henselae, formerly *Rochalimaea henselae*.
Caterpillar dermatitis. An irritating chemical is released
when the hairs of some species of caterpillars
penetrate the skin. The onset of irritation is quite
immediate. Red macular lesions, then urticarial

papules, and occasionally vesicles develop in areas exposed. Mild lesions can be gone in 12
hours, but more extensive cases can take several
days to resolve. In these more severe cases,
there occasionally can be constitutional symptoms of restlessness and headache. Therapy is
not very effective or necessary. Scotch tape
placed over the affected skin might pull out
some of the bristle-like hairs.
Causalgia. A condition characterized by burning pain aggravated by touching the neuralgic site.
Chalazion. A small cyst of the meibomian glands of the
eyelid.
Chancre, 165, 165f. *See* Primary chancre type diseases.
monorecidive. A relapsing form of syphilis characterized by the development of a lesion reduplicat-
ing the primary sore.
primary, 165
Chancre-type, primary disease. *See* Primary chancre-type
diseases
Charcot joints. A type of joint destruction in patients with
central nervous system syphilis of the paretic
type.
Chédiak-Higashi syndrome. 96. A fatal syndrome in children characterized by pigmentary disturbances,
photophobia, pyogenic infections, excessive
sweating, pale optic fundi, splenomegaly, and
lymphadenopathy.
Chilblain lupus erythematosus of Hutchinson. Subtype of
lupus erythematosus with cold induced, red, ulcerative symmetrical lesions on ears, nose, digits, knees and elbows.
Chilblains. Also called *pernio*. A cutaneous reaction, either acute or chronic, from exposure to excessive cold.
Child abuse. Cutaneous signs of this abuse include linear
bruising, loop marks, buckle marks, pinch
marks, blunt trauma lesions, burns, traumatic
alopecia, human bites, and genital tears.
CHILD syndrome. Rare disease present at birth showing
congenital hemidysplasia, ichthyosis, and limb
defects. Occurs almost exclusively in females.
Chromhidrosis. The excretion of colored sweat, usually
brownish, grayish, bluish, or yellowish.
Chrysarobin. A reducing agent that hastens keratinization when it is applied to the skin. It can be incorporated into petrolatum or chloroform but
must be used with great caution and in mild
strength such as 0.25% to 3%. Mainly used in
treatment of resistant cases of psoriasis and
tinea cruris.

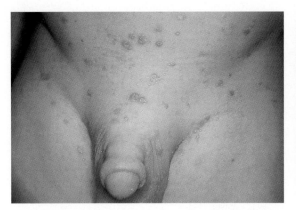

(*A*) Letterer-Siwe disease of lower abdomen in child.

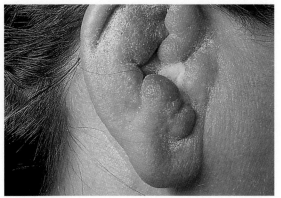

(*B*) Lymphedema (elephantiasis nostras) of ear (*Dr. M. Feldaker*).

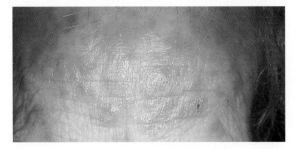

(*C*) Pseudolymphoma of Spiegler-Fendt.

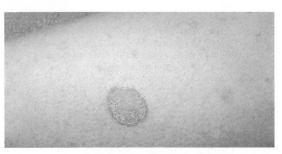

(*D*) Porokeratosis of leg (*Dr. J. Hall*).

Figure I-2. Rarer dermatoses. (*Smith-Kline-Beecham*)

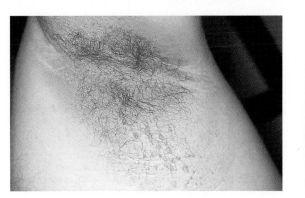

(*E*) Pseudoacanthosis nigricans of axilla.

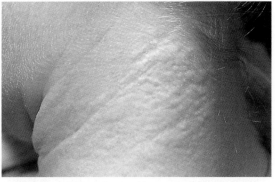

(*F*) Pseudoxanthoma elasticum of neck (*Dr. J. Hall*).

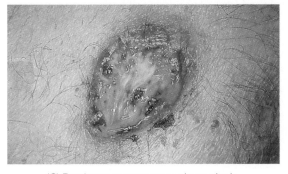

(*G*) Pyoderma gangrenosum above nipple.

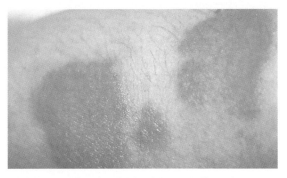

(*H*) Neutrophilic acute febrile dermatosis (Sweet's syndrome) (*Dr. J. DeSpain*).